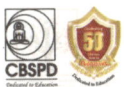

CBS
Handbooks Series

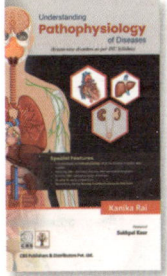

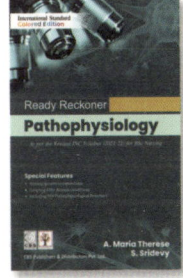

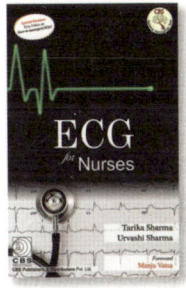

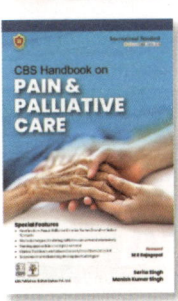

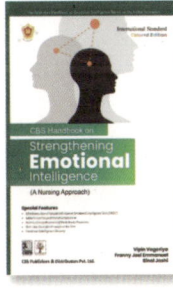

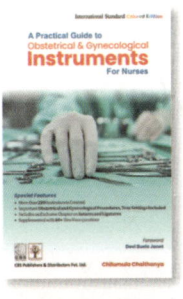

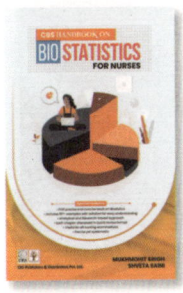

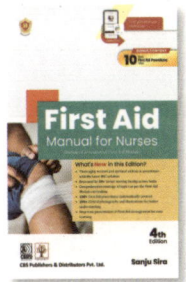

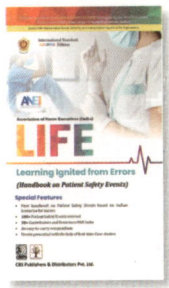

CBS Publishers & Distributors Pvt. Ltd.

New Delhi | Bengaluru | Chennai | Kochi | Kolkata | Lucknow | Mumbai
Hyderabad | Jharkhand | Nagpur | Patna | Pune | Uttarakhand

Buy Book Online at: www.cbspd.com

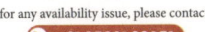

Also available at
All Medical Book Stores of India

Socially Connect with us:

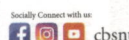 cbsnursingknowledgetree

for any availability issue, please contact:
📞 +91 95991 99051

 Scan the QR Code to access
CBS Catalogue
2025-26

CBS

Nursing Knowledge Tree
An Initiative by CBS Nursing Division

Dictionary *for* Nurses

Third Edition

Jacintha D'Souza MPhil (N)

Principal and Professor
Father Muller College of Nursing
Mangaluru, Karnataka

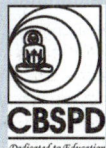

CBSPD
Dedicated to Education

CBS Publishers & Distributors Pvt Ltd

• New Delhi • Bengaluru • Chennai • Kochi • Kolkata • Lucknow
• Mumbai • Hyderabad • Jharkhand • Nagpur • Patna
• Pune • Uttarakhand

CBS
Dictionary
for
Nurses

ISBN: 978-93-90619-29-0

Copyright © Publishers

Revised Reprint: 2026

Reprint: 2025, 2024
Third Edition: 2022
Second Edition: 2017

Published by **Satish Kumar Jain** and produced by **Varun Jain** for

CBS Publishers & Distributors Pvt Ltd

4819/XI Prahlad Street, 24 Ansari Road, Daryaganj, New Delhi 110 002, India.
Ph: +91-11-23289259, 23266861, 23266867   Website: www.cbspd.com
Fax: 011-23243014
e-mail: delhi@cbspd.com; cbspubs@airtelmail.in.

Corporate Office: 204 FIE, Industrial Area, Patparganj, Delhi 110 092
Ph: +91-11-4934 4934   Fax: 4934 4935
e-mail: feedback@cbspd.com

Branches

- **Bengaluru:** Seema House 2975, 17th Cross, K.R. Road, Banashankari 2nd Stage, Bengaluru-560 070, Karnataka
  Ph: +91-80-26771678/79   Fax: +91-80-26771680
  e-mail: bangalore@cbspd.com

- **Chennai:** 7, Subbaraya Street, Shenoy Nagar, Chennai 600 030, Tamil Nadu
  Ph: +91-44-26680620, 26681266   Fax: +91-44-42032115
  e-mail: chennai@cbspd.com

- **Kochi:** 68/1534, 35, 36-Power House Road, Opp. KSEB, Cochin-682018, Kochi, Kerala
  Ph: +91-484-4059061-65   Fax: +91-484-4059065
  e-mail: kochi@cbspd.com

- **Kolkata:** Hind Ceramics Compound, 1st Floor, 147, Nilganj Road, Belghoria, Kolkata-700056, West Bengal
  Ph: +91-033-2563-3055/56   e-mail: kolkata@cbspd.com

- **Lucknow:** Basement, Khushnuma Complex, 7-Meerabai Marg, (Behind Jawahar Bhawan), Lucknow-226001, Uttar Pradesh
  Ph: +0522-4000032   e-mail: tiwari.lucknow@cbspd.com

- **Mumbai:** PWD Shed, Gala No. 25/26, Ramchandra Bhatt Marg, Next to J.J. Hospital Gate No. 2, Opp. Union Bank of India, Noor Baug, Mumbai-400009, Maharashtra
  Ph: +91-22-66661880/89   Fax: +91-22-24902342
  e-mail: mumbai@cbspd.com

Representatives

- **Hyderabad** +91-9885175004
- **Nagpur** +91-9421945513
- **Pune** +91-9623451994
- **Jharkhand** +91-9811541605
- **Patna** +91-9334159340
- **Uttarakhand** +91-9716462459

Printed at : Goyal Offset Works Pvt. Ltd. Haryana

CBS Nursing Knowledge Tree

Extends its Tribute to

Florence Nightingale

For glorifying the role of women as nurses,
For holding the title of "The Lady with the Lamp,"
For working tirelessly for humanity—
Florence Nightingale will always be
remembered for her
selfless and memorable services to the
human race.

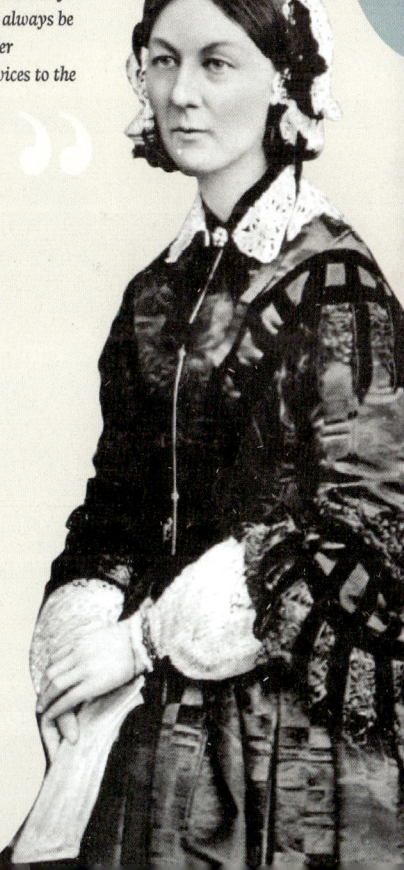

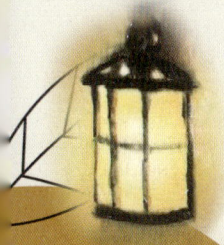

Florence Nightingale
(May 1820 – August 1910)

Dedicated to

my sisters in my religious community
who have been my constant strength,
my management which has been my great support,
and
my staff members and students, past and future,
who are my joy, satisfaction and hope.

All praise, honour and glory to my God
Whose grace has blessed me with
this day and will head me to my Home.

ANNEXURES

Annexure 1

COVID-19 Terminology

Aerosol: A tiny particle or droplet that is suspended in the air.

Antibody test: Also known as **serology test,** this checks to see if you have antibodies in your blood that show that you were previously infected with the virus.

Antibody: A protein which is made by your immune system in response to an infection. If you have antibodies for the coronavirus in your blood, it means you have been infected with this virus at some point (even if you never had any symptoms).

Antigen test: A type of **diagnostic test** that checks to see if you are currently infected. The test looks for proteins (antigens) in a sample taken from your nose or throat. Antigen tests are faster than PCR tests, but they have a higher risk of false positives (meaning that they are more likely to say you have the infection when you do not have). This may also be known as a rapid test or rapid diagnostic test.

Asymptomatic: Not showing any symptoms (signs of disease or illness).

Cluster: A grouping of disease cases in a geographic area during a set time period.

Communicable: It means "contagious." Disease that can be spread or transmitted from one person to another.

Community spread: The spread of an illness or disease within a particular location, like a neighborhood or town. During community spread, there is no clear source of contact or infection.

Confirmed case: Someone tested and confirmed to have COVID-19 disease.

Congregate settings: Public places that can get crowded and where contact with infected people can happen. Examples: malls, theaters, grocery stores, etc.

Contact tracing: A disease control measure. Public health workers known as contact tracers work with infected people to identify anyone, they had close contact with while they were contagious. The exposed contacts are then informed that they might be carrying the coronavirus and advised to stay home for 14 days while monitoring themselves for symptoms.

Convalescent plasma therapy: A treatment that involves taking blood from someone who already has antibodies to a disease, separating out the clear liquid part (plasma), and then administering it to someone who is sick with the same disease. This technique has been used to treat many different diseases but is still considered experimental for treating **COVID-19**.

Coronavirus: A family of related viruses. Many of them cause respiratory illnesses. Coronaviruses cause COVID-19, SARS, MERS, and some strains of influenza or flu.

COVID-19: Stands for coronavirus disease-19. COVID-19 is the name of the infection caused by the novel (new) strain of highly contagious coronavirus (SARS-CoV-2) that was first identified in late 2019.

Droplet: A tiny, moist particle that is released when you cough or sneeze. You may get infected with the coronavirus if you are close to someone who is carrying it and your mouth, nose, or eyes come into contact with droplets they have released.

Endemic: The baseline or expected level of a disease in a given community.

Epidemic: A significant and possibly sudden increase in the number of cases of a disease in the community.

Epidemiology: The branch of medicine that studies how diseases happen and spread in communities of people.

Flattening the curve: Refers to efforts designed to prevent too many people from getting sick around the same time, which would overwhelm the health care system.

Herd immunity: When the majority of people in an area are immune to a specific infection, even the members of the population (herd) are protected simply by being around them. Anywhere from 50% to 90% of the population would have to have antibodies to COVID-19 in order for herd immunity to kick in.

Hydroxychloroquine: A medication used to treat or prevent malaria. The FDA originally granted emergency use to treat patients with COVID-19 based on very limited data showing that it has activity against SARS-CoV-2. But the ruling was later removed because studies didn't show that the drugs worked against COVID-19 or that its benefits outweigh the risks.

Immunity: Your body's ability to resist or fight against an infection.

Immunocompromised: Someone who has an immune system that can't resist or fight off infections as in most people.

Incubation period: It refers to time it takes for someone with an infection to start showing symptoms. For COVID-19, symptoms appear 2–14 days after infection.

Infusion: A procedure that puts a medicine, blood, or fluid directly into your veins through an IV or catheter over a period of time.

N95 respirator: Unlike a surgical or cloth mask, N95 respirators are designed to prevent the wearer from breathing in tiny particles. When fit properly, they filter out at least 95% of large and small particles.

Outbreak: A sudden increase of a specific illness in a small area.

Pandemic: When a new disease or illness spreads to many countries around the world.

PCR test: Stands for polymerase chain reaction test. This is a **diagnostic test** that determines if you are infected by analyzing a sample to see if it contains genetic material from the virus.

Person under investigation (PUI): When a health provider suspects a person has the coronavirus. But no test has confirmed the infection.

PPE: It stands for personal protective equipment. This includes masks, face shields, gloves, gowns and other coverings that healthcare workers use to prevent the spread of infection to themselves and other patients.

Presumptive positive case: When a person tests positive for the coronavirus, but the CDC hasn't confirmed the case.

Quarantine: It is also called "isolation." Quarantines keep people away from each other to prevent the spread of disease. Stay-at-home orders are a type of quarantine.

Remdesivir: An antiviral drug made to treat Ebola (but never approved for that purpose), Remdesivir is the first treatment to be granted full approval by the FDA to treat COVID-19.

SARS: The coronavirus that causes COVID-19 is officially called SARS-CoV-2, which stands for severe acute respiratory syndrome coronavirus 2.

Screening: It includes asking a series of basic questions about your health condition and recent history. Screening may also include other common healthcare procedures, like taking your temperature.

Self-isolation: Also called self-quarantine. Separating yourself when you're sick from healthy individuals to prevent further spread.

Social distancing: Also called physical distancing. It means maintaining space between yourself and other people to control the spread of particular communicable illness or disease.

Swab test: A type of **diagnostic test** that involves taking sample from the back of your nasal cavity so it can be analyzed in a lab to see if it contains the virus. Also called a **viral test.**

Symptomatic: When a person shows signs or symptoms of illness. For COVID-19, that includes cough, fever or shortness of breath.

Trial: Short for **clinical trial,** this is when researchers study a medical test or treatment in a set group of people to make sure it's safe and effective before giving it to the public.

Vaccine: A kind of medicine or medication that prevents disease by training your body's immune system to fight a germ that it's never come into contact with before.

Variant: It means a change or alteration in the existing one. In the case of the coronavirus, a variant is a mutation in which the original virus has taken on new characteristics.

Ventilator: A machine that supplies oxygen to a patient with severe lung issues. A ventilator machine requires a specialist or respiratory therapist. It is more invasive than an oxygen mask. Many hospitals don't have a supply of ventilators big enough for the COVID-19 outbreak.

Viral load: Also called viral dose, viral load refers to the amount of virus you are exposed to. Someone who is exposed to a relatively small amount of the coronavirus might not develop any symptoms, while someone who is exposed to a large amount is more apt to get severe symptoms.

Viral shedding: The release of virus from an infected person into the environment, where it can infect others. In the case of COVID-19, most viral shedding occurs through the respiratory tract (often via a cough or **sneeze**), but the virus may also be shed though the gastrointestinal tract and show up in the stool.

Virus: A tiny infectious organism made up of genetic material (DNA or RNA) wrapped in a protein coat. Viruses can't multiply on their own; they reproduce by invading living cells and taking control of them.

Annexure 2

AIIMS/ICMR COVID-19 National Task Force/Joint Monitoring Group Clinical Guidance for Management of Adult COVID-19 Patients

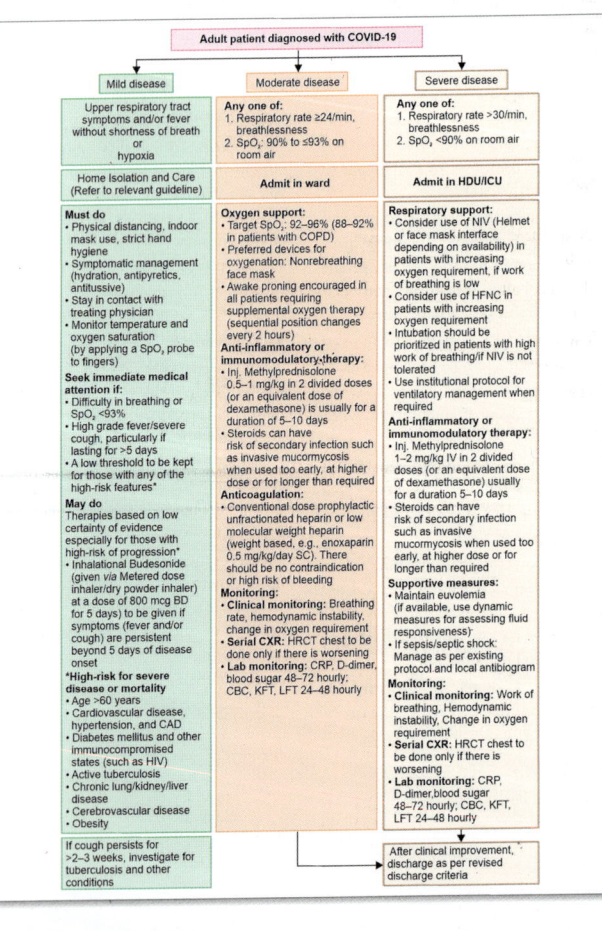

Adult patient diagnosed with COVID-19

Mild disease	Moderate disease	Severe disease
Upper respiratory tract symptoms and/or fever without shortness of breath or hypoxia	Any one of: 1. Respiratory rate ≥24/min, breathlessness 2. SpO₂: 90% to ≤93% on room air	Any one of: 1. Respiratory rate >30/min, breathlessness 2. SpO₂ <90% on room air
Home Isolation and Care (Refer to relevant guideline)	**Admit in ward**	**Admit in HDU/ICU**

Mild disease

Must do
- Physical distancing, indoor mask use, strict hand hygiene
- Symptomatic management (hydration, antipyretics, antitussive)
- Stay in contact with treating physician
- Monitor temperature and oxygen saturation (by applying a SpO₂ probe to fingers)

Seek immediate medical attention if:
- Difficulty in breathing or SpO₂ <93%
- High grade fever/severe cough, particularly if lasting for >5 days
- A low threshold to be kept for those with any of the high-risk features*

May do
Therapies based on low certainty of evidence especially for those with high-risk of progression*
- Inhalational Budesonide (given via Metered dose inhaler/dry powder inhaler) at a dose of 800 mcg BD for 5 days) to be given if symptoms (fever and/or cough) are persistent beyond 5 days of disease onset

*High-risk for severe disease or mortality
- Age >60 years
- Cardiovascular disease, hypertension, and CAD
- Diabetes mellitus and other immunocompromised states (such as HIV)
- Active tuberculosis
- Chronic lung/kidney/liver disease
- Cerebrovascular disease
- Obesity

If cough persists for >2–3 weeks, investigate for tuberculosis and other conditions

Moderate disease

Oxygen support:
- Target SpO₂: 92–96% (88–92% in patients with COPD)
- Preferred devices for oxygenation: Nonrebreathing face mask
- Awake proning encouraged in all patients requiring supplemental oxygen therapy (sequential position changes every 2 hours)

Anti-inflammatory or immunomodulatory therapy:
- Inj. Methylprednisolone 0.5–1 mg/kg in 2 divided doses (or an equivalent dose of dexamethasone) is usually for a duration of 5–10 days
- Steroids can have risk of secondary infection such as invasive mucormycosis when used too early, at higher dose or for longer than required

Anticoagulation:
- Conventional dose prophylactic unfractionated heparin or low molecular weight heparin (weight based, e.g., enoxaparin 0.5 mg/kg/day SC). There should be no contraindication or high risk of bleeding

Monitoring:
- **Clinical monitoring:** Breathing rate, hemodynamic instability, change in oxygen requirement
- **Serial CXR:** HRCT chest to be done only if there is worsening
- **Lab monitoring:** CRP, D-dimer, blood sugar 48–72 hourly; CBC, KFT, LFT 24–48 hourly

Severe disease

Respiratory support:
- Consider use of NIV (Helmet or face mask interface depending on availability) in patients with increasing oxygen requirement, if work of breathing is low
- Consider use of HFNC in patients with increasing oxygen requirement
- Intubation should be prioritized in patients with high work of breathing/if NIV is not tolerated
- Use institutional protocol for ventilatory management when required

Anti-inflammatory or immunomodulatory therapy:
- Inj. Methylprednisolone 1–2 mg/kg IV in 2 divided doses (or an equivalent dose of dexamethasone) usually for a duration 5–10 days
- Steroids can have risk of secondary infection such as invasive mucormycosis when used too early, at higher dose or for longer than required

Supportive measures:
- Maintain euvolemia (if available, use dynamic measures for assessing fluid responsiveness)
- If sepsis/septic shock: Manage as per existing protocol and local antibiogram

Monitoring:
- **Clinical monitoring:** Work of breathing, Hemodynamic instability, Change in oxygen requirement
- **Serial CXR:** HRCT chest to be done only if there is worsening
- **Lab monitoring:** CRP, D-dimer, blood sugar 48–72 hourly; CBC, KFT, LFT 24–48 hourly

After clinical improvement, discharge as per revised discharge criteria

Annexure 3

Medical Abbreviations

Abbreviation	Meaning
a.c.	before meals
add.	add let there be added
ad lib.	Latin, "at one's pleasure"; as much as one desires; freely
agit.	agitate (stir or shake)
alt. d., alt. dieb.	every other day; on alternate days
alt. h., alt. hor.	every other hour; at alternate hours
a.m.	morning, before noon
BDS, b.d.s.	twice daily
b.i.d., b.d.	twice daily
bis ind.	twice a day
bucc.	buccal (inside cheek)
cap., caps.	capsule
c.m.	tomorrow morning
c.n.	tomorrow night
DAW	dispense as written (i.e., no generic substitution)
dil.	dilute
emuls.	emulsion
garg.	gargle
gtt(s)	drop(s)

Abbreviation	Meaning
h, hr, hor.	hour
hor. alt.	every other hour (every second hour; at alternate hours)
hor. decub.	at bedtime
ID	intradermal
IJ, inj.	injection
IM	intramuscular
IN	intranasal
inf.	infusion (extraction)/ intravenous infusion
IP	intraperitoneal
IT	intrathecal
IV	intravenous
lat. dol.	to the painful side
lin	liniment
liq.	solution
lot.	lotion
mane	in the morning
mcg	microgram
mist.	mixture
mod. prescript.	in the manner directed
nebul	a spray (such as for insufflation)
noct.	at night
non rep.	no repeats (no refills)

Contd...   *Contd...*

Abbreviation	Meaning
NS	normal saline (0.9%)
1/2NS	half-normal saline (0.45%)
o.m.	every morning
o.n.	every night
p.	continue
per	by or through
p.c.	after meals
p.o.	by mouth or orally
p.r., PR	rectally
p.r.n., PRN	as needed
p.v., PV	vaginally
q.1 h, q.1°	every 1 hour (can replace '1' with other numbers)
q.a.d.	every other day
q.a.m.	every morning (every day before noon)
q.d./q.1.d.	every day
q.d.a.m.	once daily in the morning
q.d.p.m.	once daily in the evening
q.d.s.	4 times a day

Abbreviation	Meaning
q.p.m.	every evening (every day after noon)
q.h.	every hour
q.h.s.	every night at bedtime
q.i.d.	4 times a day
rep., rept.	repeats
SC	subcutaneous
SL, s.l.	sublingually, under the tongue
s.o.s., si op. sit	if there is a need
stat	immediately
supp.	suppository
susp.	suspension
syr.	syrup
tab.	tablet
t.d.s., TDS	3 times a day
t.i.d., t.d.	3 times a day
t.i.w.	3 times a week
top.	topical
TPN	total parenteral nutrition
vag.	vaginally
w/o	without

Contd...

Annexure 4

Normal Values

Vital Signs and Body Mass Index

Blood Pressure: Systolic/Diastolic (mm Hg)	
At physician's office (average 5 measurements)	<140/90
Ambulatory BP monitor	<135/85
With diabetes	<130/80
Heart Rate (HR) or Pulse (Beats/min)	
Bradycardia	<60
Normal	60–80
Tachycardia	>100
Respiration Rate (RR) (Breaths/min)	
Bradypnea	<12
Normal (eupnea)	12–18
Tachypnea	>18
Body Temperature (°C)	
Fever	>37.5
Normal	36.5–37.5 (approximate)
Hypothermia	<35
Body Mass Index (BMI) (kg/m²)	
Underweight	<18.5
Normal	18.5–24.9
Overweight	25.0–29.9
Obesity class I	30.0–34.9
Obesity class II	35.0–39.9
Obesity class III (extreme, morbid)	≥40

Contd...

Common Blood Tests with Normal Range	
Tests	**Range**
Albumin	3.5–5.0 g/dL
Alkaline phosphatase (ALP serum)	35–100 U/L
Ammonia – NH_3	20–70 µg/dL
Amylase (serum)	<160 U/L
Aspartate aminotransferase (AST)	0–35 U/L
Bicarbonate (HCO_3) **(Serum)**	24–30 mEq/L
Bilirubin serum total	1.5 mg/dL
Bilirubin, conjugated (Direct)	<0.4 mg/dL
Blood Urea Nitrogen (BUN)	7–22 mg/dL
Calcium serum total	8.7–10.3 mg/dL
Ionized	4.2–5.2 mg/dL
Carbon dioxide pressure, arterial ($PaCO_2$)	35–45 mm Hg
Chloride serum	98–106 mEq/L
Cholesterol, total desirable	<200 mg/dL
Borderline high	201–240
High	>241
Cholesterol, LDL	
High risk patients (Framingham risk score)	<77.3 mg/dL or >50% reduction
Intermediate risk patient if LDL ≥3.5	<77.3 mg/dL or 50% reduction
Low risk patient if LDL	≥5 >50% reduction from baseline
Cholesterol, HDL	
Low	<40 mg/dL
Creatine Kinase serum (CK also CPK)	5–130 U/L
Copper	70–155 µg/dL
Creatinine, serum	
Male	0.8–1.4 mg/dL
Female	0.56–1.0 mg/dL
Creatinine clearance (Adult)	75–125 mL/min
Ferritin	10–250 ng/mL
Folic Acid (Folate)	3–16 ng/mL
Gamma Glutamyl Transferase (GGT)	
Female	5–36 U/L
Male	8–61 U/L
Glucose, fasting	59–105 mg/dL
Normal	<120 mg/dL

Contd...

Common Blood Tests with Normal Range	
Glucose, postprandial	
Normal	<120 mg/dL
Glycosylated Hemoglobin – HbA1c	
Normal	4–6%
Iron	60–178 µg/dL
Iron Binding Capacity, Total – TIBC	251–460 µg/dL
Lactic Acid (Lactate plasma venous)	9–16 mg/dL
Lactate Dehydrogenase serum (LDH)	95–195 IU/L
Magnesium serum	1.82–2.31 mg/dL
Osmolality serum	280–300 mOsm/kg
Oxygen partial pressure, arterial – PaO$_2$	85–105 mm Hg
pH – arterial	7.35–7.45 pH
Phosphorus, inorganic	2.5–4.5 mg/dL
Potassium	3.5–5.0 mEq/L
Protein, total	
Plasma	6.0–8.0 g/dL
Urine	<150 mg/24 hrs
Triglyceride	<195 mg/dL
Uric Acid	3.0–7.0 mg/dL
Blood Urea Nitrogen (BUN)	7–22.4 mg/dL
Hematocrit	
Female	37–46%
Male	42–52%
Hemoglobin	
Female	12.3–15.7 g/dL
Male	14.0–17.4 g/dL
Erythrocyte Sedimentation Rate	
(ESR Westergren)	5–36 U/L
Female	<10 mm/hr
Male	<6 mm/hr
Bleeding Time (IVY)	<9 minutes
Clotting Time	5–15 minutes
Fibrinogen	175–400 mg/dL
Prothrombin Time (PT)	10–13 seconds
Partial Thromboplastin Time (PTT)	28–38 seconds
Thrombin Time	14–16 seconds

Note: *Values and units of measurement listed in these tables are derived from several resources. Substantial variation exists in the ranges quoted as 'normal' and may vary depending on the assay used by different laboratories. Therefore, these tables should be considered directional only. Some values vary by gender, age, time of day and condition.*

Annexure 5

Fever of Unknown Origin

FUO is defined as:

- Fever >38.3°C (101°F) on at least two occasions.
- Illness duration ≥3 weeks.
- No known immunocompromised state.
- Diagnosis is uncertain after thorough history taking, physical examination and obligatory investigations, including blood culture (n = 3), urine culture, CXR, abdominal ultrasound and tuberculin skin test.

Etiology	**Infectious causes (15–25%)**
	• Abscess—usually in abdomen or pelvis due to risk factors, like cirrhosis, steroid or immunosuppressive medications, recent surgery, diabetes
	• Osteomyelitis
	• Bacterial endocarditis—culture negative in 2–5%, especially in *Coxiella burnetii*, *Tropheryma whipplei*, *Brucella*, *Mycoplasma*, *Chlamydia*, *Histoplasma*, *Legionella*, *Bartonella*, HACEK organisms which required either special media or longer than usual incubation
	• Prostatitis, dental abscesses, sinusitis, and cholangitis are sources of occult fever
	• TB, HIV/AIDS, CMV, EBV, malaria, typhoid fever, dengue fever, hepatitis A, Lyme disease, syphilis, psittacosis (bird exposure) and rat-bite fever
	Neoplastic causes (<20%)
	• Lymphomas (especially non-Hodgkin's lymphoma, most common cause)
	• Solid tumors: RCC most common, also breast, liver, colon, pancreas or liver metastases
	• Malignant histiocytosis
	Collagen vascular diseases (15–25% of cases)
	• SLE
	• RA
	• Rheumatic fever
	• Vasculitis, especially temporal (giant cell) arteritis
	• Juvenile rheumatoid arthritis (JRA), Still's disease

Contd...

	Miscellaneous causes (15–20% of cases) • Drug fever: Commonly antibiotics, antihistamines, antiarrhythmics, methyldopa, phenytoin, dilatin and NSAIDs • Sarcoidosis • Inherited Familial Mediterranean fever • Factitious • Pulmonary embolism
Investigations	**Initial investigations** • **Bloodwork:** CBC with differential and smear, electrolytes, BUN, Creatinine, calcium profile, LFTs, ESR, CRP, muscle enzymes, RF, ANA, serum protein electrophoresis, Fe, transferrin, TIBC, B_{12} • **Cultures:** Blood (×2 sets), urine, sputum, stool C&S, other fluids as appropriate VDRL, heterophile Ab (mononucleosis), CMV antigenemia tests, HIV serology, PPD and CXR. *If no diagnostic clues from the above, proceed with further investigations including:* • CT chest, abdomen and pelvis with contrast • Colonoscopy *If no diagnostic clue from the above, proceed with further investigations including:* • 67-Gallium scan • 111 Indium PMN scan • FDG PET scan
Management	• Treatment is directed at the specific cause found from the above investigations. • If no diagnosis with the above, consider empiric therapy versus watchful waiting. • Prognosis for most patients with FUO persisting without a diagnosis is very good without intervention. • **Empirical therapies may include:** Anti-TB therapy, broad spectrum antibiotics, colchicine, NSAIDS, steroids.

Conceptual Diagnostic Algorithm for FUO

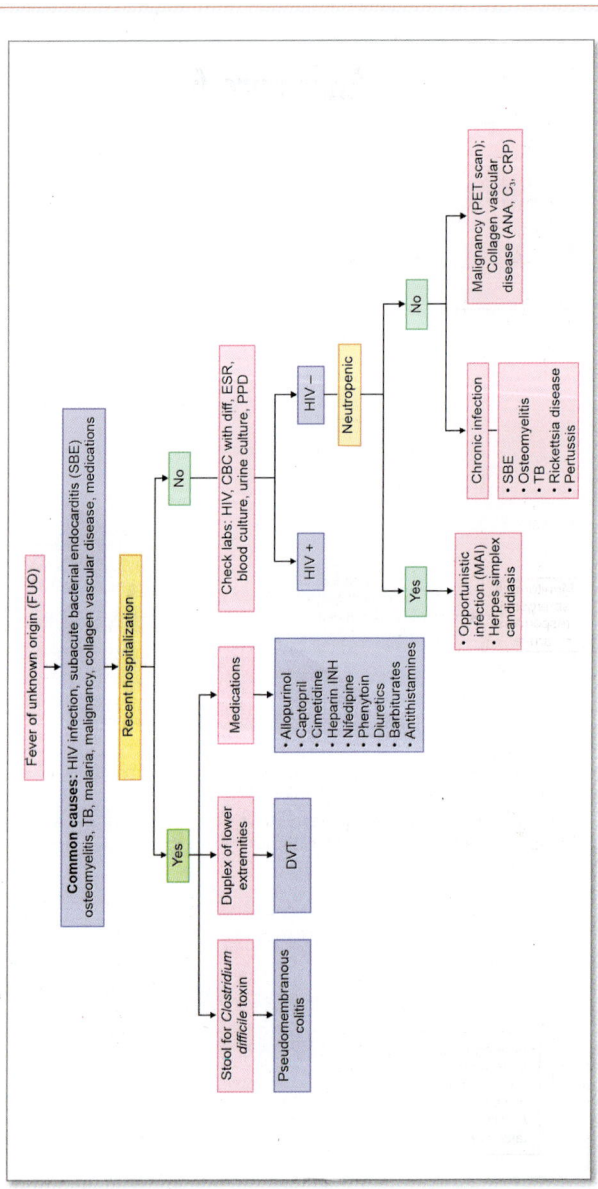

Annexure 6

Adult Basic Life Support Algorithm for Healthcare Provider

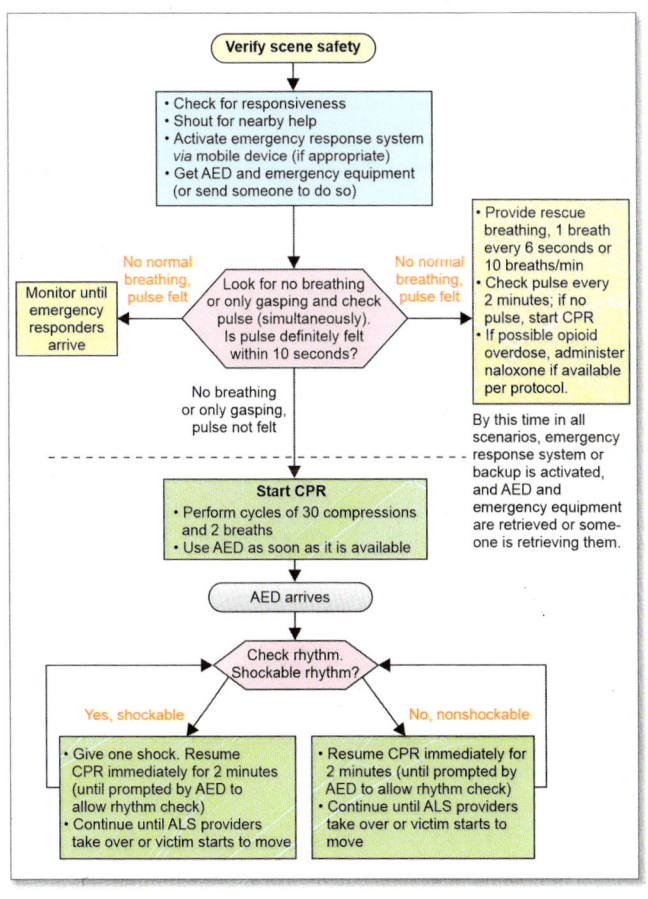

Annexure 7

Mechanical Ventilation

Silverman-Anderson scoring of respiratory distress in preterm babies

Parameter	Score 0	Score 1	Score 2
Upper chest retraction (observe if upper chest is synchronized with abdomen during inspiration)	Synchronized movement	Upper chest lags during inspiration	See-saw movement of upper chest
Lower chest retraction (observe for retractions in the rib spaces below mid-axillary line)	None	Just visible	Marked
Xiphoid retraction (observe for retractions below xiphoid)	None	Just visible	Marked
Nasal flaring	None	Minimal	Marked
Expiratory grunt	None	Audible with stethoscope	Audible with unaided ear

Downes' scoring of respiratory distress in newborn (both term and preterm babies)

Parameters	Score 0	Score 1	Score 2
Respiratory rate	<60/min	60–80/min	>80/min
Cyanosis	Nil	In room air	In >40% FiO_2
Air entry	Normal	Mild decrease	Marked decrease
Grunt	None	Audible with stethoscope	Audible with unaided ear
Retraction	Nil	Mild	Moderate

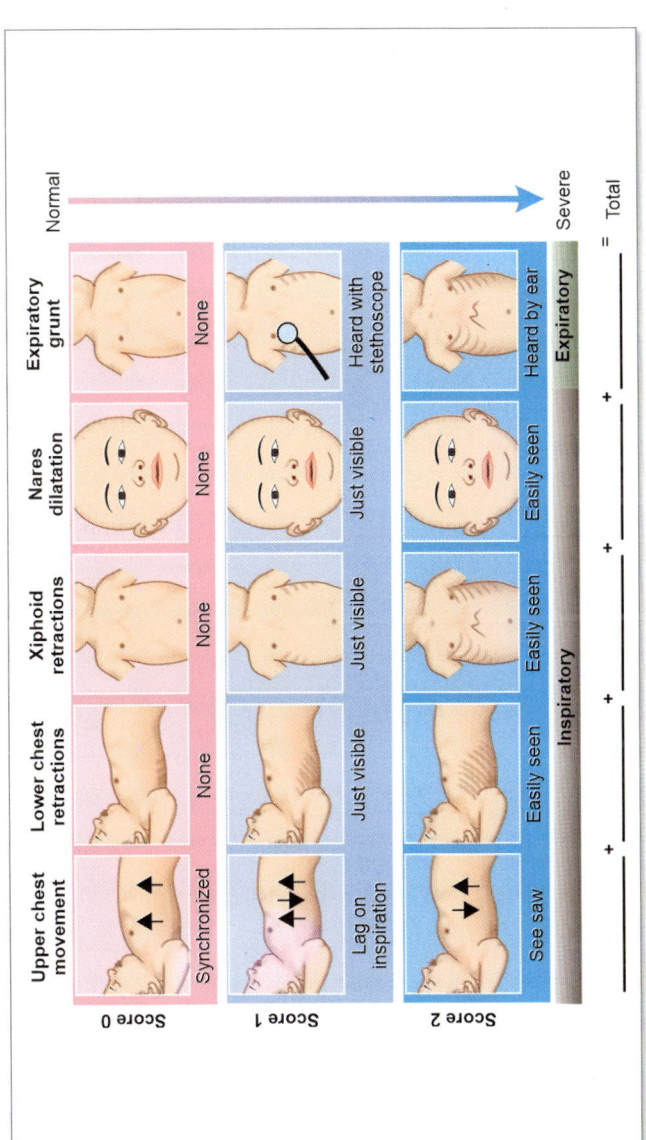

Annexure 8

Incubation Period of Various Communicable Diseases

Sl. no.	Communicable diseases	Causes	Incubation period
		Respiratory infections	
1.	Measles	Rubeola	10 days from exposure to onset of fever, and 14 days to appearance of rash (average is 7 days)
2.	Smallpox	Variola	Range 7–19 days
3.	Viral Rhinitis (Common cold)	Different viruses	12 hours–5 days (average 48 hours)
4.	Severe Acute Respiratory Syndrome (SARS)	SARS-associated corona virus	3–10 days, usually 4–6 days
5.	Chicken pox	Varicella-zoster virus	14–16 days
6.	Shingles (varicella zoster virus, second outbreak of chicken pox	Varicella-zoster virus	2–3 weeks and is usually 14–16 days
7.	Rubella (German measles)	RNA virus of the Togaviridae virus family	2–3 weeks
8.	Mumps	Myxovirus parotiditis	2–3 weeks
9.	Influenza	Influenza virus (A, B, C, D)	18–72 hours
10.	Pandemic Influenza A (H1N1 - Swine flu)	Influenza virus (A)	2–3 days
11.	Diphtheria	*Cornybacterium diphtheriae*	2–6 days

Contd...

Sl. no.	Communicable diseases	Causes	Incubation period
12.	Pneumonia	*Streptococcus pneumoniae*	12 hours or as long as 3 days after exposure to the flu virus
13.	Pertusis (whooping cough)	*B. pertussis*	7–14 days
14.	Meningococcal meningitis	*N. meningitidis*	3–4 days
15.	Respiratory tract infection	Rhinoviruses and group A streptococci	1–5 days
16.	Influenza and parainfluenza	Influenza virus and parainfluenza virus	1–4 days
17.	Respiratory syncytial disease	Respiratory syncytial virus (RSV)	1 week
18.	EBV disease	Epstein-Barr virus (EBV)	4–6 weeks
19.	Tuberculosis	*Mycobacterium tuberculosis*	3–6 weeks
Intestinal infections			
20.	Acute diarrhea, often with fever and cramps	Salmonella	Usually 6–48 hours
21.	Cholera	*Vibrio cholerae*	Few hours to 5 days
22.	Hepatitis	Hepatitis A virus	14–50 days, average 4 weeks
23.	Hepatitis	Hepatitis B virus	50–180 days, usually 2–3 months
24.	Hepatitis	Hepatitis C virus	2 weeks–6 months
25.	Hepatitis	Hepatitis E virus	3–8 weeks
26.	Hepatitis	Hepatitis D virus	Usually between 2–8 weeks In case of co-infection with hepatitis B: about 45–160 days
27.	Hepatitis	Hepatitis G virus	
28.	Poliomyelitis	Poliovirus	7–14 days
29.	Typhoid fever (Entric fever)	*Salmonella typhi*	10–14 days

Contd...

Sl. no.	Communicable diseases	Causes	Incubation period
Food poisoning			
30.	Salmonella food poisoning	*Salmonella typhimurium*	12–24 hours
31.	Staphylococcal food poisoning	*Staphylococcus aureus*	1–8 hours
32.	Botulism	*Clostridium botulinum*	18–36 hours
33.	*Clostridium perfringens* food poisoning	*Clostridium perfringens*	6–24 hours
34.	Cereus food poisoning	*Bacillus cereus*	1–6 hours
35.	Amoebiasis	*Entamoeba histolytica*	2–4 weeks
36.	Ascariasis	*Ascaris lumbricoides*	18 days to several weeks
37.	Hook worm infection	*Ancylostoma duodenale*	5 weeks–9 months
38.	Whip worm infection	*Trichuris trichiura*	60–90 days
Arthropod-borne infection			
39.	Dengue	*Aedes aegypti*	8–10 days
40.	Malaria	*Plasmodium vivax, P falciparum, P malariae, P ovale, Plasmodium knowlesi*	12 days for falciparum 14 days for vivax 17 days for ovale
41.	Lymphatic filariasis	Culex, anopheles, and aedes mosquito	8–16 months
42.	Zika virus disease	Zika virus	Few days–1 week
Zoonoses			
43.	Rabies	Rabies virus	1–3 months
44.	Monkey pox	Monkey pox virus	Usually 7–14 days but can range from 5 to 21 days
45.	Nipah virus	Paramyxoviridae	4–14 days
46.	Japanese encephalitis	Group B arbo virus	5–15 days
47.	Yellow fever	Flavi virus fibricus	3–6 days
48.	KFD	Group B flavi viruses	Between 3 and 8 days

Contd...

Sl. no.	Communicable diseases	Causes	Incubation period
49.	Chikungunya	Group A virus-aedes mosquitoes	4–7 days
50.	Brucellosis	4 species infect man-*B melitensis, B abortus, B suis, B canis*	1–3 weeks
51.	Leptosiprosis	Spirocheates	10 days
52.	Plague	Y. pestis	Bubonic plague: 2–7 days Septicaemic plague: 2–7 days Pneumonic plague: 1–3 days
53.	Human salmo-nellosis	Salmonella	6–72 hours
54.	Rickettsial zoo-noses	Rickettsiae	5–10 days
55.	Scrub typhus	*Rickettsia tsutsugamushi*	10–12 days
56.	Murine typhus	*Rickettsia typhi*	1–2 weeks
57.	Indian tick typhus	*Rickettsia conorii*	3–7 days
58.	Q fever	*Coxiella burnetii*	2–3 weeks
59.	Taeniasis	*T. saginata, T. solium, Taenia asiatica*	8–14 weeks
60.	Hydatid disease	*Echinococcus granulosus Echinococcus multilocularis*	Months to years
61.	Leishmaniasis	Leishmania	1–4 months
Surface infections			
62.	Trachoma	*Chlamydia trachomatis*	5–12 days
63.	Scabies	*Sarcoptes scabiei* (itch mite)	6 weeks before onset of itching. Re-exposure— symptoms develop in 1–4 days

Contd...

Sl. no.	Communicable diseases	Causes	Incubation period
64.	Methicillin resistant *Staphylococcus aureus* infection	Methicillin resistant *Staphylococcus aureus* (MRSA)	1–10 days
65.	Tetanus	*Clostridium tetani*	6–10 days
66.	Leprosy (Hansen's disease)	*Mycobacterium leprae*	3–5 years
67.	Conjunctivitis (pink eyes)	*Mycobacterium leprae*	24–72 hours
Sexually-transmitted diseases			
68.	Syphilis	*Treponema pallidum*	10–90 days, usually 3 weeks
69.	AIDS	Human immunodeficiency virus	<1–15 + years

Annexure 9

List of Prohibited Drugs

Manufacture and Sale through Gazette Notifications Under Section 26A of Drugs & Cosmetics Act, 1940 by The Ministry of Health and Family Welfare, Government of India

Banned Drugs

Analgin: All formulations containing Analgin for human use.

Fixed dose combination of **Flupenthixol + Malitrecen** for human use.

Pioglitazone and all formulations containing **Pioglitazone** for human use.

Dextropropoxyphene and formulations containing Dextropropoxyphene for human use.

Amidopyrine

Fixed dose combinations of vitamins with anti-inflammatory agents and tranquilizers.

Fixed dose combinations of Iron with **Strychnine, Arsenic** and **Yohimbine.**

Fixed dose combinations of **Yohimbine** and **Strychnine** with **Testosterone** and vitamins.

Fixed dose combinations of **Atropine** in **Analgesics** and **Antipyretics**.

Fixed dose combinations of **Strychnine** and **Caffeine** in tonics.

Nialamide

Fixed dose combinations of crude **Ergot** preparations except those containing **Ergotamine, Caffeine**, analgesics, antihistamines for the treatment of migraine, headaches.

Fixed dose combinations of vitamins with anti TB drugs except combination of **Isoniazid** with **Pyridoxine Hydrochloride** (vitamin B_6).

Fixed dose combinations of **Penicillin** with **Sulfonamides**.

Fixed dose combinations of **Chloramphenicol** with any other drug for internal use.

Fixed dose combinations of **Corticosteroids** with any other drug for internal use.

Fixed dose combination of **Histamine** H_2 receptor antagonists with antacids except for those combinations approved by Drugs Controller, India.

All Pharmaceutical preparations containing **Chloroform** exceeding 0.5% w/w or v/v whichever is appropriate.

Contd...   *Contd...*

Fixed dose combination containing more than one antihistamine.

Fixed dose combination of **Salbutamol** or any other drug having primarily bronchodilatory activity with centrally acting antitussive and/or antihistamine.

Fixed dose combination of **Metoclopramide** with systemically absorbed drugs except fixed dose combination of metoclopramide with **aspirin/paracetamol**.

Preparations claiming to combat cough associated with asthma containing centrally acting antitussive and/or an antihistamine.

Fixed dose combination containing **Pectin** and/or **Kaolin** with any drug which is systemically absorbed from GI tract except for combinations of Pectin and/or Kaolin with drugs not systemically absorbed.

Dover's Powder IP and Dover's Powder Tablets IP.

Antidiarrheal formulations containing **Phthalylsulfathiazole** or **Sulfaguanidine** or **Succinyl Sulfathiazole**.

Liquid oral antidiarrheals or any other dosage form for pediatric use containing **Diphenoxylate Loperamide** or **Atropine** or **Belladona** including their salts or esters or metabolites **Hyoscyamine** or their extracts or their alkaloids.

Fixed dose combination of antidiarrheals with electrolytes.

Patent and proprietary oral rehydration salts other than those confirming to the following parameters:
Patent and proprietary oral rehydration salts on reconstitution to one liter shall contain:
Sodium: 50–90 millimoles.
Total osmolarity: 240–290 millimoles.
Dextrose: Sodium molar ratio—Not less than 1:1 and not more than 3:1.

Patent and proprietary oral rehydration salts shall not contain mono or polysaccharides or saccharine sweetening agent.

Fixed dose combination of **Diazepam** and **Diphenhydramine Hydrochloride**.

Phenylpropanolamine and its formulation for human use.

Nimesulide formulations for human use in children below 12 years of age.

Fixed dose combination of a drug, standards of which are prescribed in the Second Schedule to the said Act with an Ayurvedic, Siddha or Unani drug.

Fixed dose combination of **Analgin** with any other drug.

Fixed dose combination of **Oxyphenbutazone** or **Phenylbutazone** with any other drug.

Tegaserod and its formulations for human use.

Fixed dose combinations of **Sodium Bromide/Chloral Hydrate** with other drugs.

Contd...

Contd...

Fixed dose combination of **Sedatives/hypnotics/anxiolytics** with analgesics-antipyretics.

Fixed dose combination of **Estrogen** and **Progestin** (other than oral contraceptive) containing per tablet estrogen content of >50 mcg (equivalent to **Ethinyl Estradiol**) and **progestin** content of >3 mg (equivalent to **Norethisterone Acetate**) and all fixed dose combination injectable preparations containing synthetic **Estrogen** and **Progesterone**. (Subs. By Noti. No. 743 (E) dt 10-08-1989).

Combination of anabolic **Steroids** with other drugs.

Phenacetin

Demeclocycline liquid oral preparations.

Oxytetracycline liquid oral preparations.

Methapyrilene, its salts.

Penicillin skin/eye ointment.

Tetracycline liquid oral preparations.

Methaqualone

Practolol

Fixed dose combinations of antihistaminic with antidiarrheals.

Fixed dose combinations of vitamins with analgesics.

Fixed dose combinations of any other **Tetracycline** with vitamin C.

Fixed dose combinations of **Hydroxyquinoline** group of drugs with any other drug except for preparations meant for external use.

The patent and proprietary medicines of fixed dose combinations of essential oils with alcohol having percentage higher than 20% proof except preparations given in the Indian Pharmacopoeia.

Fixed dose combination of **Ethambutol** with INH other than the following: INH Ethambutol 200 mg, 600 mg, 300 mg, 800 mg.

Fixed dose combination of any anthelmintic with cathartic/purgative except for **piperazine/santonin**.

Fixed dose combination of laxatives and/or antispasmodic drugs in enzyme preparations.

Fixed dose combination of centrally acting, antitussive with antihistamine, having high atropine like activity in expectorants.

Liquid oral tonic preparations containing **glycerophosphates** and/or other phosphates and/or central nervous system stimulant and such preparations containing alcohol >20% proof.

Chloralhydrate as a drug.

Antidiarrheal formulations containing **Kaolin** or **Pectin** or **Attapulgite** or **Activated Charcoal**.

Antidiarrheal formulations containing **Neomycin** or **Streptomycin** or **Dihydrostreptomycin** including their respective salts or esters.

Liquid oral antidiarrheals or any other dosage form for pediatric use containing halogenated **hydroxyquinolines**.

Contd...   *Contd...*

Patent and proprietary cereal-based oral rehydration salts on reconstitution to one liter shall contain:
Sodium: 50–90 millimoles.
Total osmolarity: Not >290 milliosmoles.

Precooked rice—equivalent to not <50 g and not >80 g as total replacement of **Dextrose**. Patent and proprietary oral with rehydration salts (ORS) specifications and labeled with the indication for "Adult Choleretic Diarrhea only".

Fenfluramine and **Dexfenfluramine Rimonabant Rosiglitazone.**

Sibutramine and its formulations for human use, and **R-Sibutramine** and its formulations for human use.

(*)Human Placental Extract and its formulations for human use.

Cisapride and its formulations for human use.

Mepacrine Hydrochloride (Quinacrine and its salts) in any dosage form for use for female sterilization or contraception.

Fixed dose combination of **dextropropoxyphene** with any other drug other than antispasmodic and/or nonsteriodal anti-inflammatory drugs (NSAIDs).

Gatifloxacin formulations for systemic use in humans by any route including oral and injectable.

Contd...

Prohibition revoked vide Gazette Notification GSR No. 418(E) dated May 30, 2011.

List of Drugs Prohibited for Import

Nialamide

Practolol

Methapyrilene and its salts.

Mepacrine Hydrochloride (**Quinacrine** and its Salts) in any dosage form for use for female sterilization or contraception.

Rimonabant

Chloral Hydrate as a drug.

Phenacetin

Methaqualone

Fenfluramine and **Dexfenfluramine**

Other Pharmaceutical Items Prohibited from Manufacturing, Sale and Distribution

Cosmetics Licensed as toothpaste/ tooth powder containing tobacco.

Fixed dose combination of vitamin B_1, vitamin B_6 and vitamin B_{12} for human use.

Fixed dose combination of **Pancreatin** or **Pancrelipase** containing amylase, protease and lipase with any other enzyme.

Fixed dose combination of **Phenobarbitone** with any antiasthmatic drugs.

Fixed dose combination of **Phenobarbitone** with **Ergotamine** and/or **Belladona**.

Fixed dose combination of **Nalidixic acid** with any antiamoebic including **Metronidazole**.

Fixed dose combination of **Cyproheptadine** with **Lysine** or **Peptone**.

Contd...

Valdecoxib and its formulation.

Letrozole for induction of ovulation in anovulatory infertility.

Parenteral preparations fixed dose combination of **streptomycin** with **Penicillin**.

Fixed dose combination of hemoglobin in any form (natural or synthetic).

Fixed dose combination of **Nitrofurantoin** and **trimethoprim**.

Fixed dose combination of **Phenobarbitone** with **Hyoscine** and/or **Hyoscyamine**.

Contd...

Fixed dose combination of **Haloperidol** with any anticholinergic agent including **Propantheline Bromide**.

Fixed dose combination of **Loperamide Hydrochloride** with **Furazolidone**.

Astemizole
Terfinadine
Fenformin
Rofecoxib

Diclofenac and its formulations for animal use.

Source: *https://drugs.delhi.gov.in/drugs/ banned-drugs*

Annexure 10

Administration of Drugs

Nurses administer drugs to patients/clients based on the prescription given by doctors. Drugs are administered for cure, prevention of diseases, diagnoses of health problems and to promote physical and mental well-being. Administering drugs is an important and very responsible function of the nurses. To carry out this function, nurses must:

- Know the principles of pharmacology and action and side effects of drugs to be administered and generic drug names.
- Have competencies in:
  - Calculation of doses of drugs
  - Use of different routes of drugs administration
  - Educating clients on drug consumption
  - Appropriate observation of clients before and after administrating drugs
  - Recording and reporting administration of drugs
- Practise locking safely the Narcotics and Barbiturates
- Remember not to leave drugs at bedside of clients
- Follow the rules of rights of drug administration:
  - Right drug
  - Right dose
  - Right time
  - Right route
  - Right patient
  - Right assessment of the patient before and after drug administration
  - Right documentation
  - Right of the client to refuse the consumption of drug
  - Right education of the client

Annexure 11

Code of Ethics for Nurses in India
(As per Indian Nursing Council)

1. **The Nurse Respects the Uniqueness of Individual in Provision of Care**

   Nurse
   - Provides care for individuals without consideration of caste, creed, religion, culture, ethnicity, gender, socioeconomic and political status, personal attributes, or any other grounds
   - Individualizes the care considering the beliefs, values and cultural sensitivities
   - Appreciates the place of individual in the family and community and facilitates participation of significant others in the care
   - Develops and promotes trustful relationship with individual(s)
   - Recognizes uniqueness of response of individuals to interventions and adapts accordingly

2. **The Nurse Respects the Rights of Individuals as Partner in Care and Helps in Making Informed Choices**

   Nurse
   - Appreciates individuals' right to make decisions about their care and therefore, gives adequate and accurate information for enabling them to make informed choices
   - Respects the decisions made by individual(s) regarding their care
   - Protects public from misinformation and misinterpretations
   - Advocates special provisions to protect vulnerable individuals/groups.

3. **The Nurse Respects Individual's Right to Privacy, Maintains Confidentiality, and Shares Information Judiciously**

   Nurse
   - Respects the individuals' right to privacy of their personal information
   - Maintains confidentiality of privileged information except in life-threatening situations and uses discretion in sharing information
   - Takes informed consent and maintains anonymity when information is required for quality assurance/academic/legal reasons
   - Limits the access to all personal records written and computerized to authorized persons only

4. **Nurse Maintains Competence in order to Render Quality Nursing Care**
   - Nursing care must be provided only by registered nurse
   - Nurse strives to maintain quality nursing care and upholds the standards of care

- Nurse values continuing education, initiates and utilizes all opportunities for self development
- Nurse values research as a means of development of nursing profession and participates in nursing research adhering to ethical principles

5. **The Nurse is Obliged to Practice within the Framework of Ethical, Professional and Legal Boundaries**

   Nurse
   - Adheres to code of ethics and code of professional conduct for nurses in India developed by Indian Nursing Council
   - Familiarizes with relevant laws and practices in accordance with the law of the state

6. **Nurse is Obliged to Work Harmoniously with Members of the Health Team**

   Nurse
   - Appreciates the team efforts in rendering care
   - Cooperates, coordinates and collaborates with members of the health team to meet the needs of people

7. **Nurse Commits to Reciprocate the Trust Invested in Nursing Profession by Society**

   Nurse
   - Demonstrates personal etiquettes in all dealings
   - Demonstrates professional attributes in all dealings

Annexure 12

Code of Professional Conduct for Nurses in India
(As per Indian Nursing Council)

1. Professional Responsibility and Accountability

Nurse

- Appreciates sense of self-worth and nurtures it
- Maintains standards of personal conduct reflecting credit upon the profession
- Carries out responsibilities within the framework of the professional boundaries
- Is accountable for maintaining practice standards set by **Indian Nursing Council**
- Is accountable for own decisions and actions
- Is compassionate
- Is responsible for continuous improvement of current practices
- Provides adequate information to individuals that allows them informed choices
- Practices healthful behavior

2. Nursing Practice

Nurse

- Provides care in accordance with set standards of practice
- Treats all individuals and families with human dignity in providing physical, psychological, emotional, social and spiritual aspects of care
- Respects individuals and families in the context of traditional and cultural practices, promoting healthy practices and discouraging harmful practices
- Presents realistic picture truthfully in all situations for facilitating autonomous decision-making by individuals and families
- Promotes participation of individuals and significant others in the care
- Ensures safe practice
- Consults, coordinates, collaborates and follows up appropriately when individuals' care needs exceed the nurse's competence

3. Communication and Interpersonal Relationships

Nurse

- Establishes and maintains effective interpersonal relationships with individuals, families and communities
- Upholds the dignity of team members and maintains effective interpersonal relationship with them
- Appreciates and nurtures professional role of team members
- Cooperates with other health professionals to meet the needs of the individuals, families and communities

4. Valuing Human Being

Nurse

- Takes appropriate action to protect individuals from harmful unethical practice
- Considers relevant facts while taking conscience decisions in the best interest of individuals
- Encourages and supports individuals in their right to speak for themselves on issues affecting their health and welfare
- Respects and supports choices made by individuals

5. Management

Nurse

- Ensures appropriate allocation and utilization of available resources
- Participates in supervision and education of students and other formal care providers
- Uses judgment in relation to individual competence while accepting and delegating responsibility
- Facilitates conducive work culture in order to achieve institutional objectives

- Communicates effectively following appropriate channels of communication
- Participates in performance appraisal
- Participates in evaluation of nursing services
- Participates in policy decisions, following the principle of equity and accessibility of services
- Works with individuals to identify their needs and sensitizes policy makers and funding agencies for resource allocation

6. Professional Advancement

Nurse

- Ensures the protection of the human fights while pursuing the advancement of knowledge
- Contributes to the development of nursing practice
- Participates in determining and implementing quality care
- Takes responsibility for updating own knowledge and competencies
- Contributes to core of professional knowledge by conducting and participating in research

Annexure 13

Standards for Nursing Practice
(As per Indian Nursing Council)

1. **Professional Responsibility and Accountability**

   Nursing Care is based on Quality Assurance Model

   - Demonstrates an understanding of the concept of quality assurance
   - Analyzes and identifies needs and problems
   - Uses relevant tools and processes to evaluate care
   - Takes appropriate action to improve quality

   Nursing Care is Professionally Managed and Ethically Justified

   - Demonstrates knowledge of current ethical issues in health care
   - Adheres to the code of ethics and professional conduct for nurses in India
   - Participates effectively in ethical decision making
   - Demonstrates managerial skills
   - Demonstrates a humanistic approach to management

   Nursing Care is Provided within the Legal Framework

   - Describes the legal framework for practice and its implications
   - Performs activities that are authorized within the legal boundaries
   - Recognizes breach of law related to practice and reports to appropriate authorities

   Nursing Care is Documented Accurately and Completely

   - Demonstrates an understanding of the value and implications of maintaining records
   - Maintains legible, complete and accurate records
   - Keeps record systematically and safely
   - Maintains confidentiality of records

   Nurse Accepts Responsibility and Accountability for Own Action

   - Recognizes the scope of nursing practice and own competence
   - Assumes and delegates responsibility within the scope of nursing practice and competence
   - Consults other members of nursing team when requisite nursing care beyond own competency
   - Consults other health care professionals as and when required

2. **Nursing Practice**

   Nursing Care Reflects that Practice Standards are being Adhered to

   - Demonstrates understanding of standards of nursing practice
   - Demonstrates adherence to satisfactory level of practice standards
   - Maintains records of care that are congruent with practice standards

Delivery of Nursing Care Reflects Nursing Process Approach

- Conducts systematic, comprehensive and accurate nursing assessment of individuals/groups
- Formulates a plan of care based on prioritized needs
- Collaborates with individuals and groups in formulating the plan of care
- Implements the care as per the plan
- Evaluates the outcome of actions taken and revises the plan of care

Nursing Care is provided in a Safe Environment

- Ensures safe and therapeutic environment in care settings
- Adheres to standard safety measures
- Follows guidelines for biomedical waste management
- Sensitizes coworkers, individuals and groups about the importance of safe environment

3. **Communication and Interpersonal Relationship**

Nurse Fosters Effective Interpersonal Relationship with Individuals and Families

- Establishes and maintains rapport with individuals and groups
- Demonstrates effective communication skills
- Demonstrates ability to listen attentively and patiently
- Responds empathetically and constructively to concerns expressed by individuals/groups
- Fosters a conducive environment of communication
- Engages in ethically justifiable communication
- Maintains interpersonal relationship within professional boundaries

Nurse Initiates Strategies to Promote the Learning of Individuals and Groups

- Identifies learning needs of individuals and groups
- Optimizes learning opportunities for individuals and groups
- Conducts planned and incidental teachings
- Evaluate outcome of teaching learning process

4. **Valuing Human Beings**

Nursing Care Enhances the Dignity, Individuality and Self-esteem of Individuals and Groups

- Conveys respects to individuals in all dealings
- Promotes and supports self-awareness, self-esteem and self-determination among individuals

Nursing Care Reflects Active Pursuit for Rights of All Individuals and in Particular the Vulnerable Groups

- Describes the constitutional and legal rights of individuals
- Informs and educates individuals about their rights
- Seeks consent of individuals after giving adequate and factual information
- Respects the rights of individuals and families to refuse care after ensuring that they understand the consequences of refusal as per policy
- Mobilizes support of health team members, families and communities for protection of rights of vulnerable groups

Nursing Care Reflects Gender Sensitivity toward the Needs of Women Related to their Health

- Describes cultural, social, economic and political context in which women live

- Promotes and supports self-awareness, self-esteem and self-determination among women
- Enhances the dignity of women as reflected in dealing with them
- Promotes health seeking behavior in women
- Mobilizes support for educating health team members, families and communities for rights of women

5. **Management**

Management of Nursing Services Reflects Effective Management Techniques

- Demonstrates understanding of different management techniques
- Applies appropriate management techniques based on situational analysis
- Initiates activities for enhancement of own managerial skills

Management of Nursing Services Reflects Use of Quality Assurance Model

- Appreciates the significance of quality assurance program for quality nursing care
- Demonstrates an understanding of quality assurance program and own role in implementation
- Involves team members' in development and implementation of quality assurance program

Management of Nursing Services Organizes and Utilizes Resources Efficiently

- Assesses the essential requirements of resources for delivery of quality nursing care
- Demonstrates an understanding of the system for procuring, utilizing and monitoring of resources
- Delegates responsibilities to appropriate team members for inventory control

- Ensures preventive maintenance of equipment

Management of Nursing Services Contributes to Development and Implementation of Institutional Policies in Conformity with Statutory Regulations

- Demonstrates an understanding of institution policies and statutory regulations
- Contributes to framing and renewing the institution policy as per the statutory regulations
- Communicates the policies, rules and regulations to concerned persons and ensures compliance

Management of Nursing Services Develops and Implements Staff Development and Welfare Program

- Prepares a plan for staff development program and welfare
- Facilitates implementation of staff development and welfare activities
- Participates in ongoing training activities
- Assesses the effectiveness of staff development activities
- Advocates the interest of the nurses for welfare measures

Management of Nursing Services Ensures Disaster Preparedness

- Participates in institutional plan for disaster preparedness
- Organizes training and drill for the members of the disaster management

6. **Professional Advancement**

Nursing Care Reflects the Commitment to Ongoing Education and Professional Growth of Self and Others

- Participates in continuing education program

- Reviews current literature
- Participates in professional meetings
- Seeks new information related to nursing practice from professional colleagues
- Assesses own learning needs and identifies areas of further training
- Contributes to professional growth of others
- Contributes to professional journals

Nursing Care Includes Activities which Focus on the Advancement of Profession

- Identifies the need for change in scope of nursing practice
- Participates in research activities
- Conducts nursing research and disseminates findings
- Interprets and utilizes research findings in nursing practice
- Shares information regarding advancement in nursing with administration, professional and policy makers

Annexure 14

How to do CPR on an Adult (BLS)

Five Parts: *Taking Vitals, Administering CPR, Continuing the Process Until Help Arrives, Using an AED, Putting the Patient in Recovery Position.*

Knowing how to perform both methods of CPR (cardiopulmonary resuscitation) on an adult could save a life. However, the recommended method for performing CPR has changed relatively recently, and it is important to know the difference. In 2010, the American Heart Association made a radical change to the recommended CPR process for victims of cardiac arrest after studies showed that compression-only CPR (no mouth-to-mouth breathing) is as effective as the traditional approach.

PART 1

Taking Vitals

1. **Check the scene for immediate danger.** Make sure you are not putting yourself in harm's way by administering CPR to someone unconscious. Is there a fire? Is the person lying on a roadway? Do whatever is necessary to move yourself and the other person to safety.

   ▪ If there is anything that could endanger you or the victim, see whether there is something you can do to counteract it. Open a window, turn off the stove, or put out the fire, if possible.

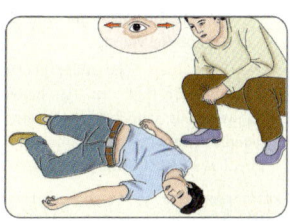

   ▪ However, if there is nothing you can do to counteract the danger, move the victim. The best way to move the victim is by placing a blanket or coat underneath his/her back and dragging it.

2. **Assess the victim's consciousness.** Gently tap his or her shoulder and ask "Are you OK?" in a loud, clear voice. If he or she responds agreement "Yeah" or such, CPR is not required. Instead, undertake *basic first aid* and *take measures to prevent or treat shock*, and assess whether you need to contact emergency services.

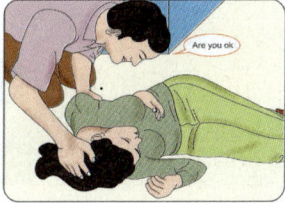

   ▪ If the victim does not respond, continue with the following steps:

- To contact emergency services, call **108** in India.
- Give the dispatcher your location, and notify him or her that you are going to perform CPR. If you are alone, get off the phone and start compressions after that. If you have someone else with you, have him or her stay on the line while you do CPR on the victim.

3. **Send for help.** The more people available for this step, the better. However, it can be done alone. Send someone to call for emergency medical services (EMS).

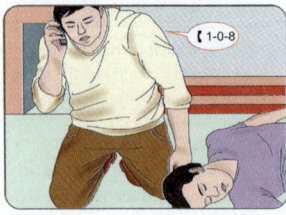

4. **Do not check for a pulse.** Unless you are a trained medical professional, odds are you'll spend too much valuable time looking for a pulse when you should be doing compressions.

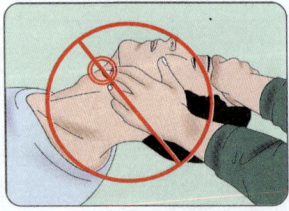

5. **Check for breathing.** And, make sure that the airway is not blocked. If the mouth is closed, press with your thumb and forefinger on both cheeks at the end of the teeth and then look inside. Remove any visible obstacle that is in your reach but never push your fingers inside too far. Put your ear close to the victim's nose and mouth, and listen for breathing. **If the victim is coughing or breathing normally, do not perform CPR.**

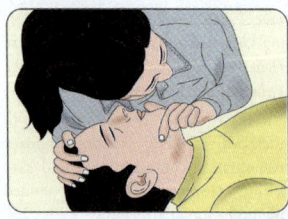

PART 2

Administering CPR

1. **Place the victim on his or her back.** Make sure he or she is lying as flat as possible - this will prevent injury while you are doing chest compressions. Tilt his head back by using your palm against the forehead and a push against his chin.

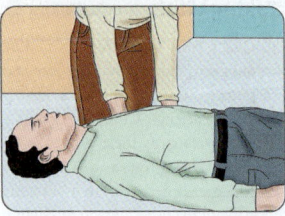

2. **Place the heel of one hand on the victim's breastbone, 2 finger-widths above the meeting area of the lower ribs, exactly between the nipples.**

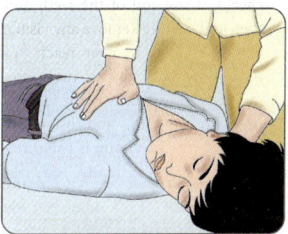

3. **Place your second hand on top of the first hand, palms-down, interlock the fingers of the second hand between the first.**

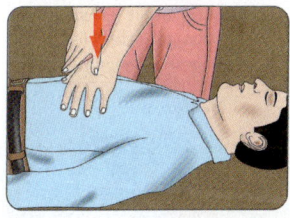

4. **Position your body directly over your hands, so that your arms are straight and somewhat rigid.** Don't flex the arms to push, but sort of lock your elbows, and use your upper body strength to push.

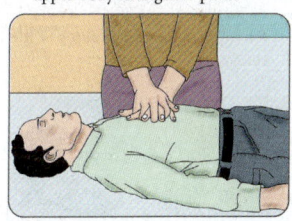

5. **Perform 30 chest compressions.** Press down with both hands directly over the breastbone to perform a compression, which helps the heart beat. Chest compressions are more critical for correcting abnormal heart rhythms (ventricular fibrillation or pulseless ventricular tachycardia, heart rapidly quivering instead of beating).

- You should press down by about 2 inches (5 cm).
- Do the compressions in a relatively fast rhythm.

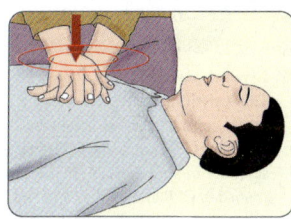

PART 3

Continuing the Process until Help Arrives

1. **Minimize pauses in chest compression that occur when changing providers or preparing for a shock.** Attempt to limit interruptions to less than 10 seconds.

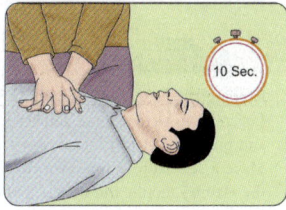

2. **Make sure the airway is open.** Place your hand on the victim's forehead and two fingers on his/her chin and tilt the head back to open the airway.

- If you suspect a neck injury, *pull the jaw forward rather than lifting the chin*. If jaw thrust fails to open the airway, do a careful head tilt and chin lift.
- If there are no signs of life, place a breathing barrier (if available) over the victim's mouth.

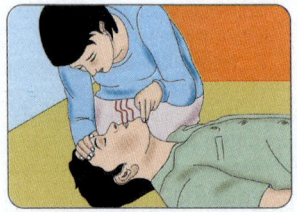

3. Give two rescue breaths (optional).
The American Heart Association no longer considers rescue breaths necessary for CPR, as the chest compressions are more important. If you are trained in CPR and totally confident, give two rescue breaths after your 30 chest compressions. If you have never done CPR before, or you are trained but rusty, stick with only chest compressions.

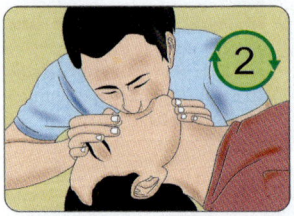

Keeping the airway open, take the fingers that were on the forehead and pinch the victim's nose closed. Make a seal with your mouth over the victim's mouth and breathe out for about one second. Make sure you breathe slowly, as this will make sure the air goes in the lungs and not the stomach.

- If the breath goes in, you should see the chest slightly rise and also feel it go in. Give a second rescue breath.

- If the breath does not go in, reposition the head and try again. If it does not go in again, the victim may be choking. *Do abdominal thrusts (the Heimlich maneuver)* to remove the obstruction.

4. Repeat the cycle of 30 chest compressions. If you are also doing rescue breaths, keep doing a cycle of 30 chest compressions, and then 2 rescue breaths; repeat the 30 compressions and 2 more breaths.

- You should do CPR for 2 minutes (5 cycles of compressions to breaths) before spending time checking for signs of life.

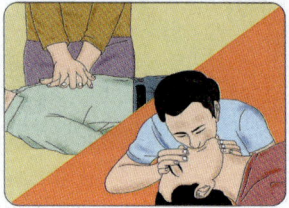

5. Continue CPR until someone takes over for you, emergency personnel arrive, you are too exhausted to continue, an automated external defibrillator (AED) is available for immediate use, or signs of life return.

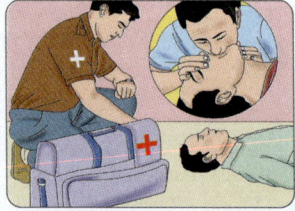

CPR Revised Guidelines: Think C-A-B

Compressions	Airway	Breathing
Push at least 2 inches on adult breastbone, 100 times per minute, to move oxygenated blood to vital organs	Open the airway and check for breathing or blockage; watch for rise of chest and listen for air movement	Tilt chin back for the unobstructed passing of air; give two breaths and resume chest compressions

Note: Those untrained in CPR can simply do chest compressions until help arrives.

Annexure 15

National Immunization Schedule

National Immunization Schedule for Infants, Children and Pregnant Women (IPHS)

Vaccine	When to Give	Dose	Route	Site
For Pregnant Women				
TT-1	Early in pregnancy	0.5 mL	Intramuscular	Upper arm
TT-2	4 weeks after TT – 1*	0.5 mL	Intramuscular	Upper arm
TT-Booster	If pregnancy occurs within three years of last TT vaccinations*	0.5 mL	Intramuscular	Upper arm
For Infants				
BCG	At birth (for institutional deliveries) or along with DPT-1	0.05 mL for infant up to 1 month	Intradermal	Left upper arm
OPV – 0	At birth if delivery is in institution	2 drops	Oral	Oral
OPV 1, 2 and 3	At 6 weeks, 10 weeks and 14 weeks	2 drops	Oral	Oral
DPT-1, 2 and 3	At 6 weeks, 10 weeks and 14 weeks	0.5 mL	Intramuscular	Outer mid-thigh (anterolateral side of mid thigh)

Contd…

Vaccine	When to Give	Dose	Route	Site
Hep B1, 2 and 3	At 6 weeks, 10 weeks and 14 weeks**	0.5 mL	Intramuscular	Outer mid-thigh (anterolateral side of mid-thigh)
Measles	9–12 months	0.5 mL	Subcutaneous	Right upper arm
Vitamin-A (1st dose)	At 9 months with measles	1 mL (1 lakh IU)	Oral	Oral
For children				
DPT Booster	16–24 months	0.5 mL	Intramuscular	Outer mid-thigh (anterolateral side of mid thigh)
OPV Booster	16–24 months	2 drops	Oral	Oral
Vitamin A 2nd to 5th	16 months with DPT/OPV booster. 24 months, 30 months and 36 months	2 mL (2 lakh IU)	Oral (dose)	Oral
DT Booster	5 years	0.5 mL	Intramuscular	Upper arm
TT	10 years and 16 years	0.5 mL	Intramuscular	Upper arm

*TT-2 or Booster dose to be given before 36 weeks of pregnancy
**For institutional deliveries, give at birth, 6 weeks and 14 weeks

A fully immunized infant is one who has received BCG, three doses of DPT, three doses of OPV and Measles before one year of age.

Annexure 16

APGAR Scoring

Parameters	Scores		
Signs	0	1	2
Respiratory effort	Absent	Slow, irregular	Good, crying
Heart rate	Absent	<100 bpm	>100 bpm
Muscle tone	Flaccid	Flexion of extremities	Active body movements
Reflex irritability	No response	Grimace	Cough or sneeze
Color	Blue, pale	Body pink, extremities blue	Complete pink

Grading

Total score = 10

No depression = 8–10

Mild depression = 5–7

Moderate depression = 3–4

Severe depression = 0–2

Reference

Textbook of Obstetrics, DC Dutta, 9th ed, 2018

Annexure 17

NAAC Assessment Criteria

NAAC Criteria: What are NAAC Accreditation Criteria?

- #1: Curricular Aspects. ...
- #2: Teaching, Learning, and Evaluation. ...
- #3: Research, Innovation, and Extensions. ...
- #4: Infrastructure and Learning Resources. ...
- #5: Student Support and Progression. ...
- #6: Governance, Leadership, and Management. ...
- #7: Institutional Values and Best Practices.

Key Indicators and Weightages

The criterion-wise differential weightages for the three types of HEIs are:

Curricular aspects	150 (U)	150 (Au)	100 (Aff UG)	100 (Aff PG)
Teaching-learning and Evaluation	200 (U)	300 (Au)	350 (Aff UG)	350 (Aff PG)
Research, innovations and extension	250 (U)	150 (Au)	110 (Aff UG)	120 (Aff PG)
Infrastructure and learning resources	100 (U)	100 (Au)	100 (Aff UG)	100 (Aff PG)
Student support and progression	100 (U)	100 (Au)	140 (Aff UG)	130 (Aff PG)
Governance, leadership and management	100 (U)	100 (Au)	100 (Aff UG)	100 (Aff PG)
Institutional values and best practices	100 (U)	100 (Au)	100 (Aff UG)	100 (Aff PG)

Annexure 18

Types of Insulin

Rapid and short-acting insulin helps reduce blood glucose levels at mealtimes and intermediate or long-acting insulin helps with managing the body's general needs. Both help manage blood glucose levels.

Insulin is grouped according to how long it works in the body. The five different types of insulin range from rapid- to long-acting. Some types of insulin look clear, while others are cloudy.

Before injecting a cloudy insulin, the pen or vial needs to be gently rolled between your hands to make sure the insulin is evenly mixed (until it looks milky). Don't use clear insulin if it appears cloudy.

Often, people need both rapid- and longer-acting insulin. Everyone is different and needs different combinations.

The five types of insulin are described here in detail:

1. Rapid-acting Insulin

Rapid-acting insulin starts working somewhere between 2.5 and 20 minutes after injection.

2. Short-acting Insulin

Short-acting insulin takes longer to start working than the rapid-acting insulin.

It begins to lower blood glucose levels within 30 minutes, so one needs to have injection 30 minutes before eating.

3. Intermediate-acting Insulin

The intermediate-acting insulin are cloudy in nature and need to be mixed well.

These insulins begin to work about 60–90 minutes after injection, peak between 4–12 hours and last for between 16–24 hours.

4. Mixed Insulin

Mixed insulin contains a pre-mixed combination of either very rapid-acting or short-acting insulin, together with intermediate-acting insulin.

5. Long-acting Insulin

Slow, steady release of insulin with no apparent peak action. One injection can last up to 24 hours. It is usually injected once a day but can be taken twice daily.

Insulin Injection Sites

Insulin is injected through the skin into the fatty tissue known as the subcutaneous layer. It shouldn't go into muscle or directly into the blood, as this changes how quickly the insulin is absorbed and works.

Absorption of insulin varies depending on where in the body it is injected. The abdomen absorbs insulin the fastest and is used by most people. The upper arms, buttocks and thighs have a slower absorption rate and can also be used.

Insulin Storage

Insulin needs to be stored correctly. This includes:

- Storing unopened insulin on its side in a fridge.

- Keeping the fridge temperature between 2°C and 8°C.
- Making sure that insulin does not freeze.
- Once opened, keeping it at room temperature (less than 25°C) for not more than one month and then disposing of it safely.
- Avoiding keeping insulin in direct sunlight.

Extreme (hot or cold) temperatures can damage insulin so it doesn't work properly. It must not be left where temperatures are over 30°C.

Color Plates

PLATE 1: **SKIN AND ITS STRUCTURES**

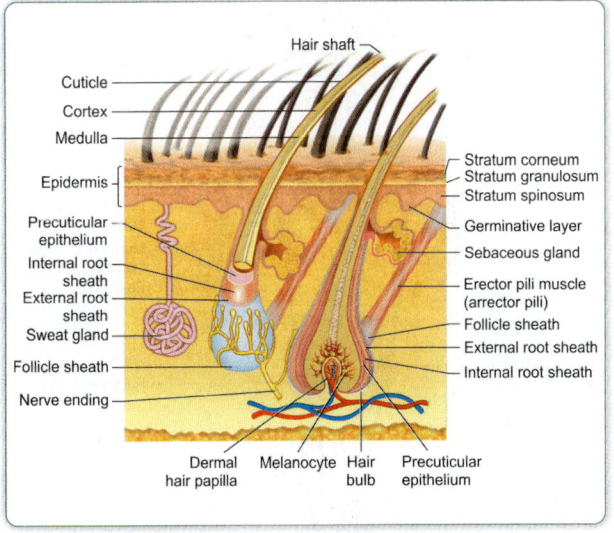

Hair shaft

Cuticle
Cortex
Medulla

Epidermis

Precuticular epithelium
Internal root sheath
External root sheath
Sweat gland
Follicle sheath
Nerve ending

Stratum corneum
Stratum granulosum
Stratum spinosum
Germinative layer
Sebaceous gland
Erector pili muscle (arrector pili)
Follicle sheath
External root sheath
Internal root sheath

Dermal hair papilla   Melanocyte   Hair bulb   Precuticular epithelium

PLATE 2: SKELETAL SYSTEM

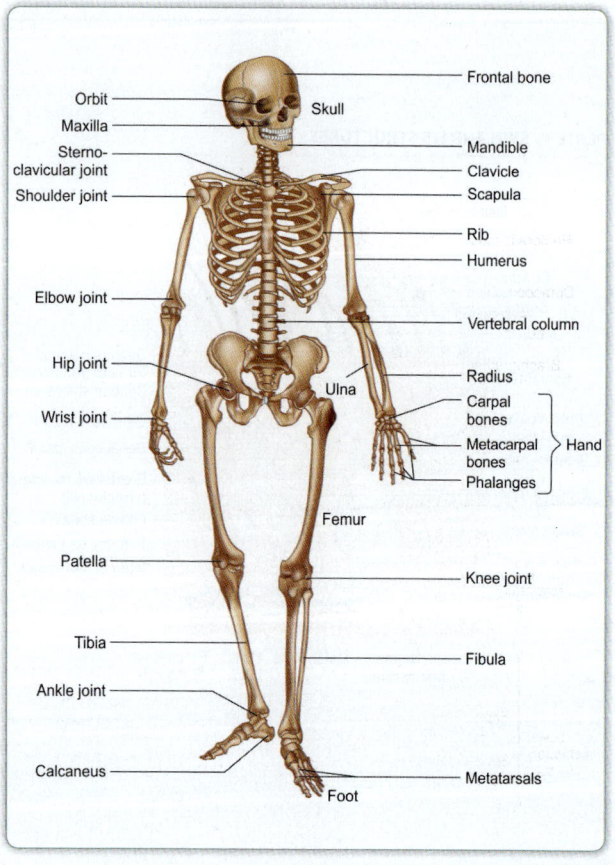

Orbit
Maxilla
Sterno-clavicular joint
Shoulder joint
Elbow joint
Hip joint
Wrist joint
Patella
Tibia
Ankle joint
Calcaneus

Skull

Ulna

Femur

Foot

Frontal bone
Mandible
Clavicle
Scapula
Rib
Humerus
Vertebral column
Radius
Carpal bones
Metacarpal bones
Phalanges
} Hand
Knee joint
Fibula
Metatarsals

PLATE 3: RESPIRATORY SYSTEM

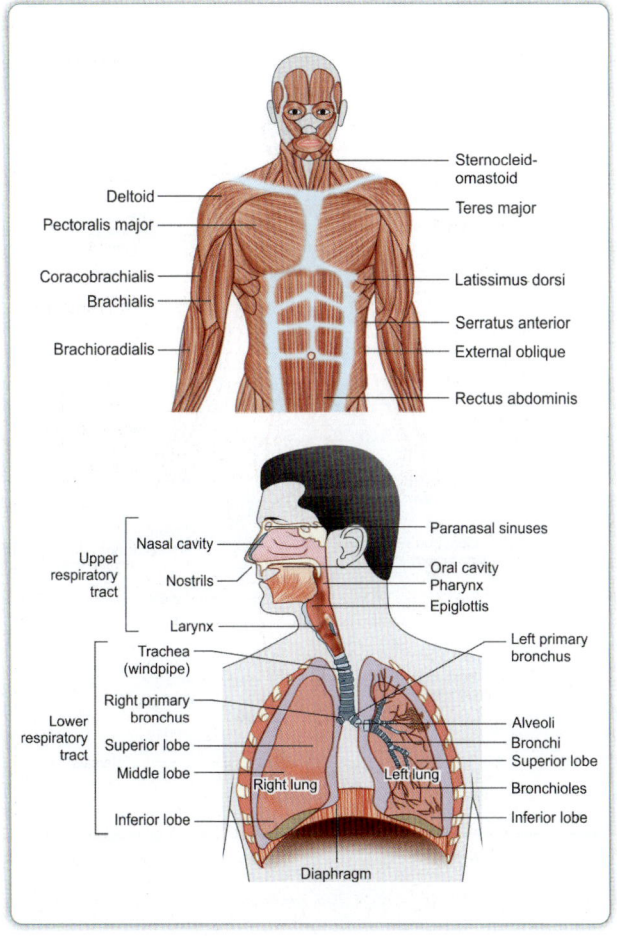

Sternocleid-
omastoid

Deltoid

Teres major

Pectoralis major

Coracobrachialis

Latissimus dorsi

Brachialis

Serratus anterior

Brachioradialis

External oblique

Rectus abdominis

Paranasal sinuses

Upper
respiratory
tract

Nasal cavity

Oral cavity

Nostrils

Pharynx

Epiglottis

Larynx

Left primary
bronchus

Trachea
(windpipe)

Right primary
bronchus

Lower
respiratory
tract

Alveoli

Superior lobe

Bronchi

Middle lobe

Superior lobe

Right lung

Left lung

Bronchioles

Inferior lobe

Inferior lobe

Diaphragm

PLATE 4: ARTERIAL SYSTEM

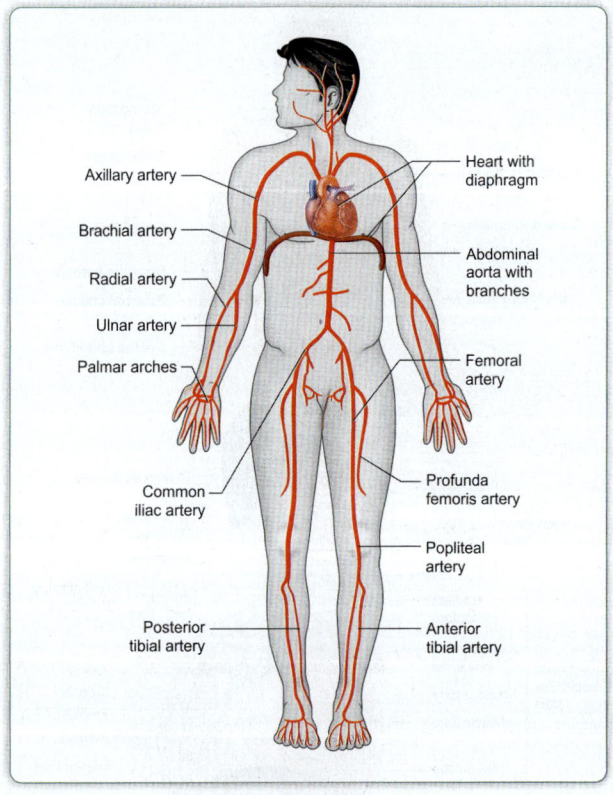

PLATE 5: VENOUS SYSTEM

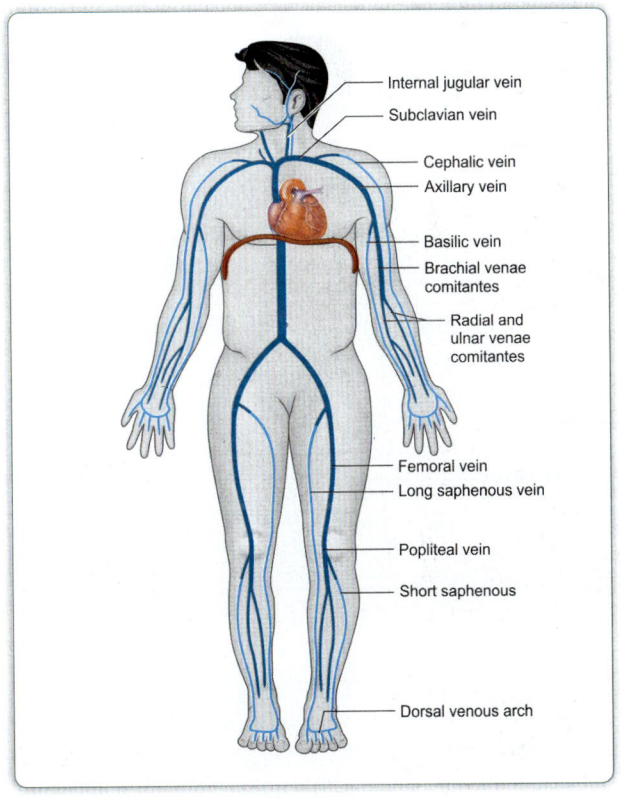

PLATE 6: LMYPHATIC SYSTEM

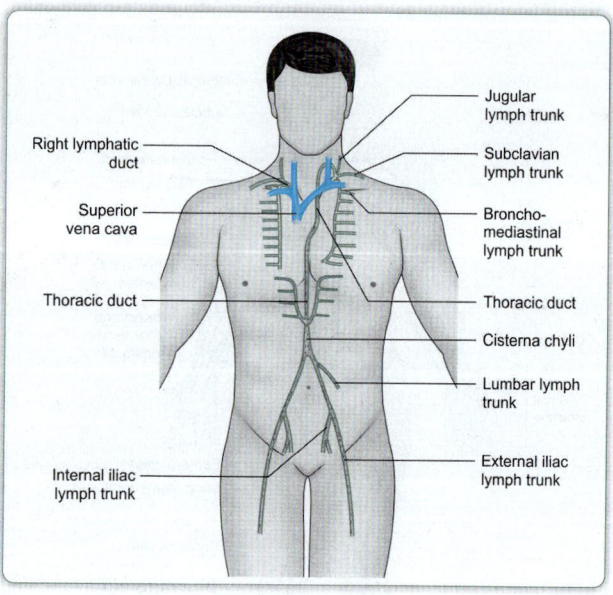

PLATE 7: DIGESTIVE SYSTEM

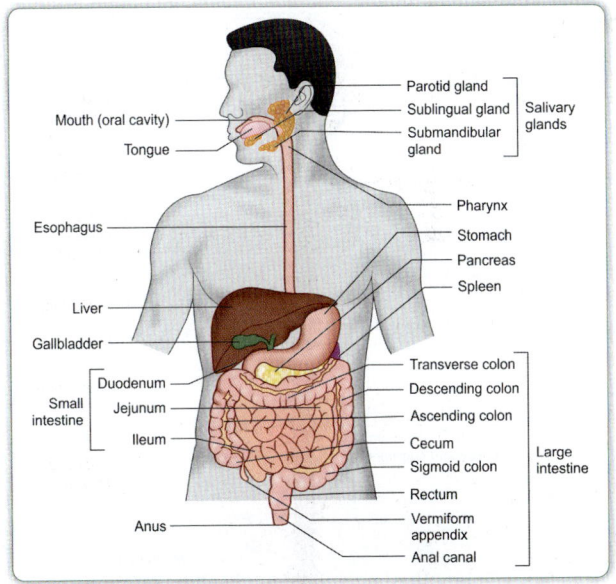

PLATE 8: CRANIAL SYSTEM

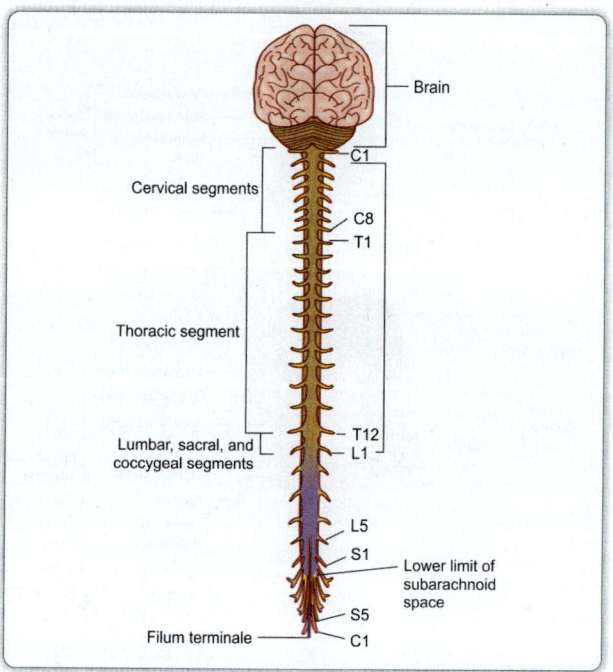

Brain

C1

Cervical segments

C8
T1

Thoracic segment

T12
L1

Lumbar, sacral, and
coccygeal segments

L5
S1

Lower limit of
subarachnoid
space

S5
C1

Filum terminale

PLATE 9: URINARY SYSTEM

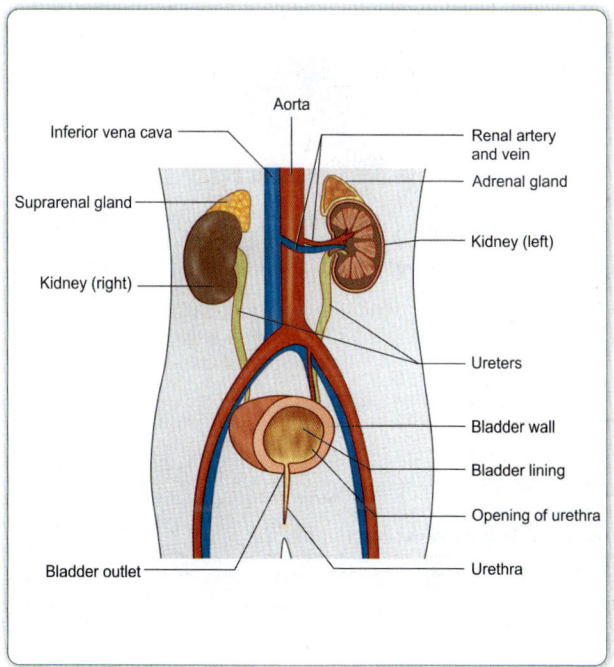

PLATE 10: MALE REPRODUCTIVE SYSTEM

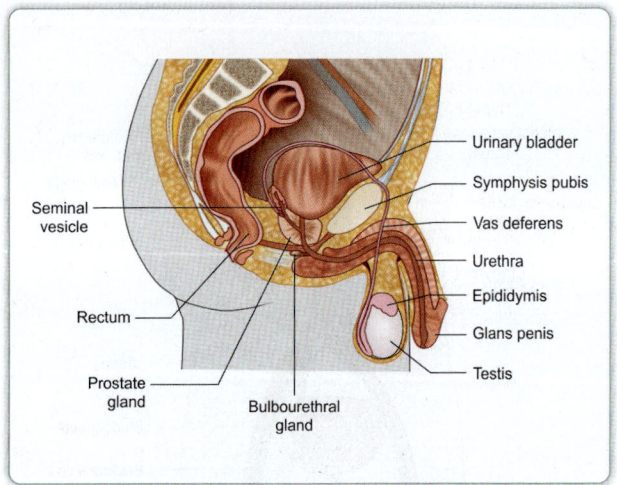

PLATE 11: FEMALE REPRODUCTIVE SYSTEM

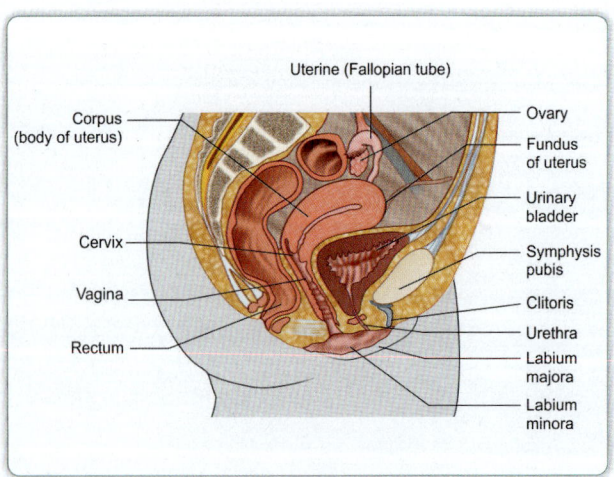

PLATE 12: ENDOCRINE SYSTEM

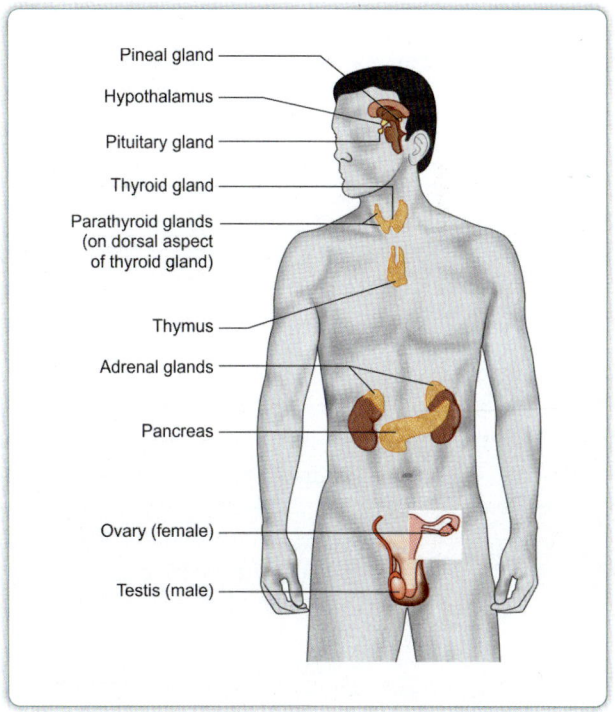

Pineal gland

Hypothalamus

Pituitary gland

Thyroid gland

Parathyroid glands
(on dorsal aspect
of thyroid gland)

Thymus

Adrenal glands

Pancreas

Ovary (female)

Testis (male)

@ at

A Accommodation; adenine; anode (anodal); anterior; axial; symbol for ampere and mass number.

A seeing eye

AAA Abdominal aortic aneurysm

A-scan Ultrasonographic display used for measuring the size and thickness of organs and tissues accurately.

Abacterial Indicating a condition not caused by bacteria.

Abadie's sign 1. A sign in tabes dorsalis in which there is loss of pain from squeezing the calcaneal tendon 2. Spasm of the levator palpebrae superioris muscles occurring frequently in thyrotoxicosis, also seen in tension and fatigue.

Aband A dark band in muscle representing overlapping of actin and myosin filaments.

Abasia Inability to walk because of motor incoordination.

Abate To lessen in force or intensity.

Abatement A decrease in the severity of a pain or a symptom.

Abdomen The cavity between the diaphragm and the pelvis, lined by a serous membrane, the peritoneum, and containing the stomach, intestines, liver, gallbladder, spleen, pancreas, kidneys, suprarenal glands, ureters and bladder. For descriptive purposes, its area can be divided into nine regions.

Acute abdomen Any abdominal condition urgently requiring treatment, usually surgical. Pendulous a. A condition in which the anterior part of the abdominal wall hangs down over the pubis.

Scaphoid (navicular) abdomen Hollowing of the anterior wall so that it presents a concave rather than convex contour.

Abdominal Pertaining to the abdomen.

Abdominal angina An acute attack of severe abdominal pain, commonly occurring after eating and often associated with weight loss, nausea, vomiting and diarrhea. It is caused by narrowing or obstruction of the mesenteric arteries, primarily atherosclerotic in origin.

Abdominal aneurysm A dilatation of the abdominal aorta.

Abdominal aorta Part of the aorta below the diaphragm.

Abdominal aponeurosis The wide tendinous expanse by which the external oblique, internal oblique and transverse muscles are inserted.

Abdominal apoplexy Infarction of an abdominal organ, usually the small intestine, resulting from vascular stenosis or occlusion.

Abdominal breathing Deep breathing; hyperpnea.

Abdominal muscles A group of four pair of muscles making up the abdominal wall: the external oblique, internal oblique, rectus abdominus and transversus abdominis.

Abdominal reflex Reflex contraction of abdominal wall muscles observed when abdominal skin is lightly stroked.

Abdominal regions For descriptive purposes, abdominal area can be divided into nine regions. It is divided by two horizontal and two parasagittal lines. The regions thus formed are: above the umbilicus - right hypochondriac, epigastric, left hypochondriac, middle - right lumbar, umbilical and left lumbar and below the umbilicus - right iliac, hypogastric or pubic and left iliac.

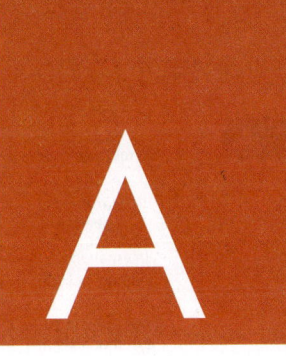

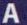

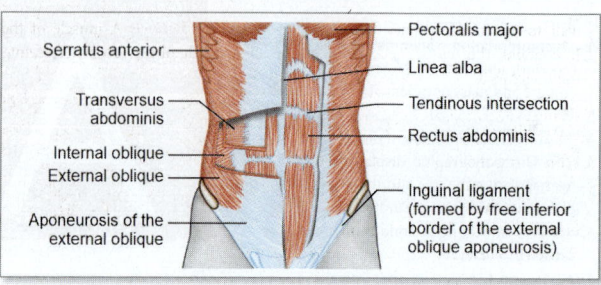

Abdominal Muscles

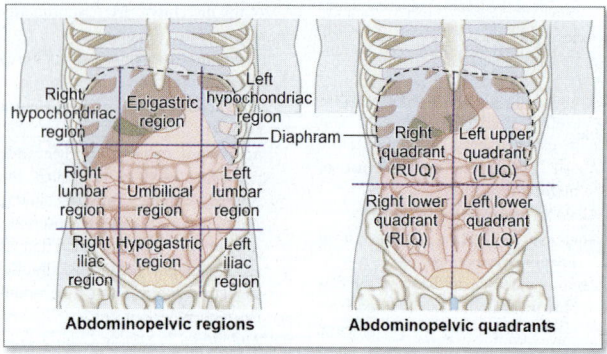

Abdominopelvic regions   **Abdominopelvic quadrants**

Abdominal Regions

Regions of the Abdomen 1. Right hypochondriac; 2. Epigastric; 3. Left hypochondriac; 4. Right lumbar; 5. Umbilical; 6. Left lumbar; 7. Right iliac; 8. Hypogastric; 9. Left iliac.

Abdominal respiration Respiration caused by the contraction of the diaphragm and the expansion and recoil of the abdominal walls.

Abdominal section Incision through the abdominal wall.

Abdominal thrusts A technique used to relieve chocking vitims

Abdominopelvic Relating to the abdomen and the pelvic cavity.

Abdominoperineal Pertaining to the abdomen and the perineum.

Abdomino-excision An operation performed through the abdomen and the perineum for the excision of the rectum or bladder. Often done as a synchronized operation by two surgeons, one working at each approach.

Abdominoplasty Also known as a tummy tuck, it is a cosmetic surgery procedure to remove fat and excess loose skin to improve the shape of the abdominal area.

Abdominoposterior Indicating a position of the fetus with its abdomen turned toward the maternal back.

Abdominovesical pouch A pouch formed by the reflection of the peritonium from the anterior abdominal wall to distended urinary bladder. It contains the lateral and medial inguinal fossae.

Abduce To abduct or to draw away.

Abducent Leading away from the midline.

Abducent muscle The external rectus muscle of the eye, which rotates it outward.

Abducent nerve A small cranial (motor) nerve supplying the blood to rectus muscle of the eye.

Abducent nucleus A nucleus lying under the floor of the fourth ventricle at the junction of the pons and medulla which gives origin to the abducent nerve.

Abduct To draw away from the median line.

Abduction Movement of a body part away from the median plane.

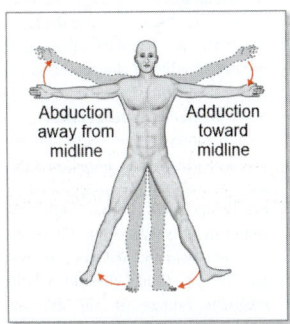

Abduction

Abduction cap An orthopedic appliance of canvas or leather to maintain abduction in case of subdeltoid bursitis.

Abductor A muscle that draws a limb away from the midline of the body. The opposite of adductor.

Abductor digiti minimi The abductor muscle of the little finger or little toe.

Abductor hallucis A muscle of the medial side of the foot inserted into the base of the metatarsal.

Abductor hallucis longus A muscle of the anterior region of the leg inserted into the base of the first metatarsal.

Abductor indicis The first dorsal interosseous muscle of the hand.

Abductor paralysis Paralysis of the abduction especially of the posterior arytenoid muscle and, thus of the vocal cords.

Abductor pollisis brevis The short abductor muscle of the thumb.

Abductor pollicis longus The long abductor muscle of the thumb.

Aberdeen formula A method of estimating the number of nurses needed in a ward based on the number and dependency of the patients. The formula: W = N (B + T) + A + D + E. (W= average workload in hours/week, N = average number of patients in the ward, B = time in hours/week required to maintain the standard of basic nursing care for a totally dependent patient, T = percentage of time spent on basic nursing, A = time/patient/week for administrative work, D = percentage of time spent on basic nursing, A = time/patient/week for domestic work, E = patient dependency factor for ward speciality.

Aberrant Taking an unusual course. Used in case of blood vessels and nerves.

Aberration Deviation from the normal. In optics, failure to focus rays of light.

Mental aberration Mental disorder of an unspecified kind. Chromosomal aberration loss, gain or exchange of genetic material in the chromosomes of a cell.

Ability The power to perform an act, either mental or physical, with or without training.

A

Innate ability The ability with which a person is born.

Abiogenesis A theory which says that living organisms can originate from nonliving matter; spontaneous generation.

Abiosis Absence of life, nonviability.

Abiotrophy Progressive loss of vitality of certain tissues or organs leading to disorders or loss of function applied specially to degenerative hereditary diseases of late onset.

Ablation Removal or destruction, by surgical or radiological means, of neoplasms or other body tissue.

Ablepsia Loss or absence of vision.

Abluent Detergent, cleansing.

Abnormal Varying from what is regular or usual. Not conforming with the natural or general rule.

ABO System The classification of human blood

Abort 1. To terminate a process or disease before it has run its normal course. 2. To remove or expel from the womb an embryo or fetus before it is capable of independent existence.

Aborticide An agent that destroys fetus and causes abortion.

Abortifacient An agent or drug that may induce abortion.

Abortion 1. Premature cessation of a normal process. 2. Emptying of the pregnant uterus before the stage of viability that is 20th week of gestation. 3. The product of nonviable birth.

Accidental abortion Abortion due to fall, blow or any other injury.

Complete abortion One in which the contents of the uterus, i.e., embryo and the membranes expelled intact.

Criminal abortion The termination of a pregnancy for reasons other than those permitted by law (i.e., danger to

mental or physical health of mother or child or family) and without medical approval.

Habitual abortion A condition in which a woman has had three or more consecutive spontaneous abortions.

Incomplete abortion One in which some part of the fetus or placenta is retained in the uterus.

Induced abortion The intentional emptying of the uterus.

Inevitable abortion Abortion where bleeding is profuse and accompanied by pains, the cervix is dilated and the contents of the uterus can be felt. There is no hope for preventing abortion.

Incipient abortion Threatened or impending abortion in which there is copious vaginal bleeding, uterine contractions and cervical dilatation.

Missed abortion One where all signs of pregnancy disappear and the fetus dies in the uterus and later the uterus discharges a blood clot surrounding a shrivelled fetus.

Septic abortion Abortion associated with infection.

Therapeutic (legal) abortion One induced on medical advice because the continuance of the pregnancy would involve risk to the life of the pregnant woman, or injury to the physical or mental health of the pregnant woman or any existing children of her family, greater than if the pregnancy were terminated; or because there is a substantial risk that if the child were born it would suffer from such physical or mental abnormalities as to be seriously handicapped (1976 Abortion Act, as amended by the Human Fertilization and Embryology Act, 1990).

Threatened abortion The appearance of signs of premature expulsion of the fetus; bleeding is slight, the cervix is closed.

Tubal abortion The termination of a tubal pregnancy caused by rupture of the uterine tube.

Abrachia Armless.

Abrachius An armless individual.

Abrasion A superficial injury, where the skin or mucous membrane is rubbed or torn.

Corneal abrasion This can occur when the surface of the cornea has been removed, e.g., by a scratch or other injury.

Abreaction An emotional release of previously repressed emotionally charged memories and experiences. It is a mental process occurring in hypnosis or narco analysis.

Abrosia Abstinence from food, fasting.

Abruption A breaking away.

Abruptio placentae Premature detachment of the placenta, prior to the delivery of the fetus, causing maternal shock.

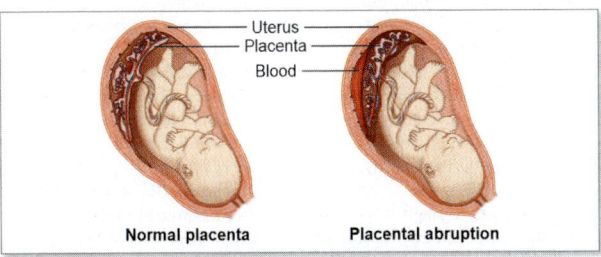

Labels: Uterus, Placenta, Blood — Normal placenta / Placental abruption

Abruptio Placentae

Abscess A collection of pus in a cavity. Caused by the disintegration and replacement of tissue damaged by mechanical, chemical or bacterial injury.

Alveolar abscess An abscess in a tooth socket.

Amebic abscess An abscess of the liver that contains ameba and may follow amebic dysentery.

Bezold's abscess A deep abscess in the neck associated with suppuration of the middle ear and purulent sinus thrombosis.

Brodie's abscess A bone abscess, usually on the head of the tibia.

Cold abscess The result of chronic tubercular infection and so called because there are few, if any, signs of inflammation.

Psoas abscess A cold abscess that has tracked down the psoas muscle from caries of the lumbar vertebrae.

Subphrenic abscess One situated under the diaphragm.

Absence attack or seizure A form of epilepsy characterized by sudden transient lapse of consciousness, by a blank stare, sometimes accompanied by minor motor activities such as blinking of eyes, stereotyped hand movement, etc.

Absolute refractory period The refractory period in which no stimulus, however strong can excite a response.

Absolute scotoma Scotoma with perception of light entirely absent.

Absolute temperature Temperature reckoned from the absolute zero estimated at approximately -273°C or –459°F.

Absolute threshold The lowest intensity as measured under optimal experimental conditions. At which a stimulus is effective or perceived.

A

Absolute zero A temperature of approximately −273.2°C or −459.8°F; the complete absence of heat.

Absorb Able to take in, or suck up and incorporate. To infiltrate into the skin.

Absorbable ligature A ligature composed of animal tissue such as catgut which can be absorbed by the tissues.

Absorbed dose In radiology, the amount of energy imparted by ionizing particles to a unit mass of irradiated material at a place of interest.

Absorbefacient An agent that promotes absorption.

Absorbent A tissue structure involved in absorption. A substance that absorbs or promotes absorption.

Absorption 1. In physiology, the taking up by suction of fluids or other substances by the tissues of the body. 2. In psychology, great mental concentration on a single object or activity. 3. In radiology, uptake of radiation by body tissues.

Absorption atelectasis Obstructive atelectasis.

Absorption band A region of the absorption spectrum in which the absorptivity passes through maximum or inflection.

Abstergent Having cleansing or purgative properties; a cleaning lotion; a purgative.

Abstinence A refraining from the use of or indulgence in food, stimulants or coitus.

Abstinence delirium Delirium occurring on withdrawal of alcohol or of a drug from one addicted to it.

Abstinence syndrome Withdrawal symptoms.

Abstract A brief, comprehensive summary of a research study or other academic report.

Abulia Loss or defect of the ability to make decisions.

Abulomania Mental disorder characterized by lack of will power and indecisiveness.

Abuse Misuse, maltreatment or excessive use.

Child abuse The nonaccidental use of physical force or the nonaccidental act of omission by a parent or other custodian responsible for the care of a child.

Drug abuse Use of illegal drugs or misuse of prescribed drugs.

Solvent abuse The deliberate inhalation of volatile chemicals with the aim of inducing intoxication.

Abusive head injury Commonly called shaken baby syndrome resulting in traumatic brain injury in infants and young children.

Acalcerosis Calcium deficiency of the diet or of the body as a result of the loss of the mineral in the excreta.

Acanthion The tip of the anterior nasal spine.

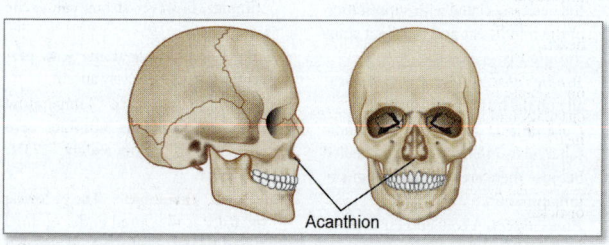

Acanthion

Acanthion

Acanthocyte A thorny or peculiarly spiny erythrocyte characterized by multiple spiny cytoplasmic projections.

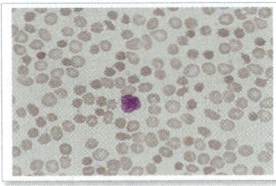

Acanthocyte

Acanthocytosis A rare condition in which as many as 70 to 80 % of the RBC's are acanthocytes.

Acanthoid Spine shaped, spinous.

Acantholysis A term used in dermal pathology to denote dissolution of the layers of the epidermis. It is seen in pemphigus vulgaris and keratosis follicularis.

Acanthoma Well differentiated keratinizing cornifying squamous cell carcinoma. The term is also used for neoplasms in the skin with little or no histologic evidence of invasion.

Acanthosis nigricans Darkened, thickened patches of skin that develop around the groin, neck and axilla. These patches can sometimes be itchy and may indicate underlying disease.

Acapnia A deficiency of carbon dioxide in the blood.

Acarbia Reduction in bicarbonate of the blood.

Acardia Congenital absence of the heart.

Acardiacus A conjoined twin parasite on its mate or utilizing the placental circulation of its mate and having no heart.

Acardiotrophia Atrophy of heart.

Acaricide An agent that destroys mites or ticks.

Acariasis Any disease caused by an acarid.

Acarid A member of the order Acarina, a mite.

Acaroid Resembling a mite; an acrus or mite.

Acarophobia fear of small parasites or small particles.

Acarus A genus of small mites.
  Acarus scabiei The cause of scabies.

Acatalepsy A mental deficiency characterized by lack of understanding.

Acataleptic Deficient in comprehension; uncertain.

Acataphasia Loss of the ability to express connected thought, resulting from a cerebral lesion.

Acataposis Difficulty in swallowing liquids.

Acathexia An abnormal loss of the secretions.

Acathexis A mental disorder in which certain objects or ideas fail to arouse an emotional response on the individual.

Accessory Supplementary.
  Accessory nerve The 11th cranial nerve. It is made up of two portions: the cranial and the spinal.

Acceleration 1. An increase in the speed or velocity of an object or reaction. 2. An increase in the fetal heartbeat of at least 15 beats per minute over the baseline rate for at least 15 seconds.

Access to health care records Patients (or in the case of deceased patients, their representative) can apply for access to health care records, unless it is not considered to cause serious physical or mental harm to them; or where information would be disclosed relating to a third party who has not consented.

Accident A sudden unexpected event or injury occurring without omen or forewarning or developing in the cause of a disease.

Accident and emergency Sometimes referred to as casualty, the emergency department or trauma medicine. A setting for dealing with problems, which require immediate attention and where patients can be directed or referred by a general practitioner or the emergency services.

Acclimatization The ability of the body to adapt physiologically to changes in the environment. Taking exercise in a hotter climate than the body is used to will lead to increased sweating with lower sodium levels in an attempt to cool the body but that may lead to dehydration. Climbing, for example, at a high altitude can produce altitude sickness with low oxygen levels in the blood, associated with increased cardiac output and respiratory effort. Athletes partic-

ipating in sports events at international venues held in hot climates or at high altitudes will require training to adapt to the physiological adjustments that will affect the athletic performance.

Accommodation Adjustment. In ophthalmology, the term refers specifically to adjustment of the ciliary muscle, which controls the shape of the lens.

Negative accommodation The ciliary muscle relaxes and the lens becomes less convex, giving long distance vision.

Positive accommodation The ciliary muscle contracts and the lens becomes more convex, giving near vision.

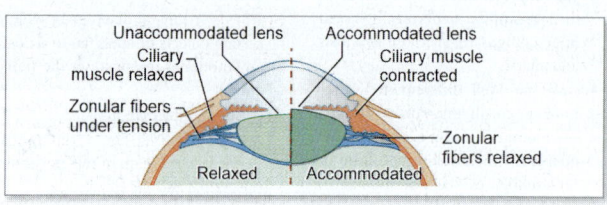

Accommodation

Accountable Liable to be held responsible for a course of action. A qualified nurse has a duty to care according to law; in nursing being accountable refers to the responsibility the qualified nurse takes for prescribing and initiating nursing care. Nurses are accountable to their patients, their peers and their employing authority, according to the Code of Professional Conduct. Registered practitioners (nurses, midwives or health visitors) are accountable at all times for their actions, on or off duty and whether engaged in current practice or not.

Accreditation A process of evaluation whereby an institution or an individual undergoes regular appraisal

against agreed criteria, which, if met, result in the individual or institution being given official recognition by the accrediting organization.

Accretion Growth. The accumulation of deposits, e.g., of salts to form a calculus in the bladder. In dentistry, the growth of tartar on the teeth.

Acculturation The process by which a person absorbs the beliefs, values and customs of another culture, usually through direct contact, e.g., migrant residents in another country.

ACE inhibitors A group of drugs used in the treatment of hypertension. Their name, angiotensin converting enzyme inhibitors, explains part of their mode of action, although it is thought that some of their other actions may also be important in reducing blood pressure.

Acebutolol Beta adrenergic blocking agent used in hypertension.

Acenesthesia Absence of the normal sensation of physical existence or of the consciousness of visceral function.

Acentric Lacking a center. Cytogenetics denoting a chromosome fragments without a centromere.

Acenocoumarol (NND) An orally effective synthetic anticoagulant of the coumarin type and with similar action.

Acestoma Exuberant granulations that are forming a cicatrix.

Acet Combining form denoting acid. From the Latin *acetum*, vinegar.

Acetabuloplasty An operation performed to improve the depth and shape of the hip socket in correcting congenital dislocation of the hip or in treating osteoarthritis of the hip.

Acetabulum The cup-like socket in the innominate bone, in which the head of the femur moves.

Acetal A clear liquid made by the imperfect oxidation of alcohol. Has been used as hypnotic.

Acetaminophen N-Acetyl-p-amino-phenol, P - acetamidophenol, a white odorless crystalline slightly bitter powder used as an antipyretic and analgesic.

Acetarsone Acetarsol (BP), used in ambiasis and as a local application in vincents angina and in *Trichomonas vaginalis*.

Acetate A salt of acetic acid.

Acetazolamide A sulfonamide compound which is an oral diuretic and is used in the treatment of congestive heart failure and of glaucoma.

Acetic Relative to vinegar; sour.

Acetoacetic acid Diacetic acid, a product of fat metabolism. It occurs in excessive amounts in diabetes and starvation, giving rise to acetone bodies in the urine.

Acetobactor A genus of the family pseudomonadaceae, containing rod shaped organisms frequently found in elongated, branched or swollen forms, polarly flagellate when motile, energy secured by oxidation of alcohol in wine cider or beer to acetic acid.

Acetolactic acid An intermediate in pyruvic acid catabolism in yeast.

Acetomorphine Heroin.

Acetonemia The presence of acetone bodies in the blood.

Acetone A colorless inflammable liquid with a characteristic odor. Traces are found in the blood and in normal urine.

Acetone bodies Ketones found in the blood and urine of uncontrolled diabetic patients and also in acute starvation as a result of the incomplete breakdown of fatty and amino acids.

Acetonuria The presence of an excess quantity of acetone bodies in the urine, giving it a peculiar sweet smell. Commonly occurs in diabetic acidosis.

Acetylcholine A chemical transmitter that is released by some nerve endings at the synapse between one neuron and the next or between a nerve ending and the effector organ it supplies. These nerves are said to be cholinergic, e.g., the parasympathetic nerves and the lower motor neurons to skeletal muscles. Acetylcholine is rapidly destroyed in the body by cholinesterase.

Acetylcholinesterase Cholinesterase, that breaks down acetyl choline into choline and acetic acid.

A

Acetyl coenzyme A (acetyl CoA) Condensation product of coenzyme A and acetic acid, symbolized as COAS—COCH₃.

Acetylcysteine Mucomyst, a mucolytic agent that reduces the viscosity of mucous secretions.

Acetyldigitoxin Acylanid, same actions and uses as digitoxin but more rapid onset and shorter duration of action.

Acetylene A colorless gas of a disagreeable odor that burns with an intense white flame. It is prepared commercially by the action of water on calcium carbide.

Acetylsalicylic acid Aspirin. An analgesic, antipyretic and antirheumatic drug. It is available in its pure form or in combination with other drugs.

Achalasia Failure of relaxation of a muscle sphincter causing dilatation of the part above, e.g., of the esophagus above the cardiac sphincter.

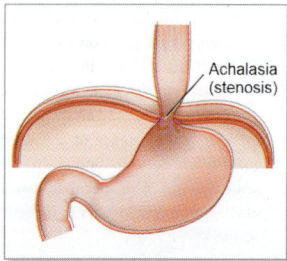

Achalasia

Ache A dull continuous pain.

Acheilia Congenital absence of the lips.

Achilles Greek mythological hero who could be wounded only in the heel.

Achilles tendon Largest and the strongest tendon of the body, formed by the union of soleus and gastrocnemius muscles of the calf to the heel bone (os calcis). Tapping the Achilles tendon normally produces the Achilles reflex or ankle jerk.

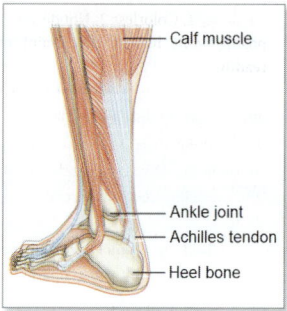

Achilles Tendon

Achiria 1. Congenital absence of the hands. 2. Anesthesia with loss of the sense of possession of one or both, a condition sometimes noted in hysteria. 3. A form of dyschiria in which the patient is unable to tell on which side of the body a stimulus has been applied.

Achirus A malformed individual without hands.

Achlorhydria The absence of free hydrochloric acid in the stomach. Maybe found in pernicious anaemia, pellagra and gastric cancer.

Achluophobia Fear of darkness.

Acholia Lack of secretion of bile.

Acholic Without bile.

Acholuria Deficiency or lack of bile in the urine.

Acholuric Pertaining to acholuria.

Acholuric jaundice Without bile in the urine.

Achondroplasia An inherited condition in which there is early union of the epiphysis and diaphysis of long bones. Growth is arrested resulting in short stature.

Achromasia 1. Lack of color in the skin. 2. Absence of normal reaction to staining in a tissue or cell.

Achromate An absolutely color blind person.

Achromatic 1. Colorless 2. Not decomposing white light 3. Not staining readily.

Achromatopsia Complete color blindness caused by disease or trauma. It maybe congenital.

Achromatosis Absence of natural pigmentation as in albinism.

Achromaturia The passing of colorless or very pale urine.

Achylia Absence of hydrochloric acid and enzymes in the gastric secretions. Absence of chyle.

Achylia gastrica A condition in which gastric secretion is reduced or absent.

Acid 1. Sour or sharp in taste. 2. A substance which, when combined with an alkali, will form a salt. Any acid substance will turn blue litmus red. Individual acids are given under their specific names.

Acid-alcohol-fast Descriptive of stained bacteria that are resistant to decolorization by both acid and alcohol.

Acid-base balance The normal ratio between the acid ions and the basic or alkaline ions required to maintain the pH of the blood and body fluids.

Acidemia Abnormal acidity of the blood, which contains an excess of hydrogen ions in which the pH of the blood falls below 7.35.

Acid fast A term denoting bacteria that are not decolorized in mineral acids after having been stained with aniline dyes. e.g., leprosy, tubercle and hay bacilli.

Acid phosphotase An enzyme found in many tissues and fluid in the body. It maybe elevated in conditions like paget's disease, oesteomalacia, hepatitis, obstructive jaundice, etc.

Acidity 1. Sourness or sharpness of taste. 2. The state of being acid.

Acidosis A condition in which the relation of alkalinity to acidity of the blood is disturbed, with an increase in the hydrogen ion concentration. It is characterized by vomiting, drowsiness, hyperpnea, acetone odor of breath (of 'new-mownhay') and acetone bodies in the urine. It may occur in diabetes mellitus owing to incomplete metabolism of fat *(See also Ketosis)*.

Acid rain Rain contaminated with sulfur dioxide and nitrogen oxide. It is harmful for aquatic and plant life.

Acid reflux disorder A condition in which acid comes from the stomach into esophagus causing discomfort and damage to the esophageal lining.

Acidotic 1. Pertaining to acidosis. 2. A person suffering from acidosis.

Aciduria 1. A condition in which acid urine is excreted. 2. Excretion of an abnormal amount of any specified acid.

Acinus A minute saccule or alveolus of a compound gland, lined by secreting cells. The secreting portion of the mammary gland consists of acini.

Acme 1. The highest point. 2. The crisis of a fever when the symptoms are fully developed.

Acne An inflammatory condition of the sebaceous glands in which blackheads (comedones) are usually present together with papules and pustules.

Acne keratitis Inflammation of the cornea associated with acne rosacea.

Acne rosacea A redness of the forehead, nose and cheeks due to chronic dilatation of the subcutaneous capillaries, which becomes permanent with the formation of pustules in the affected areas.

Acne urticata An eruption beginning as small urticarial wheals and followed by slight scarring.

Acne vulgaris Form that occurs commonly only in adolescents and young adults, affecting the face, chest and back.

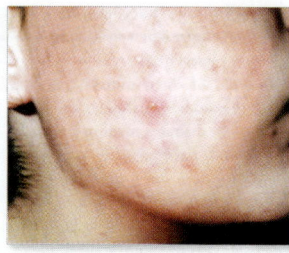

Acne

Acnegenic Pertaining to substances thought to be responsible for causing acne vulgaris.

Acneiform Resembling acne.

Acnemia 1. Atrophy of the calf muscles 2. Congenital absence of legs.

Acomia Alopecia, baldness.

Acorea Congenital absence of the pupil of the eye.

Acoria Absence of the feeling of satiety after eating.

Acousma The hearing of imaginary sounds.

Acoustic Relating to sound or the sense of hearing.

Acoustic apparatus Auditory apparatus; the anatomical structures that helps in hearing.

Acoustic area Part of the brain which lies over the vestibular and cochlear nuclei.

Acoustics The science of sounds and their perception.

Acquired Pertaining to disease, habits or immunity developed after birth; not inherited.

Acquired immune deficiency syndrome Abbreviated AIDS *(See AIDS)*.

Acrid Bitter; pungent; irritating.

Acrocentric A chromosome in which the centromere is situated at or very near to one end.

Acrocephalia Malformation of the head, in which the top is pointed (oxycephaly) due to premature closure of the sutures.

Acrocyanosis Persistent cyanosis, coldness of the hands and feet and profuse sweating of the digits, often associated with a vasomotor defect.

Acrodynia An allergic reaction to mercury in children, causing pain and erythema in the fingers and toes. Pink disease.

Acromegaly A chronic condition producing gradual enlargement of the hands, feet, and bones of the head and chest associated with over activity of the anterior lobe of the pituitary gland in adults.

Acromelalgia A vasomotor neurosis marked by redness, pain and swelling of the fingers and toes, headache and vomiting.

Acromioclavicular Pertaining to the joint between the acromion process of the scapula and the lateral aspect of the clavicle.

Acromion The outward projection of the spine of the scapula, forming the point of the shoulder.

Acropachy Hypertrophic pulmonary osteoarthropathy.

Acroparaesthesia Condition in which pressure on the nerves of the brachial plexus causes numbness, pain and tingling of the hand and forearm.

Acropathy Simple hereditary clubbing of the digits without associated pulmonary or other progressive disease.

Acrophobia Morbid terror of being at a height.

Acrosclerosis A type of scleroderma that affects the hands, feet, face or chest.

Acrosome Part of the head of a spermatozoon containing enzymes which break down the cell membrane of the ovum and allow penetration.

Acrotism Absence or imperceptibility of the pulse; pulselessness.

ACTH Adrenocorticotropic hormone; corticotropin.

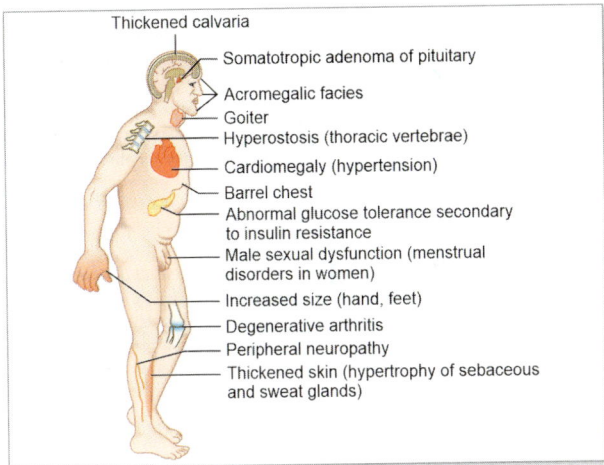

Thickened calvaria
Somatotropic adenoma of pituitary
Acromegalic facies
Goiter
Hyperostosis (thoracic vertebrae)
Cardiomegaly (hypertension)
Barrel chest
Abnormal glucose tolerance secondary to insulin resistance
Male sexual dysfunction (menstrual disorders in women)
Increased size (hand, feet)
Degenerative arthritis
Peripheral neuropathy
Thickened skin (hypertrophy of sebaceous and sweat glands)

Symptoms of Acromegaly

Actin The protein of myofibrils responsible for contraction and relaxation of muscles.

Actinic keratoses Also known as solar keratoses are rough patches of skin caused by sun exposure over a prolonged period of time.

Actinodermatitis Inflammation of the skin due to the action of ultraviolet or X-rays.

Actinomyces A genus of branching, spore-forming, vegetable parasites, which may give rise to actinomycosis and from which many antibiotic drugs are produced, e.g., streptomycin.

Actinomycin A group of cytotoxic drugs used in the treatment of malignant disease.

Actinomycosis A chronic infective disease of cattle that is also found in humans. Granulated tumors occur, chiefly on the tongue and jaws. It is caused by the ray fungus *Actinomyces (Nocardia)*.

Actinotherapy Treatment of disease by rays of light, e.g., artificial sunlight (UV light therapy).

Action Performance of any functions, the manner of such performance or its result whether mechanical or chemical, or the effect so produced.

Action research A method of undertaking social research that incorporates the researcher's involvement as a direct and deliberate part of the research, i.e., the researcher acts as a change agent.

Cumulative action The sudden and markedly increased action of a drug after administration of several doses.

Reflex action An involuntary response to a stimulus conveyed to the nervous system and reflected to the periphery, passing below the level of consciousness *(See also Reflex).*

Activator A substance, hormone or enzyme that stimulates a chemical change, although it may not take part in the change. In chemistry, a

A

catalyst. For example, yeast is the activator in the process by which sugar is converted into alcohol; the digestive secretions are activated by hormones to carry out normal digestion.

Active Causing change; energetic.

Active immunity An immunity in which individuals have been stimulated to produce their own antibodies.

Active movements Movements made by the patient, as distinct from passive movements.

Active principle The ingredient in a drug that is primarily responsible for its therapeutic action.

Activities of daily living Abbreviated ADL. Activities usually performed in the course of a person's normal daily routine, such as eating, cleaning teeth, washing and dressing.

Activities of living (ALs) Those activities which meet the physical, psychological and social needs of the individual, e.g., eating, elimination, communication, breathing, expressing sexuality, working, play, etc.

Activity theory Describes a psychosocial process whereby aging people disengage from some activities of their earlier life and replace these with other hobbies and pastimes, according to their changing physical abilities and economic situation.

Activity tolerance The amount of physical activity tolerated by a patient. It maybe assessed in patients with cardiac or chronic respiratory disease. Graded exercises, including walking, cycling and going up and down stairs, maybe used to rebuild confidence during the convalescent phase after any serious illness or injury as an important part of any rehabilitation programme.

Actomyosin Muscle protein complex; the myosin component acts as an enzyme which causes the release of energy.

Acuity Sharpness.

Acuity of hearing An acute perception of sound.

Acuity of vision Clear focusing ability.

Acupressure A system of complementary medicine in which pressure is applied to various points on the body to stimulate the innate self-healing capacity of the individual. *(See Acupuncture, Shiatsu).*

Acupuncture A Chinese medical system which aims to diagnose illness and promote health by stimulating the body's self-healing powers. The insertion of special needles into specific points along the "meridians" of the body is used for the production of anesthesia, the relief of pain and the treatment of certain conditions.

Acute A term applied to a disease in which the attack is sudden, severe and of short duration.

Acute care Medical treatment given in a hospital to the patients suffering from an acute illness or injury or recovering from surgery.

Acute respiratory distress syndrome Abbreviated ARDS. A severe form of acute lung function failure which occurs after an event such as trauma, inhalation of a toxic substance or septic shock. There is severe breathlessness and a dangerous reduction in the supply of oxygen to the blood.

Acute urethral syndrome Dysuria, urgency, frequency of micturition in absence of significant bacteriuria.

Acyclic Occurring independently of a natural cycle of events (such as the menstrual cycle).

Acyclovir An antiviral agent used to treat herpes viruses. Uses include the treatment of varicella zoster and herpes simplex. It is only active if started at the onset of the infection. May also be used as prophylaxis in the immunocompromised and for prevention of recurrence.

Acyesis 1. Sterility in the woman 2. The nonpregnant condition.

Adam's apple The laryngeal prominence, a protrusion of the front of the neck formed by the thyroid cartilage.

Adamantine Pertaining to the enamel of the teeth.

Adamantinoma A tumor of jaw, arising from enamel cells. Maybe benign or of low grade malignancy.

Adams-Strokes syndrome Black out due to sudden fall in cerebral circulation commonly after heart block.

Adaptation 1. The process of modification that a living organism undergoes when adjusting itself to new surroundings or circumstances. 2. A function of the stimulus to which the individual is exposed and of the individual's accommodation to the situation. The adaptation response may relate to physiological needs, role, "self" concept and interdependence. 3. The process of overcoming difficulties and adjusting to changing circumstances. Neuroses and psychoses are often associated with failure of adaptation. 4. Used in ophthalmology to mean the adjustment of visual function according to the ambient illumination.

Color adaptation 1. Changes in visual perception of color with prolonged stimulation. 2. Adjustment of vision to a degree of brightness or color tone of illumination.

Dark adaptation Adaptation of the eye to vision in reduced illumination.

Light adaptation Adaptation of the eye to vision in bright illumination (photopia) with reduction in the concentration of the photosensitive pigments of the eye.

Addict A person exhibiting addiction.

Addiction Habituation to some practice, withdrawal from which causes withdrawal symptoms. E.g., the taking of drugs or alcohol leading to physiological and psychological dependence with a tendency to increase use *(See Dependence and Drug addiction)*.

Addison's anaemia *T. Addison, British physician, (1793–1860).* Pernicious anaemia.

Addison's disease Deficiency disease of the suprarenal cortex; often tuberculous. There is wasting, brown pigmentation of the skin and extreme debility.

Additive A substance not essentially part of a material such as food, fuel etc., which is deliberately added to fulfill some specific purpose.

Additive effect The effect of a combination of two or more drugs that is equal to the sum of the individual drug effect.

Additives Substances added to improve, enhance or preserve something.

Food additives Used in the food industry to preserve and make the food look more attractive; these are given serial numbers, e.g., E102 (tartrazine) E200 (sorbic acid). Some additives may produce an allergic reaction in some people and few are thought to be associated with behavioral problems in children.

Adducent Leading toward the midline.

Adducent muscle The medial rectus muscle of the eye, which turns it inward.

Adduction Movement of a limb toward the central axis of the body.

Adductor A muscle that draws a limb toward the midline of the body. The opposite of abductor.

Adefovir Antiviral agent used in hepatitis B.

Adenectomy Excision of a gland.

Adenine One of the purine bases found in DNA.

Adenitis Inflammation of a gland or lymph node.

Adenocanthoma A malignant neoplasm consisting chiefly of glandular epithelium (adenocarcinoma).

Adenoblast An embryonic cell destined to proliferate into cells that will enter into the formation of a gland.

Adenocarcinoma A malignant neoplasm of epithelial cells in glandular or gland-like pattern; frequently with infiltration to adjacent tissue, metastasis, recurrence of removal; a malignant adenoma.

Adenocyst A cystic tumor developing from glandular epithelium, adenocystoma.

Adenocystoma Adenoma in which the neoplastic glandular epithelium forms cysts or cyst like structures.

Adenofibroma A benign tumor of connective tissue which contains glandular structures.

Adenohypophysis Anterior lobe of the pituitary gland.

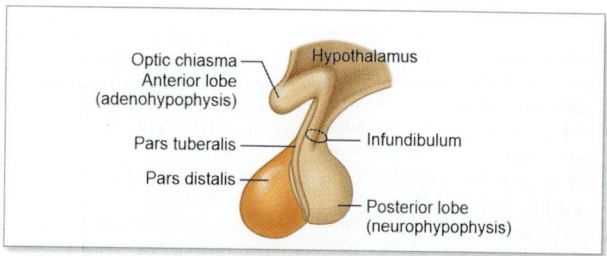

Optic chiasma
Hypothalamus
Anterior lobe (adenohypophysis)
Pars tuberalis
Infundibulum
Pars distalis
Posterior lobe (neurophypophysis)

Adenohypophysis

Adenoid Resembling a gland. Generally applied to abnormal lymphoid growth in the nasopharynx.

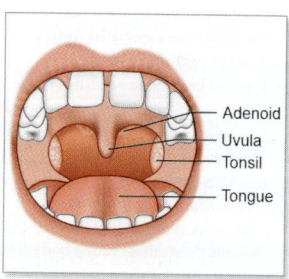

Adenoid
Uvula
Tonsil
Tongue

Adenoid

Adenoidectomy The surgical removal of adenoid tissue from the nasopharynx.

Adenoid Small lumps of tissue at the back of the nose, above the roof of the mouth. Part of the immune system.

Adenoma A nonmalignant tumor of glandular tissue.

Adenomyoma An innocent new growth involving both endometrium and muscle tissue; found in the uterus or uterine ligaments.

Adenomyosis The ectopic occurrence or diffuse implantation of adenomatous tissue in muscle as in benign invasion of myometrium by endometrial tissue.

Adenomyxoma A benign neoplasm with histologic characteristics of adenoma and myxoma.

Adenopathy Enlargement of any gland, especially those of the lymphatic system.

Adenosarcoma A malignant tumor of connective and glandular tissue.

Adenosclerosis Hardening of a gland. Usually the result of calcification.

Adenosine A nucleoside consisting of adenine and D-ribose (a pentose sugar).

Adenosine triphosphate Abbreviated ATP. A compound containing three phosphoric acids. It is present in all cells and serves as a store for energy.

Adenosis A more or less generalized glandular disease especially one involving the lymph nodes.

Adenotome An instrument for the removal of adenoids.

Adenovirus A virus of the Adenoviridae family. Many types have been isolated, some of which cause respiratory tract infections, while others are associated with conjunctivitis, epidemic kerato conjunctivitis or gastrointestinal infection.

ADH Antidiuretic hormone. Vasopressin.

Adhesion Union between two surfaces of parts. Usually the result of inflammation when fibrous tissue forms, e.g., peritonitis may cause adhesions between organs. A possible cause of intestinal obstruction.

Adhesive capsulitis Painful condition in which the movement of the shoulder becomes limited.

Adiaphoresis Absence or deficiency of perspiration.

Adiaphoretic An anhidrotic agent. A drug that prevents the secretion of sweat.

Adipocele A hernia, with the sac containing fatty tissue.

Adipose Of the nature of fat. Fatty.

Adeposia Absence of thirst.

Adiposity The state of being too fat. Obesity.

Adiposogenital dystrophy A condition occurring in adolescent boys with increased body fat accompanied by underdevelopment of the genitalia and altered secondary sexual characteristics caused by damage to the hypothalamus usually as a result of a tumor or infection. Also known as Frohlich's syndrome.

Adiposuria The presence of fat in the urine. Lipuria.

Aditus An opening or passageway; often applied to that between the middle ear and the mastoid antrum.

Adjustment In psychology, the ability of a person to adapt to changing circumstances or environment.

Adjuvant 1. Any treatment used in conjunction with another to enhance its efficacy. 2. A substance administered with a drug to enhance its effect.

ADL Activities of daily living.

Adler's theory *A. Adler, Austrian psychiatrist, (1870–1937).* The theory that neuroses develop as a compensation for feelings of inferiority, either social or physical.

Adnexa Appendages.

Uterine adnexa The ovaries and tubes.

Adolescence The period between puberty and maturity. In male, 14–25 years. In female, 12–21 years.

Adopt 1. To take a person, especially another's child, into a legal relationship as one's own. 2. To choose to follow a course of action.

Adoption The legal procedure by which a child is transferred from its natural parents to adopting parents. Regulated by law, the child's welfare is paramount. Local authorities offer advice and social work support and may act as an adoption agency, and there are also private and charitable agencies registered with the local authority.

Adrenal 1. Near the kidneys. 2. A triangular endocrine gland situated above each kidney.

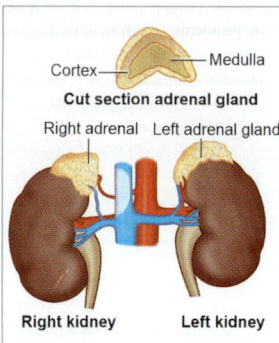

Cortex — Medulla

Cut section adrenal gland

Right adrenal   Left adrenal gland

Right kidney   Left kidney

Adrenal Glands

Adrenalectomy Surgical excision of adrenal gland.

Adrenaline A hormone secreted by the medulla of the adrenal gland. Has an action similar to normal stimulation of the sympathetic nervous system: (a) causing dilatation of the bronchioles; (b) raising the blood pressure by constriction of surface vessels and stimulation of the cardiac output; (c) releasing glycogen from the liver. It is therefore used to treat such conditions as asthma, collapse and hypoglycemia. It acts as a hemostat in local anesthetics. Trade name for epinephrine.

Adrenergic Pertaining to nerves that release the chemical transmitter nor-adrenaline in order to stimulate the muscles and glands they supply.

Adrenocorticotrophin Adrenocorticotropic hormone (ACTH); Secreted by the anterior lobe of the pituitary body; Stimulates the adrenal cortex to produce cortisol. *(See corticotrophin).*

Adrenogenital Relating to both the adrenal glands and the gonads.

Adrenogenital syndrome A condition of masculinization caused by overactivity of the adrenal cortex resulting in precocious puberty in the male infant and masculinization in the female. Both sexes are liable to Addisonian crises.

Adrenolytic A drug that inhibits the stimulation of the sympathetic nerves and the activity of adrenaline.

Adson's maneuver Test for thoracic-outlet syndrome in which there is loss of radial pulse in the arm by rotating the head to the unaffected side with extended neck following deep inspiration.

Adsorbent A substance that has the power of attracting gas or fluid to itself.

Adsorption The process of certain substances to attract molecules of gases or solutions to their surface. This phenomenon is used chromatography.

Adult Mature. A mature person.

Adulterant Impurity, additive that is considered to have an undesirable effect.

Adulteration Addition of an impure/cheap or unnecessary ingredient to cheat with, cheapen or falsify a preparation.

Advance care planning Discussions about the wishes and preferences for end-of-life care, which are documented and shared with permission with relevant agencies and individuals.

Advance decision Sometimes also referred to as advanced decision to refuse treatment, advance directive or a living will, is a written declaration made by a mentally competent person, which sets out his/her wishes with regard to life-prolonging medical interventions; if they are incapacitated by an irreversible disease or are terminally ill preventing them in making their wishes known to health professionals at the time. *(See Living Will).*

A

Advanced cardiac life support (ACLS)
Use of adjunctive measures like monitoring arrhythmia control, defibrillation, and ventilator support in patients with shock.

Advanced life support (ALS) Resuscitation techniques used during a cardiac arrest that follows on from basic life support. They include defibrillation and the administration of appropriate drugs. Pediatric advanced life support (PALS) is a structured and algorithm method of life support for children with severe medical emergencies.

Advanced trauma life support A set of protocols recommended for use by doctors and paramedics when dealing with seriously injured people at the scene of an accident. The immediate treatment of shock from reduced blood volume by the infusion of fluids is an integral component of the life support regime.

Advancement In surgery, an operation to detach a tendon or muscle and reattach it further forward. Used in the treatment of strabismus and plastic surgery.

Adventitia The outer coat of an artery or vein; the tunica adventitia.

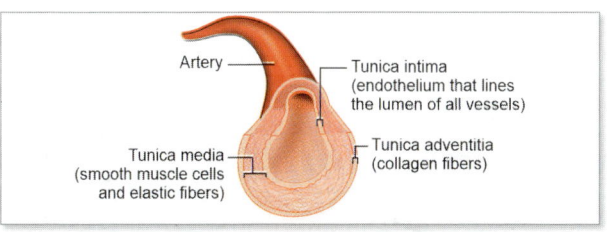

Artery
Tunica intima (endothelium that lines the lumen of all vessels)
Tunica media (smooth muscle cells and elastic fibers)
Tunica adventitia (collagen fibers)

Adventitia

Adventititous 1. Coming from without; extrinsic. 2. Accidental, 3. Relating to the adventitia of an artery or an organ.

Advocacy The process whereby a nurse provides a patient and/or the family with information to enable them to make informed decisions relating to the care situation. The nurse is then able to support the patient's decision vis-à-vis other professionals and also to incorporate the informed decisions into care planning.

Adynamia Weakness, vital debility, asthenia.

Aerobactor A genus of the tribe *Escherichia,* family enterobacteriacea, containing rod shaped Gramnegative organisms, found chiefly in the intestine.

A-EQUIP A model of clinical supervision for midwives. Full form is Advocating for Education and Quality Improvement.

Aeration Supplying with air. Used to describe the oxygenation of blood which takes place in the lungs.

Aerobe An organism that can live and thrive only in the presence of oxygen.

Aerobic exercise Physical exercises for which the degree of effort is such that it can be maintained for long periods without undue breathlessness. The aim of this form of exercising is to increase the effectiveness of the heart and lungs and the supply of oxygen to the tissues of the body.

Aerocele Refers to a cavity or pouch filled with air or gas. Aeroceles are commonly seen in connection with trachea or larynx resulting in formation of tracheocele and laryngocele respectively. An epidural aerocele is a collection of air between the dura mater and walls of the spinal column.

Aerodynamics The study of the air and other gases in motion, the forces that set them in motion, and the result of such motion.

Aerometer An apparatus for determining the density of or for weighing air.

Aeropathy Commonly called the bends (decompression sickness).

Aerophagia The excessive swallowing of air.

Aerophilia Abnormal and extreme dread of fresh air or of air in motion.

Aeroscope An instrument for the examination of air for visible impurities.

Aerosol Finely divided particles or droplets.

Aerosol Used in medicine to humidify air or oxygen, or for the administration of drugs by inhalation.

Aesculapius The god of healing in Roman mythology.

Aesthetic Description of a type of body build: a pale, lean, narrowly built person with poor muscle development.

Aetinolol Cardio selective beta blocker drug used in hypertension.

Aetiology The science of the cause of disease.

Afebrile Without fever.

Affect In psychiatry, the feeling experienced in connection with an emotion or mood.

Affection 1. A morbid condition or disease state. 2. A warm feeling for someone or something.

Affective Pertaining to the emotions or moods.

Affective psychoses Major mental disorders in which there is grave disturbance of the emotions.

Afferent Conveying toward the center.

Afferent nerves The sensory nerve fibers that convey impulses from the periphery toward the brain.

Afferent paths or tracts The course of the sensory nerves up the spinal cord and through the brain.

Afferent vessels Arterioles entering the glomerulus of the kidney, or lymphatics entering a lymph gland *(See Efferent).*

Affiliation The judicial decision about the paternity of a child with a view to the issue of a maintenance order.

Affinity In chemistry, the attraction of two substances to each other, e.g., hemoglobin and oxygen.

Affusion The pouring of water upon the body or any of its parts for therapeutic purpose.

Afibrinogenemia Absence of fibrinogen in the blood. The clotting mechanism of the blood is impaired as a result.

African tick fever Disease caused by a spirochaete, *Barrilia duttonic* transmitted by ticks *(See Relapsing fever).*

Afterbirth A lay expression used to describe the placenta, cord and membranes expelled after childbirth.

Aftercare The care and treatment provided to the patient after a period of hospital treatment.

Afterimage A visual impression that remains briefly after the cessation of sensory stimulation.

Afterpains Pain due to uterine contraction after childbirth.

After potential The small changes in electrical potential in a stimulated nerve which follow the main potential change.

Afunctional Lacking function.

Agalactia Absence of milk in the breasts after the child birth.

Agammaglobulinemia A condition in which there is no gamma-globulin in the blood. The patients are, therefore, susceptible to infections because of an inability to form antibodies.

Agamogony A sexual reproduction.

Aganglionosis A condition of the large intestine (colon) that causes difficulty passing stool.

Agar A gelatinous substance prepared from seaweed. Used as a culture medium for bacteria and as a laxative because it absorbs liquid from the digestive tract and swells, so stimulating peristalsis.

Age 1. The duration, or the measure of time, of the existence of a person or object. 2. To undergo change as a result of the passage of time.

Achievement age 1. *(See Developmental milestones)*. 2. Proficiency in study expressed in terms of the chronological age of a normal child showing the same degree of attainment. 3. Acquirement of a new skill or interest in old age or a praiseworthy accomplishment by an aged person.

Chronological age The actual measure of time elapsed since a person's birth.

Gestational age An expression of age of a developing fetus, usually given in weeks. It is measured from the date of the mother's last menstrual period, and so is approximately 2 weeks longer than time from conception.

Mental age The age level of mental ability of a person as gauged by standard intelligence tests.

Age spots With increasing age, skin blemishes appear; most commonly they are seborrheic keratoses, which are brown or yellow and can occur anywhere on the body. Also common with increasing age are freckles, red pinpoint blemishes on the trunk and solar keratoses due to overexposure to the sun. Treatment is usually unnecessary except occasionally for solar keratoses, which may eventually progress to skin cancer.

Age-associated memory impairment With age, short-term memory declines; most elderly people learn to overcome and compensate for this deficit. However, for some it maybe a considerable problem in daily living. Memory loss associated with dementia is often due to Alzheimer's disease or cerebral vascular disease. *(See Dementia and Alzheimer's Disease)*.

Ageing The structural changes that take place with time and are not caused by accident or disease.

Ageism The systematic discrimination against people on the grounds of age, based on stereotyping of the elderly as helpless, infirm, confused and requiring health care and supportive social services.

Agenda for Change The grading and pay system for NHS staff with the exception of doctors, dentists and some very senior managers.

Agenesis Failure of formation of any part.

Agent Any substance or force capable of producing a physical, chemical or biological effect.

Alkylating agent A cytotoxic preparation.

Chelating agent A chemical compound that binds metal ions.

Wetting agent A substance that lowers the surface tension of water and promotes wetting.

Ageusia Loss of the sense of taste.

Agglutinate Pertaining to a specific activity of antibody in an antigen antibody reaction, as a specific hemagglutinin as certain red blood cells.

Agglutination Collecting into clumps, particularly of cells suspended in a fluid and of bacteria affected by specific immune serum.

Agglutination test A means of aiding diagnosis and identification of bacteria. If serum containing known agglutinins comes into contact with the specific bacteria, clumping will take place *(See Widal reaction)*.

Cross agglutination Simple test to decide the group to which blood belongs *(See Blood group)*.

Agglutinative 1. Adherent or gluing together. 2. Serum that causes clumping of bacteria, e.g., in the Widal reaction.

Agglutinin Any substance causing agglutination (clumping together) of cells, particularly a specific antibody formed in the blood in response to the presence of an invading agent. Agglutinins are proteins (immunoglobulin) and function as part of the immune mechanism of the body. When the invading agents bring about the production of agglutinins the agglutinins produced bring about agglutination of the bacterial cells.

Agglutinogen Any substance that, when present in the bloodstream can cause the production of specific antibodies or agglutinins.

Aggregation The massing together of materials, as in clumping.

Familial aggregation The increased incidence of cases of a disease in a family compared with that in control families.

Platelet aggregation The clumping together of platelets, which maybe induced by a number of agents, such as thrombin and collagen.

Aggression Animosity or hostility shown toward another person or object as a response to opposition or frustration.

Aging The structural changes that take place with time and are not caused by accident or disease. Heredity is an important determinant of life expectancy, but factors such as smoking,

an excessive intake of alcohol, obesity, poor diet and insufficient exercise can all contribute to physical and mental deterioration.

A. population As the number of older people increases, the demand for health care increases. Expectations for health care delivery and provision too are changing as patients are becoming increasingly knowledgeable about their health.

Agitation 1. Shaking. 2. Mental distress causing extreme restlessness.

Agitophasia Abnormally rapid speech in which words are imperfectly spoken or dropped out of a sentence.

Aglossia Congenital absence of the tongue.

Aglutition Difficulty in the act of swallowing, aphagia, dysphagia.

Agnathia Absence of the lower jaw.

Agnosia An inability to recognize objects because the sensory stimulus cannot be interpreted, in spite of the presence of a normal sense organ.

Agonal Relating to the process of dying or the movement of death.

Agonist The prime mover. A muscle opposed in action by another (the antagonist).

Agony Extreme suffering, either mental or physical.

Agoraphobia A fear of open spaces.

Agranulocyte A white blood cell without granules in its cytoplasm. The term includes monocytes and lymphocytes.

Agranulocytosis A condition in which there is a marked decrease or complete absence of granular leukocytes in the blood, leaving the body defenseless against bacterial invasion. May result from: (a) The use of toxic drugs; (b) Irradiation. Characterized by a sore throat, ulceration of the mouth and pyrexia. It may result in severe prostration and death.

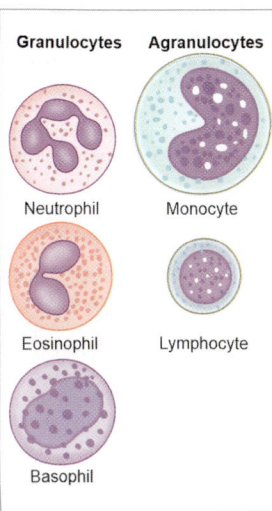

Granulocytes	Agranulocytes
Neutrophil	Monocyte
Eosinophil	Lymphocyte
Basophil	

Agranulocyte

Agraphia Absence of the power of expressing thought in writing. It arises from a lack of muscular coordination or as a result of a cerebral lesion.

Ague An intermittent fever.

AHF Antihemophilic factor (clotting factor VIII).

AHG Antihemophilic globulin (clotting factor VIII).

AHP Allied Health Professional.

AID Artificial insemination of a woman with donor semen (artificial insemination donor).

AIDS Acquired immune deficiency syndrome. It is the extreme end of the spectrum of disease caused by human immunodeficiency virus (HIV) infection, and impairs the body's cellular immune system. This may result in infection by organisms of normally no or low pathogenicity (opportunistic infections), principally.

Pneumocystis carinii pneumonia (PCP), or the development of unusual tumors, namely Kaposi's sarcoma (KS).

AIDS-related complex (ARC) Recurrent symptoms such as lymphadenopathy, night sweats, diarrhea, weight loss, malaise and chest infections. Examination of the blood may show abnormally low platelet and neutrophil counts as well as low lymphocyte counts.

AIH Artificial insemination of a woman by her husband's semen.

Ailment Any minor disorder of the body.

Air A mixture of gases that make up the earth's atmosphere. It consists of: nonactive nitrogen 79%; oxygen 21%, which supports life and combustion; traces of neon, argon, hydrogen, etc.; and carbon dioxide 0.03%, except in expired air, when 6% is exhaled as a result of diffusion that has taken place in the lungs. Air has weight and exerts pressure, which aids in syphonage from body cavities.

Air-bed A rubber mattress inflated with air.

Air embolism An embolism caused by air entering the circulatory system.

Air encephalography Radiological examination of the brain after the injection of air into the subarachnoid space.

Air hunger A form of dyspnea in which there are deep sighing respirations, characteristic of severe hemorrhage or acidosis.

Complemental air Additional air that can be inhaled with inspiratory effort.

Residual air Air remaining in the lungs after deep expiration. *Stationary air* That retained in the lungs after normal expiration.

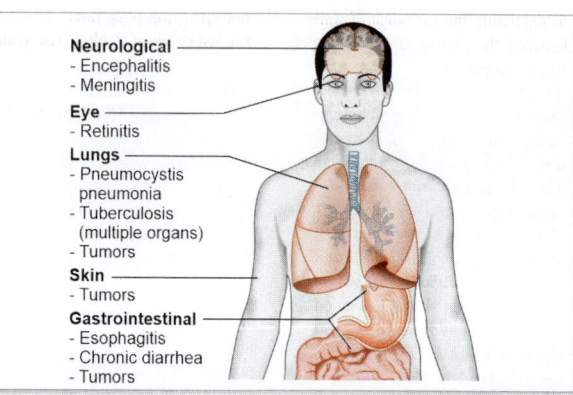

Neurological
- Encephalitis
- Meningitis

Eye
- Retinitis

Lungs
- Pneumocystis pneumonia
- Tuberculosis (multiple organs)
- Tumors

Skin
- Tumors

Gastrointestinal
- Esophagitis
- Chronic diarrhea
- Tumors

Main Symptoms of AIDS

Supplemental air The extra air forced out of the lungs with expiratory effort.

Tidal air That which passes in and out of the lungs in normal respiratory action.

Airway 1. The passage by which the air enters and leaves the lungs. 2. A mechanical device (tube) used for securing unobstructed respiration during general anesthesia or on other occasions when the patient is not ventilating or exchanging gases properly. It maybe passed through the mouth or nose. The tube prevents a flaccid tongue from resting against the posterior pharyngeal wall and causing obstruction of the airway.

Akathisia Motor restlessness.

Akinesia Loss of muscle power. This maybe the result of a brain or spinal cord lesion or, temporarily, of anesthesia.

Akinetic Relating to states or conditions where there is lack of movement.

Alacrima A deficiency or absence of secretion of tears.

Alalia Loss or impairment of the power of speech due to muscle paralysis or a cerebral lesion.

Alanine An amino acid formed by the ingestion of dietary protein.

Albers-Schonberg's disease *HE Albers-Schonberg, German radiologist, 1865–1921.* Syn.: osteopetrosis.

Albinism A condition in which there is congenital absence of pigment in the skin, hair and eyes. It maybe partial or complete.

Albino A person affected with albinism.

Albright's syndrome *F Albright, American physician. 1900–1969.* Condition in which there is abnormal development of bone, excessive pigmentation of the skin and in females, precocious sexual development.

Albumin 1. Any protein that is soluble in water and moderately concentrated salt solutions and is coagulable by heat, e.g., egg white. 2. Serum albumin; a plasma protein, formed principally in the liver and constituting about four-sevenths of the 6–8% protein concentration in the plasma. Albumin is a very important factor in regulating the exchange of water between the plasma and the interstitial compartment (space between the cells). A drop in the amount of albumin in the plasma results in an increase in tissue fluid, which, if severe, becomes apparent as edema. Albumin also serves as a transport for protein.

Albuminuria The presence of albumin in the urine, e.g., occurring in renal disease, in most feverish conditions and sometimes in pregnancy.

Orthostatic or postural albuminuria A nonpathological form that affects some individuals after prolonged standing but disappears after bed rest for a few hours.

Albumose A substance, formed during gastric digestion, intermediate between albumin and peptone.

Albuterol A sympathomimetic drug used in bronchial asthma.

Alcaine Proparacaine, a local anesthetic.

Alcohol A volatile liquid distilled from fermented saccharine liquids and forming the basis of wines and spirits. The official (British Pharmacopoeia) preparation of ethyl alcohol (ethanol) contains 95% alcohol and 5% water. Used: (a) As an antiseptic; (b) In the preparation of tinctures; (c) As a preservative for anatomical specimens. Taken internally, it acts as a temporary heart stimulant, and in large quantities as a depressant poison.

Absolute alcohol That which contains not more than 1% by weight of water.

Alcohol fast Pertaining to bacteria that, once having been stained, are resistant to decolorization by alcohol.

Alcohol withdrawal syndrome A group of symptoms that develop in a person suffering from alcoholism within 6–24 hours of taking the last drink of alcohol. The symptoms include restlessness, tremors, loss of appetite, nausea, vomiting, insomnia, disorientation, seizures and delirium tremens. Treatment involves sedation, improving nutrition, counseling and social support.

Alcoholic 1. Pertaining to alcohol. 2. A person addicted to excessive, uncontrolled alcohol consumption. This results in loss of appetite and vitamin B deficiency, leading to peripheral neuritis with eye changes and cirrhosis of the liver and to progressive deterioration in the personality.

Alcoholism The state of poisoning resulting from alcoholic addiction.

Alcoholophilia The craving for alcohol.

Alcoholuria The presence of alcohol in the urine. This maybe estimated when excess blood levels of alcohol are suspected.

Aldosterone A compound, isolated from the adrenal cortex, that aids the retention of sodium and the excretion of potassium in the body, and by so doing aids the maintenance of electrolyte balance.

Aldosteronism An excess secretion of aldosterone caused by an adrenal neoplasm. The serum potassium is low and the patient has hypertension and severe muscular weakness.

Aleukemia An acute condition in which there is an absence or deficiency of white cells in the blood.

Alexander technique A process of psychophysical postural re-education. Body posture is believed to affect physical and psychological well-being and the postural re-education process aims to assist individuals in monitoring how they consciously use their bodies to promote good health.

Alexia A form of aphasia in which there is an inability to recognize written or printed words. Word blindness.

26

A

Alfentanil Newer more potent opoid analgesic with shorter duration of action.

Algesia State of increased sensitivity, to pain sometimes provoked by stimuli not normally painful.

Algesiometer, algesimeter An instrument for measuring the degree of sensitivity to a painful stimulus.

Algid Chilly cold.

Algogenic Producing pain or lowering the body temperature.

Algolagnia *(Greek: algos + lagnia= pain + lust).* Sexual tendency in which the person derive sexual gratification either by inflicting pain to the partner or by experiencing the pain, particularly involving the erogenous zone.

Algophily A desire to suffer from pain because one derives sexual pleasure from it.

Algophobia An abnormal and persistent fear of experiencing pain.

Algor *(latin: algor=coolness)* Chill or rigor; coldness.

Algorithm A process or set of rules used in calculations, e.g., of medications, or for other problem solving. Computer programs are the most familiar examples of algorithms in everyday use.

Alienation A feeling of estrangement or separation from others or from self.

Alienation symptom of schizophrenia. Sufferers often believe that they are under the control of someone else. Depersonalization.

Alignment The state of being arranged in a line, i.e., in the correct anatomical position.

Aliment Food or nourishment.

Alimentary Relating to the system of nutrition.

Alimentary canal Alimentary tract. The passage through which the food passes, from mouth to anus.

Alimentary system The alimentary tract together with the liver and other organs concerned in digestion and absorption.

Alimentary tract Alimentary canal.

Alimentation The giving or receiving of nourishment. The process of supplying the patient's need for nutrition.

Aliphatic 1. Fatty. 2. Denoting the open chain compounds most of which belong to the fatty series.

Alkalemia An increase in the alkali content of the blood. Alkalosis.

Alkali A substance capable of uniting with acids to form salts, and with fats and fatty acids to form soaps. Alkaline solutions turn red litmus paper blue.

Alkali reserves The ability of the combined buffer systems of the blood to neutralize acid. The pH of the blood is normally slightly on the alkaline side, between 7.35 and 7.45. The principal buffer in the blood is bicarbonate; the alkali reserve is essentially represented by the plasma bicarbonate concentration.

Alkaline Having the reactions of an alkali.

Alkaline phosphatase An enzyme localized on cell membranes that hydrolyse phosphate esters, liberating inorganic phosphate, and has an optimal pH of about 10.0. Serum alkaline phosphatase activity is elevated in obstructive jaundice and bone disease.

Alkalinity 1. The quality of being alkaline. 2. The combining ALK 16 power of a base, expressed as the maximum number of equivalents of acid with which it reacts to form a salt.

Alkaloid One of a group of active nitrogenous compounds that are alkaline in solution. They usually have a bitter taste and are characterized by powerful physiological activity. Examples are morphine, cocaine, atropine, quinine, nicotine and caffeine. The term is also applied to synthetic substances that have structures similar to plant alkaloids, such as procaine.

Alkalosis An increase in the alkali reserve in the blood. It maybe confirmed by estimation of the blood carbon dioxide content and treated by giving normal saline or ammonium chloride intravenously to encourage the excretion of bicarbonate by the kidneys.

Alkaptonuria The excretion of alkapton, an abnormal product of protein metabolism, in the urine. On exposure to air, oxidation takes place, giving a dark-brown color to the urine.

Alkylating agent Cell cycle nonspecific anticancer drugs· A drug that damages the deoxyribonucleic acid (DNA) molecule of the nucleus of the cell.

All-or-none law Principle that states that in individual cardiac and skeletal muscle fibers there are only two possible reactions to a stimulus: either there is no reaction at all or there is a full reaction, with no gradation of response according to the strength of the stimulus. Whole muscles can grade their response by increasing or decreasing the *number* of fibers involved.

Allantois A membranous sac projecting from the ventral surface of the fetus in its early stages. It eventually helps to form the placenta.

Allele Allelomorph. One of a pair of genes that occupy the same relative positions on homologous chromosomes and produce different effects on the same process of development.

Allelism State of two or more genes that must occupy the same position or locus on a specific chromosome.

Allelomorph Allele.

Allen Test Used to test the blood supply to the hand, specifically the patency of the radial and ulnar arteries. It is performed prior to radial arterial sampling or cannulation.

Allergen A substance that can produce an allergy or manifestation of an immune response.

Allergic rhinitis A common condition where there is inflammation of the inside of the nose caused by an allergen such as pollen, dust, mould or animal skin.

Allergy A hypersensitivity to some foreign substances (bacteria, drug, food items, cold, pollens, etc.) that are normally harmless but which produce a violent reaction in the patient. Asthma, hay fever, angio neurotic edema, migraine, and some types of urticaria and eczema are allergic states *(See Anaphylaxis)*.

Alliesthesia also known as *Allocheiria*. A sensation or stimulus is perceived at a point on the body which is opposite to the point where the stimulus was actually applied.

Alloantigen An antigen present in the blood or tissue of a donor and not present in the recipient which triggers an immune response.

Alloarthroplasty Surgical creation of a new joint in the body using materials other than the cells and tissues from human body. An artificial joint.

Allocate To assign for a particular purpose.

Allocation The act of allocating.

Clinical allocation A period of time spent in ward/department/unit where there are patients/clients.

Patient allocation One nurse is designated as responsible for the care of one patient or a group of patients for a spell of duty.

Task allocation Patient care in a ward/unit is provided by a group of nurses. Each nurse is allocated a specific nursing activity (task), e.g., one nurse in the clinical area will be responsible for sponge bath while another will be

A

taking and recording vital signs for the same group of patients.

Allochezia Either defecation from an opening other than the anus or expulsion of nonfecal matter from the anus.

Alloeroticism Sexual attraction toward another person, as opposed to autoeroticism.

Allogamy The fertilization of the ova of one individual by the spermatozoa of another; the opposite of autogamy.

Allograft Tissue transplanted from one person to another.

Nonviable allograft Skin, taken from a cadaver, which cannot regenerate.

Viable allograft Living tissue transplanted.

Alloimmunization The immune response to donated blood, bone marrow or transplanted organ; rhesus-negative pregnant women with a rhesus-positive fetus can become alloimmunized following a sensitizing event, e.g., antepartum hemorrhage or miscarriage, through the development of antibodies that target the foreign material, causing hemolytic disease of the newborn.

Allopath One who practices medicine according to the system of allopathy.

Allopathy A therapeutic system in which a disease is treated by producing a morbid reaction of another kind or in another part by method of substitution.

Alloploidy The condition of a hybrid individual or cell having two or more sets of chromosomes derived from two different ancestral species.

Allopurinol A drug that reduces the serum and urinary levels of uric acid. Used in the long-term treatment of gout to lessen the frequency and severity of attacks.

Allosome One of the chromosomes differing in appearance or behavior from the ordinary chromosomes or autosomes and sometimes unequally

distributed among the germ cell, heterotypical chromosome.

Alma – Ata declaration A declaration made in 1978 at a conference on Primary Health Care at Alma-Ata in USSR for attaining health for all by year 2000.

Almetrine Respiratory stimulant used in COPD.

Alochia Absence of lochia.

Alopecia Baldness. Loss of hair. The cause of simple baldness is not yet fully understood, although it is known that the tendency to become bald is limited almost entirely to males, runs in certain families and is more common in certain racial groups than in others. Baldness is often associated with ageing.

Alopecia areata Hair loss in sharply defined areas, usually the scalp or beard.

Alopecia cicatrisata Irreversible loss of hair associated with scarring, usually on the scalp.

Malepattern alopecia Loss of scalp hair, genetically determined and androgen dependent, beginning with frontal recession and progressing symmetrically to leave ultimately only a sparse peripheral rim of hair.

Alveolus A small angular cavity; bony socket of a tooth; air sac of the lungs.

Alovera Skin texture enhancer and emollient.

Alpha The first letter of the Greek alphabet, α.

Alpha cells Cells found in the islet of Langerhans in the pancreas. They produce the hormone glucagon.

Alpha fetoprotein Abbreviated AFP. A plasma protein originating in the fetal liver and gastrointestinal tract. The serum AFP level is used to monitor the effectiveness of cancer treatment; the amniotic fluid AFP level is used in the prenatal diagnosis of neural tube defects.

A

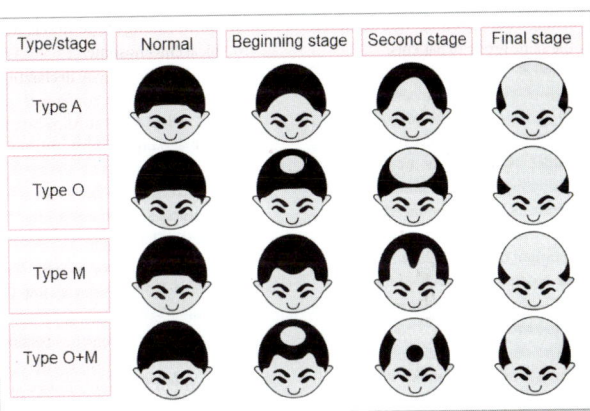

Type/stage	Normal	Beginning stage	Second stage	Final stage
Type A				
Type O				
Type M				
Type O+M				

Types of Alopecia

Alpha receptors Tissue receptors associated with the stimulation (contraction) of smooth muscle.

Alport's syndrome *AC Alport, South African physician, 1880–1959.* A hereditary disorder marked by progressive nerve deafness, progressive pyelonephritis or glomerulonephritis, and occasionally ocular defects.

Alprazolam A benzodiazepine, anxiolytic agent.

Alternating current An electrical current that runs alternately from the negative and positive poles.

Alternative medicine A form of medicine differing from conventional health care. Consists of a range of treatments essentially based upon a holistic approach to health and well-being, including homeopathy, aromatherapy, hypnosis, acupuncture and others. Generally these therapies have not been subject to scientific scrutiny but are often used when conventional treatments have failed. Commonly called complementary therapies *(See Complementary).*

Altitude sickness Condition caused by hypoxia that occurs as a result of lower oxygen pressure at high altitudes.

Altruism A sense of unconditional concern for the welfare of others.

Aluminium Symbol Al. A silver-white metal with a low specific gravity compounds of which are astringent and antiseptic.

Aluminium hydroxide Compound used as an antacid in the treatment of gastric conditions.

Alveolar Concerning an alveolus, or/ and sac of the lung.

Alveolar air Air found in the alveoli.

Alveolitis Inflammation of the alveoli.

Extrinsic allergic alveolitis Inflammation of the alveoli caused by inhalation of an antigen, such as pollen.

Alzheimer's cells *A. Alzheimer, German neurologist, 1864–1915.* 1. Giant astrocytes with large prominent nuclei found in the brain in hepatolenticular degeneration and hepatic comas. 2. Degenerated astrocytes.

A

Alzheimer's disease A progressive form of neuronal degeneration in the brain and the most common cause of dementia in people of all ages. It is more common in older than younger people and is not just a form of pre senile dementia, as was originally thought. The degeneration of neurones is accompanied by changes in the brain's biochemistry. At the moment this condition is irreversible and there is no effective treatment.

Amalgam A compound of mercury and other metals.

Dental amalgam Used for filling teeth.

Amantadine An antiviral agent used against influenza A virus; also used as an antidyskinetic in the treatment of Parkinson's disease.

Amaurosis Loss of vision, sometimes following excessive blood loss, especially after prolonged bleeding, e.g., hematuria. The visual loss maybe partial or complete, temporary or permanent.

Amaurotic Pertaining to amaurosis.

Amaurotic family idiocy Tay-Sachs disease A familial metabolic disorder starting in infancy or childhood. Characterized by progressive mental deterioration, blindness and spastic paralysis.

Ambeniniam An anti-cholinestrase agent.

Ambidextrous Equally skilful with either hand.

Ambivalence The existence of contradictory emotional feelings towards an object, commonly of love and hate for another person. If these feelings occur to a marked degree they lead to psychologic disturbance.

Amblyacousia Hearing dullness.

Ambylopia Dimness of vision without any apparent lesion of the eye. Uncorrectable by optical means.

Amblygeustia Temporary or permanent diminution in the sense of taste.

Amblyopia Dimness of vision without any apparent lesion of the eye. Uncorrectable by optical means.

Ambroxol A mucolytic.

Ambu bag A hand operated, self reinflating bag used during resuscitation. It is connected by tubing and non-rebreathing valve to a face mask or endotracheal tube and is used for artificial ventilation.

Ambulant Able to walk.

Ambulatory Having the capacity to walk.

Ambulatory treatment Health care services provided on an outpatient basis.

Amebiasis Infestation with *Entamoeba histolytica* or other pathogenic amoebas.

Amebocyte A cell such as neutrophil leukocyte having the power of ameboid movements.

Ameboid 1. Resembling an ameba in appearance or characteristics. 2. of irregular outline with peripheral projections.

Ameboma An amebic granuloma, a nodular tumor like focus of proliferative inflammation sometimes developing in chronic amebiasis especially in the wall of colon.

Ameiosis A cell division resulting in formation of gametes without reduction in chromosome number.

Amelia Congenital absence of a limb or limbs.

Amelioration Improvement of symptoms; a lessening of the severity of a disease.

Amenorrhea Absence of menstruation.

Primary amenorrhea The non-occurrence of the menses.

Secondary amenorrhea The cessation of the menses after they have been established, owing to disease or pregnancy.

Amenorrhoea Absence of menstruation.

Primary amenorrhoea The non-occurrence of the menses.

Secondary amenorrhoea The cessation of the menses, after they have been established, owing to disease or pregnancy.

Amentia Mental subnormality. Maybe due to hereditary factors, failure of development of the embryo or birth trauma.

Ames test A biological assay to assess the mutagenic potential of chemical compounds. A positive test indicates that the chemical is mutagenic and therefore may act as a carcinogen, e.g., cancer is often linked to mutation.

Amethocaine A local anesthetic effective when in contact with surfaces as well as when given by injection.

Ametropia Defective vision. A general word applied to incorrect refraction.

Amethopterin Methotrexata, a cytotoxic drug.

Amifostine Cytoprotective agent in cancer chemotherapy.

Amikacin A semisynthetic aminoglycoside antibiotic derived from kanamycin, used in the treatment of a wide range of infections due to susceptible organisms.

Amiloride A weak but potassium retaining diuretic drug.

Amino acid A chemical compound containing both NH_2 and COOH groups. The end product of protein digestion. **Essential amino acid** One required for replacement and growth but which cannot be synthesized in the body in sufficient amounts and must be obtained in the diet *(See Table)*.

Essential Amino Acids

1. Threonine
2. Lysine
3. Methionine
4. Valine
5. Phenylalanine
6. Leucine
7. Tryptophan
8. Isoleucine
9. Histidine
10. Arginine

Nonessential amino acid One necessary for proper growth but which can be synthesized in the body and is not specifically required in the diet.

Aminoacidopathy Any inborn error of amino acid metabolism producing a metabolic block that results in accumulation of one or more amino acids in the blood (amino acidemia) or excess excretion in the urine (amino aciduria) or both.

Aminoglutethimide A drug which inhibits adrenal hormone synthesis. Its use is sometimes referred to as "medical adrenalectomy". The effects are reversible when the drug is discontinued. Used to treat metastatic breast and prostate cancers.

Aminoglycoside Any of a group of bacterial antibiotics, derived from various species of *Streptomyces,* that interfere with the function of bacterial ribosomes. The aminoglycosides include gentamicin, netilmicin, streptomycin, tobramycin, amikacin, kanamycin and neomycin. They are used to treat infections caused by Gram-negative organisms and are classified as bactericidal agents because of their interference with bacterial replication. All the aminoglycoside antibiotics are highly toxic, requiring monitoring of blood serum levels and careful observation of the patient for early signs of toxicity, particularly ototoxicity and nephrotoxicity.

Aminophylline An alkaloid from camellia, it relaxes plain muscle spasm of the bronchioles and coronary arteries. It maybe given by mouth, intravenously or as a suppository, and is useful in treating asthma and heart failure.

Aminosalicylic acid An antibiotic primarily used to treat tuberculosis.

Amiodarone Antiarrythmic agent.

A

Amitosis Multiplication of cells by simple division or fission.

Amitriptyline An antidepressant drug that is chemically related to imipramine. It is useful in relieving tension and anxiety but may cause dizziness and hypotension.

Amlodipine Calcium channel blocker for hypertension.

Ammonia NH_3 A colorless pungent gas. In solution, used as a cardiac stimulant.

Ammonium A chemical group that combines to form salts similar to those of the alkaline metals.

Ammonium chloride Used as a mild diuretic. Widely used in mixtures as an expectorant.

Amnesia Partial or complete loss of memory.

Anterograde amnesia Loss of memory of events that have taken place since an injury or illness.

Retrograde amnesia Loss of memory for events prior to an injury. It often applies to the time immediately preceding an accident.

Visual amnesia Inability to recall to mind the appearance of objects that have been seen or to recognize printed words.

Amniocentesis The withdrawal of fluid from the uterus through the abdominal wall by means of a syringe and needle. It is primarily used in the diagnosis of chromosome disorders in the fetus and in cases of hydramnios.

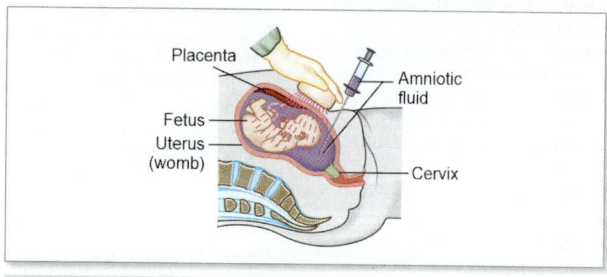

Amniocentesis

Amniography Radiography of the gravid uterus.

Amnioinfusion Infusion of normal saline into the amniotic sac to increase the amniotic fluid volume.

Amnion The innermost membrane enveloping the fetus and enclosing the liquor amnii, or amniotic fluid.

Amnioscope Instrument for examining the fetus and the amniotic fluid by means of a tube passing through the abdominal wall.

Amnioscopy Inspection of the amniotic sac using an amnioscope.

Amniotic Pertaining to the amnion.

Amniotic fluid The albuminous fluid contained in the amniotic sac. Liquor amnii.

Amniotomy Surgically breaking the amniotic sac to induce or expedite labor.

Amobarbitol White crystalline powder of a bitter taste slightly soluble in water, melting point 156°C. A central nervous system depressant, has an intermediate duration of action.

Amodiaquine hydrochloride Camoquine hydrochloride, a synthetic antimalarial drug, effective against *plasmodium vivax* in the erythrocytic phase of malaria.

Amoeba A minute unicellular Protozoon. It is able to move by pushing out parts of itself (called pseudopodia). Capable of reproduction by amitotic fission. Infection of the intestines by *Entamoeba histolytica* causes "amebic dysentery".

Amoebiasis Infection with ameba, particularly *Entamoeba histolytica*.

Amoebic Pertaining to, caused by, or of the nature of an ameba.

Amoebic abscess An abscess cavity of the liver resulting from liquefaction necrosis due to entrance of *Entamoeba histolytica* into the portal circulation in amebiasis; amebic abscesses may affect the lung, brain and spleen.

Amoebic dysentery A form of dysentery caused by *Entamoeba histolytica* and spread by contaminated food, water and flies; called also amebiasis. Amebic dysentery is mainly a tropical disease but many cases occur in temperate countries. Symptoms are diarrhea, fatigue and intestinal bleeding. Complications include involvement of the liver, liver abscess and pulmonary abscess.

Amoeboid Resembling an ameba in structure or movement.

Amorphous Without definite shape. The term maybe applied to fine powdery particles, as opposed to crystals.

Amoxapine Tricyclic anti-depressant.

Amoxil Trade name for a preparation of amoxycillin, an antibiotic.

Amoxycillin A penicillin analogue similar in action to ampicillin but more efficiently absorbed from the gastrointestinal tract and therefore requiring less frequent dosage and not as likely to cause diarrhea. It also penetrates sputum more readily than ampicillin.

Ampere Symbol A. The unit of intensity of an electrical current.

Amphetamine A synthetic drug that stimulates the central nervous system. It is addictive and is now seldom used except in the treatment of narcolepsy.

Amphiarthrosis A form of joint in which the bones are joined together by fibrocartilage, e.g., the junctions of the vertebrae.

Amphoric Pertaining to a bottle. Used to describe the sound sometimes heard on auscultation over cavities in the lungs, which resembles that produced by blowing across the mouth of a bottle.

Amphoricle *(see Amphoric)*

Amphotericin An antifungal drug which is not absorbed by the gut. The only polyene antibiotic that maybe given parenterally. Active against most yeasts and other fungi. Side effects of fever, nausea and vomiting are common when the drug is given parenterally.

Ampicillin A broad spectrum penicillin of synthetic origin, used in treatment of a number of infections. It is active against many of the Gram-negative pathogens, in addition to the usual Gram-positive ones that are sensitive to penicillin.

Ampoule A small glass or plastic vial in which sterile drugs of specified dose for injection are sealed.

Ampulla The flask-like dilatation of a canal, e.g., uterine tube.

Amputation Surgical removal of a limb or other part of the body, e.g., the breast.

Amputee A person who has had one or more limbs amputated.

Amyelia Congenital absence of spinal cord.

Amylase An enzyme that reduces starch to maltose. Found in saliva (ptyalin) and pancreatic juice (amylopsin).

Amylnitrate A vasodilator used in angina and cyanide poisoning.

Amylobarbitone One of the barbiturates, used as a short-acting hypnotic and sedative. Effects develop rapidly and the drug is eliminated more quickly than other barbiturates. Regular use may lead to habituation, and over dosage can produce narcosis and death. Classified as a controlled drug.

Amylocaine hydrochloride Benzoyl ethyldimethyl aminopropanyl hydrochloride, a local anesthetic.

Amyloid 1. Pertaining to starch. 2. A waxy starch that forms in certain tissues.

Amyloid degeneration Amyloidosis Deposits of amyloid in various organs, tissues. Four types of conditions are recognized – primary, secondary, localized mass or nodule and associated with multiple myeloma.

Amylopsin An enzyme found in the pancreas. Amylase.

Amylum [L.] Starch.

Amyotonia Atonic condition of the muscles.

Amyotonia congenita Any of several rare congenital diseases marked by general hypotonia of the muscles; called also Oppenheim's disease or floppy baby syndrome.

Amyotrophy Muscular wasting or atrophy.

Anabolic Relating to anabolism.

Anabolic compound A substance that aids in the repair of body tissue, particularly protein.

Anabolism The building up or synthesis of cell structure from digested food materials *(See Metabolism)*.

Anacidity Decrease in normal acidity.

Anaclisis Generally, reclining or leaning; typically, an emotional dependence on others.

Anaclitic Denoting the dependence of the infant on the mother or mother substitute for its sense of well-being.

Anaclitic choice A psychoanalytical term for the adult selection of a loved one who closely resembles one's mother (or another adult on whom one depended as a child).

Anaclitic depression Severe and progressive depression found in children who have lost their mothers and have not found a suitable substitute.

Anacrotism An abnormal pulse wave tracing embodying a secondary expansion.

Anaemia Deficiency in either quality or quantity of red corpuscles in the blood, giving rise especially to symptoms of anoxemia. There is pallor, breathlessness on exertion, with palpitations, lassitude, headache, giddiness and often a history of poor resistance to infection. Anaemia maybe due to many different causes. Increasingly, with the advent of electronic cell counters, anaemia is now classified according to the morphological characteristics of the erythrocytes.

Aplastic anaemia The bone marrow is unable to produce red blood corpuscles. A rare condition.

Deficiency anaemia Any type that is due to the lack of the necessary factors for red cell formation, e.g., hormones or vitamins.

Hemolytic anaemia A variety in which there is excessive destruction of red blood corpuscles caused by antibody formation in the blood *(See Rhesus factor)* by drugs or by severe toxemia, as in extensive burn.

Iron-deficiency anaemia The most common type of anaemia, due to a lack of absorbable iron in the diet. It may also be due to excessive or chronic blood loss, or to poor absorption of dietary iron.

Macrocytic anaemia A type in which the cells are larger than normal, present in pernicious anaemia.

Microcytic anaemia A variety in which the cells are smaller than normal, as in iron deficiency.

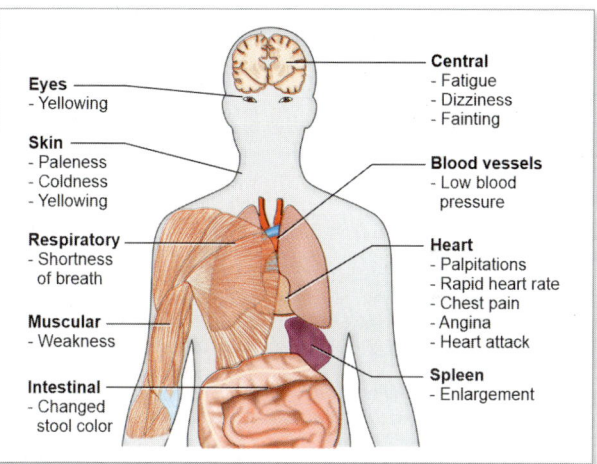

Symptoms of Anaemia

Pernicious anaemia A variety caused by the inability of the stomach to secrete the intrinsic factor necessary for the absorption of vitamin B$_{12}$ from the diet.

Sickle cell anaemia A hereditary hemolytic anaemia seen most commonly in black people living in or originating from the Caribbean islands, Africa, Asia, the Middle East and the Mediterranean. The red blood cells are sickle-shaped.

Splenic anaemia A congenital, familial disease in which the red blood cells are fragile and easily broken down.

Anaerobe A microorganism that can live and thrive in the absence of free oxygen. These organisms are found in body cavities or wounds where the oxygen tension is very low. Examples are the bacilli of tetanus and gas gangrene.

Anesthesia Loss of feeling or sensation in a part or in the whole of the body, usually induced by drugs.

Basal anesthesia Basal narcosis. Loss of consciousness, although supplemental drugs have to be given to ensure complete anesthesia.

Epidural anesthesia Injection into the extradural space between the vertebral spines and beneath the ligamentum flavum.

General anesthesia Unconsciousness produced by inhalation or injection of a drug.

Inhalation anesthesia Drugs or gas are administered by a face mask or endotracheal tube to cause general anesthesia.

Intravenous anesthesia Unconsciousness is produced by the introduction of a drug into a vein.

Local anesthesia Local analgesia. Nerve conduction is blocked by injection of a local anesthetic, or by freezing with ethyl chloride or by topical application.

Spinal anesthesia Injection of anesthetic agent into the spinal subarachnoid space.

Anaesthetic A drug causing anesthesia.

A

Anaesthetist A person who is medically qualified to administer an anesthetic and in the techniques of life support for the critically ill or injured.

Anal Pertaining to the anus.

Anal eroticism Sexual pleasure derived from anal functions.

Anal fissure A small tear in the lining of the anus.

Anal fistula An infected tunnel between the skin and the anus.

Analeptic A drug that stimulates the central nervous system.

Analgesia Insensibility to pain, especially the relief of pain without causing unconsciousness.

Patient controlled analgesia A present dose of analgesic, which the patient controls according to need. In-built safety measures prevent accidental overdose.

Analgesic 1. Relating to analgesia. 2. A remedy that relieves pain.

Analgesic cocktail An individualized mixture of drugs used to control pain.

Analogue 1. An organ with a different structure and origin but the same function as another one. 2. A compound with a similar structure to another but differing in respect of a particular element.

Analysis 1. The act of determining the component parts of a substance. 2. The breaking up of a chemical compound into its simpler elements, a process by which the composition of a substance is determined. 3. In psychiatry, a method of trying to understand the complex mental processes, experiences and relationships with other individuals or groups of individuals to determine the reasons for an individual's behavior.

Anamnesis 1. The act of remembering 2. The medical history of a patient.

Anandria Absence of masculinity.

Anaphase Part of the process of mitosis or meiosis in which the chromosomes move from the equatorial plate toward the poles of the cell.

Anaphylaxis Anaphylactic shock. A severe reaction, often fatal, occurring in response to drugs, e.g., penicillin, but also to bee stings and food allergy, e.g., nuts in sensitive individuals. The symptoms are severe dyspnea, rapid pulse, profuse sweating and collapse.

Anaplasia A change in the character of cells, seen in tumor tissue.

Anarthria Inability to articulate speech sounds owing to a brain lesion or damage to peripheral nerves innervating articulatory muscles.

Anasarca Severe generalized edema.

Anastomosis 1. In surgery, any artificial connection of two hollow structures, e.g., gastroenterostomy. 2. In anatomy, the joining of the branches of two blood vessels.

Anatomy The science of the structure of the body.

Ancylostoma A genus of nematode roundworms which may inhabit the duodenum and cause extreme anaemia.

Ancylostoma duodenale A hookworm, very wide spread in tropical and subtropical areas *(See Figure).*

Androgen One of a group of hormones secreted by the testes and adrenal cortex. They are steroids which can be synthesized and produce the secondary male characteristics and the building up of protein tissue.

Android Resembling a man.

Android pelvis A female pelvis shaped like male pelvis with a wedge-shaped entrance and narrow anterior segment.

Androgynoid A man with hermaphrodite sexual characteristics who is mistaken for a woman, a pseudohermaphrodite. Possession of masculine characteristics by a genetically pure female.

Androgynus Female pseudohermaphrodite.

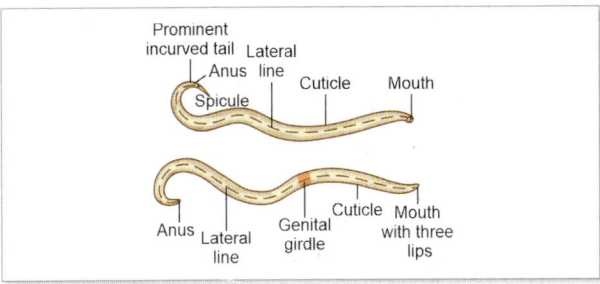

Ancylostoma

Andropathy Any disease such as prostatitis peculiar to the male sex.

Androstenedione A testosterone precursor.

Anencephaly Congenital absence of the cranial vault, with the cerebral hemispheres completely missing or reduced to small masses.

Anergy 1. Specific immunological tolerance in which T cells and B cells fail to respond normally. The state can be reversed. 2. Tiredness, lethargy, lack of energy.

Aneroid Equipment that does not utilize liquid medium for measurement of pressure. e.g., aneroid barometer.

Aneuploidy Possession of abnormal number of chromosomes.

Aneurine Thiamine. An essential vitamin involved in carbohydrate metabolism. The main sources are unrefined cereals and pork. Vitamin B_1.

Aneurysm A local dilatation of a blood vessel, usually an artery. Atherosclerosis is responsible for most arterial wall can predispose to the formation of a sac. Other diseases that can lead to an aneurysm include syphilis, certain nonspecific inflammations and a congenital defect in the artery. The pressure of blood causes it to increase in size and rupture is likely. Sometimes excision of the aneurysm or ligation of the artery is possible.

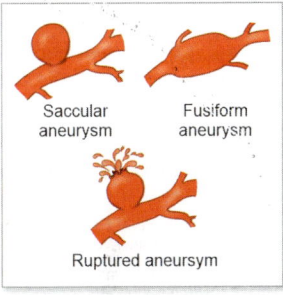

Aneurysm

Dissecting aneurysm A condition in which a tear occurs in the aortic lining when the middle coat is necrosed and blood gets between the layers, stripping them apart.

Fusiform aneurysm A spindle-shaped arterial aneurysm.

Saccular aneurysm A dilatation of only a part of the circumference of an artery.

Micotic aneurysm Aneurysm due to bacterial infection of vessel wall.

Angel's wing Posterior projection of scapula caused by paralysis of serratus anterior.

Anger The emotion of extreme displeasure to person, a situation or an object.

Angiectasia Dilatation of blood and lymph vessel.

Angititis Inflammation of a blood or lymph vessel.

Angina 1. A tight strangling sensation or pain. 2. An inflammation of the throat causing pain on swallowing.

Angina crusis Intermittent claudication. Severe pain in the leg after walking.

Angina pectoris Cardiac pain that occurs on exertion owing to insufficient blood supply to the heart muscles.

Vincent's angina Infection and ulceration of the tonsils by a spirochaete, *Borrelia vincentii* and a bacillus, *fusiforms*.

Angina abdominis Abdominal pain due to ischemia of gut.

Ludwig angina Deep infection of tissues in the floor of the mouth.

Angina prinzmetal's Angina pectoris with ST elevation due to coronary spasm.

Unstable angina Angina of recent onset, abrupt progression, occurring at rest, is due to superadded coronary thrombosis, a fore runner of impending infarction.

Variant angina Angina occurring at rest in absence of cardiac acceleration.

Angioblast The mesenchymal cell derivative which ultimately develops into blood vessels.

Angioblastoma Tumor involving blood vessels of brain and meninges.

Angiocardiogram Radiological examination of the heart and large blood vessels by means of cardiac catheterization and an opaque contrast medium.

Angiocardiography Radiological examination of the heart and large blood vessels by means of cardiac catheterization and an opaque contrast medium.

Angioectasis Abnormal enlargement of capillaries.

Angioedema An allergic condition characterized by urticaria and edematous areas of skin and mucus membrane or viscera.

Angioendothelioma A tumor with endothelial cells predominance occurring in bone.

Angiogenesis development of blood vessels.

Angiography Radiological examination of the blood vessels using an opaque contrast medium.

Cerebral angiography X-ray picture of cerebral circulation to evaluate stroke, tumor, AV malformation, aneurysm or abnormal vascular pattern.

Coronary angiography X-ray of coronary circulation to evaluate ischemic disease.

Digital subtraction angiography A computer aided "subtraction" technique that subtracts images of surrounding tissue from the contrast image to give better resolution and minor details.

Angioid streaks Dark wavy anastomosing striae lying beneath the retinal vessels.

Angiokeratoma Thickening of epidermis of feet with telangiectases warty growths.

Angiolipoma A mixed tumor containing blood vessels and fatty tissue.

Angiolith Calcareous deposits in walls of blood vessels.

Angiology Science of blood vessels and lymphatics.

Angioma A benign tumor composed of dilated blood vessels (hemangioma) or lymph vessels (lymphangioma).

Angioma capillary Congenital superficial hemangioma appearing as irregular red discoloration due to overgrowth of capillaries.

Angioma cavernous Elevated dark red tumor consisting of blood filled vascular spaces; involves submucous and subcutaneous tissue and is pulsatile.

Angioma senile Hemangioma in elderly due to capillary wall degeneration, producing a compressible mass.

Angioma serpiginous A skin disorder characterized by appearance of small red vascular dots arranged in rings due to proliferation of capillaries.

Angioma stellate Hemangioma in which telangiectatic blood vessels radiate from a central point. SYN – spider nevus.

Angiomalacia Softening of wall of blood vessels.

Angiomatosis Multiple angiomas.

Angiomyolipoma A benign growth containing vascular, muscular and fatty elements.

Angioneurosis A neurosis affecting the blood vessels, which may produce paralysis.

Angioneurotic Pertaining to angioneurosis.

Angioneurotic edema (See Oedema).

Angiopathy Any disease of blood or lymph vessel.

Angioplasty Surgery of a narrowed artery to promote the normal flow of blood. A common technique is balloon angioplasty.

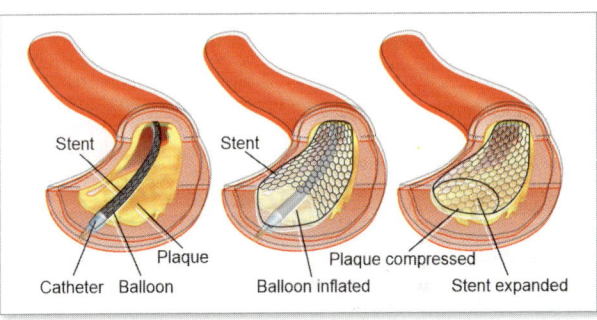

Stent | Stent | Plaque compressed
Catheter | Balloon | Plaque | Balloon inflated | Stent expanded

Angioplasty

Angiosarcoma A malignant vascular growth.

Angiospasm A spasmodic contraction of an artery, causing cramping of the muscles.

Angiotensin A substance that raises the blood pressure. It is a polypeptide produced by the action of renin on plasma globulins. Hypertension.

Angiotensinogen A serum globulin fraction formed in the liver.

Angor animi A feeling that one is dying as in angina pectoris.

Angular artery Artery at inner canthus of eye.

Anhedonia Lack of pleasure in normally pleasurable acts.

Anhidrosis Marked deficiency in the secretion of sweat.

Anhidrotic An agent that decreases perspiration. An adiaphoretic.

Anhydremia Deficiency of water in the blood.

Anhydrase Enzyme that helps in removal of water from a chemical compound.

Anhydride Compound formed by removal of water from a substance, specially an acid.

Anhydrous Containing no water.

Anicteric Without jaundice.

Aniline A chemical compound derived from coal tar, used for making antiseptic dyes. It is an important cause of serious industrial poisoning associated with bone marrow depression as well as methemoglobinemia.

Anilism Chronic aniline poisoning manifesting with vertigo, cardiac conduction defects, muscular weakness.

Anima 1. The soul. 2. Jung's term for the unconscious, or inner being, of the individual, as opposed to the personality presented to the world (persona). In Jungian psychoanalysis, the more feminine soul or feminine component of a man's personality.

Animal A living organism.

Animation State of being alive.

Anion A negatively charged ion which travels against the current toward the anode.

Aniridia Lack of part or the whole of the iris.

Anisindione Anticoagulant agent.

Anisocoria Inequality of diameter of the pupils of the two eyes.

Anisocytosis Inequality in the size of the red blood cells.

Anisodactyly Unequal length of the corresponding fingers or digits.

Anisogamy Sexual fusion of two gametes of different form and size.

Anisognathous A condition of having different sizes of maxillary and mandibular dental arches or jaws. The upper jaw is usually larger than the lower one.

Anisoleukocytosis Various forms of leukocytes are present in an abnormal ratio in the blood.

Anisomastia Condition of unequal size of breasts.

Anisometropia A marked difference in the refractive power of the two eyes.

Anisophoria Muscular imbalance in eye where horizontal visual plane of one eye is different from other.

Anisopiesis Inequality in arterial blood pressure between the two sides of the body.

Anisotropine A belladonna alkaloid derivative, spasmolytic.

Anisuria A condition where there is marked alteration in the amount of urine produced; alternating between oliguria and polyuria.

Ankle The joint between the leg and foot, formed by the tibia and fibula articulating with the talus.

Ankle jerk Plantar flexion of foot due to contraction of calf musculature following a brisk tap to tendo- achilis tendon.

Ankle-brachial pressure index (ABPI) The measurement of the ratio of systolic blood pressure at the ankle measured by a Doppler ultrasound probe to that measured at the brachial artery to quantify the degree of arterial occlusion in the leg. Forms an important part of a leg ulcer assessment regarding the patient's suitability for compression bandaging.

Ankyloblepharon Adhesions and scar tissue on the ciliary borders of the eyelids, giving the eye a distorted appearance.

Ankylocolpos Imperforated or atretic vaginal canal.

Ankyloglossia Poor tongue protrusion due to abnormally short frenulum.

Ankylosis Consolidation, immobility and stiffness of a joint as a result of disease.

Annelida A phylum of metazoan, the segmented worms, including the leeches.

Annular Ring-shaped.

Annulorophy Closure of hernial ring by suture.

Annulus A ring-shaped structure.

Anociassociation The exclusion of the pain, fear and shock in surgical operations brought about by means of local anesthetics and basal narcosis.

Anococcygeal body The muscle and fibrous tissue lying between anus and coccyx.

Anococcygeal ligament A band of fibrous tissue joining coccyx to external sphincter ani.

Anode The positive pole of an electric battery *(See Cathode)*.

Anodontia Absence of teeth.

Anodyne 1. Pain relieving or relaxing. 2. A drug or other treatment that relieves pain.

Anomaloscope Device for detection of color blindness.

Anomaly Considerable variation from normal.

Anomia Inability in naming objects.

Anomie A feeling of hopelessness and lack of purpose.

Anonychia Congenital absence of nails.

Anopheles A genus of mosquito. Many are carriers of the malarial parasite and infect human beings by their bite. Other species transmit filariasis.

Anophthalmia Congenital absence of a seeing eye. Some portion of the eye, e.g., the conjunctiva, is always present.

Anorchism Congenital absence of one or both testes.

Anorexia Loss of appetite for food.

Anorexia nervosa A condition in which there is complete lack of appetite, with extreme emaciation. It is due to psychological causes and usually occurs in young women, leading them to perceive themselves as fat and to take extreme forms of dietary control in order to lose weight.

Anorexigenic Causing loss of appetite.

Anoscope Speculum for examining anus and lower rectum.

Anosmia Loss of the sense of smell.

Anovular Applied to the absence of ovulation. Usually refers to uterine bleeding when there has been no ovulation, the result of taking contraceptive pills.

Anoxemia Complete lack of oxygen in the blood.

Anoxia Lack of oxygen in an organ or tissue.

Antabuse Trade name for a preparation of disulfiram used in the treatment of alcoholism.

Antacid A substance neutralizing acidity, particularly of gastric juices.

Antagonism Mutual opposite or contradictory action.

Antagonist 1. A muscle that has an opposite action to another, e.g., the biceps to the triceps. 2. In pharmacology, a drug that inhibits the action of another drug or enzyme, e.g., methotrexate is a folic acid antagonist. 3. In dentistry, a tooth in one jaw opposing one in the other jaw.

Ante (Prefix) meaning before.

Antecedent Something coming before; precursor.

Antecibum Before meals.

Antecubital At the bend of elbow.

Anteflexion A bending forward, as of the body of uterus *(See Retroflexion)*.

Antegrade Moving forward or direction of flow.

Antemortem Before death.

Antenatal Before birth.

Antenatal care Care provided by midwives and obstetricians during pregnancy to ensure that the fetal and maternal health are satisfactory. Deviations from normal can be detected and treated early. The mother can be prepared for labor and parenthood and health education offered.

Antepar Trade name for piperazine citrate.

Antepartum Shortly before birth, i.e., in the last three months of pregnancy.

Antepartum hemorrhage Bleeding occurring before parturition *(See Placenta previa)*.

Anterior Situated at or facing toward the front.

Anterior capsule Anterior covering of the lens of the eye.

Anterior chamber of the eye Space between the cornea in front and the iris and lens behind.

A

Anterior horn cell The nerve cells in anterior horn of spinal cord whose axons form the efferent fibers innervating the muscles.

Anterograde Tending or moving forward.

Anteroinferior In front and below.

Anterolateral In front and to one side.

Anteromedian In front and toward midline.

Anteroposterior Passing from front to rear.

Anterosuperior In front and above.

Anteversion The forward tilting of an organ, e.g., normal position of the uterus *(See Retroversion)*.

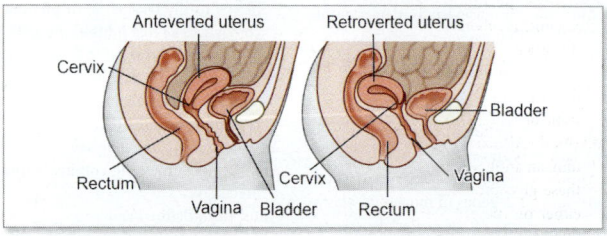

Anteverted and Retroverted Uterus

Anthelmintic (anthelminthic) 1. Destructive to worms. 2. An agent destructive to worms.

Anthracosis *SYN* – black lung. A disease of the lungs, caused by inhalation of coal dust. A form of pneumoconiosis. "Miner's lung".

Anthralin A synthetic hydrocarbon used as ointment to treat fungal infections and eczema.

Anthrax An acute, notifiable, infectious disease due to *Bacillus anthracis*, acquired through contact with infected animals or their byproducts, such as carcasses, bones or skin, usually by occupational exposure. The incubation period is 2–5 days. A worldwide zoonosis.

Anthropogeny Origin and development of man.

Anthropoid Resembling man.

Anthropoid pelvis Female pelvis in which the anteroposterior diameter exceeds the transverse diameter.

Anthropology The study of human beings that focuses on origins, historical and cultural development, and races.

Cultural anthropology The branch of anthropology that is concerned with individuals and their relationship to others and to their environment.

Medical anthropology Biocultural discipline concerned with both the biological and sociocultural aspects of human behavior, and the ways in which the two interact to influence health and disease.

Physical anthropology The branch of anthropology that concerns the physical and evolutionary characteristics of human beings.

Anthropometry The science that deals with the comparative measurement of parts of the human body, such as height, weight, body fat, etc.

Anthropomorphism Attributing human qualities to non-humans.

Anthropophilic Parasites that prefer human host rather than other animals.

Anti (Prefix) meaning against.

Antiadrenergic Counter acting or preventing adrenergic actions.

Antiagglutinin A specific antibody opposing the action of agglutinin.

Antiamebic A medicine used to treat amebiasis.

Antiandrogen Substances antagonizing the action of androgen.

Antibacterial A substance that destroys or suppresses the growth of bacteria.

Antibiosis Relationship between two organisms where one is harmful to the other.

Antibiotic Substances that inhibit or destroy microorganisms; bacteristatic or bactericidal.

Antibody Also known as immunoglobulin, an antibody is one of a group of these glycoprotein molecules found either on the cell surface of B lymphocytes where they act as antigen receptors, or produced and secreted by B lymphocytes that have been stimulated and transformed by an antigen into plasma cells. There are **five** different types, or classes of antibody, each named by the abbreviation for immunoglobulin (Ig) and a letter of the alphabet, i.e., IgM, IgG, IgA, IgD, IgE, IgG (also called GAMMAGLOBULIN) is the most abundant of the five classes of antibody and is the major immunoglobulin in the secondary humoral immune response.

Anti-D gamma-globulin Anti-rhesus antibody which is given to a rhesus negative woman within 72 hours of delivery of her infant or following termination of her pregnancy, miscarriage or invasive investigations such as anmiocentesis, to prevent hemolytic disease of the newborn in the next pregnancy *(See Rhesus factor)*.

Anti-inflammatory A drug that reduces or acts against inflammation. Maybelong to one of several groups.

Anti-rhesus serum A substance containing rhesus agglutinins produced in the blood of those who are rhesus-negative if the rhesus positive antigen obtains access to it. e.g., by blood transfusion. Hemolysis and jaundice are the result *(See Rhesus factor)*.

Anticholinergic A drug that inhibits the action of acetylcholine.

Anticholinesterase An enzyme that inhibits the action of the enzyme acetyl cholinesterase, thereby potentiate the action of acetylcholine at postsynaptic receptors in the parasympathetic nervous system, thus allowing return of normal muscle contraction.

Anticoagulant A substance that prevents blood from clotting, e.g., heparin.

Anticonvulsant A substance that will arrest or prevent convulsions. Anticonvulsant drugs such as phenytoin are used in the treatment of epilepsy and other conditions in which convulsions occur.

Anti-D immunoglobulin Anti-rhesus antibody, which is given by intramuscular injection to a rhesus-negative woman within 72 hours of delivery of her infant or following termination of her pregnancy, miscarriage or invasive investigations such as amniocentesis, to prevent hemolytic disease of the newborn in the next pregnancy. Anti-D is also available to all rhesus-negative women as antenatal prophylaxis. *(See Rhesus Factor)*.

Antidepressant One of a group of drugs which elevate mood, often diminish anxiety and increase coping behavior. Tricyclic antidepressants are most commonly used in treatment of depression. Monoamine oxidase inhibitors (MAOIs) are less commonly used because of the dietary restriction necessary and the toxic side effects.

A

Anti-discriminatory practice The professional policies, practice and provisions that actively seek to reduce institutional discrimination experienced by individuals and groups, particularly on the grounds of age, race, gender disability, social class or sexual orientation. Anti-discriminatory practice can utilize particularly the Equalities Act 2010 to challenge discrimination.

Antidiuretic A substance that reduces the volume of urine excreted.

Antidiuretic hormone Abbreviated ADH. A hormone which is secreted by the posterior pituitary gland. Vasopressin.

Antidote An agent that counteracts the effect of a poison.

Antidromic Nerve impulse traveling in opposite direction than normal.

Antiembolic Against embolism. Antiembolic hose/stockings are worn to prevent the formation/decrease the risk of deep vein thrombosis, especially in patients after surgery or those confined to bed.

Antiemetic A drug that prevents or overcomes nausea and vomiting.

Antiestrogen Substances that block or modify action of estrogen.

Antifungal A preparation effective in treating fungal infections.

Antigen Any substance, bacterial or otherwise, which in suitable conditions can stimulate the production of an immune response.

Antigen-antibody reaction Combination of antigen with specific antibody that may result in agglutination, precipitation, neutralization, complement fixation or increased susceptibility to phagocytosis.

Antihemophilic 1. Effective against the bleeding tendency in hemophilia. 2. An agent that counteracts the bleeding tendency in hemophilia.

Antihemophilic factor Abbreviated AHF. One of clotting factors, deficiency of which causes classic, sex-linked hemophilia; called also factor VIII an antihemophilic globulin (AHG). It is available in a preparation for preventive and therapeutic use.

Antihelix Inner curved ridge of external ear parallel to helix.

Antihistamine A group of drugs which block the tissue receptors for histamine. They are used to treat allergic conditions, e.g., drug rashes, hay fever and serum sickness.

Antihypertensive 1. Effective against hypertension. 2. An agent that reduces high blood pressure.

Antimalarial Against malaria. Drugs that are used both in the treatment of an attack and for prophylaxis. All visitors to malarial countries should take preventative antimalarial drugs. Expert advice should be sought regarding the appropriate drug and dose. *(See Malaria).*

Antimetabolite One of a group of chemical compounds which prevent the effective utilization of the corresponding metabolite, and interfere with normal growth or cell mitosis of the process which requires that metabolite.

Antimycotic A preparation effective in treating fungal infections.

Antineoplastic Effective against the multiplication of malignant cells.

Antinuclear antibody A group of antibodies that react against normal components of cell nucleus. They are present in SLE, PSS, scleroderma, polymyositis, etc.

Antioxidants Agents that prevent or inhibit oxidation.

Antipathy Antagonism, strong aversion.

Antiperistalsis Contrary contractions which propel the contents of the intestines backward and upward.

Antiperspirant A substance applied to the body as a lotion, cream or spray, to reduce sweating. Usage can sometimes result in irritation especially if the skin is broken.

Antiphospholipid syndrome (APS) Also known as Hughes syndrome. An immune disorder causing increased risk of blood clots.

Antiplasmin An inhibitor of fibrinolysis; its deficiency causes bleeding.

Antiplastic Preventing or inhibiting wound healing.

Antiprostaglandins Agents that interfere with prostaglandin activity; used for treatment of arthritis, dysmenorrhea.

Antiprostate Cowper's gland.

Antipruritic External application or drug that relieves itching.

Antipyretic An agent that reduces fever.

Antisepsis The prevention of infection by destroying or arresting the growth of harmful microorganisms.

Antiseptic 1. Preventing sepsis. 2. Any substance that inhibits the growth of bacteria, in contrast to a germicide, which kills bacteria outright.

Antiserum Animal or human blood serum which contains antibodies to infective organisms or to their toxins. The serum donor must have previously been infected with the identified organism.

Antisocial Against society.
Antisocial behavior In psychiatry, the refusal of an individual to accept the normal obligations and restraints imposed by the community upon its members.

Antispasmodic Any measure used to prevent or relieve the occurrence of muscle spasm.

Antisudorific Agent that inhibits perspiration.

Antithrombin III A protein synthesized in liver. Its concentration is lowered in nephritic syndrome leading to renal veins thrombosis.

Antitoxin A substance produced by the body cells as a reaction to invasion by bacteria which neutralizes their toxins *(See Immunity)*.

Antitrypsin A substance that inhibits actions of trypsin.

Antitussive 1. Effective against cough. 2. An agent that suppresses coughing.

Antivenin An antitoxic serum to neutralize the poison injected by the bite of a snake or insect.

Antiviral 1. Acting against viruses. 2. A drug that is effective against viruses causing disease, e.g., acyclovir.

Antrectomy Excision of an antrum.

Antroatticotomy Operation to open the maxillary sinus and the attic of tympanum.

Antrocele Fluid accumulation causing a cystic swelling of antrum.

Antrostomy Surgical opening of an antrum, particularly the maxillary antrum for drainage purposes.

Antrum A cavity or chamber especially in a bone.
Mastoid antrum The tympanic antrum, which is an airconditioning cavity in the mastoid portion of the temporal bone.
Maxillary antrum The air sinus in the upper jawbone.

Annulus A ring shaped structure.

Anuria Cessation of the secretion of urine.

Anus The extremity of the alimentary canal, through which the feces are discharged.
Imperforate anus One where there is no opening because of a congenital defect.

Anxiety A chronic state of tension, which affects both mind and body.

Anxiety neurosis A mental disorder with excessive anxiety not restricted to specific situation or objects and is associated with somatic symptoms like palpitation, tremor, dryness of throat, headache.

A

Anxiolytic A substance, such as diazepam, used for relief of anxiety. Anxiolytics may quickly cause dependence and are not suitable for long-term administration. Also called anti-anxiety agent and minor tranquilizer.

Aorta The large artery rising out of the left ventricle of the heart and supplying blood to all the body parts.

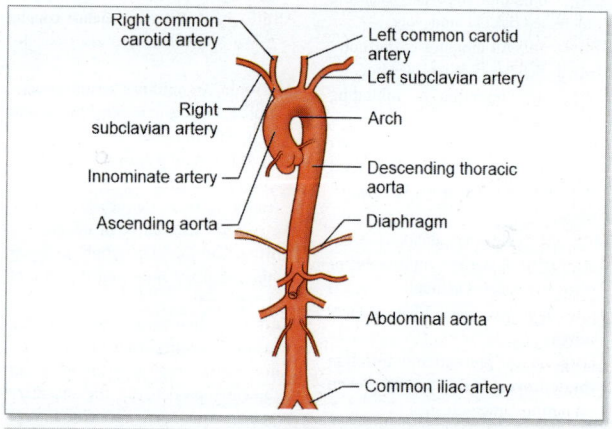

Right common carotid artery
Left common carotid artery
Left subclavian artery
Right subclavian artery
Arch
Innominate artery
Descending thoracic aorta
Ascending aorta
Diaphragm
Abdominal aorta
Common iliac artery

Aorta

Abdominal aorta The part of the artery lying in the abdomen.

Arch of the aorta The curve of the artery over the heart.

Thoracic aorta The part which passes through the chest.

Aortic Pertaining to the aorta.

Aortic bodies Chemoreceptors present in wall of aorta to monitor oxygen saturation.

Aortic incompetence Owing to previous inflammation the aortic valve has become fibrosed and is unable to close completely, thus allowing backward flow of blood into the left ventricle during diastole.

Aortic regurgitation Leakage of blood from aorta into left ventricle during diastole.

Aortic stenosis A narrowing of the aortic valve.

Aortic valve The valve between the left ventricle of the heart and the ascending aorta, which prevents the backward flow of blood through the artery.

Aortitis Inflammation of the aorta, commonly syphilitic or of unknown origin.

Aorto coronary bypass Surgical procedure to direct blood from root of aorta to coronary vessels by putting a sphenous vein graft or internal mammary arteries; a modality of treatment for coronary obstruction.

Aortography Radiographic examination of the aorta. A radiopaque contrast medium is injected into the blood to render visible lesions of the aorta or its main branches.

Aortolith Calcareous deposits in the aortic wall.

APACHE II Acute Physiology and Chronic Health Evaluation II is a severity-of-disease classification, applied within 24 hours of admission of the patients to the ICU.

Apareunia Inability to accomplish sexual intercourse.

Apathy An appearance of indifference, with no response to stimuli or display of emotion.

Apatite The deceptive stone, a mineral containing calcium and phosphorus ions.

APEL 1. To officially recognize someone who is having particular status or being qualified to perform particular activity. 2. An acknowledgement of a person's responsibility or achievement of something 3.The granting of approval to an institution, which meets a satisfactory level of organizational achievement. Accreditation for Prior Experiential Learning (APEL) credit gained for non-academic work (clinical or work experience) can be used to give credit to academic course work and programmes of study in colleges and universities. Accreditation for Prior Learning abbreviated APL or APCL (Accreditation for Prior Certificated Learning) is a system used by academic institutions and other establishments to grant credit for previous academic achievements. It is usually used to gain credit transfer between institutions leading to academic qualifications.

Aperient A drug that produces an action of the bowels. A laxative.

Aperistalsis Lack of peristaltic movement of the intestines.

Aperitive Appetite stimulant.

Apert's syndrome *E Apert, French pediatrician, 1868–1940.* A congenital abnormality in which there is fusion at birth of all the cranial sutures, in addition to syndactyly (webbed fingers).

Aperture An orifice or opening.

Apex The top or pointed end of a cone-shaped structure.

Apex beat The beat of the heart against the chest wall which can be felt during systole.

Apex of the heart The end closing the left ventricle.

Apex of the lung The extreme upper part of the organ.

Apgar score *V Apgar, American anesthetic, 1909–1974.* A system used in the assessment of the newborn: reflex, irritability and color. The Apgar score is assessed 1 min after birth and again at 5 min. Most healthy infants score 9 at birth. A score below 7 would indicate cause for concern.

APH Antepartum hemorrhage.

Aphagia Loss of the power to swallow.

Aphakia Absence of the lens of the eye.

Aphasia A communication disorder due to brain damage; characterized by complete or partial disturbance of language comprehension, formulation or expression. Partial disturbance is called dysphasia.

Amnestic aphasia Loss of memory for words.

Anomic aphasia Forgetful for naming.

Broca's aphasia Disorder in which verbal output is impaired, and in which verbal communication maybe affected as well. Speech is slow and labored and writing is often impaired.

Developmental aphasia A childhood failure to acquire normal language when deafness, learning difficulties, motor disability or severe emotional disturbance are not causes.

Jargon aphasia Use of disconnected words.

Motor aphasia Inability to use muscles controlling speech production.

Semantic aphasia Inability to understand meaning of words.

Syntactic aphasia Lack of proper grammatical composition.

A

Aphephobia Morbid fear of being touched.

Apheresis Technique of separating blood into its components.

Aphonia Inability to produce sound. The cause maybe organic disease of the larynx or maybe purely functional.

Aphrasia Inability to speak or understand phrases.

Aphrodisiac A drug which excites sexual desire.

Aphthae Small ulcers surrounded by erythema on the inside of the mouth (aphthous ulcers).

Apical Pertaining to the apex of a structure.

Apicectomy Excision of the root of a tooth. Root resection.

Apicitis Inflammation of tooth/lung apex.

Aplanatic lens A lens that corrects spherical aberration.

Aplasia Incomplete development of an organ or tissue or absence of growth.

Aplastic Without power of a development.

Aplastic anaemia *(See Anaemia).*

Apnea Temporary cessation of respiration.

Apnea mattress A mattress designed to sound an alarm if the infant lying on it ceases breathing.

Apnea monitors Designed to give an audible signal when a certain period of apnea has occurred.

Apnea of prematurity Apneic periods occurring in the respiration of newborn infants in whom the respiratory center is immature or depressed.

Cardiac apnea The temporary cessation of breathing caused by a reduction of the carbon dioxide tension in the blood, as seen in Cheyne- Stokes respiration.

Sleep apnea Transient attacks of failure of autonomic control of respiration, becoming more pronounced sleep.

Apneumatosis Congenital atelectasis.

Apneusis Abnormal respiration with sustained inspiratory effort; caused by pontine lesion.

Apochromatic lens Lens that corrects both spherical and chromatic aberration.

Apocrine Pertaining to modified sweat glands that develop in hair follicles these are mainly found in the axillary, pubic and perineal areas.

Apoenzyme The protein portion of an enzyme.

Apoferritin The protein that combine with iron to form ferritin.

Apomorphine A derivative of morphine which produces vomiting.

Aponeurosis A sheet of tendon-like tissue which connects some muscles to the parts that they move.

Apophysis A prominence or excrescence, usually of a bone.

Apophysitis Inflammation of apophysis.

Apoplexy A sudden fit of insensibility, usually caused by rupture of a cerebral blood vessel or its occlusion by a blood clot. The symptoms are coma, accompanied by stertorous breathing and a varying degree of paralysis of the opposite side of the body to the lesion.

Apoptosis Disintegration of cells into membrane bound particles, that are then phagocytosed by other cells, an important process for limitation of tumor growth.

Apparatus 1. A mechanical device or appliance used in operations or experiments. 2. A group of structures or organs that work together to perform function, e.g., *an auditory, a biliary, a lacrimal.*

Apparition A hallucinatory vision, usually the phantom appearance of a person. A specter.

Appendectomy Appendicectomy.

Appendicectomy Surgical removal of the vermiform appendix.

Appendicitis Inflammation of the vermiform appendix.

Chronic appendicitis follows acute attack with inflammatory adhesions, and formation of a lump.

Gangrenous appendicitis Acute appendicitis involving blood vessels with their occlusion and development of gangrene and its vulnerability for rupture.

Appendicolysis Operation to free appendix from adhesions.

Appendicostomy Operation in which opening is made in vermiform appendix to irrigate cecum and colon.

Appendix A supplementary or dependent part.

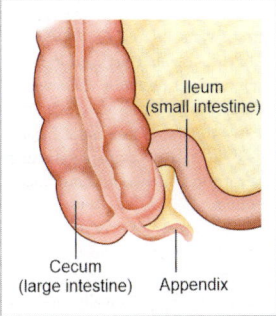

Ileum
(small intestine)

Cecum
(large intestine)   Appendix

Appendix

Appendix atrial Muscular pouch attached to left and right atria; the sites for atrial thrombi.

Appendix epiploicae Small tag-like structure of peritoneum containing fat which are scattered over the surface of the large intestine, especially the transverse colon.

Vermiform appendix A worm-like tube with a blind end, projecting from the cecum in the right iliac region. It maybe from 2.5 to 15 cm long.

Apperception Conscious reception and recognition of a sensory stimulus.

Appestat Area of brain controlling appetite.

Appetite The desire for food. It is stimulated by the sight, smell or thought of food and accompanied by the flow of saliva in the mouth and gastric juice in the stomach. The stomach wall also receives an extra blood supply in preparation for the digestive activity. Appetite is psychologically dependent on memory and associations, as compared with hunger, which is physiologically aroused by the body's need for food, appetite can be discouraged by unattractive food, surroundings or company and by emotional states such as anxiety, irritation, anger and fear *SYN* - pica.

Appetizer Substance that promotes appetite.

Applanation A technique for flattening the cornea to determine the intraocular pressure or detect the presence of glaucoma.

Applanometer Device for measuring intraocular pressure.

Apple picker's disease Respiratory involvement due to fungicides used in apple harvesting.

Appliance A device used for performing a particular function.

Applicator Any device used to apply medication or treatment to a particular part of the body.

Apposition The bringing into contact of two structures, e.g., fragments of bone in setting a fracture.

Appraisal A formal review, usually annually, of a health care professional's performance by a trained appraiser in order to provide feedback on past performance, identification of progress made and setting of future goals and objectives.

Apprehension A feeling of dread or fear.

A

Approach 1. Surgical procedure for exposing any organ or tissue. 2. Draw near.

Approved name The non-proprietary or generic name for a drug. The approved name should always be used in prescribing except where the bioavailability may vary between brands.

Apraxia The inability to perform correct movements because of a brain lesion and not because of sensory impairment or loss of muscle power in the limbs.

Amnestic appraxia Patient cannot understand the action asked to perform even though ability to perform the act is intact.

Constructional appraxia Inability to construct two- or three-dimensional figures due to lack of ability to integrate perception into kinesthetic images.

Motor appraxia Inability to perform an action although the components of it are understood.

Oral appraxia Inability to perform volitional movements of the tongue and lips in the absence of paralysis or paresis. Involuntary movements may, however, be observed, e.g., patients may purse their lips in order to blowout a match.

Aprosody Absence of normal variations in pitch, rhythm and stress in the pitch.

Aptitude The natural ability or capacity to acquire mental and physical skills.

Aptitude test The evaluation of a person's ability for learning certain skills or carrying out specific tasks.

Aptyalism Deficient secretions of saliva.

Apyrexia The absence of fever.

Aqua [L.] Water.

Aqua aerata Carbonated water.

Aqua calcariae Lime water.

Aqua destillata Distilled water.

Aqua fervens Hot water.

Aqua Fontana Spring water.

Aqua fortis Nitric acid.

Aquanaut Persons working under water for carrying out research.

Aquaphobia Morbid fear of water.

Aquapuncture Subcutaneous injection of water to produce counter irritation.

Aqueduct A canal for the passage of fluid.

Aqueduct cochleae Canal connecting subarachnoid space and the cochlear perilymphatic space.

Aqueduct of Sylvius The canal connecting the third and fourth ventricles of the brain.

Aqueduct vestibular Passage from vestibule to petrous part of temporal bone.

Aqueous Watery.

Aqueous humor The fluid filling the anterior and posterior chambers of the eye.

Arachis A genus of leguminous plants used in various preparations such as ear wax softeners and skin medications.

Arachidonic acid An essential fatty acid, precursor for prostaglandins, thromboxane and leukotrienes.

Arachnodactyly Abnormally long and thin fingers and toes. A congenital condition.

Arachnoid 1. Resembling a spider's web. 2. A web-like membrane covering the central nervous system between the dura and pia mater.

Arborization The branching terminations of many nerve fibers and processes.

Arbovirus One of a large group of viruses transmitted by insect vectors (arthropod borne), e.g., mosquitoes, sandflies or ticks. The diseases caused include many types of encephalitis, also yellow, dengue, sandfly and rift valley fevers.

Arc A structure or projected path having a curved or bow-like outline.

Arch Any anatomic structure with a curved or bow-like outline. For example, aortic arch.

Architis Inflammation of the anus.

Arcuate Shaped like an arc.

Arcus [L.] Bow, arch.

Arcus senilis An opaque circle appearing round the edge of the cornea in old age.

Ardor A burning sensation during urination.

ARDS Acute respiratory distress syndrome.

Area Well-defined space with defined boundaries.

Areflexia Absence of reflexes.

Areola 1. A space in connective tissue. 2. A ring of pigmentation, e.g., that surrounding the nipple.

Arena virus A group of viruses that include lymphocytic choriomeningitis viruses and lassa fever viruses; mostly arthropod borne.

Areolar glands (Montegomery's glands) Large modified sweat glands beneath the areola secreting a lipoid material that lubricates the nipple.

Areometer Device for measuring specific gravity of fluids.

Arformeterol Betagonist for inhalation in asthma.

Argentaffinoma An argentaffin tumor secreting serotonin that may arise in intestinal tract, bile ducts, pancreas, bronchus or ovary.

Argentum [L.] Silver.

Arginase An enzyme of the liver that splits arginine into urea and ornithine.

Arginine An essential amino acid produced by the digestion of protein. It forms a link in the excretion of nitrogen, being hydrolysed by the enzyme arginase.

Argon Symbol Ar. An inert gaseous element; less than 0.1% in the atmosphere.

Argyll Robertson pupil D *Argyll Robertson, British ophthalmologist, 1837–1909 (See Pupil).*

Argyria Bluish discoloration of skin and mucus membranes from prolonged administration of silver.

Argyrol Mild silver protein used as an antiseptic for eye, nose, throat and urethral irrigation.

Argyrophil Cells that bind to silver salts producing brown or black stain.

Aristogenics *SYN* - Eugenics. The science dealing with genetic and prenatal influences affecting expression of certain characteristics in offspring.

Arm board Board placed under the arm for stabilization during IV administration.

Armamentarium The total utilities at disposal like drugs, instruments, books, supplies.

Arnold-Chiari deformity *Arnold, German pathologist, 1835–1915; H. Chiari, German pathologist, 1851–1916.* Herniation of the cerebellum and elongation of the medulla oblongata; occurs in hydrocephalus associated with spina bifida.

Arnold-Chiari malformation J. Arnold, German pathologist, 1835-1915; H Chiari, German pathologist, 1851-1916. Herniation of the cerebellum and elongation of the medulla oblongata; occurs in hydrocephalus associated with spina bifida. Also known as Chiari Malformation.

Aroma Pleasant odor.

Aromatherapy The therapeutic use of specially prepared essential or aromatic oils obtained from the different parts of plants, including the flowers, leaves, seeds, wood, roots and bark. The oils maybe diluted for use in massage, baths or infusions.

Aromatic 1. Having a spicy fragrance. 2. A stimulant spicy medicine.

Arousal A state of alertness and increased response to stimuli.

A

Arrector pili A small muscle attached to the hair follicle of the skin. When contracted it causes the hair to become erect, producing the appearance known as gooseflesh.

Arrest A cessation or stopping.

Cardiac arrest Cessation of ventricular contractions.

Developmental arrest Discontinuation of a child's mental or physical development at a certain stage.

Respiratory arrest Cessation of breathing.

Arrhenoblastoma A rare ovarian tumor that causes masculinization in women, with male distribution of hair and coarsening of the skin.

Arrhythmia Variation from the normal rhythm, e.g., in the heart's action.

Sinus arrhythmia an abnormal pulse rhythm due to disturbance of the sinoatrial node, causing quickening of the heart on inspiration and slowing on expiration.

Arsenic Symbol As. a metaliic element, organic preparations of which were used in medicine in the past.

Arterial blood gases (ABGs) Normally present in arterial blood including oxygen, carbon dioxide and nitrogen. Measurements of the partial pressures of oxygen and carbon dioxide together with the pH of the blood provide important information on the oxygen saturation of the hemoglobin and acid-base state of the blood indicating the adequacy of ventilation in critical care situations.

Arterial line A method of hemodynamic monitoring where catheter is put into an artery for recording blood pressure, arterial gas analysis.

Art therapy The use of art as a medium to encourage patients to express their feelings when unable to do so verbally.

Arteriectomy The removal of a portion of artery wall, usually followed by anastomosis or a replacement graft *(See Arterioplasty).*

Arteriogram X-ray of an artery after injection of radiopaque material.

Arteriography Radiography of arteries after the injection of a radiopaque contrast medium.

Arteriole A minute artery that leads into capillary.

Arterioplasty The reconstruction of an artery by means of replacement surgery.

Arteriorrhaphy Ligature of an artery.

Arteriosclerosis A gradual loss of elasticity in the walls of arteries due to thickening and calcification. It is accompanied by high blood pressure, and precedes the degeneration of internal organs associated with old age or chronic disease.

Arteriotomy An incision into an artery.

Arteriovenous Both arterial and venous; pertaining to both artery and vein, e.g., an arteriovenous aneurysm, fistula, or shunt for hemodialysis.

Arteriovenoussis A gradual loss of elasticity in the walls of arteries due to thickening and calcification. It is accompanied by high blood pressure, and precedes the degeneration of internal organs associated with old age or chronic disease.

Arteritis Inflammation of an artery.

Giant cell arteritis A variety of polyarteritis resulting in partial or complete occlusion of a number of arteries. The carotid arteries are often involved.

Temporal arteritis Occlusion of the extracranial arteries, particularly the carotid arteries.

Artery A tube of muscle and elastic fibers, lined with endothelium, which distributes blood from the heart to the capillaries throughout the body.

Artesunate An antimalarial for resistant falciparum malaria.

Arthralgia Neuralgic pains in a joint.

Arthrectomy Excision of a joint.

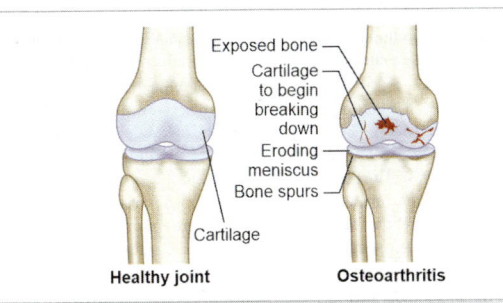

Healthy joint   **Osteoarthritis**

Exposed bone
Cartilage to begin breaking down
Eroding meniscus
Bone spurs
Cartilage

Arthritis

Arthritide A skin eruption caused by arthritis.

Arthritis Inflammation of one or more joints. Movement in the joint is restricted, with pain and swelling.

Acute rheumatic arthritis Rheumatic fever.

Osteoarthritis A degenerative condition attacking the articular cartilage and aggravated by an impaired blood supply, previous injury or over weight, mainly affecting weight-bearing joints and causing pain.

Rheumatoid arthritis A chronic inflammation, usually of unknown origin. The disease is progressive and incapacitating, owing to the resulting ankylosis and deformity of the bones. Usually affects the elderly. A juvenile form is known as Still's disease.

Arthrocentesis Puncture of a joint to drain joint fluid for analysis.

Arthroclasia The breaking down of adhesions in a joint to produce freer movement.

Arthrodesis The surgical immobilization of a joint; artificial ankylosis.

Arthrodynia Painful joints. Arthralgia.

Arthrography The examination of a joint by means of X-rays. An opaque contrast medium maybe used.

Arthrogryposis Fixation of a joint in a flexed or contracted position.

Arthrolysis Restoration of mobility of an ankylosed joint.

Arthropathy Any joint disease.

Arthroplasty Plastic surgery for the reorganization of a joint. *Charnley's arthroplasty (See Mckee Farrar a.).*

Cup arthroplasty Reconstruction of the articular surface, which is then covered by a vitallium cup.

Excision arthroplasty Excision of the joint surfaces affected, so that the gap thus formed then fills with fibrous tissue or muscle.

Girdlestone arthroplasty An excision arthroplasty of the hip.

McKee Farrar arthroplasty Replacement of both the head and the socket of the femur; *Charnley's a.* Is similar.

Replacement arthroplasty Partial removal of the head of the femur and its replacement by a metal prosthesis.

Arthroscope An endoscope for examining the interior of a joint.

Arthroscopy Keyhole surgery used to diagnose and treat joint problems.

Arthrotome Knife for making incision into joint.

Arthrotomy An incision into a joint.

Arthus reaction An immediate hypersensitivity reaction due to preformed antibody to injected antigen.

A

Articular Pertaining to a joint.

Articulation 1. A junction of two or more bones. 2. The enunciation of words.

Artefact Something that is man-made or introduced artificially.

Artificial Not natural.

Artificial feeding 1. The giving of food other than by placing it directly in the mouth. It maybe provided via the mouth, using an esophageal tube; the food maybe introduced into the stomach through a fine tube via the nostril (the nasal route); an opening through the abdominal wall into the stomach (i.e., a gastrostomy) may allow direct introduction; or food maybe injected intravenously *(See Parenteral)*. 2. In reference to the feeding of infants, giving food other than human milk.

Artificial insemination The insertion of sperm into the uterus by means of syringe and cannula instead of coitus. The husband's (AIH) or donor (AID) semen maybe used.

Artificial kidney A dialysis machine to remove unwanted waste materials from the patient with acute or chronic renal failure *(See Hemodialysis)*.

Artificial respiration Means of resuscitation from asphyxia.

Artificial tears Sterile solutions designed to maintain the moisture of the cornea when the latter is abnormally dry due to inadequate tear production. Methylcellulose is a common ingredient.

Artisan's cramps Muscle cramps involving muscles used in prolonged spells of writing, sewing, telegraphing, etc.

Aryepiglottic Pertaining to arytenoids cartilage and epiglottis.

Arytenoid Resembling the mouth of a pitcher.

Arytenoid cartilages Two cartilages of the larynx; their function is to regulate the tension of the vocal cords attached to them.

Asafetida A gum resin with strong odor and garlic taste.

Asbestos A fibrous noncombustible silicate of magnesium and calcium that is a good nonconductor of heat.

Asbestosis A form of pneumoconiosis (chronic lung disease), due to the inhalation of asbestos fibers causing scarring of the lung tissue. It results in breathlessness and may lead to respiratory failure.

Ascariasis The condition in which roundworms are found in the gastrointestinal tract.

Ascaris lumbricoides A genus of round worm. Some types may infest the human intestine, often producing dyspepsia, intestinal obstruction, biliary colic and appendicitis.

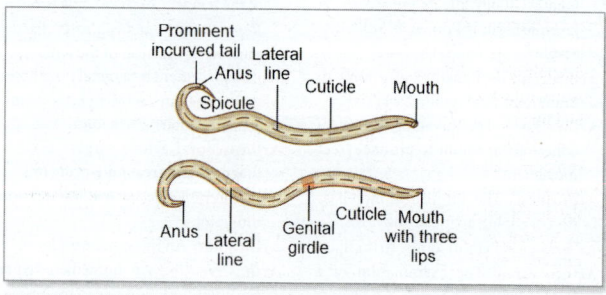

Ascaris lumbricoides

Aschheim-Zondek test A pregnancy test where patients' urine is injected into female mice to induce ovulation.

Aschner's phenomenon Slowing of pulse following carotid sinus massage or pressure on eyeball.

Aschoff's cells Large multinucleated cell with vesicular nucleus and basophilic cytoplasm.

Aschoff's nodules or bodies *KAL Aschoff, German pathologist, 1866–1942.* The nodules present in heart muscle in rheumatic myocarditis.

Ascites Free fluid in the peritoneal cavity. It maybe the result of local inflammation or venous obstruction, or be part of a generalized edema.

Ascorbic acid Vitamin C. This acid is found in many vegetables and fruits and is an essential dietary constituent for humans. Vitamin C is destroyed by heat and deteriorates during storage. It is necessary for connective tissue and collagen fiber synthesis and promotes the healing of wounds. Deficiency causes scurvy.

Asepsis Freedom from pathogenic microorganisms.

Aseptic Free from sepsis.

Aseptic technique A method of carrying out sterile procedures so that there is the minimum risk of introducing infection. Achieved by the sterility of equipment and a non-touch technique.

Asexual Without sex.

Asexual reproduction The production of new individuals without sexual union, e.g., by cell division or budding.

Asilone Trade name for a proprietary compound antacid mixture.

Asparaginase An enzyme that catalyses the deamination of asparagine; used as an antineoplastic agent against cancers, e.g., acute lymphocytic leukemia, in which the malignant cells require exogenous asparagines for protein synthesis.

Aspartame A synthetic compound of two amino acids (L-aspartyl- L-phenylalanine methyl ester) used as a low-calorie sweetener. It is 180 times as sweet as sucrose (table sugar); the amount equal in sweetness to a teaspoon of sugar contains 0.1 calorie (4.21). Aspartame does not promote the formation of dental caries. The amount of phenylalanine in aspartame must be taken into account in the low-phenylalanine diet for patients with phenylketonuria.

Aspartate transaminase (AST) An enzyme released when the liver or muscles are damaged. Levels of AST are measured as markers of liver health.

Aspect Part of a surface facing in a particular direction.

Dorsal aspect That facing and seen from the back.

Ventral aspect That facing and seen from the front.

Aspergillosis A bronchopulmonary disease in which the mucous membrane is attacked by the fungus, *Aspergillus.*

Aspergillus A genus of fungi.

Aspergillus fumigatus A common cause of aspergillosis, found in soil and manure.

Aspermia Absence of sperm.

Aspersion Sprinkling of an affected part with water, a form of hydrotherapy.

Asphyxia A deficiency of oxygen in the blood and an increase in carbon dioxide in the blood and tissues. Symptoms include irregular and disturbed respirations, or a complete absence of breathing, and pallor or cyanosis. Asphyxia may occur whenever there is an interruption in the normal exchange of oxygen and carbon dioxide between the lungs and the outside air. Common causes are drowning, electric shock, lodging of a foreign body in the air passages, inhalation of smoke and poisonous gases and trauma to or disease of the lungs or air passages. Treatment includes immediate remedy of the situation *(See Respiration artificial)* and removal of the underlying cause whenever possible.

Asphyxiant An agent, especially gas producing asphyxia.

Asphyxiate To cause asphyxia.

Aspirate To draw in or out by suction.

Aspiration 1. The act of inhaling. 2. The drawing off fluid from a cavity by means of suction.

Aspirator Any apparatus for withdrawing fluid or gases from a cavity of the body by means of suction.

Aspirin Acetylsalicylic acid. It reduces temperature, relieves pain and is an antiplatelet agent to reduce the tendency of the blood to clot within the circulation.

Soluble aspirin A combination of aspirin with citric acid and calcium carbonate.

Assault Unlawful personal attack or trespass upon another person including threatening words.

Assay A quantitative examination to determine the amount of a particular constituent of a mixture, or of the biological or pharmacological potency of a drug.

Assent Agreement to undergo medical care and treatment that is obtained from an adult or child who is legally incompetent to consent.

Assertiveness A form of behavior characterized by a confident declaration or affirmation of a statement without need of proof. To assert oneself is to compel recognition of one's rights or position without either aggressively transgressing the rights of another and assuming a position of dominance, or submissively permitting another to deny one's rights or rightful position. *Assertiveness training* Instruction and practice in tech-

niques for dealing with interpersonal conflicts and threatening situations is an assertive manner, avoiding the extremes of aggressive and submissive behavior.

Assessment 1. The critical analysis and evaluation or judgment of the status or quality of a particular condition, situation or other subject of appraisal. In the nursing process, assessment involves the gathering of information about the health status of the patient/client, analysis and synthesis of the data, and the making of a clinical nursing judgment *(See Nursing process)*. The outcome of the nursing assessment is the establishment of a nursing diagnosis, the identification of the nursing problems. 2. An examination set by an examining authority to test a candidate's nursing skills and knowledge.

Assimilation The process of transforming food so that it can be absorbed and utilized as nourishment by the tissues of the body.

Associate nurse A nurse who, as a member of the primary nursing team, is responsible for effecting a patient's care plans on behalf of the primary nurse *(See Primary nursing)*.

Association Coordination of function of similar parts.

Association fibers Nerve fibers linking different areas of the brain.

Association of ideas A mental impression which a thought or any sensor impulse will call to mind another object or idea connected in some way with the former.

Free association Method employed in psychoanalysis in which the patient is encouraged to express freely whatever comes to mind. By this method material that is in the unconscious can be recalled.

Associative play Form of play in which a group of children participate in similar activities without formal organization direction.

Astasia Inability to stand or sit erect due to motor incoordination.

Astasia abasia A form of hysterical ataxia with inability to stand or walk although all leg movements can be performed while sitting or lying down.

Astereognosis Inability to recognize objects or forms by touch.

Asterion The junction of lamboid, occipitomastoid and parietomastoid sutures.

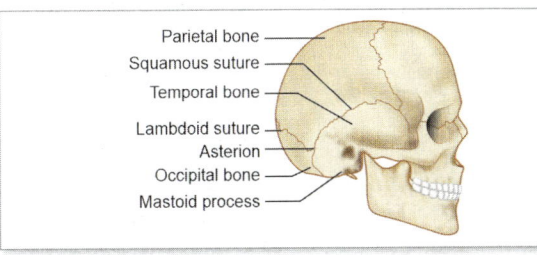

Parietal bone —
Squamous suture —
Temporal bone —
Lambdoid suture —
Asterion —
Occipital bone —
Mastoid process —

Asterion

Asterixis Transient lapses of muscle tone with involuntary jerky movements especially of hands as in hepatic failure.

Asthenia Want of strength. Debility. Loss of tone.

Asthenia neurocirculatory A psychosomatic disorder characterized by mental and physical fatigue, dyspnea, giddiness, etc.

Asthemic Description of a type of body build; a pale, lean, narrowly built person with poor muscle development.

Asthenopia Eye strain giving rise to an aching, burning sensation and headache. Likely to arise in longsighted people when continual effort of accommodation is required for close work.

Asthma Paroxysmal dyspnea characterized by wheezing and difficulty in expiration.

Bronchial asthma Attacks of dyspnea in which there is wheezing and difficulty in expiration due to muscular spasm of the bronchi. The attack maybe precipitated by hypersensitivity to foreign substances, air pollution, exertion or infection, or associated with emotional upsets. There is often a family history of asthma or other allergic condition. Treatment is with bronchodilators with or without corticosteroids, usually via an aerosol or a powder inhaler.

Cardiac asthma Attacks of dyspnea and palpitation, arising most often at night, associated with left-sided heart failure and pulmonary congestion.

Extrinsic asthma Asthma due to environmental allergens.

Intrinsic asthma Asthma where no external cause is identified.

Renal asthma Dyspnea occurring in kidney disease, which maybe a sign of developing uremia. It is unrelated to true asthma.

Astigmatism Inequality of the refractive power of an eye, due to curvature of its corneal meridians. The curve across the front of the eye from side to side is not quite the same as the curve from above downward. The focus on the retina is then not a point but a diffuse and indistinct area.

Maybe congenital or acquired.

Astraphobia Fear of thunder and lightening.

Astringent An agent causing contraction of organic tissues, thereby checking secretions and hemorrhage, e.g., silver nitrate, tannic acid.

Astrocyte Star shaped neuroglial cell with many branching processes.

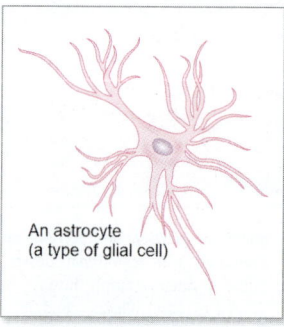

An astrocyte
(a type of glial cell)

Astrocyte

Astrocytoma A malignant tumor of the brain or spinal cord. It is slow growing.

Astrophobia Morbid fear of stars and celestial bodies.

Astrup machine An apparatus for ascertaining the pH value of arterial blood.

Asymmetry Inequality in size or shape of two normally similar structures or of two halves of a structure normally the same.

Asymptomatic Without symptoms.

Asynclitism An oblique presentation of fetal head during labor.

Asynergy Lack of coordination of structures which normally act in harmony.

Asystole Absence of heartbeat. Cardiac arrest.

At risk Whereby an individual or population maybe vulnerable to a particular disease, hazard or injury. At risk situations are those involving possible problems that maybe preventable with appropriate intervention, or, if they should occur, treatment.

Ataractic 1. Pertaining to or characterized by ataraxia. 2. An agent that induces ataraxia. A tranquillizer.

Ataraxia A state of detached serenity with depression of mental faculties or impairment of consciousness.

Ataxia, ataxy Failure of muscle coordination resulting in irregular jerky movements, and unsteadiness in standing and walking from a disorder of the controlling mechanisms in the brain, or from inadequate input to the brain from joints and muscles.

Alcoholic ataxia Ataxia sue to loss of proprioception in chronic alchoholism.

Brun's ataxia Ataxia of bilateral frontal lobe lesions with a tendency to stagger and fall backward.

Cerebellar ataxia Motor ataxia of cerebellar disease, often with a nystagmus, tremor, scanning speech and dysmetria.

Hereditary ataxia (Friedreich's ataxia). An inherited disease manifesting in childhood or adolescence. There is degeneration of lateral and dorsal columns of spinal cord. Peripheral neuropathy, high arch palate, kyphoscoliosis are often associated.

Ataxia sensory Ataxia due to loss of proprioceptive impulses.

Ataxia telangiectasia IgA deficiency state of congenital origin manifesting with cerebellar ataxia, telangiectasia and recurrent sinopulmonary infections.

Atelectasis A collapsed or airless state of the lung, which maybe acute or chronic and may involve all or part of the lung: (a) from imperfect expansion of pulmonary alveoli at birth *(congenital atelectasis)*, (b) as the result of disease or injury.

A

Atherogenesis Formation of atheromata in the wall of arteries.

Atheroma An abnormal mass of fatty or lipid material with a fibrous covering, existing as a discrete, raised plaque within the intima of an artery.

Atherosclerosis A condition in which the fatty degenerative plaques of atheroma are accompanied by arteriosclerosis, a narrowing and hardening of the vessels.

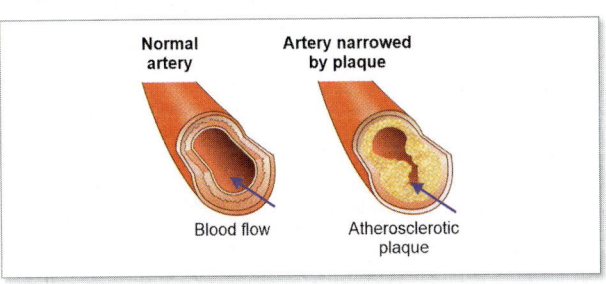

Normal artery — Blood flow

Artery narrowed by plaque — Atherosclerotic plaque

Atherosclerosis

Athetosis A recurring series of slow, writhing movements of the hands, usually due to a cerebral lesion.

Athlete's foot A fungal infection between the toes, easily transmitted to other people. Tinea pedis.

Atlantoaxial Pertaining to first and second cervical vertebrae.

Atlas The first cervical vertebra, articulating with the occipital bone of the skull.

Atmosphere 1. The gases that surround the earth, extending to an altitude of 16 km. 2. The air or climate of a particular place, e.g., a smoking atmosphere. 3. Mental or moral environment, tone or mood.

Atmospheric pressure Pressure exerted by the air in all directions. At sea level it is about 100 kPa.

Atom The smallest particle of an element that retains all the properties of that element. It is made up of a central positively charged nucleus and, moving around it in orbit, negatively charged electrons.

Atomizer An instrument by which a liquid is divided to form a fine spray or vapor (nebulizer).

Atony Lack of tone, e.g., in a muscle.

Atopy A state of hypersensitivity to certain antigens. There is an inherited tendency that includes asthma, eczema and hay fever.

Atorvastatin Lipid lowering agent.

ATP Adenosine triphosphate.

Atracurium A muscle relaxant with a relatively short duration of action used in anesthesia.

Atresia Absence of a natural opening or tubular structure, e.g., of the anus or vagina; usually a congenital malformation.

Atrial Relating to the atrium.

Atrial fibrillation Over stimulation of the atrial walls so that many areas of excitation arise and the atrioventricular node is bombarded with impulses, many of which it cannot transmit, resulting in a highly irregular pulse.

Atrial flutter Rapid regular action of the atria. The atrioventricular node transmits alternative impulses of one in three or four. The atrial rate is usually about 300 beats per minute.

A

Atrial septal defect The nonclosure of the foramen ovale at the time of birth, giving rise to a congenital heart defect.

Atrichosis Congenital absence of hair.

Atrioventricular Pertaining to the atrium and ventricle.

Atrioventricular bundle (See *Bundle of His*).

Atrioventricular node A node of neurogenic tissue situated between the atrium and ventricle and transmitter impulses.

Atrioventricular valves The bicuspid and tricuspid valve on the left and right sides of the heart respectively.

Atrium Pl. atria 1. A cavity, entrance or passage. 2. One of the two upper chambers of the heart. Formerly called auricle.

Atrophy Wasting of any part of the body, due to degeneration of the cells, from disuse, or lack of nourishment or nerve supply.

Acute yellow atrophy Massive necrosis of liver cells. A rare condition that may follow acute hepatitis or eclampsia or be precipitated by certain drugs.

Disuse atrophy Atrophy resulting from lack of use of muscles.

Optic atrophy Degeneration of optic nerve head, primary or secondary.

Progressive muscular atrophy Motor neurons disease, degeneration of the motor neurons with wasting of muscle tissue.

Sudeck's atrophy Acute atrophy of bone at the site of injury, possibly due to local vasospasm.

Atropine The active principle of belladonna. An alkaloid which inhibits respirator and gastric secretions, relaxes muscle spasm and dilates the pupil.

Atropinization Administration of atropine till desired effect is obtained.

Attack An episode or onset illness.

Attack rate Number of cases of a disease in a particular group, e.g., a school, over a given period related to the population of that group.

Transient ischemic attack Brief attack (a few hours or less) of cerebral dysfunction of vascular origin, without lasting neurological deficit.

Attention deficit syndrome A disorder of childhood characterized by marked failure of attention, impulsiveness and increased motor activity. Affects more boys than girls. Treatment involves medication usually with methyl phenidate, behavior therapy and social support.

Attenuation A bacteriological process by which organisms are rendered less virulent by culture in artificial media through many generations, exposure to light, air, etc.; it is used for vaccine preparations.

Attic The middle ear cavity above the tympanic membrane.

Attitude 1. A posture or position of the body; in obstetrics, the relation of the various parts of the fetal body to one another. 2. A pattern of mental views established by cumulative prior experience.

Atypical Irregular; not conforming to type.

Audible sound Sound with frequency of 15–15,000 Hz.

Audiogram A graph produced by an audiometer.

Audiologist An allied health professional specializing in audiology, who provides services that include: (a) Evaluation of hearing function to detect hearing impairment and, if there is a hearing disorder, to determine the anatomical site involved and the cause of the disorder; (b) Selection of appropriate hearing aids; and (c) Training in lip reading, hearing aid use and maintenance of normal speech.

Audiology The science concerned with the sense of hearing, especially the evaluation and measurement of impaired hearing and the rehabilitation of those with impaired hearing.

Audiometer An instrument for testing hearing, whereby the threshold of the patient's hearing can be measured.

Audit Systematic review and evaluation of records and other data to determine the quality of the services or products provided in a given situation. It is also now a government requirement for the financial review. *Audit monitor* An adaptation for system of assessing quality of care. It consists of "checklists" for quality, leading to a scoring system. *Medical audit* The systematic critical analysis of the quality of medical treatment and nursing care, including the procedures for diagnosis and treatment, the use of resources, outcomes and the resultant quality of life for the patient. *Nursing audit* An evaluation of structure, process and outcome as a measurement of the quality of nursing care. Concurrent audits are conducted at the time the care is being provided to clients/patients. They maybe conducted by means of observation and interview of clients/patients, review of open charts, or conferences with groups of consumers and providers of nursing care. Retrospective audits are conducted after the patient's discharge. Methods include the study of closed patient's charts and nursing care plans, questionnaires, interviews, and surveys of patients and families.

Audito-oculogyric reflex Sudden turning of eyes and head toward direction of loud sound.

Auditory Relating to the ear or to the sense of hearing.

Auditory bulb The membranous labyrinth and cochlea.

Auditory evoked response An objective method of assessing hearing where the hearing stimulus as traverses along its path to auditory cortex produces characteristic electric potentials recorded across the cortex.

Auditory reflex Any reflex produced by stimulation of auditory nerve like blinking of eyes in response to sudden sound.

Auer bodies Rod shaped intracytoplasmic structure present in myeloblasts in acute myeloblastic leukemia.

Auerbach's plexus A plexus formed by sympathetic nerve fibers in muscular coats of GI tract.

Augmentin Amoxycillin-clavulanic acid.

Aura The premonition, peculiar to an individual, which often precedes an epileptic fit.

Aural Referring to the ear.

Auricle 1. The external portion of the ear. 2. Obsolete term for the atrium.

Auriculopapebral reflex Closure of eye resulting from tactile or thermal stimulation of external auditory meatus. *SYN* Kisch's reflex.

Auriscope An instrument for examining the drum of the ear. An otoscope.

Aurum [L.] Gold.

Aurotherapy Treatment with gold salts, e.g., rheumatoid arthritis.

Auscultation Examining the internal organs by listening to the sounds that they give out. In direct or immediate auscultation the ear is placed directly against the body. In mediate auscultation a stethoscope is used.

Austin flint murmur Diastolic mitral regurgitation in a aortic insufficiency mimicking mitral stenosis but without the opening snap or presystolic accentuation.

62

A

Australia antigen Hepatitis B surface antigen found in the blood of a patient with serum hepatitis or who is a carrier of the virus. Dilute concentrations of the antigen can cause the disease and health care personnel must take adequate precautions to avoid inoculation accidents. Blood banks routinely screen for the antigen to exclude infected blood donations.

Autism Self-absorption. Abnormal dislike of the society and others.

Infantile autism Failure of a child to relate to people and situations, leading to complete withdrawal into a world of private fantasies.

Autistic Pertaining to autism.

Autistic spectrum disorder Also known as autism spectrum disorder. It is a range of conditions, which encompass the previous diagnosis of autism, Asperger's syndrome, pervasive developmental disorder and childhood disintegrative disorder.

Auto-agglutination 1. Clumping or agglutination of cells by an individual's own serum, as in auto- hemagglutination. Auto-agglutination occurring at low temperature is called cold agglutination. 2. Agglutination of particulate antigens, e.g., bacteria, in the absence of specific antigens.

Autoanalyzer Device that analyzes multiple samples automatically.

Autoantibody An antibody formed in response to, and reacting against, an antigenic constituent of the individual's own tissues.

Autoantigen A tissue constituent that stimulates production of autoantibodies in the organism in which it occurs.

Autoclave A steam-heated sterilizing apparatus in which the temperature is raised by reducing the air pressure inside; steam is injected under pressure, bringing about efficient sterilization of instruments and dishes treated in this way.

Autodigestion Dissolution of tissue by its own secretions.

Autoeroticism Sexual pleasure derived from self-stimulation of erogenous zones (the mouth, the anus, the genitals and the skin).

Autogenic therapy A complementary therapy combining self-hypnosis and relaxation.

Autogenous Generated within the body and not acquired from external sources.

Autograft The transfer of skin or other tissue from one part of the body to another to repair some deficiency.

Autohemolysis Hemolysis of one's blood by persons own serum.

Autohemotherapy Injection of patients' own blood.

Autoimmunity Condition in which antibodies are produced against body's own tissues.

Autoimmune disease Condition in which the body develops antibodies to its own tissues, e.g., in autoimmune thyroiditis (Hashimoto's disease).

Autoimmunization The formation of antibodies against the individual's own tissue.

Autoinfection Self-infection, transferred from one part of the body to another by fingers, towels, etc.

Autoinfusion Forcing blood from extremities to body core by applying tight bandages.

Autoinoculation Inoculation with a microorganism from the body itself.

Autointoxication Poisoning by toxins generated within the body itself.

Autologous Related to self; belonging to the same organism.

Autologous blood transfusion Abbreviated ABT. The patient donates blood before elective surgery for transfusion postoperatively. ABT may also be obtained as a blood salvage procedure during operation or postoperatively. Avoids cross-matching, compatibility and transfusion infection problems.

Autolysis A breaking up of living tissues, e.g., as may occur if pancreatic ferments escape into surrounding tissues. It also occurs after death.

Automated auditory brainstem response (AABR) One of two hearing tests in the Newborn Hearing Screening Programme that records brain activity in response to clicking sounds via sensors placed on the infant's head. Those infants who fail to respond to this test are referred for a full auditory diagnostic assessment.

Automatic Performed without the influence of the will.

Automatism Performance of non-reflex acts without apparent volition, and of which the patient may have no memory afterwards, as in somnambulism.

Postepileptic automatism Automatic acts following an epileptic fit.

Autonomic Self governing.

Autonomic nervous system The sympathetic and parasympathetic nerves that control involuntary muscles and glandular secretion, over which there is no conscious control.

Autonomy The right of personal freedom of action, which is regarded as one of the hallmarks of a profession.

Autoplasty 1. Replacement of missing tissue by grafting a healthy section from another part of the body. 2. In psychoanalysis, instinctive modification within the psychic systems in adaptation to reality.

Autoregulation A phenomena where the involved tissue regulates events like blood flow into/through it according to its requirement. e.g., as in brain.

Autopsy Postmortem examination of a body to determine the cause of death.

Autosome Any chromosome other than the sex chromosomes. In humans there are 22 pairs of autosomes and 1 pair of sex chromosomes.

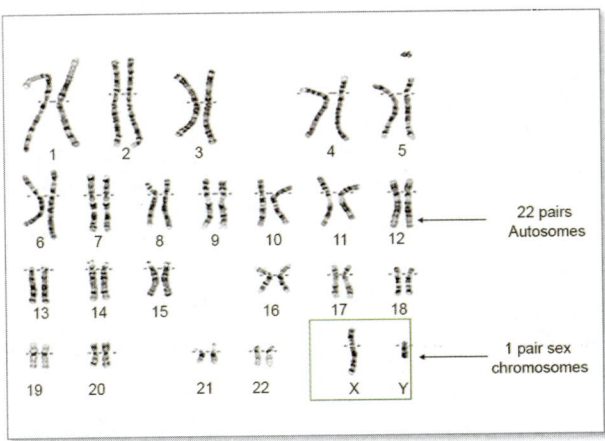

1 2 3 4 5
6 7 8 9 10 11 12
13 14 15 16 17 18
19 20 21 22 X Y

22 pairs Autosomes

1 pair sex chromosomes

Autosome

Autosplenectomy Multiple infarcts of spleen that cause it to shrink as in sickle cell anaemia.

Autotrophic Self nourishing.

Autosuggestion Suggestion arising in one's self. Uncritical acceptance of an idea arising in the individual's own mind.

Autotransfusion Reinfusion of a patient's own blood.

Autotransplantation Transfer of tissue from one part of the body to another part.

A-V block A block in atrioventricular node whereby impulses arising from atria cannot reach ventricles or are delayed; divided into first degree, second degree and third degree (A-V block).

Avascular Not vascular. Bloodless.

Avascular necrosis Death of bone owing to deficient blood supply, usually following an injury.

Average 1. The value or score that is typical of a group. The result is obtained by adding several amounts together and then dividing the total by the number of amounts. Sometimes also referred to as the mean. 2. A colloquial term used to mean 'usual' or 'ordinary'

Aversion Intense dislike.

Aversion therapy A method of treating addictions by associating the craving for what is addictive with painful or unpleasant stimuli. It is rarely used.

Avian influenza Commonly known as bird flu, a disease of poultry and other birds caused by strains of the influenza virus that can occasionally infect people who are in close contact with infected birds. The severity of the disease depends upon the strain of the virus involved; the strain caused by the H5N1 virus is particularly virulent. Presently, normal influenza vaccines do not protect against the H5N1 virus. *(See Orthomyxovirus and swine influenza).*

Aviation medicine A statement or proposition that can be accepted without evidence as it is obviously true.

Avidin A protein of egg white inhibiting biotin.

Avitaminosis A condition resulting from an insufficiency of vitamins in the diet. A deficiency disease.

Avoidance A conscious or unconscious defence mechanism whereby an individual seeks to escape or avoid certain situations, feelings or conflicts.

Avulsion The tearing away of one part from another.

Phrenic avulsion A tearing away of the phrenic nerve. It paralyses the diaphragm on the affected side.

Axanthopsia Yellow blindness.

Axial line A line running in the main axis of the body. The axial line of hand runs through second digit.

Axilla An armpit.

Axiom A statement or proposition that can be accepted without evidence as it is obviously true.

Axis 1. A line through the center of a structure. 2. The second cervical vertebra.

Axis traction Traction made on the fetus in the direction of long axis of birth canal.

Axon The process of a nerve cell along which electrical impulses travel. The nerve fiber.

Axoneme Axial thread of a chromosome.

Axonometer Device for determining axis of astigmatism.

Axonotmesis Nerve injury characterized by disruption of the axon and myelin sheath but with preservation of the connective tissue fragments, resulting in degeneration of the axon distal to the injury site; regeneration of the axon is spontaneous.

A

Azathioprine An immunosuppressive drug widely used for transplant recipients and also as treatment for autoimmune conditions.

Azoospermia Absence of spermatozoa in the semen.

Azotemia Increased blood urea.

Azotobacter Gram-negative rod-shaped, non-pathogenic bacteria that fix atmospheric nitrogen.

AZT Azidothymidine; *(See Zidovudine)*.

Azygos Something that is unpaired.

Azygos vein An unpaired vein that ascends the posterior mediastinum and enters the superior vena cava.

⊙ ⊙ ⊙

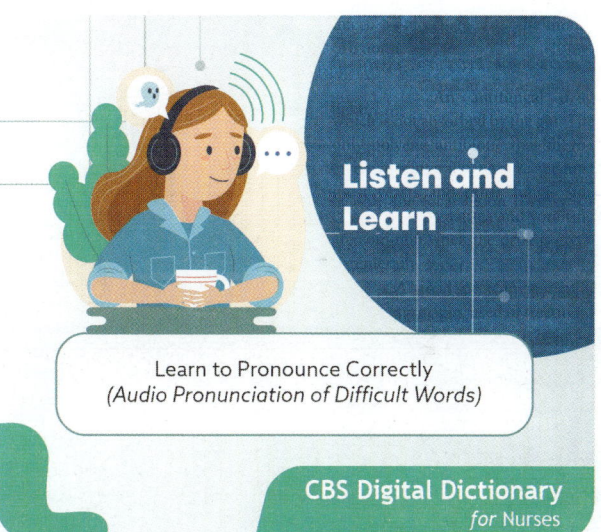
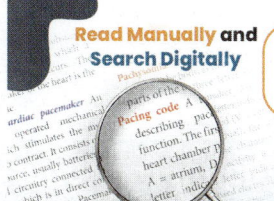

Dil Mange More Content

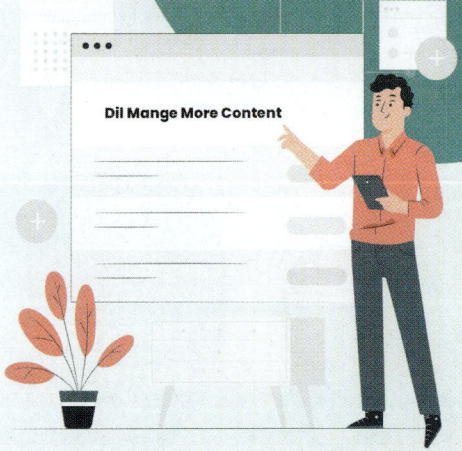

Dil Mange More Content

- Get additional explanations of Important Terminologies
- Word Quiz on Day-To-Day Basis on Scientific and General Terminology (One New Word Every Day with example)
- **50+** Animated & Interactive Videos on various important Topics and Concepts on nursing students' day-to-day interactions/daily needs.
- 4 Hybrid Updates (Every Quarter) covering New Words, Recent Topics & Interactive Videos

CBS Digital Dictionary
for Nurses

Ba Symbol for barium.

Babcock sentence for test This is a test for dementia. This test aims at testing the patient's memory by asking him to repeat a complicated sentence.

Babesia A genus of the order Haemosporidia found in the cattle, sheep, horse, dogs and other vertebrate animals transmitted by tick.

Babesia microti Principally manifesting with fever, chills and hemoglobinuria.

Babesiosis A disease caused by intraerythrocytic protozoan parasite.

Babinski reflex or sign *J.F.F Babinski, French neurologist, 1857–1932*. On stroking the sole of the foot, the great toe bends upwards instead of downwards (dorsal instead of plantar flexion). Presenting disease or injury to the upper motor neuron. Babies who have not walked react in the same way, but normal flexion develops later.

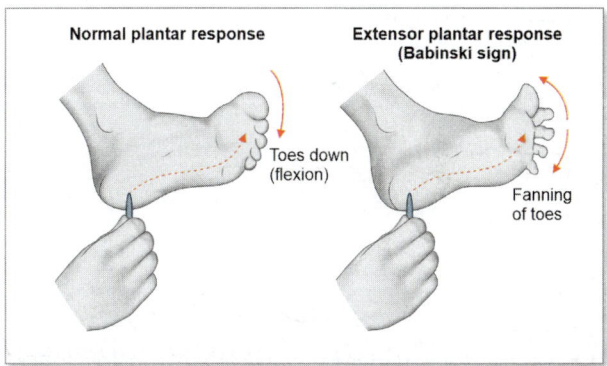

Babinski sign

Baby An infant or young child who is not walking.

Battered baby One suffering from the result continued violence; extensive bruising, fractures of limbs, rib and skull, or an internal trauma may found.

Blue baby One suffering from cyanosis at birth as a result of atelectasis or congenital heart malformation.

Baby blues The transient feelings of unhappiness and tearfulness that affect many women after the birth of their baby.

Baby friendly' initiative Abbreviated BFI of global campaign by the World Health Organization and the United Fund to ensure that all mothers are facilitated in breast-feeding to enable babies to benefit from the health and social advantages.

Bach flower remedies A system of complementary medicine, devised by Dr Edward Bach and based on homeopathic principles. Flower remedies can be used to treat emotional and psychological disorders. There are 38 flower remedies *(See also Homeopathy)*.

Bacampicillin A long acting ampicillin.

Bacillemia The presence of bacilli in the blood.

Bacilluria Presence of bacilli in the urine.

Bacillus A genus of aerobic, spore-bearing gram-positive bacteria. Any rod-shaped microorganism, e.g., *Escherichia coli*, the colon bacillus.

Bacillus Calmette-Guerin A strain of *Mycobacterium bovis* made a virulant by serial cultivation on bile glycerol potato medium, used in BCG vaccine for prevention of tuberculosis.

Back Dorsum. Posterior trunk from neck pelvis.
Back bone The vertebral column.
Back slab Plaster or plastic splint in which a limb is supported.
Hunch back Kyphosis.

Backache Any pain in the back, usually the lower part. The pain is often dull and continuous, but sometimes sharp and throbbing. Backache is one of the most common ailments and can be caused by a variety of disorders. Nurses are at particular risk and one in six is thought to experience back pain.

Baclofen GABA inhibitor used to reduce muscle spasticity.

Bacteria Any microorganism of the class Schizomycetes; can be spherical or ovoid (cocci); rod shaped (bacilli) or spiral.

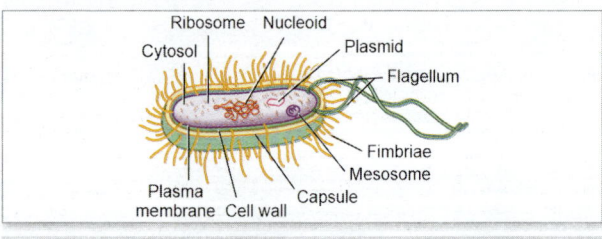

Structure of Bacteria

Bacteremia The presence of bacteria in the bloodstream.

Bacterial Pertaining to bacteria.

Bactericidal Capable of killing bacteria, e.g., disinfectants, great heat, intense cold or sunlight.

Bactericide An agent that kills bacteria.

Bacteriocin Protein produced by certain bacteria which is lethal to other bacteria.

Bacteriocinogen A plasmid that produces bacteriocin.

Bacteriologist One who is qualified in the science of bacteriology.

Bacteriology The scientific study of bacteria.

Bacteriolysin An antibody in blood to assist in the destruction of bacteria. The action is specific.

Bacteriolysis The dissolution of bacteria by a bacteriolytic agent.

Bacteriolytic Capable of destroying or dissolving bacteria.

Bacteriophage A virus that only infects bacteria. Many strains exist, some which are used for identifying types of staphylococci and salmonellae.

Bacteriostat An agent that inhibits the growth of bacteria.

Bacteriostatic Inhibiting the growth of bacteria.

Bacterium A general name given to a minute vegetable organism which may live on organic matter. There are many varieties, only some of which are pathogenic to man, animals and plants. Each bacterium consists of a single cell and, given favourable conditions, multiplies by subdivision. Bacteria are classified according to their shape: (a) bacilli, rod-shaped; (b) cocci, spherical, subdivided into (i) streptococci, in chains; (ii) staphylococci, in groups; (iii) diplococci, in pairs; (c) spirilla, spirochaetes, spiral.

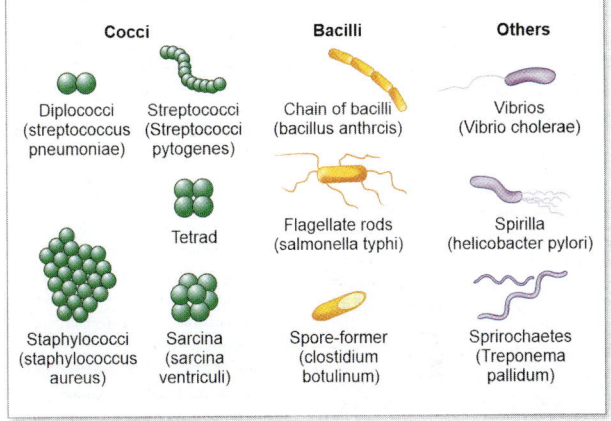

Cocci		Bacilli	Others
Diplococci (streptococcus pneumoniae)	Streptococci (Streptococci pytogenes)	Chain of bacilli (bacillus anthrcis)	Vibrios (Vibrio cholerae)
	Tetrad	Flagellate rods (salmonella typhi)	Spirilla (helicobacter pylori)
Staphylococci (staphylococcus aureus)	Sarcina (sarcina ventriculi)	Spore-former (clostidium botulinum)	Sprirochaetes (Treponema pallidum)

Shapes of Bacteria

Pathogenic bacterium One whose growth in the body gives rise to disease, either by destruction of tissue or by formation of toxins, which circulate in the blood. Pathogenic bacteria thrive on organic matter in the presence of warmth and moisture.

Bacteriuria The presence of bacteria in the urine.

Bag A sac or pouch.

Bag of waters The membranes enclosing the amniotic fluid and the developing fetus in utero.

Colostomy bag A receptacle worn over the stoma by the patient, to receive the fecal discharge.

Douglas bag A receptacle for the collection of expired air, permitting measurement of respiratory gases.

Ice bag A rubber or plastic bag half filled with pieces of ice and applied near or to a part of the body.

Ileostomy bag Any of various plastic or latex pouches attached to the stoma for the collection of fecal material after ileostomy.

Politizer bag A soft bag of rubber for inflating the pharyngotympanic tube.

Urine bag A receptable used for urine by ambulatory patients with urinary incontinence.

B

Bacteroides A genus of non-spore forming, gram negative, anaerobic bacteria frequently found in necrotic tissue.

Begasosis Hypersensitive pneu-monitis due to inhalation of bagasse dust, the moldy fibrous waste of sugar-cane.

Brainbridgereflex An increase in the heart rate caused by an increase in right atrial pressure.

Baker's cyst Synovial cyst in popliteal fossa.

Balance The ability to remain upright and to move without falling over. In physiological terms, the harmonious relationship between parts and organs of the body and their functions or between substances in the body. *(See Acid-base Balance).*
B. of probabilities Is the standard of proof required in civil proceedings.

Balanced diet A varied diet that contains all the nutritional elements in the correct quantities required for growth and repair of body tissues.

Balanced salt solution (BSS) A solution that is made to a physiological pH with appropriate concentrations of salts and electrolytes. Used during intraocular surgery to replace intraocular fluids.

Balanitis Inflammation of the glans penis and of the prepuce, usually associated with phimosis. Balanoposthitis.

Balantidiasis A rare form of colitis or dysentery caused by intestinal infestation by *Balantidium coli*, a protozoon.

Baldness Absence of hair, especially from the scalp. Alopecia.

Balanoplasty Plastic surgery repair of glans penis.

Balanoposthitis Inflammation of glans and prepuce.

Balanus This is the glans of the penis or clitoris.

Ballance's sign This is a sign indicative of ruptured spleen. In this sign there is presence of a dull percussion note in both the flanks. The dullness on the left side is due to the presence of coagulated blood, whereas that on the right side is due to the fluid blood. Dullness on the left flank remains constant. However, with the change of position to the right side, the hemorrhagic fluid moves to the right flank resulting in dullness.

Ballottement [Fr.] A method of testing for a floating object, e.g., abdominal palpation of the uterus when testing for pregnancy. The uterus is pushed upward by a finger in the vagina, and if a fetus is present it will fall back again like a heavy body in water.

Balneology Science of baths and bathing.

Balsam An aromatic vegetable juice.
Friar's balsam a compound containing tincture of benzoin, used for steam inhalations.
Peru balsam Used externally as an antiseptic ointment.
Tolubalsam Used as an expectorant. A constituent of friar's balsam.

Balser's fatty necrosis Gangrenous pancreatitis with fatty necrosis of pancreas and often of bone marrow.

Bamboo spine Spinal column in radiograph resembling bamboo stalk as in ankylosing spondylitis.

Banding Placing a band round a vessel to restrict the flow from it.
Pulmonary arterial banding A palliative operation used in treating infants ventricular septal defects.

Bank An institution offering services, or a store of donated human tissues for use in the future by other individuals, e.g., blood bank, human milk bank, sperm bank.
Nurse bank A group of nurses who are known to the employing authority available for employment on an on-call basis.

B

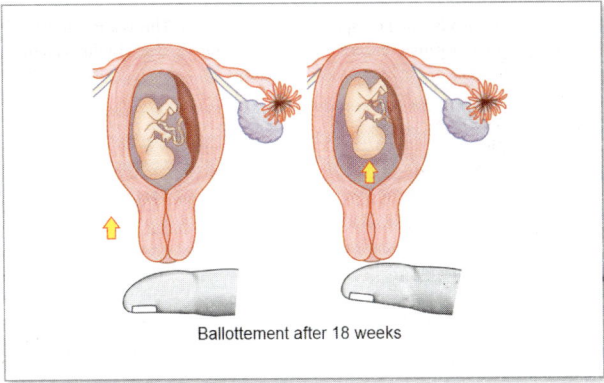

Ballottement after 18 weeks

Ballottement

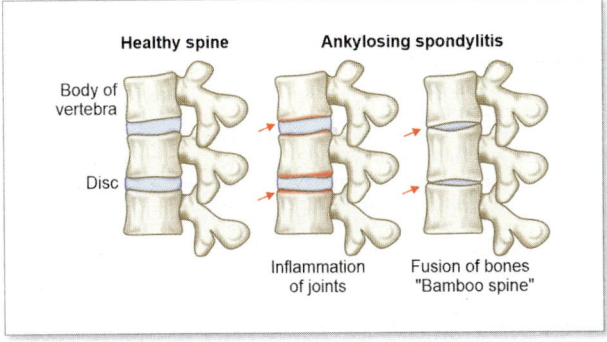

Healthy spine **Ankylosing spondylitis**

Body of vertebra

Disc

Inflammation of joints

Fusion of bones "Bamboo spine"

Bamboo Spine

Bandl's ring Ring like thickening at the junction of upper and lower uterine segments.

Bankart's operation *A. S. B. Bankhart, British orthopedic surgeon, 1879–1951.* An operation to repair a defect in the glenoid cavity that causes repeated dislocation of the shoulder joint.

Bandage 1. A strip or roll of gauze or other material for wrapping or binding any part of the body. 2. To cover by wrapping with such material.

Bandages maybe used to stop the flow of blood, to provide a safeguard against contamination, or to hold a dressing in place. They may also be used to hold a splint in position or otherwise immobilize an injured part of the body to prevent further injury and to facilitate healing.

Banti's disease *G. Banti, Italian pathologist, 1852–1925.* A clinical syndrome characterized by splenomegaly, cirrhosis of the liver, anemia, leukopenia and gastrointestinal bleeding.

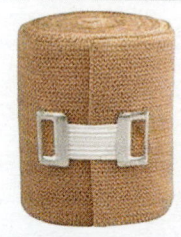 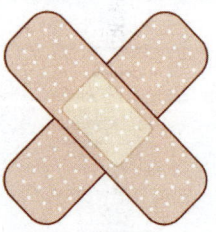

Bandage

Barber's itch Folliculitis of face mostly by *Staphylococcus aureus*.

Barbiturates A large group of sedative and hypnotic drugs derived from barbituric acid, e.g., phenobarbitone, amylobarbitone. Prolonged use may lead to addiction.

Barbotage [Fr.] A method of spinal anesthesia by which some of the anesthetic is injected, followed by partial withdrawal and then re-injection with more of the drug. This process is repeated until the full amount has been given, allowing dilution and mixing with the cerebrospinal fluid.

Baresthesia Pressure sense.

Bariatrics A branch of medicine, surgery and dietetics that deals with obesity, its effects, treatment and control *(See Obesity)*.

Baritosis Barium dust induced pneumoconiosis.

Barium Symbol Ba. a soft silvery metallic element.

Barium sulphate A heavy mineral salt that comparatively impermeable to X-rays and can, therefore, be used as a contrast medium, given as a meal or as an enema. Used to demonstrate abnormality in the stomach or intestines, and to show peristaltic movement.

Barium sulphide The chief constituent of depilatory preparations, i.e., those which remove hair.

Barium enema Enema in which a suspension of barium sulphate is injected into the rectum to render the lower GI tract radio-opaque, in order to diagnose the intestinal (colonic or small intestinal) lesions.

Barium meal Solution of barium sulphate that is swallowed by a patient in order to aid the radiographic diagnosis of stomach and duodenum.

Barium swallow Solution of barium sulphate swallowed by the patient for the radiographic diagnosis of the esophagus.

Barlow's disease Vit. C. deficiency state.

Barrett's esophagus Metaplasia of the lower esophageal squamous epithelial lining to goblet cells (usually found in the lower gastrointestinal tract) *(See Figure)*.

Barognosis The ability to estimate weigh.

Baroreflex Reflex mediated by pressure changes within great vessels through stimulation of mechanoreceptors.

Baroreceptors The sensory branches of the glossopharyngeal and vagus nerves that influence the blood pressure. The receptors are situated in the walls of the carotid sinus and aortic arch.

Barotrauma Injury due to pressure, such as to structures of the ear, owing to differences between atmospheric and intratympanic pressures.

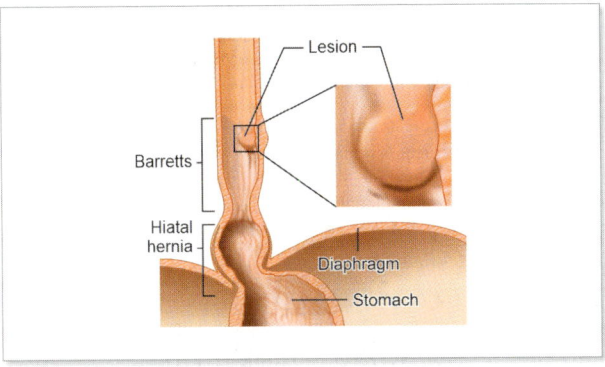

Barrett's Esophagus

Barr body *M.L. Barr, Canadian anatomist (1908).* Small, dark-staining area underneath the nuclear membrane of female cells. Represents an inactive X chromosome.

Barre-Guillain syndromes *(See Guillain- Barre syndrome).*

Barrel chest Rounded chest due to air trapping as in emphysema. In normal chest AP diameter is more than transverse, hence elliptical shape.

Barrier An obstruction.

Barrier contraceptive Mechanical barrier preventing the sperm from entering the cervical canal, e.g., diaphragm, sheath.

Barrier nursing Precautions taken by nurses to prevent infection from a patient spreading to other and/or staff. This normally involves nursing the patient in a separate room or cubicle.

Bloodbrain barrier The selective barrier which separates the circulating blood from the cerebrospinal fluid.

Placental barrier Semipermeable membrane between maternal and fetal blood.

Protective barrier Radiation-absorbing shield, e.g., lead, to protect the body against ionizing radiations.

Reverse barrier nursing A technique used by nurses to prevent the transmission of infection to the patient who maybe especially vulnerable, e.g., the immunosuppressed patient.

Barthel index A widely used index for the functional assessment of a person's ability to perform the daily activities like feeding, grooming, controlling bowel and bladder functions, etc.

Bartholin's duct Duct of sublingual salivary gland that runs parallel with Wharton's duct and opens with it.

Bartholin's glands *C.T. Bartholin. Danish anatomist, 1655–1738.* Two glands situated in the labia majora, with ducts opening inside the vulva.

Bartonellosis Infection due to *Bartonella bacilliformis* (oroya fever) characterized by fever and hemolysis; transmitted by female sand flies and treated with chloramphenicol.

Bartter's syndrome Hyperplesia of Juxtaglomerular cells with hypokalemia, hyper aldosterionism but without rise in blood pressure.

Basal 1. Fundamental. 2. Referring to a base.

Basal body temperature chart Daily temperature charting to predict ovulation.

Basal ganglia The collections of nerve cells or grey matter in the base of the cerebrum. They consist of the caudate nucleus and putamen, forming the corpus striatum, and the globus pallidus. Such cells are concerned with modifying and coordinating voluntary muscle movements.

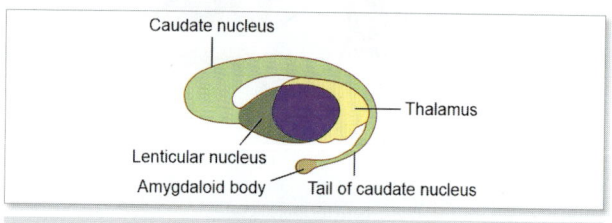

Caudate nucleus

Thalamus

Lenticular nucleus

Amygdaloid body   Tail of caudate nucleus

Basal Ganglia

Basal metabolic rate Abbreviated BMR. An indirect method of estimating the rate of metabolism in the body by measuring the oxygen intake and carbon dioxide output on breathing. The age, gender, weight and size of the patient have to be taken into account.

Base 1. lowest part or foundation. 2. The main constituent of a compound. 3. An alkali or other substance that can unite with an acid to form a salt.

Basement membrane A thin layer of modified connective tissue supporting layers of cells, found at the base of the epidermis and underlying mucous membranes.

Base pair In double stranded helical DNA the connecting chemicals, i.e., base pairs adenine-thymine, guanine-cytosine bind the strands.

Basilar Situated at the base.

Basilar artery Midline artery at the base of the skull, formed by the junction of the vertebral arteries.

Basilic Prominent.

Basilic vein A large vein on the inner side of the arm.

Basion Mid point of anterior border of foramen magnum.

Basiphobia Fear of walking.

Basisphenoid An embryonic bone that becomes the lower portion of sphenoid.

Basophil Adj. basophilic 1. Any structure, cell or histological element staining readily with basic dyes. 2. A granular leukocyte with an irregularly shaped, relatively pale-staining nucleus that is partially constricted into two lobes, and with cytoplasm containing coarse bluish black granules of variable size. 3. A beta cell of the adenohypophysis.

Basophilia 1. affinity of cells or tissues for basic dyes. 2. The reaction of relatively immature erythrocytes to basic dyes whereby the stained cells appear blue, grey grayish blue, or bluish granules appear. 3. Abnormal increase of basophilic leukocytes in the blood. 4. Basophilic leukocytosis.

Bassini's operation Surgical repair of inguinal hernia.

Batchelor plaster *J.S. Batchelor; British surgeon.* A double abduction splint used in the correction of congenital dislocation of the hip.

B

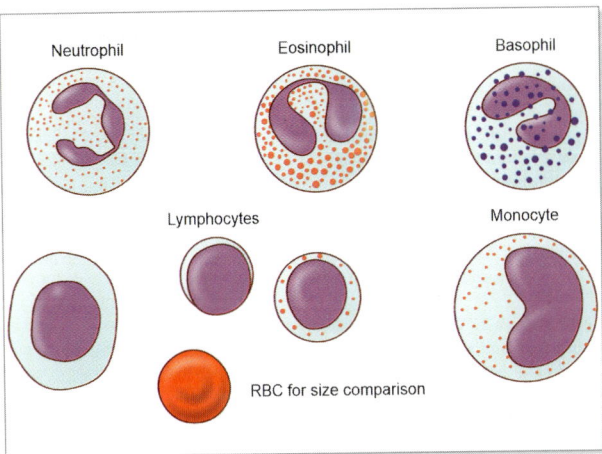

Basophil

Battered child syndrome Physical injuries inflicted upon children.

Battery Unlawful touching of a patient without consent, justification; battery occurs if a surgical or medical procedure is done without prior consent.

Battery sign Swelling behind the ear in fracture base of skull.

Bath 1. A medium, e.g., water, vapour, sand or mud, with which the body is washed or in which the body wholly or partially immersed for therapeutic or cleansing purposes; application of such a medium to the body. 2. The equipment or apparatus in which a body or object maybe immersed.

Bed bath Washing a patient in bed.

Emollient bath A bath in a soothing and softening liquid, used in various skin disorders. It is prepared by soothing agents such as gelatin, starch, bran or similar substances to the bath water, for the purpose of relieving skin irritation and pruritis. The patient is dried by patting rather than rubbing the skin. Care must be taken to avoid chilling.

Hot bath One taken in water at 36–44°C. Care must be taken to avoid faintness.

Sponge bath one in which the patient's body is not immersed but is wiped with a wet cloth or sponge. Sponge baths are most often employed for reduction of body temperature in the presence of a fever, in which case the water used is tepid and may contain alcohol to increase evaporation of moisture from the skin.

Tepid bath One taken in water at 30–33°C.

Warm bath One taken in water at 32–40°C.

Whirlpool bath (Jacuzzi) One in which the water is kept in constant motion by mechanical means. It has a gentle massaging action that promotes relaxation.

Baxter's formula This is a commonly used formula to calculate the fluid requirements, particularly in case of burn victims. According to this formula 4 mL of ringer lactate solution is administered per kilogram body weight percent of body surface area burnt.

Bazin's disease Erythema induratum.

B Cells Bone marrow derived lymphocytes, which when stimulated by antigen, transform to antibody producing plasma cells.

BCG vaccine Bacille Calmette Guerin vaccine, a tuberculosis vaccine containing live, attenuated bovine tubercle bacillis *(Mycobacterium bovis).*

Bearing down 1. The expulsive pains in the second stage of labour. 2. A feeling of heaviness and downward strain in the pelvis, present with some uterine growths or displacements.

Beaker Wide mouthed glass vessel.

Beat Pulsation of the heart or an artery.
Apex beat Pulsation of the heart felt over its apex. The beat of the heart is felt against the chest wall.
Dropped beat occasional loss of a ventricular beat.
Ectopic beat One that originates somewhere other than the sinoatrial node.

Beau's line White lines on finger nails.

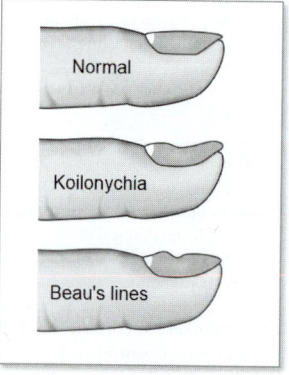

Beau's Line

Beck inventory of depression Abbreviated BID. A self-scoring system used to determine the presence and severity of depression.

Beck scale for suicide ideation (BSS) An assessment tool used to identify the potential and risk of suicide in vulnerable patients.

Beclomethasone dipropionate Aglucocorticoid administered by aerosol inhalation or spinhaler to patients who require corticosteroids for control of bronchial asthma or hay fever symptoms.

Becquerel Abbreviated Bq. The SI unit of radioactivity equal to the quantity of material undergoing one disintegration per second; 3.7×10^{10} becquerels is equal to 1 curie.

Bed 1. A supporting structure or tissue. 2. A couch or support for the body during sleep.
Bed cradle A frame placed over the body of a bed patient *(See Cradle).*
Capillary bed The capillaries of a tissue, area or organ collectively, and their volume capacity.
Fracture bed A bed for the use of patients with broken bones. *King's Fund bed* A bed fitted with jointed springs, which maybe adjusted to various positions.
Nail bed The area of modified epidermis beneath the nail over which the nail plate slides as it grows.

Bed-wetting Enuresis; involuntary voiding of urine *(See also Enuresis).*

Bedboard A rigid board placed beneath the mattress of a bed to give firm support to the patient lying upon it.

Bedbug A bug of the genus *Cimex,* a flattened, oval, reddish insect that inhabits houses, furniture and neglected beds, and feeds on humans, usually at night.

Bedlam Asylum for insane.

Bedpan A shallow vessel used for defecation or urination by patients confined to bed.

Bedrest Limiting the patient to staying in bed for a prescribed period for therapeutic reasons.

Bedsore An ulcer-like sore caused by prolonged pressure of the patient's body. Pressure sore is now the preferred term, as these sores are primarily due to pressure and can also occur in patients who are not confined to bed. A decubitus ulcer.

Bee sting Injury caused by the venom of a bee. Symptoms of a severe allergic reaction, such as collapse or swelling of the body, indicate anaphylaxis and require medical help.

Behaviour The way in which an organism reacts to an internal or external stimulus.

Behaviour disorders May take many forms, such as truancy, stealing, temper tantrums.

Behaviour modification An approach to correction of undesirable behavior that focuses on changing observable actions. Modification of the behaviour is accomplished through systematic manipulation of the environmental and behavioural variables related to the specific behaviour to be changed.

Behaviour therapy A therapeutic approach in which the focus is on the patient's observable behaviour, rather than on conflict and unconscious processes presumed to underline the maladaptive behaviour. This is accomplished through systematic manipulation of the environmental and behavioural variables related to the specific behaviour to be modified; operant conditioning, systematic desensitization, token economy, aversive control, flooding and implosion are examples of techniques that maybe used in behaviour therapy.

Incongruous behaviour Behaviour that is out of keeping with the person's normal reaction or has the opposite effect to that consciously desired.

Behavioural sciences The application of scientific principles to study the behavior of organisms, e.g., sociology, psychology and anthropology, etc.

Behaviourism The purely objective study and observation of the behaviour of individuals.

Behcet's syndrome *H. Behcet, Turkish dermatologist, 1889–1948.* A chronic condition of unknown origin, resulting in painful, recurring mouth and genital ulcers, arthritis, skin lesions and inflammation of the eyes.

Bejel A non-venereal but infectious form of syphilis caused by a *Treponema* indistinguishable from that causing syphilis. Occurs mainly in children of Africa and the Middle East. The primary lesion is on the mouth, spreading to the trunk, arms and legs. Treated with penicillin.

Belching The noisy expulsion of gas from the stomach through the mouth. Eructation.

Beliefs Thoughts, ideas and concepts developed by an individual over a period of time from cultural influences, education, religion, parents and family.

Health beliefs Those beliefs held by an individual regarding the maintenance of his or her state of physical well-being, which maybe at variance with those beliefs held by health care practitioner, possibly leading to conflict and non-compliance with prescribed treatment.

Belladonna A drug from the deadly nightshade plant. Used as an antispasmodic in colic, to check secretions and to dilate the pupil of the eye.

Belle indifference [Fr.] An indication of conversion hysteria, in which the patient describes symptoms, appearing not to be distressed by them.

Bell's palsy *Sir C. Bell, British physiologist, 1774–1842.* Facial paralysis due to edema of the facial nerve.

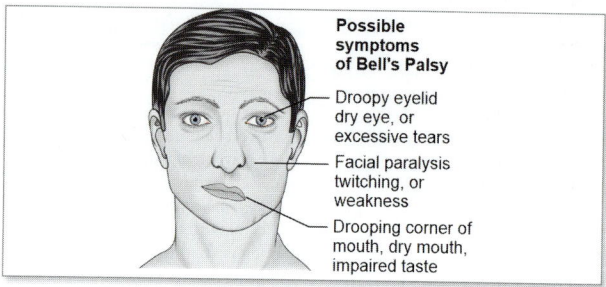

Possible symptoms of Bell's Palsy

- Droopy eyelid dry eye, or excessive tears
- Facial paralysis twitching, or weakness
- Drooping corner of mouth, dry mouth, impaired taste

Symptoms of Bell's Palsy

Bellini's tubule The straight connecting tubule of the kidney.

Bence-Jones protein A low molecular weight protein that disappears when urine is boiled to above 60°C but reappears once urine is cooled, commonly seen in multiple myeloma.

Benchmarking Comparing 'like with like' in order to identify best practice; or a process whereby organizations identify the best performers in order to improve their own performance. A scoring system is used that enables one hospital, department or other health care facility to compare their practices and services with another similar to their own. A quality-assurance technique.

Benedict's sol A solution of copper-sulfate, sodium citrate and sodium carbonate, used for testing the presence of reducing sugars in urine.

Benedict's test 8 drops of urine is added to 5 mL. of benedicts solution and boiled to see for green, yellow, orange and red precipitate.

Benedipine A calcium channel B-blocker for hypertension.

Beneficence The duty to do good, to avoid harm to other people and to protect the weak and the vulnerable. In the health care setting, this involves the staff acting in the best interests of their patients, and if necessary acting as advocate for them.

Bendrofluazide An oral diuretic of the thiazide group. Used primarily to treat mild hypertension and cardiac failure.

Bends A colloquial term for caissondisease. Decompress sickness.

Benign 1. The opposite to malignant. 2. Describes a noninvasive condition or illness that is not serious even though treatment maybe required for health or cosmetic reasons.

Benign prostatic hypertrophy (BTH) Prostatic enlargement in elderly due to hyperplasia causing obstruction of prostatic urethra.

Benorylate An ester of paracetamol and aspirin used as an anti-inflammatory and analgesic.

Benoxynate HCl Topically used ophthalmic local anesthetic.

Benserazide Inhibitor of amino acid decarboxylase, used in parkinsonism.

Bentonite Hydrated almino silicate, used as a suspending agent.

Benzalkonium chloride A quaternary ammonium compound used as a surface disinfectant and detergent, and as a topical antiseptic and antibiotic preservative. Incompatible with soap.

Benzapril An ACE inhibitor for hypertension.

Benzafibrate Lipid lowering agent.

Benzalkonium chloride An antimicrobical preservative, used as detergent and germicide.

Benzathine penicillin A long-acting antibiotic. Used in treatment of gram-positive infections. Maybe given orally or intramuscularly.

Benzene Benzol. A coal tar derivative widely used as a solvent.

Benzhexol An antispasmodic drug that helps to overcome the tremors and rigidity of Parkinson's disease.

Benzidine Used for test of occult blood in stool (to a solution of benzidine in glacial acetic acid is added 3% H_2O_2 and the stool sample. Appearance of blue color indicates presence of blood).

Benznidazole A nitroimidazole for Chaga's disease.

Benzobromarone Uricosuric agent used in gout.

Benzocaine A surface anesthetic used for the relief of pain or to anesthetize the oropharynx or anus. Available as lozenges or ointment.

Benzodiazepine Psychotropic agents with potent hypnotic and anti anxiety effects.

Benzoic acid Antifungal agent.

Benzoin A plant resin used as inhalant or protective coating for ulcers.

Benzoyl peroxide Keratolytic agent (for acne).

Benzthiazide Diuretic of thiazide group.

Benztropine mesylate Anti - parasympathomimetic agent for treatment of parkinsonism.

Benzyl benzoate An emulsion used in the treatment of scabies.

Bephenium hydroxynaphthoate Anthelmintic for hookworm and mixed infestation.

Benzyl penicillin A widely used soluble penicillin that is quickly absorbed. High blood levels can, therefore, be obtained.

Beraud's valve A fold of mucus membrane at the mouth of lacrimal duct in the lid.

Bereavement The experience of suffering loss, usually of a loved one by death or separation, but may also include the loss of previous good health, position wealth. Produces a psychological reaction that has recognized 'stages' that may overlap; these include anger, denial, disbelief and finally acceptance. Collectively recognized as mourning.

Beriberi A deficiency disease due to insufficiency of vitamin B_1 in the diet. The disease is more common in areas where refined rice is the main staple in the diet. It is a form of neuritis, with pain, paralysis and edema of the extremities.

Berylliosis An industrial lung disease due to the inhaling of the metallic element beryllium. Interstitial fibrosis arises, impairing lung function.

Bestiality Sexual intercourse with animals.

Beta The second letter in the Greek alphabet, β.

Beta blockers Drugs used to block the action of adrenaline on beta-adrenergic receptors in cardiac muscle, decreasing the workload of the heart.

Beta cells Insulin-producing cells found in the islets of Langerhans in the pancreas.

Beta rays Electrons used therapeutically for treatment of lesions of the cornea and iris.

Beta receptors Associated with the (relaxation) of smooth muscle. They also bring an increase in the force of contraction and rate of the heart.

B

Beta adrenergic receptors Specific receptors in blood vessels, heart, bronchi, intestine, etc. for action of adrenaline and noradrenaline.

Beta adrenergic receptor blockers Drugs that block both Beta-1 and Beta-2 receptors.

Betadine Trade name for preparations of povidone-iodine, which have a longer antiseptic action than most iodine solutions.

Betalactamase An enzyme produced by certain bacteria that inactivates antibiotics.

Betamethasone A synthetic glucocorticoid which is the most active of the anti-inflammatory steroids.

Betatron Electron accelerator that produces high energy electrons or X-rays.

Bethanecol A derivative of choline like substance, used in the treatment of abdominal distension and urinary retention. Hypotension and dyspnea may occur as side effects.

Bethanidine An adrenergic blocking agent used in the treatment of hypertension.

Betnovate Trade name for preparations containing betamethasone. Used in the treatment of severe inflammatory skin disorders unresponsive to less potent corticosteroids.

Betz cells Giant pyramidal cells in the motor cortex whose axons form pyramidal tract.

Bezoar A mass of hair, fruit or vegetable fibres sometimes found in the stomach or intestines.

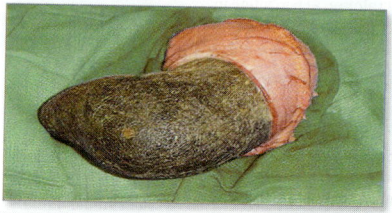

Bezoar

Bevacizumab Monoclonal antibody for colon cancer.

Bhang, bang The dried leaves of *Cannabis sativa*, the hemp plant from which marijuana is derived.

Bias In research, any tendency for results to differ from the true value in some consistent way.

Bicarbonate Any salt containing the HCO_3 anion.
Blood bicarbonate, plasma bicarbonate The bicarbonate of the blood plasma, an important parameter of acid-base balance *(See Acid)* measured in blood gas analysis.

Biblio mania Obsession with collection of books.

Bicellular Composed of two cells.

Biceps A muscle with two heads; a flexor of the arm; one of the hamstring muscles of the thigh.

Biconcave Pertaining to a lens or other structure with hollow or depression on each surface.

Biconvex Pertaining to a lens or other structure that protrudes on both surfaces.

Bicornuate Having two horns.
Bicornuate uterus A congenital malformation in which there is a partial or complete vertical division into two parts of the body of the uterus.

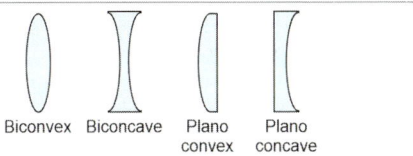

Biconvex & Biconcave Lens

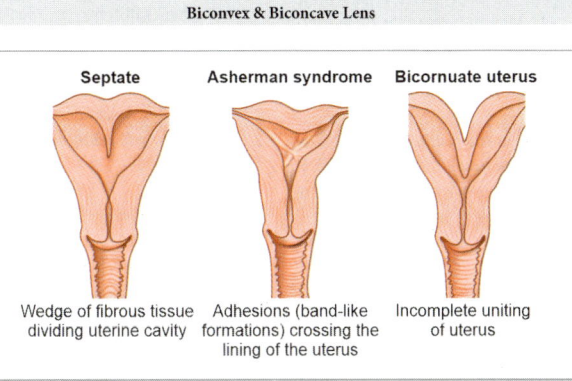

Bicornuate Uterus

Bicornis Uterus with two horns due to incomplete union of mullerian ducts.

Bicuspid Having two cusps or projections.

Bicuspid teeth The premolars.

Bicuspid mitral valve valve of the heart between the left atrium and ventricle.

Bicycle ergometer Stationary bicycle used for cardiac exercise, i.e., MUGA testing/intra operative exercise test.

Bidet A low narrow basin on a stand for washing the perineum and genitalia.

Bifid Divided or cleft into two parts.

Bifidus factor Present in human milk; promotes growth of gram-positive bacteria in gut flora, particularly Lactobacillus bifidus. This microorganism reduces the pH in the gut preventing the multiplication of pathogens.

Bifocal Having two foci, as with spectacles in which the lenses have two different foci.

Bifonazole An imidazole with antifungal activity.

Bifurcate To divide into two branches; arteries bifurcate frequently, thereby getting smaller.

Bifurcation The junction where a vessel divides into two branches, e.g., where the aorta divides into the right and left iliac vessels.

Bigeminal Double.

Bigeminal pulse Two pulse beats which occur together, regular in time and force. A regular irregularity.

Bigemini Group of two beats separated by a long pause. Commonly due to regular extrasystoles, (e.g., digitalis toxicity).

Biguanides Oral hypoglycemic agents for treating diabetes. They exert their effect by decreasing gluconeogenesis in muscle tissue. Only effective in those diabetics with functioning Islets of Langerhans cells. Most commonly used in non-insulin-dependent diabetics, especially those who have muscles of the thigh overweight.

Bilateral Pertaining to both sides.

Bile A secretion of the liver, greenish yellow to brown in colour. It concentrates in the gallbladder and passes into the small intestine, where it assists in digestion by emulsifying fats and stimulates peristalsis.

Bile ducts The canals or passage ways that conduct bile. The hepatic and cystic ducts join to form the common bile duct.

Bile pigments Bilirubin and biliverdin, produced by hemolysis in the spleen. Normally these colour the feces only, but in jaundice the skin and urine may also become coloured.

Bile salts Sodium taurocholate and sodium glycocholate, cause the emulsification of fats.

Biticyanin A blue or purple pigment, an oxidation product of biliverdin.

Bilharzia *TM Bilharz, German physician, 1825–1862.* A genus of blood fluke now known as Schistosoma.

Bilharziasis Schistosomiasis.

Biliary Pertaining to bile.

Biliary colic Spasm of muscle walls of the bile duct causing excruciating pain when gallstones are blocking the tube. Pain is in the right upper quadrant of the abdomen and referred to the shoulder.

Biliary fistula An abnormal opening between the gallbladder and the surface of the body.

Billroth's operation BI: Excision of pylorus and gastroduodenal anastomosis.

BII; Partial gastrectomy followed by side to side gastrojejunal anastomosis.

Biliousness A symptom complex comprising nausea, abdominal discomfort, headache and constipation.

Bilirubin An orange bile pigment-produced by the breakdown of haem and reduction of biliverdin; it normally circulates in plasma and is taken up by liver cells and conjugated to form bilirubin diglucuronide, the water soluble pigment

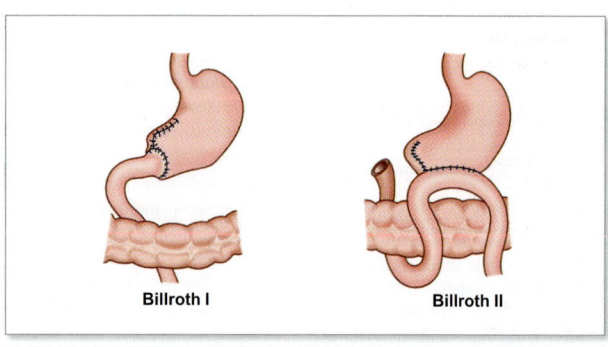

Billroth I   **Billroth II**

Billroth's I and II Operations

excreted in the bile. Bilirubin maybe classified as indirect ('free' or unconjugated) while en route to the liver from its site of formation by reticuloendothelial cells, and direct (diglucuronide) after its conjugation in the liver with glucuronic acid. Normally, the body produces a total of about 260 mg of bilirubin per day. Almost 99% of this is excreted in the feces; the remaining 1% is excreted in the urine as urobilinogen. The typical yellowness of jaundice is caused by the accumulation of bilirubin in the blood and body tissues.

Bilirubinemia The presence of bilirubin in the blood.

Biliuria Bile or bile salts in the urine.

Biliverdin A green pigment, the oxidized form of bilirubin.

Billings method A method of contraception, now rarely used. Ovulation time is estimated by observing changes in the cervical mucus that occur during the menstrual cycle.

Bimanual Using both hands.

Bimanual examination Examination with both hands. Used chiefly in gynecology, when the internal genital organs are examined between one hand on the abdomen, and the other hand or a finger within the vagina.

Bimodal Means a graphic presentation with two peaks.

Binary Made up of two parts.

Binary fission The multiplication of cells by division into two equal parts.
Binary scale One used in calculating, in which only two digits, 0 and 1, are used. Digital computers use this scale.

Binaural Pertaining to both ears.

Binaural stethoscope (See Stethoscope).

Binet's test *A. Binet, French physiologist, 1857–1911.* A method of ascertaining the mental age of children or young person by using a series of questions standardized on the capacity of normal children at various ages.

Bing test *A. Bing, German otologist, 1844–1922.* A vibrating tuning fork is held to the mastoid process and the auditory meatus is alternately occluded and left open; an increase and decrease in loudness (positive Bing) is perceived by the normal ear and in sensorineural hearing impairment, but in conductive hearing impairment no difference in loudness is perceived (negative Bing).

Binge eating disorder (BED) An eating disorder characterized by frequent and recurring binge eating associated with negative psychological and social problems, without subsequent purging (vomiting). An alternative term for bulimia.

Binocular Relating to both eyes.

Binovular Derived from two ova.

Binovular twin Twins, who may or may not be of different sexes.

Bioassay Biological assay. The use of animals or an isolated organ preparation to determine the effect of the active power of a sample of a drug. Comparison is made with the effect of standard preparation.

Bioavailability The rate and extent to which an active drug or metabolite enters the general circulation to be available at the acting site.

Biochemical screening Tests in pregnancy when the maternal serum is analyzed for biochemical markers that identify babies with fetal Down's syndrome or inherited metabolic disorders. The newborn blood-spot screening test screens for nine conditions and also relies on biochemical markers to identify those infants with cystic fibrosis.

Biochemistry The chemistry of living matter.

B

Biofeedback Visual or auditory evidence provided to an individual of the satisfactory performance of an autonomic body function, e.g., sounding a tone when blood pressure is at a satisfactory level, so that, through conditioning, the patient may assert control over that function.

Biogenesis 1. The origin of life. 2. The theory that living organisms can originate only from those already living and cannot be artificially produced.

Biogenic amines Chemical compounds important in neuro-transmission, e.g., dopamine, norepinephrine, serotonin and histamine.

Biohazard Any hazard arising from inadvertent human biological processes, e.g., accidental inoculation, needle-stick injury.

Biokinetics Study of growth changes and movements in developing organisms.

Biology The science of living organisms, dealing with their structure, function and relations with one another.

Biomechanical engineering The application of engineering knowledge and methods to the functions of the body. Used both as a means of explanation of bodily functions and in the treatment of disorders of the body. Practical applications include the use of artificial joints, electronic hearing aids and pacemakers.

Biometrics, Biometry 1. Anthropometry. 2. The use of statistics in biological science.

Biomicroscopy A microscopic examination of living tissues, e.g., of the structures of the anterior of the eye during life (*See Slit lamp*).

Bionursing The utilization of knowledge from the life sciences in the theory and practice of nursing.

Biophysics Application of physical laws to biological processes and function.

Biophysical profile A non-invasive test of fetal well-being using ultrasound to measure fetal heart rate, fetal tone, somatic movements, breathing movements and amniotic fluid volume. Each factor is scored to obtain a total biophysical score, which is an accurate predictor of fetal death in high-risk pregnancies. The score maybe affected by gestation, maternal illness, therapeutic medication, substance abuse or abnormality.

Bioplasm Protoplasm. The active principle in matter which produces living organisms.

Biopsy The removal of some tissue or organ from the living body, e.g,. a lymph gland, for examination to establish a diagnosis.

Aspiration biopsy Biopsy in which the tissue is obtained by suction through a needle and syringe.

Cone biopsy Biopsy in which an inverted cone of tissue is excised, as from the uterine cervix.

Excisional biopsy Removal of an entire lesion and significant portion of normal-looking tissue for examination.

Needle biopsy Tissue obtained by the puncture of a lesion with a needle. Rotation of the needle removes tissue within the lumen of the needle.

Punch biopsy Tissue obtained by a punch.

Biorhythm Any biological event, e.g., sleep cycle and menstrual cycle, affecting daily life.

Biosensors Noninvasive instruments that measure the result of biological processes, e.g., body temperature.

Biostatistics The branch of biometry that deals with the data and laws of human mortality, morbidity, natality and demography; also called vital statistics.

Biosynthesis The creation of a compound within a living organism.

Biot's breathing Short breaths in succession followed by long apnea as seen in raised intracranical pressure.

Biotin Formerly termed vitamin H, now part of the vitamin B complex and present in all normal diets.

Biparietal Pertaining to both parietal eminences or bones.

Biparous Giving birth to two infants as allowing mothers to give birth a time.

Bipolar With two poles.

Bipolar nerve cells Cells having two nerve fibres, e.g., ganglionic cells.

Birefringence It is also known as double refraction. It is the decomposition of a ray of light into two rays—ordinary ray and the extraordinary ray due to the polarization of light.

Birnberg bow This is an effective intrauterine contraceptive device.

Birth The act of being born.

Birth control Limiting the size of the family by abstention from sexual intercourse or the use of contraceptives.

Birth mark A nevus present from birth.

Birth plan A plan prepared by the expectant mother, usually in conjunction with her partner and midwife which records her preferences for care during and after labour.

Birth rate The number of births during one year per 1000 total estimated mid-year population (crude birth rate), per 1000 mid-year female population (refined birth rate), or per 1000 estimated mid-year female population of child-bearing age (true birth rate) that is, between the ages of 15 and 45.

Birth registration It is the notification of the birth of a child with the concerned local authority. In India according to 'Registration of Birth and Death Act 1969', it is mandatory to register the birth of a child within 21 days.

Premature birth One taking place before term.

Birthing chair A specially designed-chair for use in labour and delivery to promote greater mobility for the mother.

Birthing pool A specially designed pool allowing mothers to give birth underwater.

Bisacodyl A laxative that acts directly on the rectum. Given as tablets or in the form of suppositories.

Bisacromial Pertains to two acromial processes.

Bisexual 1. Having gonads of both sexes. 2. Hermaphrodite 3. Having both active and passive sexual interests characteristics. 4. Capable of the function of both sexes. 5. Both heterosexual and homosexual. 6. An individual who is both heterosexual and homosexual. 7. Of, relating to or involving both sexes, as in bisexual reproduction.

Bismuth Symbol Bi. A grayish metallic element. Certain of its salts are used as gastric sedatives.

Bisoprolol Betablocker.

Bistoury A slender surgical knife, sometimes curved.

Bite 1. To seize with the teeth. 2. A wound made by biting. 3. An impression made by the teeth on a thin sheet of malleable material such as wax.

Bitewing radiograph X-ray showing crown and upper third root of upper and lower teeth.

Bitot's spots P.A. Bitot, French physician, 1822–1888. Collection of epithelium, microorganisms, etc. forming shiny, greyish spots on the cornea. A sign of vitamin A deficiency.

Bivalve 1. Having two valves, as the shells of molluscs, such as oysters. 2. To cut a plaster cast into an anterior and a posterior section.

Bivalve speculum A vaginal speculum with two blades that can be adjusted for easy insertion.

Bjerrum's screen used for mapping the field of visions especially central and paracentral scotomas.

Black eye Brusing, discoloration and swelling of eyelids following trauma.

Blackhead A comedo.

Black measles Also called hemorrhagic measles implying a severe hemorrhagic measle eruption.

Blackout Momentary failure of vision and unconsciousness due to cerebral circulatory insufficiency.

Blackwater fever A form of malignant malaria in which severe hemolysis causes a dark discoloration of the urine.

Bladder A membranous sac for holding fluid or gas.

Atonic bladder A condition in which there is lack of tone in the bladder wall, which maybe the result of incomplete emptying over a long period.

Bladder worm A cysticercus.

Irritable bladder A condition in which there is frequent desire to micturate.

Urinary bladder The reservoir for urine.

Blalock-Taussig operation *A. Blalock, American surgeon, 1899–1964; H.B. Taussig, American pediatrician. 1898–1986.* Operation in which the subclavian artery is anastomosed to the pulmonary artery.

Blanch To loose colour. In blanching test, the nail is pressed quickly and then released. When circulation is good, colour returns within 5 seconds.

Bland Non-stimulating.

Bland fluids Mild and non-irritating fluids such as barley water and milk.

Bland diet Diet without irritant foods, e.g., milk, cream, prepared cereals, eggs, lean meat, fish, cheese, custard, cookie, etc.

Blandin's glands Glands on each side of frenulum of tongue.

Blast 1. An immature cell. 2. A wave of high air pressure caused by an explosion.

Blastocyst Blastula.

Blastoderm The germinal cells of the embryo consisting of three layers: the ectoderm, mesoderm and endoderm.

Blastolysis The destruction of germ substance.

Blastoma Neoplasm composed of immature undifferentiated cells.

Blastomere One of the cells resulting from cleavage of a fertilized ovum.

Blastomyces A genus of yeast like budding fungi pathogenic to man.

Blastomycosis A fungal infection, which, after invasion of the skin, may cause granulomatous lesions in the mouth, pharynx and lungs.

Blastula blastocyst An early stage in the development of the fertilized ovum. This stage precedes the gastrula.

Bleb Blister.

Bleaching powder Calcium hypochlorite or chlorinated lime.

Bleeder 1. A popular name for one who suffers from hemophilia. 2. A vessel that is difficult to seal at operation.

Bleeding 1. Escape of blood from an injured vessel. 2. Venesection.

Bleeding time The time taken for oozing to cease from a sharp prick of the finger or earlobe. The normal value is 1–3 min.

Functional bleeding Bleeding from the uterus when no organic lesion is present.

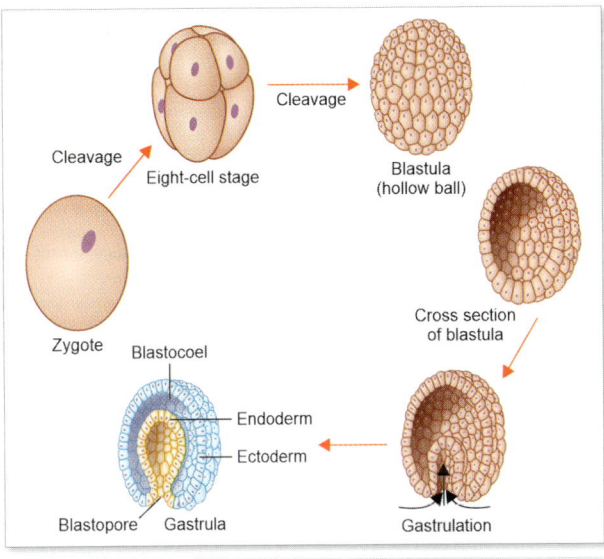

Stages of Formation of Blastula

Blennorrhagia 1. An excessive discharge of mucus, e.g., leukorrhoea. 2. Gonorrhoea.

Blennorrhea Blennorrhagia.

Bleomycin An antitumour antibiotic drug especially effective against squamous cell carcinoma.

Blepharitis Inflammation of the eyelids.

Allergic blepharitis That associated with response to drugs or cosmetics applied to the eye or eyelids.

Squamous blepharitis That associated with dandruff of the scalp.

Blepharon The eyelid.

Blepharoconjunctivitis This is the inflammation of both the conjunctiva and eyelids.

Blepharodiastasis Excessive separation of eyelids.

Blepharophimosis Abnormal narrowing of the aperture between the eyelids. Usually congenital but may arise from chronic inflammation.

Blepharospasm Prolonged spasm of the orbicular muscles of eyelids.

Blind Without sight.

Blind spot The point where the optic nerve leaves the retina which is insensitive to light. Punctum cecum.

Blind loop syndrome A stasis in the small intestine, which aids bacterial multiplication, leading to diarrhea and salt deficiencies. The cause maybe intestinal obstruction or surgical anastomosis.

Blindness Lack or loss of ability to see; lack of perception of visual stimuli.

Legally, blindness is defined as less than 6/60 vision with glasses (vision of 6/60 is the ability to see only at 6 meters what the normal eye can see at 60 meters).

B

Blister A bleb or vesicle. A collection of serum between the epidermis and the skin.

Blood blister A blister containing blood, usually caused by a pinch or bruise.

Block A stoppage or obstruction. The term is used to describe (a) Various forms of regional anesthesia, e.g., epidural block, (b) Obstruction to the passage of a nervous impulse due to disease, e.g., heart block *(See Heart)*, (c) An interruption of mental function.

Blood The fluid that circulates through the heart and blood vessels, supplying nutritive material to all parts of the body and carrying away waste products. Blood is a red viscid fluid and consists of plasma in which are suspended erythrocytes (red blood cells), leukocytes (white blood cells) and lymphocytes, and platelets or thrombocytes. (a) The red corpuscles or erythrocytes contain hemoglobin, which combines with oxygen in passing through the lungs. This oxygen is released into the tissues from the capillaries and oxidation takes place, (b) The white corpuscles or leukocytes defend against microorganisms, which they have power to destroy, (c) Blood platelets or thrombocytes are concerned with the clotting of blood. Plasma also contains many other specialized substances that have important roles to play in immunity and clotting of blood.

Blood bank 1. A place of storage for blood. 2. An organization that collects, processes, stores and transfuses blood. In most hospitals, the blood bank is located in the pathology laboratory.

Blood-borne viruses Viruses that are transmitted by blood and some other body fluids (e.g., semen, amniotic fluid), such as hepatitis B virus, hepatitis C virus and human immunodeficiency viruses (HIV-1, HIV-2).

Blood-brain barrier Abbreviated BBB. The membranous barrier separating the blood from the brain. It is permeable to water, oxygen, carbon dioxide, glucose, alcohol, general anesthetics and some drugs.

Blood casts Casts of coagulated red blood formed in the renal tubules and found in the urine.

Blood clotting Coagulation. The formation of a jelly-like substance over the ends or within the walls of a vessel, with resultant stoppage of the blood flow. Clotting is one of the natural defence mechanisms of the body when injury occurs. A clot will usually form within 5 min of a blood vessel being damaged. The exact process of clotting is not known but it is believed that the mechanism is triggered by the platelets, which disintegrate as they pass over rough places in the injured surface. If normal amounts of calcium, platelets and tissue factors are present, prothrombin will be converted to thrombin. Thrombin then acts as a catalyst for change of fibrinogen into a mesh of insoluble fibrin, in which are erythrocytes and leukocytes and small amounts of fluid (serum). Plasma coagulation factors are:

    I. Fibrinogen
    II. Prothrombin
    III. Tissue thromboplastin
    IV. Calcium ions
    V. Proaccelerin
    VII. Proconvertin
    VIII. Antihemophilic factor (AHF)
    IX. Christmas factor
    X. Stuart factor (Power factor)
    XI. Plasma thromboplastin antecedent (PTA)
    XII. Hageman factor
    XIII. Fibrin stabilizing factor

B

Stage I:
Platelets attach
to the endothelium
(blood vessel wall)

Platelet

Stage II:
Platelets start to release
fibrin and begin to seal
the endothelium

Endothelium
(blood vessel wall)

Stage III:
The fibrin network traps
the RBC, and completely
seal the endothelium

Fibrin polymers

Red blood
cells (RBC)

Connective
tissue

Blood Clotting

Blood count The number of blood cells in a given sample of blood, usually expressed as the number of cells per litre of blood (as the red blood cell, white blood cell or platelet count). A differential white cell count determines the number of various types of leukocyte in a sample of blood.

Blood dyscrasia Any abnormality of the blood cells or of the clotting elements.

Blood group ABO system *(See Table)*. In clinical practice, there are four main blood types: A, B, O and AB. In addition to this major grouping there is a rhesus (Rh) system that is important in the prevention of hemolytic disease of the newborn resulting from incompatibility of blood groups in mother and fetus. In determining blood group, a sample of blood is taken and mixed with specially prepared sera. One serum, anti-A agglutinin, causes blood of group A to agglutinate; another serum, anti-B agglutinin, causes blood of group B to agglutinate. Thus, if anti-A serum alone causes clumping, the blood is group A; if anti-B serum alone causes clumping, the blood group is B. If both cause clumping, the blood group is AB, and if it is not clumped by either, it is identified as group O. Transfusion with an incompatible ABO group will cause severe hemolytic reaction and death may occur.

Blood pressure Abbreviated BP. The pressure exerted on the artery walls by the blood as it flows through them. It can be measured in millimeters of mercury (mm Hg) using a sphygmomanometer. Two readings are made. Arterial pressure fluctuates with each heartbeat and one measure records the pressure while the heart is in systole (when the heart is ejecting blood into the arteries) and is the higher, or systolic pressure. The other records while the heart is in diastole (when the aortic and pulmonary valves are closed and the heart is relaxed) and is the lower, or diastolic pressure. The range of normal blood pressure recording varies according to age and body size, but in the normal young adult is approximately 100–120/70–80 mm Hg.

	Group A	Group B	Group AB	Group O
Red blood cell type	A	B	AB	O
Antibodies in plasma	Anti-B	Anti-A	None	Anti-A and Anti-B
Antigens in red blood cell	A antigen	B antigen	A and B antigens	None

Classifiction of Blood Groups

Blood sugar The amount of glucose present in the blood. The normal range is 2.5–4.7 mmol/L. When the amount exceeds 10 mmol/L, glucose is excreted in the urine, as in diabetes mellitus.

Blood transfusion Introduction of blood from the vein of one person (donor) or from a blood bank into the vein of another (recipient) in cases of severe loss of blood, trauma, septicemia, etc. It is used to supplement the volume of blood and also to introduce constituents, such as clotting factors or antibodies, that are deficient in the patient. Clotting must be prevented in the transition stage. This is usually done by admixture with sodium citrate (1 g) to 459 mL of blood. Too much sodium citrate tends to produce a reaction: rigor and shock may occur.

Blood urea Excretory product of protein present in the blood. The normal range is 3–7 mmol/litre; this increases in renal failure when the kidneys cease to function normally.

Blue baby syndrome (See Fallot's tetralogy).

Blumenbach's sign Sign indicative of peritonitis, pain is experienced while pressure is relieved, on the abdomen by examining hand.

Blush Glowing redness of the face, usually a reaction to emotion or heat.

BMR Basal metabolic rate.

Boa's point A tender spot left of 12th dorsal vertebra, in patients with gastric ulcer.

Bobath technique An approach to the treatment of neurological conditions.

Bochdalek's ganglion Ganglion of plexuses of dental nerve in the maxilla above the canine tooth.

Body 1. The trunk, or animal frame, with its organs. 2. The largest and most important part of any organ. 3. Any mass or collection of material.

Body dysmorphic disorder An anxiety disorder that causes a person to have a distorted view of how they look and to worry excessively about their appearance.

Body image The total concept of the body, including conscious and unconscious feelings, thoughts and perceptions that a person has of it as an object in space, which is dependent and apart from other objects.

Body-ketone They are acetone, aceto acitic acid and betahydroxy butyric acid.

Body amygdaloid Almond shaped gray matter in the lateral wall and roof of third ventricle of brain concerned with memory.

Body Aschoff Microscopic areas of central fibrinoid degeneration with surrounding chronic inflammatory cell infiltration seen in rheumatic fever.

Body Carotid Flat structure at bifurcation of common carotid, containing baroreceptors.

Body Donovan Chlamydia granulomatis, causative organism of granuloma inguinale.

Body Negri Inclusion bodies in nerve cells of CNS in patients with rabies.

Body language The expression of thoughts or emotions by means of posture or gestures. Body language may include unintended 'signs' as well as intended communication. Detailed studies of human nonverbal communication have been documented by several observers.

Body mass index Abbreviated BMI. The weight (kg) divided by the square of the height (m) (W/Hm^2). An index for estimating obesity.

Body rocking Rhythmic purposeless body movements.

Body substance isolation Abbreviated BSI. An infection control system, developed in 1987, that further elaborated universal precautions and focused on the isolation of all moist and potentially infectious body substances (blood, feces, urine, sputum, saliva, wound drainage and other body fluids) from all patients, regardless of their presumed infection status, primarily through the use of gloves. This concept has now been further developed and is known by the term standard precautions.

Boeck's sarcoid Older name for sarcoidosis.

Boil An acute staphylococcal inflammation of the skin and subcutaneous tissues round a hair follicle. It causes a painful swelling with a central core of dead tissue (slough), which is eventually discharged. A furuncle.

Bolus 1. A large pill. 2. A rounded mass of masticated food immediately before being swallowed or one passing through the intestines. 3. A quantity of a drug injected directly to raise its concentration in the blood to a therapeutic level.

Bombesin A neuropeptide present in gut and brain.

Bonding The attachment process that occurs between an infant and its parents, especially the mother, during the first hours and days following birth. Bonding is a reciprocal process and is a biological need for the future development, both physical and emotional, of the infant.

Bone The dense connective tissue forming the skeleton. It is composed of cartilage or membrane impregnated with mineral salts, chiefly calcium phosphate and calcium carbonate. This is arranged as an outer hard compact tissue and an inner network of cells (cancellous tissue), in the spaces of which is red bone marrow. In the shaft of long bones is a medullary cavity containing yellow marrow. Microscopically, the bone tissue is perforated with minute Haversian canals containing blood vessels and lymphatics for the maintenance and repair of the cells. Bone is covered by a fibrous membrane, the periosteum, containing blood vessels and by which the bone grows in girth.

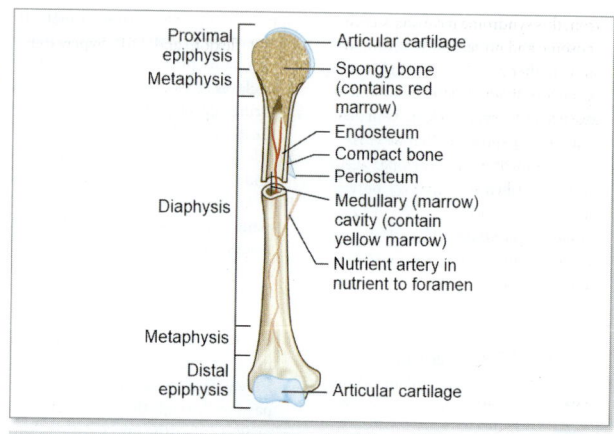

Proximal epiphysis — Articular cartilage
Metaphysis — Spongy bone (contains red marrow)
— Endosteum
— Compact bone
— Periosteum
Diaphysis — Medullary (marrow) cavity (contain yellow marrow)
— Nutrient artery in nutrient to foramen
Metaphysis
Distal epiphysis — Articular cartilage

Stucture of Bone

Bone graft Transplantation of a healthy piece of bone to replace missing or repair defective bone.

Bone marrow Substance which fills the marrow cavities of bones. Basically, there are two types: yellow and red marrow. The red marrow is responsible for producing the blood cells. The yellow is mostly fatty connective tissue.

Bone marrow aspiration Bone marrow aspiration or bone marrow biopsy is a medical procedure in order to obtain the bone marrow sample for the purpose of pathological examination. Bone marrow aspiration is used for the diagnosis of numerous hematological conditions including leukemia, multiple myeloma, anemia, hematological malignancies, etc. The common sites for bone marrow aspiration include *the sternum and posterior iliac crest*.

Bone marrow transplantation autologous Cryopreservation of patient marrow and its re-infusion for marrow hypoplasia following cancer chemotherapy.

Bone marrow transplantation A procedure used to treat aplastic anemia, acute leukemia and some rare congenital disorders, with varying success. Healthy bone marrow is taken from the donor and infused into the bloodstream of the recipient; from here it 'homes' in on the bone marrow, where it will grow. Histocompatibility between the donor (usually a sibling) and recipient is essential.

Bone age Estimation of biological age based on development of ossification centers of wrist and long bones.

Bone alveolar Bone of maxilla and mandible supporting the teeth.

Sesamoid bone Bone found embedded in tendons and joint capsule.

Bone densitometry Method of determining bone density by radiographic or ultrasonic means for diagnosis of osteoporosis.

Bong A water pipe used for smoking cannabis and other drugs.

Bonnevie-Ullrich syndrome This is another name for Turner's syndrome. The individuals suffering from this syndrome have one X chromosome and no second sex chromosome (either X or Y). The phenotype of such individuals is female due to absence of Y chromosome. The individuals may show the following features: Growth retardation, webbed neck, infertility, short stature, development delay, learning disabilities, lymphedema, etc. The external genitalia is of female type. Though uterus and fallopian tubes are present, both overies and testis are absent.

Borax Sodium borate, used as water softner, and weak antiseptic.

Borborygmus A rumbling sound caused by gas in the intestines.

Bordetella A genus of bacteria.

Bordetella pertussis The causal agent of whooping cough.

Boric acid A mild antiseptic.

Bornholm's disease An epidemic myalgia with pleural pain due to Coxsackie virus infection. It is named after the Danish island of Bornholm where there was an outbreak in 1930.

Bottle mouth syndrome Dental caries caused in infants when they take a bottle filled with liquid other than water.

Botulin The neurotoxin responsible for botulism.

Botulism An extremely severe form of food poisoning due to a neurotoxin (botulin) produced by *Clostridium botulinum,* sometimes found in improperly canned or preserved foods. The symptoms include vomiting, abdominal pain, headache, weakness, constipation and nerve paralysis, which cause difficulty in seeing, breathing and swallowing. Death is usually due to paralysis of the respiratory organs.

Bougie A flexible cylindrical instrument used to dilate a stricture, as in the esophagus or urethra.

Medicated bougie A soluble form impregnated with a medicinal substance. Used for urethral treatment.

Boutonniere deformity Proximal IP joint flexion and DIP hyperextension, characteristic of rheumatoid deformity.

Bovine Relating to the cow or ox.

Bovine tuberculosis That caused by infection from infected cows' milk, usually affecting glands and bones.

Bowel The intestine.

Bowel sounds Relatively high-pitched abdominal sounds caused by the propulsion of the intestinal contents through the lower alimentary canal.

Bowen's disease A very early form of skin cancer affecting the squamous cells. The main symptom is a red, scaly patch on the skin.

Bowleg Deformity where there is an outward curvature of one or both legs near the knee. This results in a gap between the knees on standing. Genu varum.

Bowman's capsule *Sir WP. Bowman, British physician, 1816–1892.* The expanded end of the kidney tubule, which surrounds the glomerulus.

Bowman's membrane Thin homogeneous membrane separating corneal epithelium from corneal substance.

Boyle's law The law states that at a constant temperature, the volume of gas varies inversely with pressure.

Brace 1. A support used in orthopedics to hold parts of the body in their correct positions. 2. An orthodontic appliance to correct the alignment of teeth.

Brachial Relating to the arm.

Brachial artery The continuation of the axillary artery along to inner side of the upper arm.

Brachial plexus A network of nerves at the root of the neck supplying the upper limb.

Brachium pontis Middle cerebellar peduncle.

Brachychilia Abnormally short lips.

B

Brachydactyly Abnormally short fingers and toes.

Brachytherapy Radiotherapy delivered into or adjacent to a tumour by means of an intracavitary or interstitial radioactive source.

Bradford frame This is a rectangular metallic frame having canvas or webbing straps used for immobilizing the spine and pelvis. It is often used to support individuals with diseases or fractures of the spine, hip or pelvis. This device is named after its inventor, an *American orthopedic surgeon Edward H Bradford*.

Bradycardia Abnormally low rate of heart contractions and consequent slow pulse.

Bradyarrhythmia Slow and irregular heart rate.

Bradycephaly A common condition affecting babies, also known as flathead syndrome where the back of the head is flattened as a result of spending a lot of time lying on their backs. The head widens and the forehead may bulge. The head shape will generally improve over time. *(See also Plagiocephaly).*

Bradykinesia Slowness of movement (parkinsonism).

Bradykinin Peptide formed from the degradation of protein by enzymes. It is a powerful vasodilator that also causes contraction of smooth muscle.

Bradyphasia Slowness of speech.

Bradypnea Abnormally slow respiration.

Braille A method of printing developed by *Louis Braille (1809–1852)* for the blind. Letters of the alphabet are represented by patterns of raised dots. These dots are read by passing the fingertips over them.

Brain That part of the central nervous system contained in the skull. It consists of the cerebrum, midbrain, cerebellum, medulla oblongata and pons varolii.

Brain death Isoelectric EEG for atleast 30 minutes with no change in response to sound and pain stimuli; absent respiration and all reflexes (barbiturate, diazepam, methaqualone can produce short periods of isoelectgric EEG).

Brainstem The lower part of the brain that is connected with the spinal cord and controls the automatic functions of the body, e.g., heart and respiratory rate. This consists of the midbrain, pons Varolii and medulla oblongata.

Brainstorming Or 'thought showering' is an approach to problem solving through the encouragement of intensive discussion in a group, generating ideas and solutions about an issue.

Bran The husk of grain, i.e., the coarse outer coat of cereals. High in roughage vitamins of the B complex, bran is frequently recommended as a dietary component both for those with alimentary disorders and for those in normal health.

Branchial Relating to the clefts (branchia) that are present in the neck and pharynx in the developing embryo. Normally, they disappear.

Branchial cyst A cystic swelling arising from a branchial remnant in the neck.

Branchial sinus (lateral cervical sinus) A tract leading from the posterior cervical region which opens in the lower neck in front of sternomastoid muscle.

Branchial clefts Openings between branchial arches.

Brand – Andrews maneuver Expulsion of placenta from uterus during third stage of labour by gentle traction on cord by one hand, the other hand pressing uterus backwards and upwards.

Braun's frame *H.F.W. Braun, German surgeon, 1862–1934.* A metal frame which incorporates one or more pulleys and is used to elevate the lower limb and to apply skeletal traction for a compound fracture of tibia and fibula.

Braxton contractions Braxton Hicks, *British gynaecologist, 1823–1897.* Painless uterine contractions occurring during pregnancy, becoming increasingly rhythmic and intense during the third trimester. Sometimes called 'false labour'.

Braxton Hicks contractions J. Braxton Hicks, British gynaecologist, 1823-1897. Painless uterine contractions occurring during pregnancy, becoming increasingly rhythmic and intense during the third trimester. Sometimes called 'false labor'.

BRCA genes (BRCA1 and BRCA2) Genes that produce tumor-suppressor proteins. When either gene is faulty, DNA damage may not be repaired properly and cells are more likely to develop additional alterations that can lead to cancer, particularly of the breast and ovary. Mutations can be inherited and account for around 5%–10% of breast cancers and 15% of ovarian cancers.

Break bone fever Dengue fever (group B arbovirus).

Breast 1. The anterior or front region of the chest. 2. The mammary gland.

Breast abscess Formation of pus in the mammary gland.

Breast bone The sternum.

Breast cancer The breast is the most common site of malignant tumours in women. Although the survival rates for breast cancer continue to increase, albeit slowly, the incidence of the disease in the world is also increasing. Improvement in these survival rates has come from public awareness, breast self-examination, breast screening programmes and improved methods of treatment. Women should train themselves to perform a simple self-examination of the breasts, described in the following *Figure.* The best time for this is just after-menstruation when the breasts are normally soft. If any lump in the breast can be felt, a doctor should be consulted immediately. More than 90% of breast cancers are discovered by the patients themselves.

Breastfeeding The method of feeding a baby with milk directly from the mother's breasts. Midwives and pediatricians agree that breast-feeding is usually better for the baby and the mother, both physically and emotionally.

Breast pump Apparatus for removal of milk from the breast.

Pigeon breast Prominent sternum, a deformity resulting from rickets.

BREAST SELF-EXAMINATION (BSE)

→ Any change in the shape and size of either breast or nipple should first be noted by looking in the mirror.

→ Lying down with a pillow or towel placed under the shoulder helps to spread the breast tissue for easier self-examination.

→ In front of the mirror and with arms raised, view the breasts from different angles.

→ Rotate fingers in small circles and trace a spiral route around the breast to check for any lumps or unusual thickening.

→ Squeeze each nipple gently, noting any discharge or bleeding.

→ Finally, examine the armpits using the spiral technique and note any unusual findings.

B

TEN STEPS TO SUCCESSFUL BREASTFEEDING

- Breastfeeding policy available which is communicated to all staff.
- All health-care staff trained to implement the policy.
- All pregnant mothers informed of the benefits and management of breastfeeding.
- Mothers assisted to commence breastfeeding within half an hour of delivery.
- Education of mothers for breastfeeding and maintenance of lactation even if they are separated from their babies.
- Neonates to be given nothing other than breast milk unless medically necessary.
- 24-hour rooming-in.
- On-demand breastfeeding.
- No teats or pacifiers to be given to breastfeeding babies.
- Establishment of breast-feeding support groups.
  (**Source:** UNICEF UK Baby Friendly Initiative.).

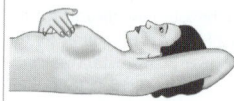

1. Lie down and put your left arm under your head. Use your right hand to examine your left breast. With your 3 middle finger flat, move gently in small circular motions over the entire breast, checking for any lump, hard knot, or thickening. Use different level of pressure-light, medium, and firm-over each area of your breast. Check the whole breast, from your collar bone above your breast down to the ribs below your breast. Switch arms and repeat on the other breast.

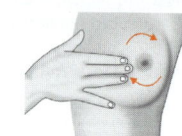

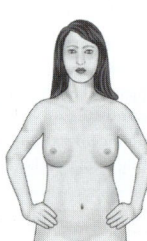

2. Look at your breasts while standing in front of a mirror with your hands on your hips. Look for lumps, new difference in size and shape, and swelling or dimpling of the skin.

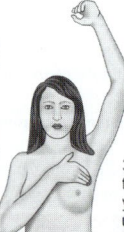

3. Raise one arm, then the other, so you can check under your arms for lumps.

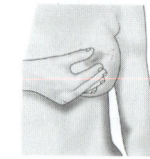

4. Squeeze the nipple of each breast gently between your thumb and index finger. Report to your healthcare provider right away any discharger or fluid from the nipples or any lumps or changes in your breast.

Breast Self-Examination

Breath The air taken in and expelled by the expansion and contraction of the thorax.

Breath holding When a young child cries, holds its breath and goes blue.

Breath sounds The sounds heard when a stethoscope is placed over the lungs during respiration.

Breathing The alternate inspiration and expiration of air into and out of the lungs *(See also Respiration)*.

Breech The buttocks.

Breech presentation A position of the fetus in the uterus such that the buttocks present.

Bregma The anterior fontanelle. The membranous junction between the coronal and sagittal sutures.

Breisky's disease Kraurosis vulvae.

Brennerman's ulcers This can be described as meatitis, meatal ulceration and meatal stenosis of the urinary meatus in circumscribed males. Circumcision results in removal of foreskin which makes the meatus prone to infection, thereby resulting in the development of ulceration.

Brenner's tumor Benign fibro-epithelioma of ovary.

Bretylium Anti-arrhythmic agent.

Bridge In dentistry, an irremovable prosthesis carrying false teeth that bridges gaps left when natural teeth are extracted.

Bright's disease Bright's disease was a term used to describe different forms of kidney disease in accordance with the older classification system of renal diseases. This usually referred to the inflammation of kidneys, what is now commonly known as nephritis.

Brimonidine Anti-glaucoma eye drop.

Briquet's syndrome A personality disorder with alcoholism and somatization disorder.

British National Formulary (BNF) A publication produced twice a year by the British Medical Association and the Pharmaceutical Society of Great Britain, containing details of nearly all the drugs currently available on prescription in the UK. Also available electronically. The Nurse Prescribers' formulary is published as an addendum to the BNF.

British Pharmacopoeia Abbreviated BP. The official publication containing the list of drugs and other medicinal substances in use in the United Kingdom. The book gives details of how these substances are obtained or prepared, and their dosages and methods of administration. It is compiled under the auspices of the General Medical Council and is regularly revised and brought up – to – date.

Brittle diabetes Changing and unpredictable response to insulin leading to ketosis, particularly in childhood diabetes.

Broca's area of speech *P. P. Broca, French surgeon, 1824–1880.* The motor center for speech, situated in the left cerebral hemisphere. Damage to the nerve cells contained in it can impair speech.

Brodie's abscess *Sir B.C. Brodie, British surgeon, 1783–1862.* A chronic abscess of bone.

Broad ligaments Folds of peritoneum extending from the uterus to the sides of the pelvis, and supporting the blood vessels to the uterus and uterine tubes.

Brodmann's area Division of cerebral cortex into 47 areas, now classified according to their function.

Bromhexine Mucolytic agent.

Bromocryptine mesylate A dopaminergic ergot derivative that is used in hyper-prolactinemia.

Bromhidrosis Offensive and fetid sweat.

Bromide A compound of bromine. Bromides are sedatives that are strongly depressant and cumulative in action.

Bromocriptine A dopamine agonist used in the treatment of Parkinsonism in cases where levodopa is not well tolerated.

Brompton cocktail Name given to mixtures containing various combinations of morphine, diamorphine and cocaine. These mixtures often contain gin and / or chlorpromazine. They were used in the relief of pain in terminal care. They have now been replaced by a simple solution morphine in chloroform water.

Bromsulphthalein A dye used in certain tests for liver function.

Bronchi Plural of bronchus.

Bronchiectasis Chronic dilatation of the bronchi and bronchioles with secondary infection, usually involving the lower lobes of the lung. The condition may occur as a congenital malformation of the alveoli with resultant dilatation of the terminal bronchi. Most often it is an acquired disease secondary to partial obstruction of the bronchi with necrotizing infection. The symptoms include a chronic cough and purulent sputum.

Bronchocele Circumscribed dilatation of bronchus.

Bronchiole One of the smallest of the subdivisions of the bronchi.

Bronchiolitis Inflammation of bronchioles, commonly in small children.

Bronchitis Inflammation of the bronchi.

Acute bronchitis A short- infection, common in young children and the elderly. It is a descending infection from common cold, influenza, measles and other upper respiratory conditions.

Chronic bronchitis A chronic infection, usually associated with infection of the upper respiratory tract. It may in time lead to emphysema.

Bronchoadenitis Inflammation of the bronchial glands.

Bronchodilator Any agent that causes dilatation of the bronchi.

Broncholith A calculus in the bronchus.

Bronchography Radiography of the bronchial tree after introduction of a radiopaque medium.

Bronchomycosis An industrial disease chiefly affecting agricultural and stable workers, etc., and due to inhalation of micro fungi which infect the air passages. Causes can be *Actinomyces* or *Aspergillus* species. Symptoms are similar to those of pulmonary tuberculosis.

Bronchophony Resonance of the voice as heard in the chest over the bronchi on auscultation.

Bronchopneumonia A descending infection starting around the bronchi and bronchioles *(See also pneumonia)*.

Bronchopulmonary Relating to the lungs, bronchi and bronchioles.

Bronchopulmonary dysplasia Abbreviated BPD. A chronic respiratory condition occurring in babies who have been ventilated for long periods or have needed prolonged oxygen therapy. It results in serious disruption of lung growth. Examination of radiographs and lung specimens reveals patches of collapse and fibrosis. Following ventilation, these babies usually require supplementary oxygen for several weeks or even months to keep the arterial oxygen tension above 55 kPa.

Bronchorrhea An excessive discharge of mucus from the bronchi.

Bronchoscope An endoscope that enables the operator to see inside the bronchi. It can also be used to wash out the bronchi, to remove foreign bodies or to take a biopsy.

Bronchoscopy Examination of the bronchi by means of a bronchoscope.

Bronchospasm Difficulty in breathing caused by the sudden constriction of plain muscle in the walls of the bronchi. This may arise inasthmaor chronic bronchitis.

Bronchospirometer An instrument used to measure the capacity of one lung or of one lobe of the lung, or of each lung separately.

Bronchotracheal Relating to both the trachea and the bronchi.

Bronchotracheal suction The removal of mucus with the aid of suction.

Bronchovesicular Sounds intermediate between bronchial and alveolar sounds.

Bronchus Any of the larger passages conveying air to (right or left principal bronchus) and within (lobar and segmental bronchi) the lungs.

Brooke's formula This is one of the most commonly used formula for calculating the amount of fluid to be administered within the first twenty-four hours following burns injury in a patient with burns involving more than 50% of the surface area. It calls for administration of ringer's lactate solution at the rate of 2 mL/kg/%burn.

Broviac catheter Trade name for a special catheter used to provide a central venous line.

Brow The forehead.

Brow presentation A position of the fetus such that the forehead appears at the cervix first.

Brown fat Special type of adipose tissue found in the newborn infant, and which is widely distributed throughout the body. The tissue is highly vascular and owes its colour to the large number of mitochondria found in the cytoplasm of its cells. It allows the infant to increase its metabolic rate and thus its heat production when subjected to cold. At the time the fat itself is used up.

Brown-Sequard's syndrome *C.E. Brown-Sequard French physiologist, 1818–1894.* Paralysis and loss of discriminatory and joint sensation on one side of the body and of pain and temperature sensation on the other, due to a lesion involving one side of the spinal cord.

Browser A computer program used to access the internet.

Brucella A genus of bacteria primarily pathogenic in animals but which may affect humans.

Brucellosis A generalized infection involving primarily the reticulo-endothelial system marked by remittent undulant fever *(See Below)*, malaise, headache and anemia. It is caused by various species of *Brucella* and is transmitted to humans from domestic animals such as pigs, goats and cattle, especially through infected milk or contact with the carcass of an infected animal. The disease is also called undulant fever because one of the major symptoms in humans is a fever that fluctuates widely at regular intervals. Prevention is best accomplished by the pasteurization of milk and a programme of testing, vaccination and elimination of infected animals. Also called Malta fever, abortus fever and Mediterranean fever.

Bruch's membrane The membrane lying between choroid membrane and the pigmented epithelium of retina.

Brudzinski's sign *Brudzinski, Polish physician, 1874–1917.* 1. Passive flexion of one thigh causing spontaneous flexion of the opposite thigh. 2. Flexion of the neck causing bilateral flexion of the hips and knees. These are indicative of meningeal irritation.

Brugada syndrome A rare but serious hereditary condition resulting in cardiac arrhythmias that can be life-threatening.

Bruise A superficial injury to tissues produced by sudden impact in which the skin is unbroken. A contusion.

Bruit [Fr.] Abnormal sound or murmur heard on auscultation of the heart and large vessels.

Brunner's glands Compound glands of duodenum and upper jejunum secreting mucus.

Brush border Hollow microvilli in the renal tubules and intestinal epithelium.

Brushfield spots Gray or pale yellow spots present at the periphery of iris in Down's syndrome.

Bruxism Teeth clenching, particularly during sleep. This occurs in persons under tension and may cause headaches as a result of muscle fatigue.

Bryant's traction Traction applied to lower leg vertically in treating femur fracture in children.

Bubo Inflammation of the lymphatic glands of the axilla or groin. Typical of bubonic plague *(See Plague)* and venereal infections.

Buccal Pertaining to the cheek or to the mouth.

Buck's traction Traction of lower extremity applied in line with long axis of the leg.

Buclizine Antihistamine used for motion sickness.

Budesonide A corticosterioid used as bronchial spray in asthma.

Budd-Chiari syndrome G. Budd, *British physician, 1808–1882; H. Chiari, Austrian pathologist, 1851–1916.* A condition in which thrombosis of the hepatic vein causes vomiting, jaundice, enlargement of the liver and ascites.

Buerger's disease L. Buerger, *American physician, 1879–1943.* Thromboangiitis obliterans.

Buffalo hump Excess fat deposition in cervical and upper thoracic region due to cortisone excess.

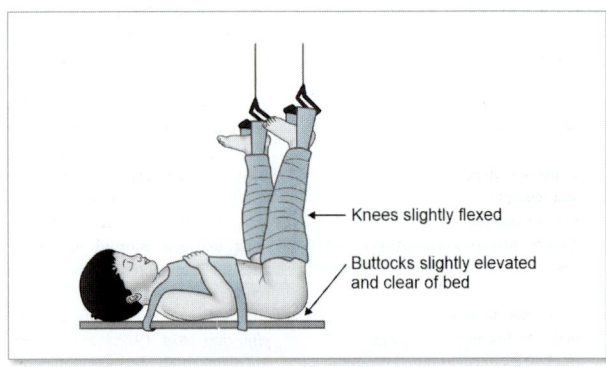

← Knees slightly flexed

Buttocks slightly elevated and clear of bed

Bryant's Traction

Buffer 1. A physical or physiological system that tends to oppose change within that system, e.g., the reflexes involved in blood pressure homeostasis. 2. A chemical system that acts to prevent change in the concentration of another chemical substance. Sodium bicarbonate is the chief buffer of the blood and tissue fluids. 3. Anything that is used to reduce shock or jarring upon contact.

Buffy coat A light coloured layer containing white cells that forms when blood is centrifused or is allowed to stand in a test tube.

Buggery Anal intercourse, either heterosexual or homosexual. In law the term also includes sexual contact with an animal. Also known as sodomy.

Bulb Any rounded or globular structure.

Bulbar Pertaining to the medulla oblongata.
Bulbar paralysis (See Paralysis).

Bulbitis Inflammation of urethra in its bulbous portion, e.g., posterior portion of corpus spongiosum found between the two crura of penis.

Bulbocavernosus reflex Contraction of bulbocavernosus muscle on percussing the dorsum of penis.

Bulbomimic reflex Contraction of facial muscles following pressure on eyeball.

Bulbourethral Relating to the bulb of the urethra (bulb of the penis).
Bulbourethral glands Small glands opening into the male urethra. Cowper's glands.

Bulimia Abnormal increase in the sensation of hunger.
Bulimia nervosa A pattern of 'binge eating', or episodes of uncontrolled and compulsive overeating occurring in response to stress. Bulimic 'binges' often occur in anorexia nervosa.

Bulk-forming agent An antidiarrheal agent that makes the feces less fluid by absorbing water.

Bulla A large, fluid-containing blister.

Bullying Tormenting others by repeated verbal harassment, physical assault or other subtle methods of coercion such as manipulation or sending hurtful or scary messages or phone calls, SMS text, emails or other social media messages. Bullying is widespread and occurs in settings where people interact. This includes schools and workplaces. These settings have a responsibility to create an environment where children and adults feel safe. In recent years, steps have been taken to develop policies against bullying. *(See also Harrasment).*

Bulaquine An antimalarial.

Bumetanide A quick-acting diuretic drug which prevents the resorption of urine from Henle's loop in the renal tubule.

Bundle A collection of nerve fibres all running in the same direction.
Bundle branch Block the delay in conduction along either branch of the atrioventricular bundle of the heart. The abnormality is detected by an ECG recording.

Bundle of His *L.His Jr, German physiologist, 1863–1934.* The band of neuromuscular fibres which, passing through the spectrum of the heart, divides at the apex into two parts, these being distributed into the walls of the ventricles. The impulse of contraction is conducted through the structure. Atrioventricular bundle.

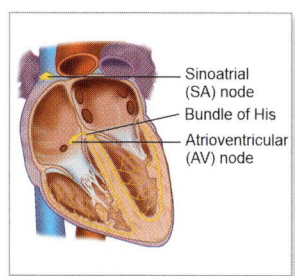

Sinoatrial (SA) node
Bundle of His
Atrioventricular (AV) node

Bundle of His

Bunion A prominence of the head of the metatarsal bone at its junction with the great toe, caused by inflammation and swelling of the bursa at that joint. Usually, due to shoes that distort the natural shape of the foot.

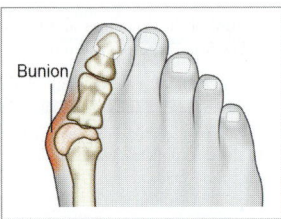

Bunion

Buphthalmos Abnormal enlargement of the eyes in congenital glaucoma.

Buprenorphine Semisynthetic morphine analog, very potent analgesic.

Burkitt's tumour *D.P. Burkitt, Irish surgeon, b. 1911.* African lymphoma. A lymphosarcoma, frequently of the jaw, occurring almost exclusively in children living in low-lying moist areas. Occurs in New Guinea and Central Africa. The Epstein-Barr virus (EB virus), a herpes virus, has been isolated from Burkitt's lymphoma cells in culture, and has been implicated as a causative agent.

Burn An injury to tissues caused by: (a) Physical agents, the sun, excess heat or cold, friction, nuclear radiation; (b) Chemical agents, acids or caustic alkalis; (c) Electrical current. Burns are described as being partial thickness (involving only the epidermis) or full thickness (involving the dermis and underlying structures). Clinically, emphasis is placed on the percentage of the body affected by the burn. The treatment of shock and prevention of infection and malnutrition need special attention.

Burnett's syndrome Milk–alkali syndrome.

Burning foot syndrome Burning in the sole of feet due to vitamin deficiency and chronic renal failure.

Burnout A term used to describe the result of chronic stress amongst workers and commonly in members of the professions. Burnout is characterized by chronic low energy, defensiveness and emergence of manoeuvres designed to create distance between helper and patient/ client. Dissatisfaction and tension maybe carried over from the work situation into the personal one and self-esteem and confidence may suffer badly.

Burr A bit for a surgical drill, used for cutting bone or teeth.
  Burr hole A circular hole drilled in the cranium to permit access to the brain or to release raised intracranial pressure.

Bursa A small sac of fibrous tissue, lined with membrane and containing synovial fluid. It is situated between parts that move upon another at a joint to reduce friction.

Bursitis Inflammation of the bursa. It produces pain and may impede movement of the joint.
  Prepatellar bursitis Housemaid's knee.

Bursolith Calculus formed in bursa.

Burton's line A blue line along the margin of the gum visible in chronic lead poisoning.

Buspirone Antianxiety agent.

Buscopan Trade name for a preparation of hyoscinebutylbromide. An antispasmodic that relaxes smooth muscle in the gastrointestinal tract.

Busulphan A cytotoxic drug that depresses the bone marrow and maybe used to treat myeloid leukemia.

Butenafine An antifungal.

Butobarbitone An intermediate-acting barbiturate, formerly much used as a sedative. Now used only in severe insomnia.

Buttock Either of the two prominences formed by the flesh covered gluteal muscles at either side of the lower spine.

Butorphenol Morphine conzener, acts like pentazocine.

Butterfly rash Skin rash on both cheeks joined by an extension across the bridge of nose.

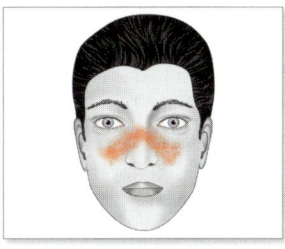

Butterfly rash

Butoxamine Beta$_2$ adrenergic antagonist.

Butyric acid A fatty acid used in disinfectants, emulsifying agent.

Butyrophenone A chemical class of major tranquillizers, especially useful in the treatment of manic and moderate to severe agitated states and in control of the utterances and tics of Gilles de la Tourete's syndrome.

Byler's disease Inherited disease with cirrhosis and mental retardation in children.

Bypass Diversion of flow. Formation of a shunt.
　Aortocoronary bypass Diversion of flow from the aorta to the coronary arteries via a saphenous vein or artificial graft.
　Femoropopliteal bypass Diversion of flow from the femoral to the popliteal artery to overcome an occlusion.

Byssinosis An industrial disease caused by inhalation of cotton or linen dust in factories. A type of pneumoconiosis.

Byte The storage space in the memory of a computer allocated to one character or letter, usually composed of a sequence of eight bits.

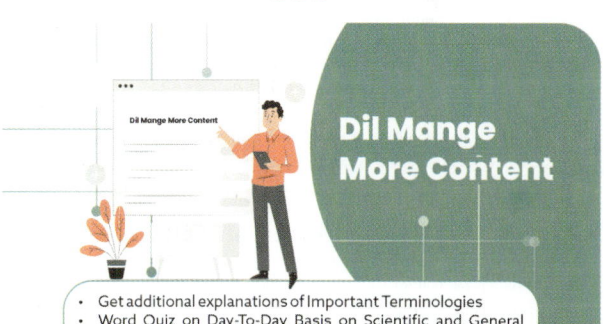

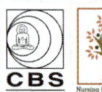

CBS
Dedicated to Education

Nursing Knowledge Tree

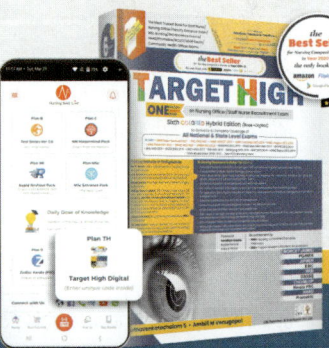

TARGET HIGH
6th Colored *Hybrid* *Edition*
(Book + Digital)

Muthuvenkatachalam S • Ambili M Venugopal

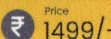
Price
₹ 1499/-

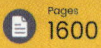
Pages
1600

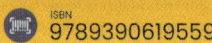
ISBN
9789390619559

- A thoroughly Revised & Updated Ed. (up to August 2021) with all Recent Papers, Topics & Current Affairs.
- Includes 6K New Qs (Book +App) & 200 Pages of New Content
- Covers about 21K Qs. (Book +App) including 5K MCQs with Rationale, 15k Practice Qs, 600 IBQs, 30+ VBQs, 300 Clinical-Based Qs in 13 Subjects covering 1000+ Topics
- 3000 Golden Points for Last Minute Revision in Book & Podcast Form
- 100+ Previous Year (2021-2010) Papers covering 25+ Exams of National & State Levels (Book+App)
- 73+ Appendices (Book+App) on Most Recent Topics, e.g. Tuberculosis, Mucormycosis, Management of COVID-19 in pregnancy, etc.
- Special and updated Section on COVID-19 management
- Attractive Layout with Integrated Approach Theory + Imp MCQs side by side
- MCQs categorized in Subject wise cum Topic wise format
- 600+ Pages of Synopses covering all Subjects, thoroughly Revised Synopses of FON, CHN, Pediatric Nursing, Midwifery & Gynecological Nursing, and Medical Surgical Nursing
- 1000+ Important Tables, Illustrations & Images for clarity of concepts.
- Strong Digital Support with plenty of ADD-ON Content, Only Genuine Buyer of TH 6th Ed. can unlock the content *(Refer to the front inside cover for detailed information)*

12 Strong Reason to refer to TARGET HIGH 6th colored Hybrid Edition

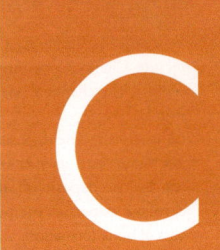

C Symbol for carbon; centigrade or Celsius; cytosine.

© Symbol for copyright

Ca Symbol for calcium.

Cabergoline Dopamine receptor agonist used in hyper-prolactinemia.

Cachet Used for administering medicines with a bitter taste.

Cachexia A condition of extreme debility. The patient is emaciated, the skin being loose and wrinkled from rapid wasting, but shiny and tense over bone. The eyes are sunken, the skin yellowish, and there is a gray "muddy" complexion. Mucous membranes are pale and anemia is extreme. The condition is typical of the late stages of chronic diseases.

Cacogenesis Abnormal development or growth.

Cacogeusia Unpleasant taste in the mouth.

Cacosmia Unpleasant odor (olfactory hallucination).

Cadaver A corpse. The dead body used for dissection.

Cadence Rythmic movements.

Cadwell Iuc operation Also known as maxillary antrostomy, this procedure involves opening the maxillary sinus by giving an incision in the buccal cavity over the canine teeth. This procedure helps in the drainage of this sinus.

Caecostomy The making of a surgical fistula into the cecum by incision through the abdominal wall.

Cecum The blind pouch forming the beginning of the large intestine. The vermiform appendix is attached to it.

Cesarean Section delivery of a fetus by an incision through the abdominal wall and uterus. Performed for the safety of either the mother or the infant.

Cesium Symbol Cs. A metallic element. *C.-137* Radioactive Cesium; a fission product from uranium. Sealed in a suitable container, it can be used instead of cobalt for beam therapy; sealed in needles, tubes or applicators, it can be used for local application.

Cafcass An independent service, which supports and represents children in family court cases. Stands for Children and Family Court Advisory and Support Service.

Café-au-lait spot Pigmented macules of a distinctive light-brown colour, like coffee with milk, as in neurofibromatosis and Albright's syndrome.

Caffeine An alkaloid of tea and coffee which acts as a nerve stimulant and diuretic. Mixed with aspirin and codeine it is often used as an analgesic.

Caffery's disease This disease is also known as infantile cortical hyperostosis and is characterized by subperiosteal new bone formation over commonly involved include mandible, clavicle and shafts of long bones. There could be appearance of fever.

Caffeinism An agitated state due to the excessive ingestion of caffeine.

Caisson's disease Decompression sickness.

Calabar A parasitic infection mainly seen in Africa, characterized by presence of lumps in the subcutaneous tissue, particularly anterior chamber of eyes.

Calamine Preparation of zinc carbonate or zinc oxide colored pink with ferric oxide. It is an astringent and antipruritic, used in lotion or ointment form for skin diseases.

Calcaneum The heel bone. Calcaneus.

Calcereus Chalky. Containing lime.

Calciferol The chemical name for vitamin D.

Calcification 1. The deposit of lime in any tissue, e.g., in formation of callus. 2. The deposit of lime salts in cartilage as part of the normal process of bone formation.

Dystrophic calcification The deposition of calcium in abnormal tissue, such as scar tissue or atherosclerotic plaques, without abnormalities of calcium.

Calcitonin A polypeptide hormone, produced by the parafollicular or C cells of the thyroid gland, which regulates blood calcium levels.

Calcitriol A sterol of Vitamin D activity, very potent.

Calcium Symbol Ca. A metallic element necessary for the normal development and functioning of the body. Calcium is the most abundant mineral in the body; it is a constituent of bones and teeth. Deficiency or excess of serum calcium causes nerve and muscle dysfunctions and abnormalities in blood clotting. The correct concentration is regulated by hormones.

Calcium carbonate Chalk.

Calcium gluconate Used as an antacid. A compound that is easily absorbed and can be given by intramuscular or intravenous route to raise the blood calcium.

Calcium lactate A compound that increases the coagulability of blood; used orally as a calcium supplement.

Calcium channel blockers A group of drugs that act by slowing the influx of calcium ions into muscle cells resulting in decreased arterial resistance and decreased myocardial O_2 demand.

Calcium dobesilate Endothelium stabilizer for hemorrhoid.

Calculus 1. A stony concretion which maybe formed in any of the secreting organs of the body or their ducts. 2. A calcified deposit that forms on the surface of the teeth leading to tooth decay and gum disease.

Caldicott guardian All NHS organizations must appoint a Caldicott guardian to safeguard the confidentiality of patient information, as all local councils with a social service responsibility. They must be either a member of the organization's management board or senior health professional with responsibility of promoting clinical governance in the organization. The Caldicott principles apply in addition to the requirements of data protection legislation.

Calf Fleshy muscular back part of leg formed by gastrocnemius and soleus.

Calibrator 1. An instrument for measuring the size of openings. 2. An instrument used to dilate a tube, e.g., in urethral stricture.

Caliper A two-pronged instrument that maybe used to exert traction on a part.

Walking caliper An appliance fitted to a boot or shoe to give support to the lower limb. It maybe used when the muscles are paralyzed or in the repair stage of fractures.

Calipers Compasses for measuring diameters and surface.

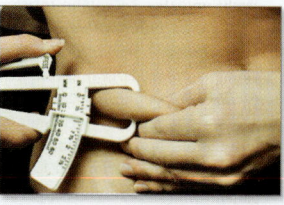

Calipers

Skinfold calipers An instrument used in nutritional assessment for determining amount of body fat.

A fold of skin and subcutaneous tissue, usually over the triceps muscle, is pinched away from the underlying muscle using the thumb and forefinger.

Calisthenics Mild gymnastics for developing the muscles and producing a graceful carriage.

Callosity The plaques of thickened skin often seen on the soles of the feet or the palms of the hand, areas subject to friction.

Callous Hard and thickened.

Callus 1. A callosity. 2. The tissue that grows round fractured ends of bone and develops into new bone to repair the injury.

Calmodulin Intracellular proteins that combine with calcium and activate a variety of cellular responses.

Calmette-Guérin bacillus *AL C Calmette, French bacteriologist, 1863–1933; C. Guérin, French bacteriologist, 1872–1961.* A deactivated tuberculosis bacillus from which the antituberculosis vaccine, BCG vaccine, is made.

Calor [L.] Heat: one of the signs of inflammation.

Caloric Pertaining to heat or calories.

Caloric test A test for vestibulo-ocular reflex. It involves irrigating cold or warm water into the external auditory canal. In a patient with intact cerebrum, the irrigation of cool water causes the eyes to turn toward the ipsilateral ear with horizontal nystagmus in the contralateral ear. Warm water, on the other hand, causes the eyes to turn toward the contralateral ear with horizontal nystagmus in the ipsilateral ear. In patients with absent vestibulo-ocular reflex, the nystagmus component of the test would be absent with both hot and cold water.

Calvaria The dome like superior portion of cranium.

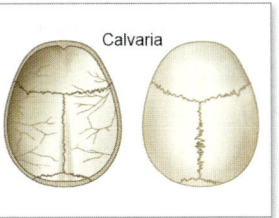

Calvaria

Calorie Symbol cal. A unit of heat. Used to denote physiological values of various food substances, estimated according to the amount of heat they produce on being oxidized in the body *(See Oxidization)*. A calorie (or kilocalorie) represents the heat required to raise 1 kg (1,000 g) of water by 1°C. A small calorie equals the heat produced in raising 1 g of water by 1°C. In the SI system the calorie is replaced by the Joule (1 cal = 4.18 kJ).

Calorific Heat-producing.

Calorimeter An apparatus for measuring the heat that is produced or lost during a chemical or physical change.

Calvé-Perthes disease Aseptic necrosis of femoral head epiphysis.

Calx Calcium oxide or lime. The basis of slaked lime, bleaching powder and quicklime.

Calyx Any cup-shaped vessel or part. *Calyx of kidney* The cup-like termination of the ureter in the renal pelvis surrounding the pyramids of the kidney.

Camphor A crystalline substance prepared from the camphor laurel. It is used internally as a carminative.

Camphorated oil 1 part camphor to 4 parts of oil, prepared for external application as a rubefacient.

Campylobacter A genus of bacteria, family spirillacea, made up of Gram-negative, nonspore forming, spirally curved rods. Causes an intestinal illness lasting several days. Usually associated with unpasteurized milk, partially cooked meat and poultry.

Canal A tubular passage.

Alimentary canal The passage along which the food passes on its way through the body.

Canal of Schlemm That which drains the acqueous humor.

Cervical canal That through the cervix of the uterus.

Semicircular canal One of the three canals in the middle ear responsible for maintenance of balance.

Canaliculus A small channel or canal.

Cancellous Being porous or spongy. Applied to the honey comb type of bone tissue in the ends of long bones and in flat and irregular bones.

Cancer A general term to describe malignant growths in tissue, of which carcinoma is of epithelial and sarcoma of tissue origin, as in bone and muscle. The basic etiology of cancer remains unknown but many potential causes are now recognized, e.g., cigarette smoking, ionizing radiation exposure to certain chemicals and over exposure to the sun. Hereditary factors also play an important part in its development. A cancerous growth is one that is not encapsulated, but infiltrates surrounding tissues, the cells of which it replaces on its own. It is spread by the lymph and blood vessels and causes metastases in other parts of the body. Death is caused by destruction of organs to a degree incompatible with life, by extreme debility and anemia or by hemorrhage. For early warning signs of cancer, *(See Table).*

Cancer phobia An irrational fear of cancer.

EARLY WARNING SIGNS OF CANCER

☞ Any lump or thickening, especially in the breast, lip or tongue.

☞ Any irregular or unexplained bleeding. Blood in the urine or bowel movements.

☞ Blood or bloody discharge from the nipple or any body opening. Unexplained vaginal bleeding or discharge, or any bleeding after the menopause.

☞ A sore that does not heal, particularly around the mouth, tongue or lips, or anywhere on the skin.

☞ Noticeable changes in the color or size of a wart, mole or birthmark.

☞ Loss of appetite or continual indigestion.

☞ Persistent hoarseness, cough or difficulty in swallowing.

☞ Persistent change in normal elimination (bowel habits).

Special note: (Pain is not usually an early warning sign of cancer).

Cancroid 1. Resembling cancer 2. A skin tumor or moderate degree of malignancy.

Cancrum oris Gangrenous stomatitis. An ulceration of the mouth which is a rare complication of measles in debilitated children. Noma.

Candida A genus of small fungi, formerly called yeast.

Monilial candida albicans The variety that causes candidiasis.

Candidiasis Infection by the *Candida* fungus. Occurs particularly in moist areas, such as mouth, vagina and skin folds. Popularly known as thrush. Candidiasis can occur as a result of a debilitating illness or immunosuppressive therapy and/or cytotoxic drugs. The infection may also occur as a result disturbed intestinal flora, and in pregnancy. Oral infection maybe due to poor hygiene caries teeth or badly fitting dentures.

Cane sugar Sucrose.

Canker Ulceration of mouth and lips.

Canine 1. Pertaining to a dog. 2. An 'eye tooth'. There are two in each jaw between the incisors and the molars.

Cannabis An illegal drug which maybe swallowed or smoked. It produces hallucinations and a temporary sense of well-being; followed by extreme lethargy. Alternative terms for cannabis include marijuana, hashish, blow, draw, hash, grass, pot, the weed, ganja, kaya, kif and bhang.

Cannibalism Eating of human flesh (kuru).

Cannon waves These refer to the large 'a' waves present on jugular venous pulse. These waves usually result when the right atrium has to contract against an increased resistance, e.g., tricuspid atresia or stenosis or right atrial myxoma.

Cannula A hollow tube for insertion into the body by which fluids are introduced or removed. Usually a trocar is fitted into it to facilitate its introduction.

Canthus The angle formed by the junction of the upper and lower eyelids.

Canthoplasty Enlargement of palpebral fissure by division of external canthus.

Canthridin Keratolytic for removal of warts.

CAPD Continuous ambulatory peritoneal dialysis.

Cap Protective covering,.

Cap enamel cap like structure of enamel organ developed during third month of fetal development.

Cap Phrygian the cholecystographic appearance of gallbladder showing kinking between body and fundus.

Cap of zinn a prominence of pulmonary arc representing dilated pulmonary artery in PA view in patent ductus arteriosus.

Capacity 1. Volume or potential volume of material. 2. Power or ability to hold, retain or contain.

Diffusion capacity the ability of alveolocapillary membrane to transfer gas.

Forced vital capacity volume of gas that can be expelled with maximum effort.

Functional residual capacity volume of gas in the lungs after quiet expiration.

Iron-binding capacity Capacity of serum transferring to bind iron.

Total lung capacity volume of air in the lungs at the end of maximal inspiration.

Vital capacity volume of gas that can be expelled after full inspiration.

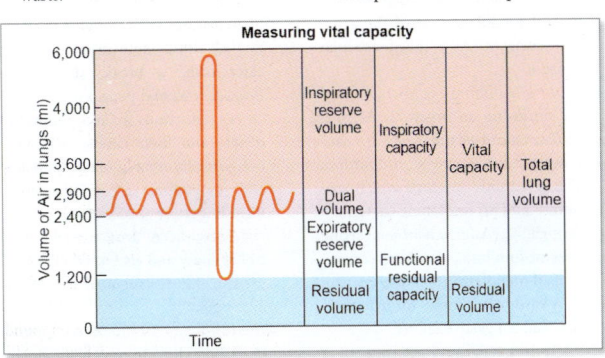

Measurement of Vital Capacity

Capeline bandage A cap-like covering of two interwoven bandages used for protecting the head or a limb stump.

Capillarity The action by which a liquid will rise upward in a fibrous substance or in a fine tube. Capillary attraction.

Capillary 1. Hair like 2. A minute vessel connecting an arteriole and a venule. 3. A minute vessel of the lymphatic system.

Capitulum Rounded articular end of bone.

Caplan's syndrome Rheumatoid arthritis with progressive massive lung fibrosis in pneumoconiosis.

Capreomycin A polypeptide antibiotic produced by *Streptomyces capreolus*, which is active against human strains of *Mycobacterium tuberculosis* and has four microbiologically active components.

Capsid Protein covering around the central core of virus particle protecting the virus particle from destructive enzymes.

Capsofungin Potent antifungal.

Capsular Relating to a capsule.
Capsular ligaments Those that completely surround a movable joint, forming a capsule which loosely encloses the bones and is lined with synovial membrane which secretes a fluid for lubrication of the articular surfaces. Also called articular capsule.

Capsule 1. A fibrous or membranous sac enclosing an organ. 2. A small soluble case of gelatin in which a nauseous medicine maybe enclosed. 3. The gelatinous envelope which surrounds and protects some bacteria.

Captopril Angiotensin-converting enzyme inhibitor, blocking conversion of angiotensin I to angiotensin II. A vasodilator useful for hypertension and congestive failure.

Capsulectomy Surgical excision of a capsule.

Capsulitis Inflammation of the capsule of a joint.

Capsulotomy The incision of a capsule, particularly that of a joint or of the lens of the eye.

Caput Head.
Caput succedaneum A transient soft swelling on an infant's head, due pressure during labor, which disappears within the first few days of life.

Caramel Flavoring and coloring agent made by heating sugar or glucose, destroying the sweet taste in the process.

Carbachol Drug related to and acting like acetylcholine, but more stable. It causes contraction of plain muscle and relaxation of the voluntary sphincter, so relieving postoperative retention of urine. Also occasionally used in the treatment of glaucoma.

Carbamate Ester of carbonic acid – the insecticides and parasiticides that act by inhibiting choline esterase. For example, Aldicarb, Aminocarb, Carbaril, Carbofuran, Dimetilan, Methomyl, Propoxur.

Caries The decay or death of bone which becomes soft discolored and porous.

Caring about Carers A national strategy supporting an estimated 6 million carers in England and Wales. Its main features are: (a) grants to allow English local authorities to help carers take a break; (b) credits towards a second pension; (c) council tax reductions for more disabled people and their carers; (d) more care-friendly employment policies; and (e) support for young carers including those at school.

Carbamazepine A drug used to control epilepsy and also to relieve pain; used in the treatment of trigeminal neuralgia.

Carbaminohemoglobin A compound of carbon dioxide and hemoglobin present in the blood.

Carbasone Contains 28% arsenic, antiamebic agent.

Carbenicillin A synthetic penicillin which is principally used in the treatment of serious infections caused by *Pseudomonas aeruginosa* and other Gram-negative organisms. Large doses, which need to be given intravenously, are required to obtain sufficiently high concentrations in the blood and tissues to be effective. Carbenoxolone, an anti inflammatory drug used in the treatment of gastric ulcers.

Carbidopa An inhibitor of the decarboxylation of levodopa (Ldopa) in peripheral tissues, which does not cross the blood-brain barrier. It is used in combination with levodopa to control the symptoms of Parkinson's disease. In the presence of carbidopa, levodopa enters the brain in larger quantities, thus avoiding the need for excessively high doses.

Carbimazole An antithyroid drug that is used to stabilize a patient with thyrotoxicosis.

Carbocistine Antithyroid drug.

Carbohydrate A compound of carbon, hydrogen and oxygen. Carbohydrates are classified into mono-, di-, tri-, poly- and heterosaccharides. In food they are an important and immediate source of energy for the body; 1 g of carbohydrate yields 17 kJ (14 kcal). They are synthesized by all green plants. In the body they are absorbed immediately or stored in the form of glycogen.

Carbolic Acid phenol.

Carbon Symbol C. A nonmetallic element.

Carbon dioxide A gas which, dissolved in water, forms weak carbonic acid. As a product of metabolism by the oxidation of carbon, it leaves the body via the lungs. It can be compressed until it freezes, and then forms a solid (carbon dioxide snow, also known as dry ice) used as an escharotic in various skin conditions. Inhalations of the gas in a 5–7% mixture with oxygen are useful for stimulating the depth of respiration.

Carbon monoxide A colorless gas that is very poisonous. It is a major constituent of coal gas and is usually present in the exhaust gases from petrol and diesel engines. In poisoning there is vertigo, flushed face with very red lips, loss of consciousness, and convulsions. The blood is bright red because of formation of carboxyhemoglobin.

Carbon tetrachloride A powerful anthelmintic used in treating hookworm and whipworm. Also used in cleaning fluids; the inhalation of vapors in solvent abuse can depress central nervous system activity and degeneration of the liver and kidneys.

Carbonic anhydrase An enzyme that catalyses the decomposition of carbonic acid into carbon dioxide and water, facilitating transfer of carbon dioxide from tissues to blood and from blood to alveolar air.

Carboplatin Antineoplastic agent.

Carboxyhemoglobin The combination of carbon monoxide with hemoglobin in the blood in carbon monoxide poisoning.

Carbodylase An enzyme that catalyzes the removal of carboxyl group (COOH) from amino acids in the presence of vitamin B_1 acting as an coenzyme.

Carboxylation Replacement of hydrogen by a carboxyl (COOH) molecule.

Carboxylic acid Organic acid with COOH group.

Carbuncle An acute staphylococcal inflammation of subcutaneous tissues, which causes local thrombosis in the veins and death of tissue with several discharging sinuses. In appearance, it resembles a collection of boils.

Carbutamide An oral hypoglycemic agent.

Carcinoembryonic antigen (CEA) A class of antigen in fetus and expressed by colonic tumors. CEA level returns to normal after complete removal of colonic tumor.

Carcinogen Any substance or agent that can produce a cancer.

Carcinogenic Pertaining to substances or agents that produce or predispose to cancer.

Carcinoid Tumor of Argentaffin cells in the GI tract, bronchi, ovary, secreting serotonin.

Carcinoid syndrome A rare condition associated with certain tumors, which spread to other parts of the body. Marked by attacks of severe cyanotic flushing of the skin and by diarrhea, bronchoconstrictive attacks, pain, serious heart damage, sudden drops in blood pressure, oedema and ascites. Symptoms are caused by serotonin, prostaglandins and other biologically active substances secreted by the tumor.

Carcinoma A malignant growth of epithelial tissue. Microscopically, the cells resemble those of the tissue in which the growth has arisen.

Adenoic carcinoma Adeno carcinoma.

Basal cell carcina A rodent ulcer *(See Ulcer)*.

Epithelial carcinoma Epithelioma.

Squamous cell carcinoma One arising from the squamous epithelium of the skin.

Carcinomatosis The condition in a carcinoma has given rise to widespread metastases.

Carcinophilia Having affinity for cancer cells.

Carderlli's sign Pulsating movement of trachea with aortic aneurysm.

Cardia The cardiac orifice of the stomach.

Cardiac 1. Pertaining to the heart. 2. Pertaining to the cardia.

Cardiac arrest The cessation of the heart beat.

Cardiac asthma *(See Asthma).*

Cardiac atrophy Fatty degeneration of the heart muscle.

Cardiac bed One that can be manipulated to form a chair shape for those who are comfortable only when sitting up.

Cardiac catheterization A procedure whereby a radiopaque catheter is passed from an arm vein to the heart. Its passage through heart can be watched on a screen. Also blood pressure readings and specimens can be taken, thus aiding diagnosis of heart abnormalities.

Cardiac cirrhosis Cirrhosis of liver secondary to a cardiac cause. Commonly constructive pericarditis.

Cardiac cycle The sequence of events, lasting about 0.8s, during which the heart completes one contraction.

Cardiac failure Condition resulting from inability of heart to pump sufficient blood to meet the body needs.

Cardiac massage Rhythmic compression of the heart performed in order to reestablish circulation of the blood in cardiac arrest.

Cardiac monitor (cardiorator) Equipment used to monitor and visually record the cardiac cycle.

Cardiac output Blood ejected from left/right ventricle per minute, usually 3 lit/m^2.

Cardiac pacemaker An electrical device that stimulates the heart muscle to maintain myocardial contractions *(See Pacemaker).*

Cardiac plexus Branches of vagus and sympathetic trunk encircling base of heart.

Cardiac position A position of comfort for the patients of asthma and cardiac diseases, who are unable to breathe easily in lying-down position. The patient is propped up in sitting position with the means of back rest and pillows and an over bed table is placed in front with a pillow on it, so that the patient can lean forward and take rest.

Cardiac reflex Slowing of heart rate from stimulation of sensory nerve endings in the walls of carotid sinus from a rise in arterial blood pressure (Marey's law).

Cardiac reserve The capacity of heart to increase cardiac output and raise blood pressure to meet body requirements.

Cardiac stimulant A pharmacological agent that increases the action of the heart. Cardiac glycosides, e.g., digoxin and digitalis, increase myocardial contractions and decrease the heart rate and conduction velocity, thus allowing more time for the ventricles to relax and fill with blood.

Cardiectasis Dilatation of heart.

Cardiff count-to-ten chart Method of evaluating the intrauterine well-being of the fetus in which the pregnant woman records fetal movements during her normal activities. If the count is less than 10, further medical evaluation is recommended.

Cardialgia Pain in the region of the heart. Cardiodynia.

Cardice A solid form of carbon dioxide used primarily as a coolant. Also known as dry ice.

Cardinal of first importance. Fundamental.

Cardinal ligaments Deep transverse cervical ligaments. Mackenrodt's ligaments.

Cardiocele Hemitation of heart through an opening in the phragm or chest wall.

Cardiocentesis Puncture of heart.

Cardiodynia Pain in the heart

Cardioesophageal reflux Reflux of gastric contents in the esophagus.

Cardiogenesis Formation and growth of embryonic heart.

Cardiogenic Originating in the heart. *Cardiogenic shock* Shock caused by disease or failure of heart action.

Cardiogram Recording of electrical activity of heart.

Cardiography The recording of the force and movements of the heart.

Cardiolipin An extract of beef heart used for test of syphilis.

Cardiologist A medically qualified person skilled in the diagnosis of heart disease.

Cardiology The study of the heart; how it works and its diseases.

Cardiomegaly Enlargement of heart.

Cardiomyopathy A chronic disorder of the heart muscle not resulting from atherosclerosis.

Cardilomyopexy Stitching of pectoral muscle to cardiac muscle in order to augment vascular supply to heart muscle.

Cardiomyoplasty Reinforcement of cardiac muscle contractility by transfer of lattimus dorsi to surround the heart and to contract synchronously with cardiac muscle.

Cardiomyotomy Surgical therapy of achalasia in which the muscle surrounding cardio esophageal junction is cut but the mucus membrane is left intact.

Cardiopathy Any disease of the heart.

Cardioplegia Deliberate arrest of cardiac function by use of hypothermia, potassium, etc.

Cardiopulmonary Relating to the heart and lungs.

Cardiopulmonary bypass The use of the heart-lung machine to oxygenate and pump the blood round the body while the surgeon operates on the heart.

Cardiopulmonary resuscitation Emergency medical care to a person whose heart and lung function is going to stop or has recently stopped. Artificial respiration and cardiac massage are the two principal components of CPR. *(See Annexure)*

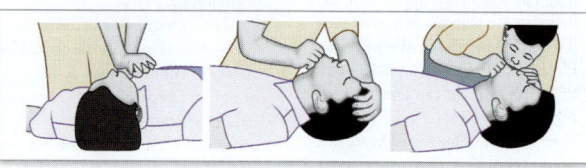

Cardiopulmonary Resuscitation

Cardiorrhexis Rupture of heart.

Cardioscope A flexible instrument with a lens and illumination attachment; used for examining the inside of the heart.

Cardiospasm Spasm of the sphincter muscle at the cardiac end of the stomach. It may result in dilatation of the esophagus, difficulty in swallowing solids and liquids, and regurgitation of undigested food. Achalasia.

Cardiothoracic Pertaining to the heart and thoracic cavity. A specialized branch of surgery.

Cardiotocography The simultaneous recording of the fetal heart rate, fetal movements and uterine contractions in order to discover possible lack of oxygen (hypoxia) to the fetus. Fetal monitoring.

Cardiotomy Surgical incision into the heart or the cardia.

Cardiotomy syndrome An inflammatory reaction after heart surgery. There is pyrexia, pericarditis and pleural effusion.

Cardiotoxic Anything that has a deleterious or poisonous effect on the heart. Cardiovascular Concerning the heart and blood vessels.

Cardiovascular system The heart together with the two chief networks of blood vessels: the systemic circulation and the pulmonary circulation.

Cardioversion A method of restoring an abnormal heart rhythm to normal (as in atrial fibrillation) by means of an electric shock.

Cardioverter Defibrillator that delivers electric shockwaves for treating cardiac arrhythmia/ventricular standstill.

Carditis Inflammation of the heart.

Care The provision of welfare and protection to children, the elderly in need, the sick and other vulnerable people. An important component of nursing practice (and that of other health care professionals) that extends the concept to include psychosocial and physical care interventions.

C. certificate A set of introductory skills, knowledge and behaviors that enables entrants new to health and social care to provide compassionate, safe and high-quality care and support. The care certificate is based on 15 standards, which must all be completed before the care certificate can be awarded.

C. contact time Part of the safer-staffing initiative developed by the Chief Nursing Officer for England providing guidance for organizations about the amount of time nurses spend in direct contact with patients, and the capacity and capability of their workforce.

C. hours per patient day (CHPPD) Measures the hours of direct care given per patient by nurses and health care support workers in acute settings.

C. pathway An integrated approach or pathway, which determines and utilizes locally agreed multidisciplinary practice based on guidelines and evidence for a specific patient or client group.

C. plan and individualized plan for the care of a patient Nursing information in this document includes data from the patient assessment regarding the patient's needs and nursing diagnosis, the specific nursing interventions outlined, the desired goals stated and the priorities set. *(See Nursing (Care Plan)).*

Care Act 2014 Gives the right to ask for an assessment from social services to the people in England, who provide substantial care on a regular basis. Local councils have a duty to promote the wellbeing of carers. In Wales, Scotland and Northern Ireland, there is country-specific legislation to cover carers' rights.

Care in the community Policy whereby patients with continuing medical and social care needs are cared for in a community or domestic, rather than institutional, setting. Care in the community is part of the UK Government agenda to give patients and clients more right to choose and be involved in their care.

Care pathway An integrated approach or pathway which determines and utilizes locally agreed multidisciplinary practice based on guidelines and evidence for a specific patient or client group. It may form part or all of the clinical record; it documents the care given and facilitates the evaluation of outcomes.

Care plans *(See Nursing care plan).*

Care Programme Approach (CPA) A way that services are assessed, planned, co-ordinated and reviewed for someone with mental health problems or a range of related complex needs.

Care Quality Commission (CQC) The regulator of health and adult social care in England. It monitors, inspects and rates care services to ensure they are safe, caring, effective, responsive and well led on an on-going basis. This includes services provided by the NHS, local authorities, private companies and voluntary organizations – whether in hospitals, GP surgeries, clinics, care homes or people's own homes.

Caregiver Strain Index (CSI) Measure used by community and mental health nurses to assess caregiver strain for those carers who are providing care for a family member or partner in the home. The results of the questionnaire answered by the caregiver provide a crude analysis of how well the carer is coping in the care situation.

Carer A nonprofessional who provides care for someone in need at home; most commonly a member of the individual's family.

Caries Suppuration and subsequent decay of bone, corresponding to ulceration in soft tissues. In caries, the bone dissolves; in necrosis it separates in large pieces and is thrown off.

Dental caries Decay of the teeth due to penetration of bacteria through the enamel to the dentine.

Spinal caries Tuberculosis of the spine. Pott's disease.

Cariogenic Conducive to dental caries formation.

Carisoprodol A muscle relaxant, acting through CNS.

Carminative An aromatic drug that relieves flatulence and associated colic. Cloves, ginger, cardamon and peppermint are examples.

Carmustine Antineoplastic agent.

Carnal Related to desires or appetite of flesh.

Carneous Fleshy.

Carneous mole tumor of organized blood clot surrounding a dead fetus in the uterus *(See Abortion)*.

Carnett's sign Method of determining the source of pain while evaluating a surgical abdomen, when the patient raises his head after being in supine position. It is positive, if the pain increases or remains the same and indicates that the source of origin lies in the abdominal wall and not the viscera.

Carnitine A chemical important in metabolism of palmitic and stearic acid. Used therapeutically in treatment of myopathy due to carnitine deficiency.

Carnivorous Flesh eating.

Carotene The coloring matter in carrots, tomatoes and other yellow foods and in fats. It is a provitamin capable of conversion into vitamin A in the liver.

Carotenemia A benign condition with high blood carotene level causing yellow coloration of skin but not of conjunctiva.

Carotid The principal artery on each side of the neck.

Carotid bodies Chemoreceptors in the bifurcation of both carotid arteries which monitor the oxygen content of the blood.

Carotid sinuses Dilated portions of the internal carotids containing the baroreceptors that monitor blood pressure.

Carotid siphon The S shaped terminal portion of internal carotid artery.

Carotinase Enzyme that converts carotene into Vitamin A.

Carpal Relating to the carpus or wrist.

Carpel tunnel The canal beneath flexor retinaculum of wrist in which flexor tendons and median nerve pass.

Carpel tunnel syndrome (CTS) Compression of the median nerve at the wrist causing numbing and tingling in the fingers.

Carphology Involuntary picking at bed clothes, muttering, etc. the signs of impending end.

Carpopedal Relating to the wrist and foot.

Carpopedal spasm Spasm of the hands and feet occurs in tetany and hyperventilation.

Carpus The bones forming the wrist and arranged in two rows: (a) Scaphoid, lunate, triquetral, pisiform; (b) Trapezium, trapezoid, capitate, hamate.

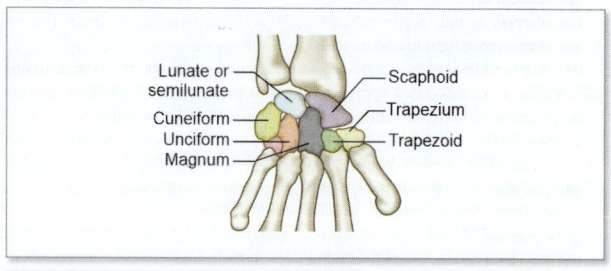

Lunate or semilunate
Cuneiform
Unciform
Magnum
Scaphoid
Trapezium
Trapezoid

Carpus

Carr-Hill formula A resource formula used to distribute funding to general practices based on costs of delivering routine primary care services to a practice population.

Carrier 1. A person who harbors the microorganisms of an infectious disease but is not necessarily affected by it, although that person may infect others. 2. One who carries and passes on a hereditary abnormality.

Cartilage A specialized, fibrous connective tissue present in adults and forming most of the temporary skeleton in the embryo. The three most important types are hyaline cartilage, elastic cartilage and fibrocartilage. Also, a general term for a mass of such tissue in a particular site in the body.

Elastic cartilage Cartilage containing elastic fibers and forming the pinna of the ear, the epiglottis and part of the nasal septum.

Fibro-cartilage Cartilage in which bundles of white fibers predominate, forming the intervertebral disks and costal cartilage.

Hyaline cartilage Flexible, somewhat elastic, semitransparent cartilage with an opalescent bluish tint, composed of a basophilic fibril containing substance with cavities in which the chondrocytes occur.

Cartilaginous of the nature of cartilage.

Caruncle A small fleshy swelling.

Lacrimal caruncle A small reddish body situated at the medial junction of the eyelids.

Urethral caruncle A small fleshy growth occurring at the urinary orifice in females and giving rise to great pain on micturition.

Carvedilol Beta blocker.

Cascara A laxative prepared from the bark of the Californian buckthorn. It maybe prepared as an elixir or tablets.

Case A particular instance of disease, as in a case of leukemia, sometimes used incorrectly to designate the patient with the disease.

Case conference A meeting of professionals involved in the care of a particular person (often a child), to agree patterns of action and to monitor progress.

Case control study An epidemiological study in which the characteristics of cases of disease are compared with a matched control group of persons without the disease. Also called retrospective study, case reference study.

Case fatality rate The number of persons dying of a particular disease expressed as a proportion of the total contracting the disease; usually expressed as a percentage.

Case history The collected data concerning an individual and that person's family and environment, including the medical history and any other information that maybe useful in analyzing and diagnosing the health issues or for instructional or research purposes.

Case load A system of care whereby a nurse, midwife or health visitor is responsible for a group of patients or clients.

Case mix Database computerized record system which combines all the data received from patient administration systems and operational systems to provide a comprehensive set of information about all the treatment and services received by each patient/client during an episode of care. The information helps to develop normal care profiles for different groups, to analyze and compare different treatments, etc. It may also be used as part of the medical audit process.

Caseation Degeneration of diseased tissue into a cheesy mass.

Casein The chief protein of milk. It forms a curd from which cheese is made.

Casein hydrolysate A predigested-concentrated protein; a useful supplement for a high-protein diet.

Casoni's test Appearance of wheal surrounded by erythematous zone following intradermal injection of sterile hydatid fluid. The test is false positive in 40% cases in diagnosis of *Echinococcus granulosus*.

Cast 1. A positive copy of an object, e.g., a mold of a hollow organ (a renal tubule bronchiole, etc.), formed of effused plastic matter and extruded from the body, as in a urinary cast; named, according to constituents, as epithelial, fatty, waxy, etc. 2. A positive copy of the tissues of the jaws, made in an impression, over which denture bases or other restorations maybe fabricated. 3. To form an object in a mold. 4. A stiff dressing or casing, usually made of plaster of Paris, used to immobilize body parts. 5. Strabismus.

Castellani's paint Composed of phenol, resorcinol, used as disinfectant for skin and as an antifungal.

Castle factor Also known as Castle's intrinsic factor, it is a small mucoprotein secreted by the gastric parietal cells. This factor is required to facilitate adequate absorption of vitamin B_{12} by the stomach. Deficiency of this factor can result in pernicious anemia.

Castor oil A vegetable oil. Internally it is a purgative. Externally it is protective and soothing and maybe used in ointments or in eye drops.

Castration The removal of the testes in the male or the ovaries in the female.

Casuality Accident/injury/death.

CAT Computerized axial tomography.

Cat-scratch disease (fever) A benign, subacute, regional lymphadenitis resulting from a scratch or bite of a cat or a scratch from a surface contaminated by a cat. No specific causative agent has been isolated but a viral etiology is suspected.

Catabolism The chemical breakdown of complex substances in the body to form simpler ones, with a release of energy *(See Metabolism)*.

Catalase An enzyme found in body cells, including red blood cells and liver cells.

Catalepsy A trance like state with diminished responsiveness but often intact perception.

Catalysis Enhancement of a chemical reaction by a catalyst.

Catalyst A substance that hastens or brings about a chemical change without itself undergoing alteration; for example, enzymes act as catalysts in the process of digestion.

Catamenia Menstruation.

Cataphasia Involuntary repetition of same word.

Cataphoria Tendency of visual axes to incline below the horizontal plane.

Cataplasm A poultice. It acts as a counter-irritant. Materials of which it can be made are linseed, bread and bran, but kaolin is more frequently used.

Cataplexy Sudden recurrent loss of muscle power without unconsciousness, often associated with narcolepsy. It maybe produced by any strong emotion.

Catapres Clonidine, an antihypertensive agent.

Cataract Opacity of the crystalline lens of the eye causing partial or complete blindness. It maybe congenital or maybe due to senility, injury or diabetes.

Catarrh Chronic inflammation of a mucous membrane accompanied by an excessive discharge of mucus.

Catatonia A syndrome of motor abnormalities occurring in schizophrenia, but less commonly in organic cerebral disease, characterized by stupor and the adoption of strange postures, or outbursts of excitement and hyperactivity. The patient may change suddenly from one of these states to the other.

Catchment area A specific geographical area for which a trust or health center is responsible for providing the health care services.

Catecholamines A group of compounds that have the effect of sympathetic nerve stimulation. They have an aromatic and an amine portion and include dopamine, adrenaline and noradrenaline.

Catgut A substance prepared from the intestines of sheep and used in surgery for sutures and ligatures. It is gradually absorbed in the body at a variable rate, according to the preparation.

Catharsis 1. A cleansing or purgation. 2. The bringing into consciousness and the emotional reliving of a forgotten (repressed) painful experience as a means of releasing anxiety and tension.

Cathartic A purgative drug.

Catheter A tubular, flexible instrument, passed through body channels for withdrawal of fluids from (or introduction of fluids into) a body cavity. Catheters are made of a variety of materials including plastic, metal, rubber and gum-elastic.

Angiographic catheter One through which a contrast medium is injected for visualization of the vascular system of an organ.

Arterial catheter One inserted into an artery utilized as part of a catheter-transducer-monitor system to continuously observe the blood pressure of critically ill patients. An arterial catheter also maybe inserted for radiological studies of the arterial system and for delivery of chemo-

therapeutic agents directly into the arterial supply of malignant tumors.

Cardiac catheter A long fine catheter specially designed for passage, usually through a peripheral blood vessel, into the chambers of the heart under fluoroscopic control.

Central venous catheter A long, fine catheter inserted into a vein for the purpose of administering, through a large blood vessel, parenteral fluids (as in parenteral nutrition), antibiotics and other therapeutic agents. This type of catheter is also used in the measurement of central venous pressure *(See Central venous pressure).*

Self-retaining catheter A catheter made in such a way that after introduction the blind end expands so that it can remain in the bladder. Useful for continuous or intermittent drainage or where frequent specimens are required.

Ureteric catheter A fine gum elastic catheter passed up the ureter to the renal pelvis and used to insert a contrast medium in retrograde urography.

Cathexis The emotional or mental energy used in concentrating on an object or idea.

Catheterization The insertion of a catheter into a body cavity.

Cathode 1. The negative electrode or pole of an electric current. 2. The negative pole of a battery *(See Anode).*

Cation A positively charged ion, which moves toward the cathode when an electric current is passed through an electrolytic solution, e.g., hydrogen (H^+), sodium (Na^+) *(See Anion).*

Cauda A tail-like appendage.

Cauda equina The bundle of coccygeal, sacral and lumbar nerves with which the spinal cord terminates.

Caudal Referring to a cauda.

Caudal block A local anesthetic agent injected into the sacral canal so that operations maybe carried out in the peritoneal area without a general anesthetic.

Caudate Possessing a tail.

Caul The amnion, which occasionally does not rupture but envelops the infant's head at birth.

Causalgia An intense burning pain which persists after peripheral nerve injuries.

Caustic A substance, usually a strong acid or alkali, capable of burning organic tissue. Silver nitrate (lunar c), carbolic acid and carbon dioxide snow are those most commonly used.

Cauterization The destruction of tissue with cautery.

Cautery 1. The application of searing heat by a hot instrument, an electric current or other means such as a laser. 2. An agent so used.

Cold cautery Cauterization by carbon dioxide, called also cryocautery.

Cavalry bone Sesamoid bone in adductor longus of thigh in riders.

Cavernitis Inflammation of corpus cavernosum of penis.

Cavernoma Cavernous hemangioma.

Cavernous Having caverns or hollows.

Cavernous breathing Sounds heard on auscultation over a pulmonary cavity.

Cavernous sinus A venous channel lying on either side of the body of the sphenoid bone through which pass the internal carotid artery and several nerves.

Cavernous sinus thrombosis A serious complication of any infection of the face, the veins from the orbit draining into the sinus and carrying the infection into the cranium.

Cavitation The formation of cavities, e.g., in the lung in tuberculosis.

Cavitis Inflammation of vena cava.

Cavity A confined space or hollow or potential hollow within the body or one of its organs, e.g., the abdominal cavity or a decayed hollow in a tooth.

Cavity preparation Artificial cavity prepared in teeth for tooth restoration, e.g., root canal treatment.

CCG Clinical commissioning group

CCU Critical care unit; coronary care unit.

Cecotomy Surgical removal of cecum.

Cecopexy Surgical fixation of cecum to abdominal wall.

Cecum The first portion of large intestine, 6 cm in length, 7.5 cm in width with appendix arising at its lower end.

Cefadroxil Long acting oral cephalosporin.

Cefdinir Oral cephalosporin.

Cefotaxime A third generation cephalosporin antibiotic having a broad spectrum of activity, used to treat infra-abdominal infections, bone and joint infections, gonorrhea, and other infections due to susceptible organisms, penicillinase-producing strains.

Cefoxitin A semisynthetic cephalosporin antibiotic, effective against Gram-negative organisms, with strong resistance to degradation by β-lactamase.

Cefpodoxime Oral third generation cephalosporin.

Celiac disease Intestinal malabsorption syndrome mostly gluten induced.

Celiac plexus Sympathetic plexus near origin of celiac artery.

Celevac Trade name for methylcellulose.

Cell 1. The basic structural unit of living organisms. A microscopic mass of protoplasm consisting of a nucleus surrounded by cytoplasm and enclosed in a cell membrane, from which all organic tissues are constructed. Each cell can reproduce itself by mitosis. 2. A small, more or less enclosed, space.

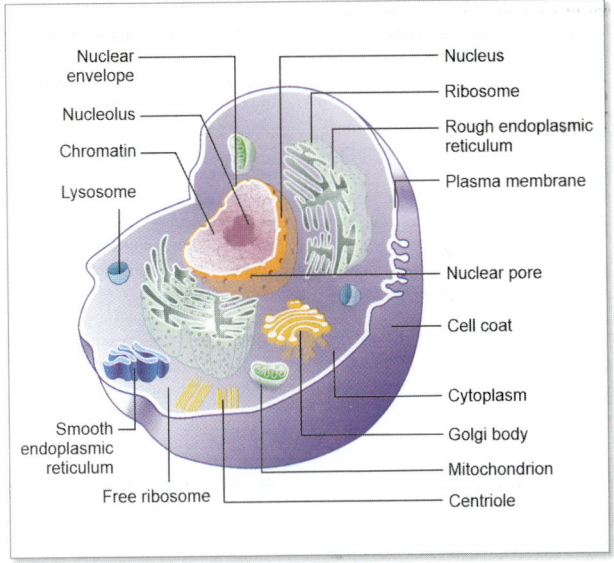

Nuclear envelope
Nucleus
Ribosome
Nucleolus
Rough endoplasmic reticulum
Chromatin
Plasma membrane
Lysosome
Nuclear pore
Cell coat
Smooth endoplasmic reticulum
Cytoplasm
Golgi body
Mitochondrion
Free ribosome
Centriole

Structure of Eukaryotic Cell

Cell kinetics The study of growth and division of cells.

Cell membrane The envelop surrounding cell, composed of carbohydrate, lipid and protein.

Cell organelle Structures in the cytoplasm like mitochondria, golgi complex, endoplasmic recticulum, ribosomes, etc.

Cellophane Thin transparent waterproof sheet of cellulose acetate, used as dialysis membrane.

Cellular immunity T-cell mediated immune reaction, basis of organ transplant rejection, lepromin test and BCG vaccination.

Cellulitis A diffuse inflammation of connective tissue, especially of subcutaneous tissue, which causes a typical browny, edematous appearance of the part.

Cellulose A carbohydrate forming the covering of vegetable cells, i.e., vegetable fibers. Not digestible in the alimentary tract of humans but gives bulk and, as "roughage", stimulates peristalsis.

Celsius scale *A Celsius, Swedish astronomer. 1701–1744.* A temperature scale with the melting point of ice set at 0° and the boiling point of water at 100°. The normal temperature of the human body is 36.9ºC. Formely known as the centigrade scale *(See Fahrenheit scale)*.

Cement Material that makes one substance bind to another.

Cementitis Inflammation of dental cementum.

Cementoblast Cells lining the developing tooth depositing cementum.

Cementoclast Multinucleated large cells that remove cementum *(i.e., odontoclasts)*.

Cementoma A benign fibrous connective tissue growth usually at root of tooth containing small masses of cementum.

Cementum Cement. Connective tissue with a bone-like structure which covers the root of a tooth and supports it within the socket.

Censor 1. A member of a committee on ethics or for critical examination of a medical or other society. 2. The psychic influence that prevents unconscious thoughts and wishes coming into consciousness.

Censorship In psychiatry, the process of selecting, accepting or rejecting conscious ideas, memories and impulses arising from the individual's subconscious.

Center A group of nerve cells in CNS subserving special function.

Apneustic center Center in brainstem regulating breathing.

Auditory center Center for hearing in the anterior part of transverse temporal gyri.

Autonomic center Center controlling autonomic functions located in hypothalamus, brainstem and spinal cord.

Cardioaccelerator center and cardioinhibitor center Both present in medulla oblongata, innervating the heart through sympathetic and parasympathetic fibers.

Broca's center Center in inferior frontal gyrus (area) controlling speech.

Ciliospinal center Center in spinal cord giving rise to sympathetic fibers dilating the pupil.

Defecation center Two centers located in medulla oblongata and in S2-S4 segments of spinal cord.

Deglutition center Center in medulla oblongata on the floor of fourth ventricle that controls swallowing.

Heat regulating center A heat loss and a heat production center located in medulla.

Micturition center Located in S2-S4 medulla and hypothalamus controlling micturition.

Pneumotaxic center Center in pons that rhythmically inhibits inspiration.

Respiratory center The inspiratory, expiratory and pneumotaxic centers in medulla oblongata controlling the respiratory movements.

Satiety center An area in ventromedial thalamus that modulates eating behavior.

Census Enumeration of a population. The national census is taken every 10 years. It usually records name, address, age, gender, occupation, marital status and other social information.

Centers for disease control Abbreviated CDC. An agency which serves as a center for the control, prevention and investigation of diseases.

Centigrade *(See Celsius scale)*.

Centigram Hundredth of gram, 10 mg.

Centiliter Hundredth of liter, 10 mL.

Centimeter Hundredth of meter, 10 mm.

Centile *(See Percentile)*.

Centipede Arthropod with long flat segmented body each with a pair of legs.

Central Pertaining to the center or midpoint.

Central nervous system Abbreviated CNS. The brain and spinal cord.

Central venous pressure The pressure recorded by the introduction of a catheter into the right atrium in order to monitor the condition of a patient after a major operative procedure, such as heart surgery.

Central sterile supplies and disinfection unit (CSSD) A hospital sterilization and disinfection unit or department.

Central core disease A form of benign familial polymyopathy characterized by hypotonia and nonpressive muscle weakness.

Central venous catheter/line A special catheter that is inserted into a large central vein either through a peripheral vein or a skin tunnel for the administration of drugs, the infusing of hypertonic fluids and to measure pressures. The catheter/line also allows long-term access for the administration of medications, nutritional support and blood products.

Centrifugal Conveying away from a center, such as from the brain to the periphery. Efferent; the reverse of centripetal.

Centrifuge An apparatus that rotates at high speed. If a test tube, for example, is filled with a fluid such as blood or urine and rotated in a centrifuge, any bacteria, cells or other solids in it are precipitated.

Centrilobular concerning The center of a lobule.

Centriole A minute organelle consisting of a hollow cylinder closed at one end and open at the other. During mitosis the centrioles migrate to opposite poles of the cell to which spindle fibers are attached.

Centripetal Conveying from the periphery to the center. Afferent; the reverse of centrifugal.

Centromere The region(s) of the chromosomes which become(s) allied with the spindle fibers at mitosis and meiosis.

Centrosome A body in the cytoplasm of most animal cells, close to the nucleus. It divides during mitosis, one half migrating to each daughter cell.

Centrosphere The cell center, in an area of clear cytoplasm near the nucleus.

Cephalexin A cephalosporin antibiotic that maybe administered orally.

Cephalgia Headache, pain in the body.

Cephalhematoma A swelling beneath the pericranium, containing blood, which maybe found on the head of the newborn infant. Caused by pressure during labor. Gradually reabsorbed within 2–3 months.

Cephalic index Maximal length of head divided by maximal breadth × 100.

Cephalocele Cerebral hernia *(See Hernia)*.

Cephalography Radiographic examination of the contours of the head.

Cephalometry Measurement of the dimensions of the head of a living person either directly or by radiography *(See also Pelvimetry)*.

Cephaloridine An antibiotic that is effective against a wide range of organisms.

Cephalosporin Any one of a group of broad spectrum antibiotics derived from the mold *Cephalosporium.*

Cephradine A cephalosporin antibiotic similar in action to cephaloridine.

Cercaria A free swimming stage in the development of fluke or trematode.

Cerclage [Fr.] Encircling of a part with a ring or loop, as for correction of an incompetent cervix uteri or fixation of the adjacent ends of a fractured bone *(See Shirodkar's suture)*.

Cerebellum The portion of the brain below the cerebrum and above the medulla oblongata. Its functions include the coordination of fine voluntary movements and posture.

Cerebral Relating to the cerebrum.

Cerebral cortex The outer layer of the cerebrum, composed of neurons.

Cerebral hemorrhage Rupture of a cerebral blood vessel. Likely causes are aneurysm and hypertension *(See Apoplexy)*.

Cerebral hernia (See Hernia).

Cerebral irritation A condition of general nervous irritability, abnormality, often with photophobia, which maybe an early sign of meningitis, tumor of the brain, etc. It is also associated with trauma.

Cerebral palsy A condition caused by injury to the brain during or immediately after birth. Coordination of movement is affected, and may cause the child to be flaccid or athetoid, in which condition there is constant random and uncontrolled movement *(See Spastic).*

Cerebration Mental activity.

Cerebromalacia Softening of cerebrum.

Cerebroside A lipid constituent of nerve tissue.

Cerebrospinal Relating to the brain and spinal cord.

Cerebrospinal fever Inflammation of brain and meninges.

Cerebrospinal fluid Abbreviated CSF. The fluid made in the choroids plexus of ventricles of the brain and circulating from them into the subarachnoid space around the brain and spinal cord.

Cerebrovascular Pertaining to the arteries and veins of the brain.

Cerebrovascular accident A disorder arising from an embolus, thrombus or hemorrhage in the cerebrum.

Cerebrovascular disease Any disorder of the blood vessels of the brain and its meninges.

Cerebrum The largest part of the brain, occupying the greater portion of the cranium and consisting of the hemispheres divided by the longitudinal fissure. Each hemisphere is divided into right and left hemisphere, contains a lateral ventricle. The internal substance is white and the convoluted surface is gray. The center of the higher functions of the brain.

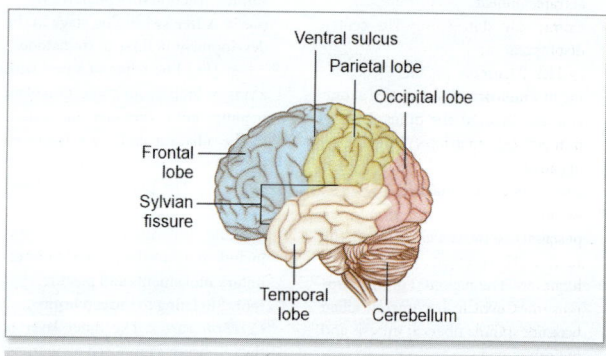

Ventral sulcus
Parietal lobe
Occipital lobe
Frontal lobe
Sylvian fissure
Temporal lobe
Cerebellum

Cerebrum

Ceruloplasmin Copper transporting glycoprotein in blood.

Cerumen A waxy substance secreted by the ceruminous glands of the auditory canal. Ear wax.

Ceruminosis Excessive secretion of cerumen.

Cervical Pertaining to the neck or the constricted part of an organ, e.g., uterine cervix.

Cervical canal The passage through the uterine cervix.

Cervical cancer Cancer of the uterine cervix.

Cervical collar A rigid or semi-rigid immobilizing support for the neck.

Cervical rib A short, extra rib, often bilateral, which sometimes occurs on the seventh cervical vertebra and may cause pressure on an artery or nerve.

Cervical smear A test for disorders of the cervical cells; material is scraped from the uterine cervix and examined microscopically.

Cervical spondylosis A degenerative disease of the intervertebral joints and disks of the neck.

Cervical vertebra One of the seven bones forming the neck portion of the spinal column.

Cervicitis Inflammation of the neck of the uterus.

Cervix A constricted portion or neck.

Cervix uteri The neck of the uterus; it is about 2 cm long and projects into the vagina. Capable of wide dilatation during childbirth.

CESDI Confidential enquiry into Stillbirths and Deaths in Infancy *(See Confidential enquiry).*

Cesarean section Delivery of fetus by giving incision on uterus, either extraperitoneal or intraperitoneal. Commonly done in cephalopelvic disproportion, breech presentation and fetal distress.

Cestode Tapeworm.

Cesium 137 Cs an radioactive isotope of metal cesium issued for radiation of cancer tissue.

Cestoda A subclass that includes tapeworms that have a scolex and a chain of segments (proglottids).

Cetirizine H$_1$ receptor blocker antiallergic.

Cetrimide Cetyltrimethyl ammonium bromide (CTAB). A detergent and antiseptic widely used for preoperative skin preparation and the cleansing of wounds.

Chaddock's reflex 1. Extension of great toe when outer edge of dorsum of foot is stroked 2. Flexion of wrist and fanning of fingers when tendon of palmaris longus is pressed; positive in corticospinal tract lesions.

Chadwick's sign Also known as Jacquemier's sign, this is a sign of pregnancy. This sign is associated with bluish discoloration of cervix, vagina and vulva due to venous congestion.

Chafe Irritation of the skin as caused by the friction between skin folds. Occurs particularly in moist areas.

Chafing Erythema, maceration and fissuring of skin due to friction of clothing in axilla, groin, between digits.

Chaga's disease African trypanosomiasis.

Chalasia Relaxation of sphincters.

Chalazion A meibomian or tarsal cyst. A swollen sebaceous gland in the eyelid. A small, hard tumor may develop.

Chalicosis Pneumonoconiosis associated with inhalation of dust produced during stone cutting.

Challenge In immunology, administration of specific antigen to an individual known to be sensitive to that antigen in order to produce an immune response.

Chamber Closed space or compartment.

Chamber anterior, posterior Anterior and posterior chambers of eye containing aqueous humor, lying between cornea and iris, iris and lens respectively.

Chamber Boyden Chamber used to measure chemotaxis.

Chamber hyperbaric Closed chamber with high internal air pressure, e.g., hyperbaric oxygen chambers for treatment of frost bite, gangrene decompression sickness.

Chamber pulp The chamber within crown of tooth containing nerve endings and blood vessels.

Chancre 1. The initial lesion of syphilis developing at the site of inoculation. 2. A papular lesion occurring at the site of infection in tuberculosis or in sporotrichosis.

Chancroid Soft chancre. A venereal ulceration, due to *Haemophilus ducreyi* accompanied by inflammation and suppuration of the local glands.

Character The combination of traits and qualities distinguishing the unique nature of the individual.

Character change Indicates alteration in a person's recognized behavior to one alien to the person's normal manner of conduct.

Character disorder A chronic state in which the person exhibits maladaptive and unacceptable forms of behavior and social response.

Charcoal Activated charcoal used for absorption of gas and poisonous alkaloids in GI tract.

Charcot's disease or joint *JM Charcot, French neurologist, 1825 – 1893.* A chronic progressive, degenerative disease of the stress-bearing portion of one or more joints. The disease is the result of an underlying neurological disorder, e.g., diabetic neuropathy, or tabes dorsalis from syphilis, or leprosy.

Charcot's triad Nystagmus, intention tremor and scanning speech. A trio of signs of disseminated sclerosis.

Charcot-Leyden crystal Colorless, hexagonal, double pointed and often needle like crystals found in sputum of asthmatic patients and in feces of patients of intestinal amebiasis.

Charcot-Marie-Tooth disease A form of hereditary progressive neuromuscular atrophy usually developing in childhood, commonly males. (SYN-peroneal muscular atrophy).

Charcots triad Nystagmus, intention tremor and scanning speech. A trio of signs of disseminated sclerosis.

Charle's Law At constant pressure, a given amount of gas will expand in direct proportion to absolute temperature.

Charnley's arthroplasty *Sir I Charnley. British orthopedic surgeon, 1911–1982.* The replacement of the hip joint using a plastic acetabulum and a steel femoral head *(See Arthroplasty)*.

Chart A record in graphic or tabular form.

Genealogical chart A graph showing various descendants of a common ancestor, used to indicate those affected by genetically determined disease.

Reading chart A chart with material printed in gradually increasing type sizes, used in testing acuity of near vision.

Reuss'c's Charts with colored letters printed on colored backgrounds, used in testing color vision.

Snellen chart A chart printed with block letters in gradually decreasing sizes, used in testing visual acuity.

Charting The keeping of a clinical record of the important fact about a patient and the progress of his or her illness. The patient's chart usually contains a medical history, a nursing history, results of physical examinations, laboratory reports, results of diagnostic tests, and the observations of the nursing staff. Medical treatments and nursing approaches are also recorded in the patient's chart *(See also Problem oriented record)*.

Chèdiak-Higashi syndrome AR disease in which neutrophils contain peroxidase positive inclusion bodies. Partial albinism, photophobia and pale optic fundi are the clinical features. Children usually die between 5 and 10 years of age due to lymphoma like disease.

Cheilitis Inflammation of lips.

Cheilosis Maceration at the angles of the mouth; fissures may also occur. It maybe associated with general debility or riboflavin deficiency.

Cheiropompholyx A skin disease characterized by vesicles on the palms and soles.

Chelate A chemical compound in which an atom of a metal is held in a molecular ring.

Chelating agent A drug that has the power of combining with certain metals and so aiding excretion to prevent or overcome poisoning *(See Dimercaprol and Penicillamine)*.

Chelation Red lips, with fissured angles of mouth commonly due to riboflavin deficiency.

Chemabrasion Use of chemicals to destroy superficial layers of skin to treat scars, tattoos, abnormal pigmentation.

Chemical change This differs from physical change as a profound alteration in properties results, usually permanently and usually accompanied by use of energy in a new substance, e.g., hydrogen (two atoms) plus oxygen produces water.

Chemical compound Any substance produced by chemical change, which may then be broken up into its components only by chemical means, unlike a mixture, which can usually be separated mechanically.

Chemical warfare Warfare with toxic chemical/biological agents. The chemicals used are nerve gases/disease producing organisms.

Chemiluminescence Light produced by chemical reactions without production of heat, e.g., light production during bacterial killing by neutrophils, fire flies.

Chemistry The science of dealing with the elements, the atoms which compose them and the compounds that they form.

Chemodectoma Tumor of chemoreceptor system, e.g., para ganglioma.

Chemoprophylaxis Use of drugs to prevent occurrence of disease.

Chemoreceptor A sensory nerve ending or group of cells that is sensitive to chemical stimuli in the blood.

Chemosis Swelling of the conjunctiva due to the presence of fluid; an edema of the conjunctiva.

Chemosurgery The destruction of tissue by chemical agents for therapeutic purposes, originally applied to chemical fixation of malignant, gangrenous or infected tissue with use of frozen sections to facilitate systematic microscopic control of its excision.

Chemotaxis The reaction of living cells to chemical stimuli. These are either attracted (positive c.) or repelled (negative c.) by acids, alkalis or other substances.

Chemotherapy The specific treatment of disease by the administration of chemical compounds.

Chemotherapeutic index The ratio of the toxicity of the drug, expressed as maximum tolerated dose/kg body weight to the minimal curative dose/kg of body weight.

Chemotropism Ability of impulse to progress or turn in certain direction in response to certain stimuli.

Chenodeoxycholic acid Used for dissolution of gallstones.

Cherry red spots Red spot in retina of Tayasch's disease.

Chest The thorax.

Barrel chest One more rounded than usual, with raised ribs and, usually, kyphosis. It is often present in emphysema.

Chest leads Leads applied to the chest during the course of an electrocardiographic recording.

Flail chest One where part of the chest wall moves in opposition to respiration as a result of multiple fractures of the ribs.

Pigeon chest A chest with the sternum protruding forward.

Cheyne-Stokes respiration *J Cheyne, British physician. 1776– 1836; W Stokes, British physician. 1804–1878.* Tidal respiration. A form of irregular but rhythmic breathing with temporary cessations (apnea). It is likely to be present in cerebral tumor, in narcotic poisoning and in advanced cases of arteriosclerosis and uremia.

Chiari malformations Structural defects in the cerebellum sometimes causing hydrocephalus as a result of obstruction of the cerebral spinal fluid. These malformations can also cause headaches, difficulty in concentrating and thinking and a range of other symptoms.

Chiari-Frommel syndrome Persistent amenorrhea and lactation following childbirth due to hyperprolactinemia.

Chiasma A crossing point.

Optic chiasma The crossing point of the optic nerves.

Chikungunya An arboviral infection with fever, joint pain and rash.

Chickenpox Varicella.

Chilblain A condition resulting from defective circulation when exposure to cold causes localized swelling and inflammation of the hands or feet, with severe itching and burning sensations.

Child The human young, from infancy to puberty.

Child abuse The non-accidental use of physical force or the non-accidental act of omission by a parent or other custodian responsible for the care of a child. Child abuse encompasses malnutrition and other kinds of neglect through ignorance, as well as deliberate withholding from the child of the necessary and basic physical care, including the medical and dental care necessary for the child to grow. Examples of physical abuse range from burns and exposure to extreme cold, to beating, poisoning, strangulation, and withholding food and water. If a child is seen to be in danger of suffering significant harm, from physical, sexual, emotional or neglectful causes, the child maybe registered on the Child Protection Register. If a nurse, health visitor or midwife has reasonable cause to suspect the abuse of a child, appropriate action must be taken in order to protect that child *(See also Children Act, 1989)*.

Deprived child A vague term usually implying that the child in question has been raised in a situation lacking in love, affection and consistent parenting responses from adults. Sometimes used to suggest that the child has experienced a generalized deficit of life opportunities, both interpersonal and social.

Child sexual abuse The subjection of a child to sexual activity likely to cause physical or psychological harm.

Child care Any matter associated with the upbringing and welfare of children, both familial and in relation to welfare and social services.

Child officer A social worker who has a responsibility to investigate any situation where a child is thought to be at risk of harm due to neglect, injury or desertion, and in those situations where the child is considered "beyond control" by the parents/ guardians or is offending.

Child development The stages of physical, psychological and social growth and attainment that occur from birth to adulthood.

Child health clinic A center which infants and preschool children attend on a regular basis to ensure normal progress and development. A medical officer and a health visitor are in attendance. Immunizations against infectious diseases, screening and health promotion information are also provided.

Child minder A person who is registered with the local authority social services department and who is approved by the department to mind an agreed number of children aged from birth to 5 years during the day.

Childbirth The act or process of giving birth to a child. Parturition.

Children Act 2004 Act of Parliament bringing together comprehensive law relating to children defining their rights, identifying parental responsibilities and detailing procedures to protect them. The Children Act is responsible for promoting awareness of views and interests of children, having regard to the United Nations Convention on the Rights of the Child. Agencies involved in children's services have a duty to cooperate to improve wellbeing of children and young people. Children's services authorities must establish Local Safeguarding Children Boards to protect children from harm; local authorities must ascertain feelings of children when making decisions about services for children in need, and providing accommodation for children under the Act.

Children Act, 1989 The main principles of this legislation for the care and welfare of children are as follows: (a) The welfare of children is the prime consideration and wherever possible they should be cared for within their own families. Parents with children in need should be helped and supported by the local authorities, and in partnership with other agencies, to bring up their children themselves. Parents should be informed of their right to complain if they are not satisfied with the services offered, (b) Children should be kept safe and protected by effective intervention if they are in danger but this should be open to parental challenge through the courts, (c) The courts, when dealing with children, should avoid any delays when processing their cases, and should only make an order if to do so is better for the child than making no order at all. (d) Children should be kept informed of any decisions taken in their interests and should participate as far as possible in any decisions or actions taken, (e) Parents should continue to have responsibility for their children, even when they are no longer living with them. Parents should be kept informed of and invited to participate in any decisions about their children's future, (f) Local authorities are required to take account of children's racial origins, culture, linguistic background and religion when making decisions about them.

Children's centers Responding to local community needs, providing child and family services, childcare advice and early learning specialist services.

Chill Shivering with sensation of coldness and pallor of skin.

Chinese medicine A traditional system based on the principles of Yin and Yang, combining acupuncture with a range of medications from herbal and animal sources.

Chinese restaurant syndrome Transient arterial dilatation due to ingestion of monosodium glutamate, which is used in seasoning Chinese food; marked by throbbing head, light-headedness, tightness of the jaw, neck and shoulders, and backache.

Chiropodist Podiatrist.

Chiropody The study and care of the feet and the treatment of foot diseases.

Chiropractic A system of treatment employing manipulation of the spine and other bony structures.

Chi-square (χ^2) A statistical test to determine the similarity of the number of occurrences being investigated to the expected occurrences.

Chlamydia A genus of bacteria comprising two species: *Chlamydia trachomatis* which causes lymphogranuloma venereum, trachoma, conjunctivitis and nongonococcal urethritis; and *Chlamydia psittaci* which causes psittacosis (parrot fever).

Chloasma A condition in which there is brown, blotchy discoloration of the skin of the face, especially during pregnancy.

Chloral An oily liquid formed by the reaction of chlorine and alcohol. Used in the production of chloral hydrate, a drug used as a hypnotic; it is well tolerated by children and old people.

Chloral hydrate Colorless, caustic hypnotic agent.

Chlorambucil An alkylating drug used in treating chronic leukemia. A cytotoxic drug.

Chloramphenicol An antibiotic. It gives rise to agranulocytosis and is used only for serious infectious diseases, such as typhoid fever, and in drops and ointment for eye infections.

Chlorobutanol Antiseptic and local anesthetic used in dentistry and as a preservative.

Chlorcyclizine An antihistamine used for travel sickness.

Chlorodane An insecticide.

Chlorodantion Topical antifungal agent.

Chlorodiazepoxide A benzodiazepine, used to treat anxiety, alcohol withdrawal syndrome, etc.

Chloremia Increased chloride concentration in blood.

Chlorhexidine An antibacterial compound used for surgical scrub, preoperative skin preparation and cleansing skin wounds.

Chlorinated lime Calcium hypochlorite and calcium chloride, used as bleaching agents and antiseptic.

Chlorine Symbol Cl. A yellow, irritating poisonous gas. A powerful disinfectant, bleach and deodorizing agent. Used in hypochlorites for sterilization purposes.

Chlorite A salt of chlorous acid, used as disinfectant and bleaching agent.

Chlormethiazole A hypnotic and sedative drug used to treat insomnia, chiefly in elderly people.

Chlormezanone Antianxiety sedative agent.

Chloroacetone Chloracetone. Tear gas.

Chlorocresol A coal tar product with a bacterial action more powerful than phenol and with a lower toxicity. Used as an antiseptic and as a preservative in injection fluids.

Chloroform A colorless volatile liquid administered through inhalation as a general anesthetic. Now rarely used.

Chloroguanide Antimalarial agent.

Chloroma A tumor having a greenish color, usually found in skull bones. It is associated with myeloid leukemia.

Chlorophane Green-yellow pigment in retina.

Chlorophenothane An insecticide known as DDT.

Chlorophyll The green pigment of plants which absorbs solar energy for the synthesis of complex materials from the carbon dioxide and water taken in by the plant.

Chlorophene A phenol, disinfectant.

Chlorpheniramine An antihistamine agent.

Chlorphenoxamine Drug for parkinsonism.

Chlorpromazine Tranquilizer used in psychosis.

Chlorpropamide Oral hypoglycemic agent of sulfonyl urea group.

Chlorprothixene Anti-depressant.

Chlortetracycline Bacteriostatic antibiotic of tetracycline group.

Chlorthalidone Diuretic.

Chloroquine An antimalarial drug that has a strong suppressant action and is also used in the treatment of amebic hepatitis, rheumatoid arthritis and lupus erythematosus.

Chlorothiazide An oral diuretic used in the treatment of fluid retention and hypertension.

Chlorotrianisene A long-acting estrogen used in the treatment of menopausal symptoms and in cancer of the prostate.

Chloroxylenol An antiseptic that is less irritating to the skin and mucous membranes than cresol and has a powerful disinfectant action.

Chlorpheniramine An antihistamine drug used in the treatment of allergies such as hay fever and urticaria.

Chlorpromazine A sedative antiemetic drug widely used to treat anxiety, agitation and vomiting, particularly in the elderly, and in the management of psychiatric patients. It is also hypotensive and enhances the effect of analgesics and anesthetics.

Chlorpropamide An oral hypoglycemic agent used in the treatment of mild diabetes.

Chlorprothixene A tranquilizer used in the treatment of schizophrenia, psychoneuroses and behavior disorders.

Chlortetracycline A broad-spectrum antibiotic effective in treating many bacterial and protozoal infections.

Chlorthalidone A diuretic used in the treatment of edema, hypertension and diabetes.

Chlorthiazide A diuretic.

Chlorzoxazone Muscle relaxant.

Choana Funnel shaped opening especially on the posterior nares.

Choking Obstruction within respiratory passage or constriction in the neck, obstructing breathing and circulation to brain.

Cholagogues An agent which promotes increased bile flow.

Cholangiectasis Dilatation of bile ducts.

Cholangiography Radiography of the hepatic, cystic and bile ducts after the insertion of a radiopaque contrast medium.

Cholangioma Tumor of bile ducts.

Cholangitis Inflammation of the bile ducts.

Cholecystectomy Excision of the gallbladder.

Cholecystitis Inflammation of the gallbladder.

Cholecystoduodenostomy An anastomosis between the gallbladder and the duodenum.

Cholecystoenterostomy The formation of an artificial opening from the gallbladder into the intestine. An operation performed in cases of irremovable obstruction of the bile duct.

Cholecystitis Inflammation of gallbladder manifesting with fever, chills, upper abdominal pain and mild jaundice; caused by gall stones.

Cholecystography Radiography of the gallbladder after administration of a radiopaque contrast medium.

Cholecystokinin A hormone, released by the presence of fats in the duodenum, which causes contraction of the gallbladder.

Cholecystolithiasis The presence of stones in the gallbladder.

Cholecystostomy An incision into the gallbladder, usually to remove gallstones.

Choledocholithiasis The presence of stones in the bile duct.

Choledocholithotomy Incision into the bile ducts to remove stones.

Choledochostomy Opening and draining the common bile duct.

Cholelithiasis Presence of gallstones in the gallbladder or bile ducts.

Cholemia Hyperbilirubinemia.

Cholera An acute, notifiable, infectious enteritis endemic and epidemic in Asia and, more recently, also in Africa. Caused by *Vibrio cholerae*, it is marked by profuse diarrhea, muscle cramp, suppression of urine and severe prostration; it is often fatal. Travellers to areas where cholera is endemic should protect themselves by vaccination, though this only provides partial immunity. The local drinking water should be boiled or sterilized and uncooked foods avoided.

Choleriform Resembling cholera.

Cholestasis Arrest of the flow of bile due to obstruction of the bile ducts.

Cholesteatoma A small tumor containing cholesterol. It may occur in the middle ear or in the meninges, central nervous system or bones of the skull.

Cholesterol A sterol found in nervous tissue, red blood corpuscles, animal fat and bile. It is a precursor of bile acids and steroid hormones, and occurs in the most common type of gallstone, in atheroma of the arteries, in various cysts and in carcinomatous tissue. Most of the body's cholesterol is synthesized, but some is obtained in the diet.

Cholesterolosis A chronic form of cholecystitis when the mucosa of the gallbladder is studded with deposits of cholesterol.

Cholestyramine A drug that causes the excretion of bile salts by binding with them. Given to lower blood levels of cholesterol and other fats.

Cholic acid A bile acid.

Choline An essential amine, found in the blood, cerebrospinal fluid and urine, which aids fat metabolism. Formerly classified as a vitamin of the B complex.

Choline theophyllinate An antispasmodic drug used in respiratory conditions.

Cholinergic Pertaining to nerves that release acetylcholine, as the chemical stimulator, at their nerve endings.

Cholinergic drugs Drugs that inhibit cholinesterase and so prevent the destruction of acetylcholine.

Cholinesterase An enzyme that rapidly destroys acetylcholine.

Choluria Presence of bile salts and/or pigments in the urine and is usually indicative of jaundice.

Chondrin Gelatin like material obtained by boiling of cartilage (the basic substance of cartilage).

Chondritis Inflammation of cartilage.

Chondroblast An embryonic cell that forms cartilage.

Chondrodysplasia Multiple exostoses of epiphysis especially of long bones, metacarpals and phalanges.

Chondrogen Basal substance of cartilage and corneal tissue, which changes to chondrin on boiling.

Chondroitin Substance present in connective tissue, including cornea and cartilage.

Chondroma An innocent new growth arising in cartilage.

Chondromalacia A condition of abnormal softening of cartilage.

Chondrosarcoma A malignant new growth arising from cartilaginous tissue.

Chorda A sinew or cord.

Chordae tendinea Tendinous cords connecting free edges of A-V valves to papillary muscles.

Chordee Downward curvature of the penis caused by congenital anomaly (common in hypospadias) or urethral infection.

Chorditis Inflammation of the vocal or spermatic cords.

Chordoma A tumor along vertebral column composed of embryonic nerve tissue.

Chordotomy An operation on the spinal cord to divide the anterolateral nerve pathways for relief of intractable pain cordotomy.

Chorea A symptom of disease of the basal ganglia when the individual suffers from spasmodic, involuntary, rapid movements of the face, shoulders and hips.

Huntington's chorea (or Huntington's disease) A rare hereditary disorder which manifests itself in early middle age. The individual also suffers from progressive dementia, which often precedes a premature death.

Sydenham's chorea St Vitus's dance. Occurs in childhood and is associated with rheumatic fever.

Choreiform Resembling chorea.

Choreoathetosis Jerky bizarre involuntary muscle contraction, usually more proximal than distal.

Chorioadenoma Adenoma of chorion, the outer membrane enclosing the fetus.

Chorioamnionitis Inflammation of membranes covering fetus, i.e., amnion & chorion.

Choriocarcinoma Formerly known as chorioepithelioma. A highly malignant neoplasm usually arising from the trophoblast of a hydatidiform mole *(See Hydatidiform mole)*. It may develop after an abortion or the evacuation of a hydatidiform mole or even in normal pregnancy. Metastases usually develop rapidly but the disease normally carries a good prognosis if early treatment is given.

Choriomeningitis Inflammation of meninges. Choriomeningitis lymphocytic is of viral origin.

Chorioepithelioma Choriocarcinoma.

Chorion The outer membrane enveloping the fetus; the placenta.

Chorionic Pertaining to the chorion.

Chorionic gonadotrophin Human chorionic gonadotrophin (HCG).

Chorionic villi Small protrusions on the chorion from which the placenta is formed. They are in close association with the maternal blood and, by diffusion, inter change of nutriment, oxygen and waste matters is affected between the maternal and the fetal blood.

Chorionic villus biopsy Tissue removed from the gestational sac early in pregnancy so that chromosomal and other inherited disorders can be identified. Can be carried out at an earlier stage than amniocentesis.

Chorioretinitis Choroidoretinitis.

Choroid The pigmented and vascular coat of the eyeball, continuous with the iris and situated between the sclera and retina. It reduces the amount of light which falls upon the retina.

Choroid plexus Specialized cells in the ventricles of the brain which produce cerebrospinal fluids. There is one choroid plexus in each ventricle.

Choroideremia X-linked choroid degeneration manifesting as night blindness progressing to absolute blindness.

Choroiditis Inflammation of the choroid.

Choroidoretinitis An inflammatory condition of both the choroid and retina of the eye.

Christian-Weber disease Nodular, nonsuppurating panniculitis with fever.

Christmas disease A hereditary bleeding disease similar to hemophilia. The name is derived from that of the first patient to be studied.

Christmns factor A thromboplastin activator present in plasma.

Chromaffin cells Pigment cells of adrenal medulla and paraganglia containing granules that stain with chromium salts.

Chromatin It is a DNA structure present in the cell nucleus. Males are chromatin negative and femals are chromatin positive (inactivated X-chromosome).

Chromatography A method of chemical analysis by which substances in solution can be separated as they percolate down a column of powdered absorbent or ascend an absorbent paper by capillary traction. A definite pattern is produced and substances maybe recognized by the use of appropriate color reagents. Amino acids can be identified in this way.

Chromatometry The measurement of colour perception.

Chromatophore A pigment bearing cell.

Chromic acid A strong caustic sometimes used for the removal of warts.

Chromicize To impregnate with chromic acid, e.g., chromicized catgut, which is particularly strong and durable.

Chromoblasts An embryonic cell that becomes a pigment cell.

Chromolysis Dissolution of chromophil substance (Nissl bodies) in neurons in certain pathological conditions.

Chromomycosis Fungal infection of skin marked by warty plaques.

Chromophil Easily staining cell of anterior pituitary which is actually secretory.

Chromosome In animal cells, a structure in the nucleus, containing a linear thread of deoxyribonucleic acid (DNA), which transmits genetic information and is associated with ribonucleic acid (RNA) and histones. During cell division the material composing the chromosome is compactly coiled. Each organism of a species is normally characterized by the same number of chromosomes in its somatic cells, 46 being the number usually present in humans: 22 pairs of autosomes, and two sex chromosomes (XX or XY), which determine the sex of the organism. In the mature gamete (ovum or spermatozoon) the number of chromosomes is halved as a result of meiosis.

Chronic of long duration; the opposite of acute.

Chronic fatigue syndrome It can be described as a debilitating disorder or disorders of uncertain causation. Symptoms usually include muscle and joint pain, cognitive difficulties and severe mental or physical exhaustion in a previously healthy and active person. It is also sometimes known as myalgic encephalomyelitis.

Chronic granulomatous disease A disease of children characterized by inability of neutrophils to kill ingested organisms.

Chronological Description of an event in natural sequence according to time.

Churg-strauss syndrome Also known as eosinophilic granulomatosis with polyangiitis. A type of vasculitis that mainly affects adults aged 30-45 years.

Chvostek's sign F Chvostek, Austrian surgeon, 1835–1884. A spasm of the facial muscles which occurs in tetany. It can be elicited by tapping the facial nerve.

Chyle Digested fats which, as a milky fluid, are absorbed into the lymphatic capillaries (lacteals) in the villi of the small intestine.

Chylemia Chyle in peripheral circulation.

Chylomicron Small particles of fat rich in triglycerides.

Chylothorax The presence of effused chyle in the pleural cavity.

Chyluria Presence of chyle or fat globules in urine.

Chyme The semiliquid acid mass of food that passes from the stomach to the intestines.

Chymopapain An enzyme related to papain.

Chymotrypsin An enzyme secreted by the pancreas. It is activated by trypsin and aids in the breakdown of proteins.

Ci Symbol for curie.

Cicatrix The scar of a healed wound (See Keloid).

Cicatrization Healing by scar formation.

Ciclesonide Topical steroid for rhinitis.

Ciclopirox Locally applied antifungal agent.

Cilia 1. The eyelashes. 2. Microscopic filaments projecting from some epithelial cells, known as ciliated membranes, as in the bronchi, where cilia wave the secretion upward.

Ciliary Hair-like.

Ciliary body A structure just behind the corneoscleral margin, composed of the ciliary muscle and processes.

Ciliary muscle The circular muscle surrounding the lens of the eye.

Ciliary processes The fringed part of the choroid coat arranged in a circle in front of the lens.

Ciliary reflex Normal contraction of pupil during process of accommodation.

Ciliospinal center Center in spinal cord that controls dilatation of pupil.

Ciliospinal reflex Dilatation of pupil following stimulation of the skin of the neck.

Cilostazol A vasodilator.

Cimetidine A histamine H_2 receptor antagonist which reduces gastric acid secretion; used in the treatment of peptic ulcers.

Cimex A genus of blood sucking bugs.

Cimex lectularius The common bedbug.

Cinchona Dried bark of cinchona tree containing quinine, cinchonine.

Cinahl *(See Cumulative Index To Nursing and Allied Healh Literature).*

Cinchocaine A local anesthetic agent used mainly as a spinal anesthetic.

Cinchophen Old agent for gout frequently producing fatal hepatitis.

Cineangiocardiography Angiography using a cine camera to show the movements of the heart and blood vessels.

Cineradiography The making of a motion picture record of successive images appearing on a fluoroscopic screen.

Cingulotomy Excision of anterior half of cingulated gyrus for control of intractable pain.

Cingulum A band of association fibers in the cingulated gyrus extending from anterior perforated substance to hippocampal gyrus.

Cinnarizine An antihistamine drug which may also be used to treat nausea, vertigo, labyrinthine disorders and motion sickness.

Cinoxacin A quinolone, antibacterial agent.

Ciprofloxacin A quinolone with broad spectrum antibacterial activity.

Circadian Denoting a period of 24 hours.

Circadian rhythm The rhythm of certain biological activities that take place daily.

Circinate Having a circular outline.

Tinea circinata is ring worm.

Circle of Willis *T Willis, British physician and anatomist, 1621–1675.* An anastomosis of arteries at the base of the brain, formed by the branches of the internal carotid and the basilar arteries.

Circulation Movement in a circular course, as of the blood.

Collateral circulation Enlargement of small vessels establishing adequate blood supply when the main vessel to the part has been occluded.

Coronary circulation The system of vessels that supplies the heart muscle itself.

Extracorporeal circulation 1. Removal of the blood by intravenous cannulae, passing it through a machine to oxygenate it, and then pumping it back into circulation. 2. The "heart-lung" machine or pump respirator, used in cardiac surgery.

Lymph circulation The flow of lymph through lymph vessels and glands.

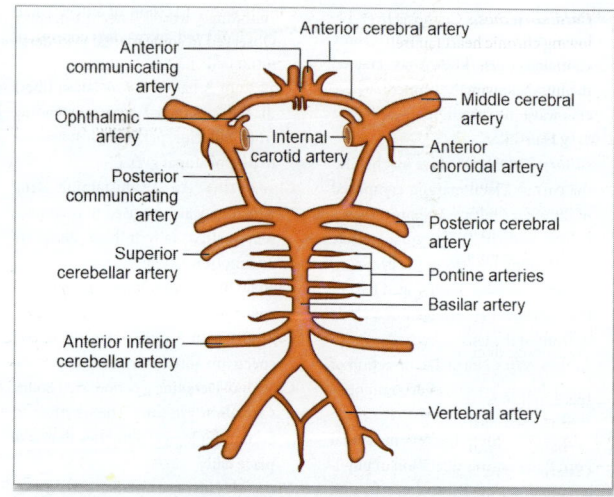

Anterior cerebral artery

Anterior communicating artery

Ophthalmic artery

Internal carotid artery

Posterior communicating artery

Superior cerebellar artery

Anterior inferior cerebellar artery

Middle cerebral artery

Anterior choroidal artery

Posterior cerebral artery

Pontine arteries

Basilar artery

Vertebral artery

Circle of Willis

Portal circulation The passage of blood from the alimentary tract, pancreas and spleen, via the portal vein and its branches through the liver and into the hepatic veins.

Pulmonary circulation The passage of the blood from the right ventricle via the pulmonary artery through the lungs and back to the heart by the pulmonary veins.

Systemic circulation The flow of blood throughout the body. The direction of flow is from the left atrium to the left ventricle and through the aorta, with its branches and capillaries. Veins then carry it back to the right atrium, and so into the right ventricle.

Circumcision Excision of the prepuce of foreskin of the penis. An operation performed for religious reasons, or sometimes for phimosis or paraphimosis.

Female circumcision Excision of the labia minora and/or labia majora, and sometimes the clitoris; still

performed ritualistically in certain countries, the extent of the surgery varying from one culture to another.

Circumduction Moving in a circle, e.g., the circular movement of the upper limb.

Circumoral Around the mouth.

Circumoral pallor A pale area around the mouth contrasting with the flushed cheeks, e.g., in scarlet fever.

Circumflex Winding around.

Circumvallate Surrounded by a wall or raised ring.

Circumvallate papilla (See Papilla).

Cirrhosis A degenerative change that can occur in any organ, but especially in the liver. Maybe due to viruses, microorganisms or toxic substances (portal cirrhosis). Fibrosis results and interferes with the working of the organ. In the liver it causes portal obstruction, with consequent ascites.

Alcoholic cirrhosis The result of chronic alcoholism and nutritional deficiency which occurs in the liver.

Cardiac cirrhosis Cirrhosis liver following chronic heart failure.

Posthepatic cirrhosis Cirrhosis of the liver following hepatitis.

Pulmonary cirrhosis Cirrhosis of the lung tissue.

Cisapride Agent to improve GI motility.

Cisplatin An antineoplastic drug, containing platinum, used in the treatment of ovarian carcinomas and testicular teratomas.

Cisterna A space or cavity containing fluid.

Cisterna chyli The dilated portion of the thoracic duct containing chyle.

Cisterna magna The subarachnoid space between the cerebellum and medulla oblongata.

Cisternal Concerning the cisterna.

Cisternal puncture Insertion of a hollow needle into the cisterna magna to withdraw cerebrospinal fluid.

Cisvestitism Wearing of clothes contrary to ones profession.

Citalopram An antidepressant.

Citric acid Acid found in the juice of lemons, limes, etc. An antiscorbutic.

Citric acid cycle (Kreb's cycle) The cycle involving oxidative metabolism of pyruvic acid to CO_2 and H_2O, releasing energy (36 ATP).

Citrovorum factory Folinic acid used with dihydrofolate reductase inhibitors.

Citrulline Amino acid formed from ornithine, present in water melons.

CJD Creutzfeldt-Jakob disease.

Cl Symbol for chlorine.

Clairvoyance Extrasensory perception. The act or power of knowing about objects or events without the use of senses.

Clamp A metal surgical instrument used to compress any part of the body.

Clang association Rhyming speech. A way of speaking where similar sounding words are associated. Observed in some mental disorders.

Clapping In physiotherapy, rhythmic beating with cupped hands. Frequently used over the chest to aid expectoration.

Clark's rule A formula for calculating pediatric dose, i.e., weight of the child in lb. x adult dose/150.

Clasmatocyte A large wandering uninucleated cell with many branches, a fixed macrophage of loose connective tissue.

Class 1. A system that divides members of a society into sets based upon social or economic status and is based upon cultural characteristics in common. 2. A group of objects that have a common characteristic.

Claude's syndrome Third cranial nerve palsy, contralateral ataxia and tremor, caused by lesion around red nucleus.

Claudication Lameness.

Intermittent claudication Limping, accompanied by severe pain in the leg on walking, which disappears with rest. A sign of occlusive arterial disease.

Claustrophilia Dread of being in an open space, a morbid desire to remain within with windows shut.

Claustrophobia Fear of confined spaces, such as small rooms.

Claspkniferigidity Passive flexion of the joint causes increased resistance of the extensors. This gives way abruptly if flexon is continued, a sign of pyramidal tract lesion.

Clavicle The collar bone. A long bone, part of the shoulder girdle.

Clavus A corn.

Clavulanic acid Beta lactamase inhibitor.

Clawfoot Excessively high longitudinal arch of foot with dorsal contracture of toes.

Clawhand A deformity in which the fingers are bent and contracted, giving a claw-like appearance.

Clean catch method Contamination free urine specimen collection.

Cleavage Splitting a complex molecule into two or more simple ones.

Cleft A fissure or longitudinal opening.

Cleft lip A congenital fissure in the upper lip, often accompanied by cleft of palate.

Cleft palate A congenital defect in the roof of the mouth due to failure of the medial plates of the palate to meet. Often associated with cleft lip.

Client 1. A recipient of a professional service. 2. A recipient of health care, regardless of the person's state of health and where the service is delivered. 3. A patient.

Climacteric The period of the menopause in women. Also used to denote the decline in sexual drive in men.

Clemastine Antihistaminic agent.

Clenching With the teeth in contact, forcible repeated contraction of jaw muscles.

Cleptomania Impulsive stealing in which motive is not related to value of stolen object.

Clidinium bromide Parasympathetic inhibitor used for treatment of peptic ulcer.

Climacteric Menopause or end of woman's reproductive ability. Male climacteric points to lessening male sexual activity.

Climax 1. The stage when a disease is at its greatest intensity. 2. The stage in sexual intercourse when orgasm occurs.

Clindamycin An antibiotic active against Gram-positive cocci and many anaerobes.

Clinic 1. Instruction of students at the bedside. 2. A department of a hospital devoted to the treatment of a particular type of disease.

Clinical Relating to bedside observation and the treatment of patients.

Clinical governance A framework through which organizations are accountable for continuously improving the quality of their services and for safeguarding high standards of care by creating an environment in which excellence in care will flourish.

Clinical nurse specialist A qualified nurse who has acquired advanced knowledge and skills in a specific area of clinical nursing.

Clinical risk index for babies Abbreviated CRIB. A professional scoring tool used in assessing the initial neonatal risks for babies, and also for comparing the performance of one neonatal intensive care unit with another.

Clinical risk management The means by which adverse events occurring in organizations and usually related to the delivery of patient care are systematically assessed and reviewed in order to seek ways for prevention of future incidents.

Clinical skills Skills required by clinicians (doctors, nurses, dentists and other clinical professionals). Clinical skills vary depending on specialty but core skills remain constant, e.g., communication skills, history-taking skills, record keeping, basic physical examination, etc.

Clinical supervision An exchange between practising professionals to enable the development of professional skills. Has a vital role in sustaining and developing professional practice in nursing, midwifery and health visiting.

Clinocephaly Congenital flatness or saddle-shape of the top of the head caused by bilateral premature closure of the sphenoparietal sutures.

Clinoid processes Three pairs of prominences on upper surface of sphenoid bone.

Clip A metal device for holding the two edges of a wound together or for controlling the flow through a tube.

Clithrophobia Morbid fear of being locked in.

Clitoridectomy Excision of the clitoris.

Clitoridotomy Removal or splitting of the clitoral hood. This is also a type of female genital mutilation.

Clitoris A small organ, formed of erectile tissue, situated at the anterior junction of the labia minora in the female.

Clitoris crises Involuntary orgasm in female in tabes dorsalis.

Clitorism Recurring painful erection of clitoris, akin to priapism in male.

Clivulus A surface that slopes as in sphenoid bone.

Cloaca 1. The common intestinal and urogenital opening present in many vertebrates. 2. Opening through newly formed bone from a diseased area so that pus may escape *(See Involucrum)*.

Clobazam A benzidiasepine.

Clobetasol A locally applied steroid.

Clofazimine Antileprotic agent that stains skin.

Clofibrate Lipid lowering agent, maybe carcinogenic and causes gall stones.

Clomiphene A nonsteroidal agent to stimulate ovulation in females and spermatogenesis in males.

Clonazepam An anticonvulsive drug.

Clone Cells which are genetically identical to each other and have descended by asexual reproduction from the parent cell, to which they are also genetically identical.

Clonic Having the character of clonus. The second stage of a grand mal fit; also referred to as a tonic-clonic seizure *(See Epilepsy)*.

Clonic spasm Spasm marked by repeated muscular contraction followed by relaxation.

Clonidine An antihypertensive drug which is also used to treat migraine.

Clonus Muscle rigidity and relaxation which occurs spasmodically.

Ankle clonus Spasmodic movements of the calf muscles when the foot is suddenly pushed upward, the leg being extended.

Clonorchiasis Liver fluke caused by chlonorchis sinensis which infects bile duct of man. Infection contracted by eating uncooked fresh water fish containing larvae. Treatment is with praziquantel.

Clopidogrel Antiplatelet agent.

Clostridium A genus of anaerobic spore-forming bacteria, found as commensals of the gut of animals and humans and saprophytes of the soil. Pathogenic species include *Clostridium botulinum* (botulism), *Clostridium tetani* (tetanus) and *Clostridium perfrillgells* (also known as *Clostridium welchii*) (gas gangrene).

Clot A semisolid mass formed in a liquid, such as blood or lymph, by coagulation.

Clotrimazole An antifungal drug clotting coagulation. The formation of a clot; *(See Blood clotting)*.

Clotrimazole time Coagulation time. The length of time taken for shed blood to coagulate.

Clotting coagulation The formation of a clot *(See Blood Clotting)*

C. time Coagulation time The length of time taken by shed blood to coagulate.

Cloxacillin An antibiotic drug effective against penicillin-resistant staphylococci.

Clubbing Broadening and thickening of the tips of the fingers (and toes) due to bad circuiation. It occurs in chronic disease of the heart and respiratory system, such as congenital cardiac defect and tuberculosis.

Clubfoot Talipes.

Clumping The collecting together into clumps. The reaction of bacteria and blood cells when agglutination occurs.

Cluster headache Nocturnal headache, 2-3 hours after falling asleep, continuing for months associated with watering from eyes.

Clutton's joint Hydrarthrosis of knee joint often associated with interstitial keratitis, seen in congenital syphilis.

Co Symbol for cobalt.

Co-trimoxazole An antibiotic drug, taken orally and used mainly to treat urinary infections.

Coaching A form of non-directive interaction in which the coach supports the coachee to identify goals and solutions to challenges. The coachee might be a professional but increasingly profession

Coagulase An enzyme formed by pathogenic staphylococci that causes coagulation of plasma. Such bacteria are termed *coagulase positive.*

Coagulation Clotting *(See Blood clotting).*

Coagulation factor concentrate 1. Effective against the bleeding tendency in hemophilia. 2. An agent that counteracts the bleeding tendency in hemophilia. Factor VIII is one of the clotting factors, deficiency of which causes the more frequent, classic, sex-linked hemophilia. It is available in a recombinant (manufactured rather than from humans) preparation for preventive and therapeutic use.

Coagulum The mass of fibrin and cells formed when blood clots; the mass formed when other masses coagulate, e.g., milk curd.

Coal tar A byproduct obtained in the destructive distillation of coal; used in ointment or solution in the treatment of eczema and psoriasis.

Coarctation A condition of contraction or stricture.
Coarctation of aorta A congenital malformation characterized by deformity of the aorta, causing narrowing, usually severe, of the lumen of the vessel. Surgical resection of the stricture maybe performed.

Coat's disease Development of large white masses in blood vessels of retina.

Cobalt Symbol Co. A metallic element, traces of which are necessary in the diet to prevent anemia.
Radioactive cobalt, cobalt-60 Used as a source of gamma irradiation in radiotherapy.

Cocaine A colorless alkaloid, obtained from coca leaves, which has a powerful but brief stimulant action. Formerly used as a local anesthetic, cocaine has been replaced by less addictive preparations like procaine, lignocaine and amethocaine. It is now a major "recreational" drug, producing euphoria with many behavioral and social effects. It is addictive and usually taken by snorting. Also known, in its various forms, as "crack", "coke"/"snow"., "charlie". or "c".

Cocainism Addiction to cocaine. Long-term abuse is associated with a toxic psychosis similar to that caused by amphetamines.

Coccus A bacterium of spheroidal shape.

Coccidioidomycosis A coccidioidal granuloma.

Coccygeal body Small arteriovenus anastomosis at the level of coccyx.

Coccydynia Persistent pain in the region of the coccyx.

Coccyx The terminal bone of the spinal column, in which four rudimentary vertebrae are fused together to form a triangle.

Cochlea The spiral canal of the internal ear.

Cochlear implant An electronic device that receives sounds and transmits the resulting electric signals to implanted electrodes in cochlea so that the sound is perceived. *SYN*– Cochlear prosthesis.

Cochlear nerve 8th cranial nerve supplying cochlea with nucleus at pons and medulla.

Cochleo-palpebral reflex Contraction of orbicularis oculi from sudden noise near the ear.

Cochrane database Database of systematic reviews of published research. An international multidisciplinary collaboration of health professionals, consumers and researchers who review randomized controlled clinical trials.

Cochrane library A. Cochrane, 1909-1988. Collection of systematic reviews of published research. An international multidisciplinary collaboration of health professionals, consumers and researchers who review randomized controlled clinical trials.

Cocktail Any beverage or product containing several ingredients.

Cod liver oil Purified oil from the liver of the codfish; valuable source of vitamins A and D.

Code 1. A set of rules governing one's conduct. 2. A system by which information can be communicated.

Genetic code The arrangement of nucleotides in the polynucleotide chain of a chromosome that governs the transmission of genetic information.

Code of ethics A written code of professional conduct for the nurse, midwife and health visitors in their respective countries.

Codeine An alkaloid of opium. A mild analgesic and antitussive.

Codman's exercise Mild exercises to restore the motion and function in the arms or shoulders after injury or immobilization.

Coeliac Relating to the abdomen.

Celiac disease Gluten enteropathy. A condition of early childhood occurring soon after the child has been weaned onto cereals; characterized by steatorrhea, distended abdomen and failure to grow. The failure of carbohydrate and fat metabolism appears to be due to the gluten in wheat and rye. The condition may continue into adult life. It is treated by giving a gluten-free diet.

Celiac plexus Nerve complex that supplies the abdominal organs.

Coenzyme An organic molecule activator to a larger protein enzyme.

Coenzyme A A precursor for biosynthesis of fatty acids and sterols.

Cogan's syndrome Interstitial keratitis associated with tinnitus, vertigo and usually deafness.

Cognition The action of knowing. Cognitive function of the conscious mind in contrast to the effective (feeling) and conative (willing).

Cogwheel Combination of tremor and rigidity as in extrapyramidal disease, i.e., Parkinson's disease.

Cohabit 1. To live together and have a sexual relationship without being married. 2. To coexist.

Coherent Sticking together, adhesiveness.

Cohort A group of people possessing a common characteristic, such as being born in the same year or of the same gender, used in research to make generalizations derived from quantitative data.

Cohort study Concerning a specific group or subpopulation in a research study.

Coil *(See Intrauterine Device).*

Coin test A test for pneumothorax, a coin placed on chest is struck with another coin. A metallic ringing sound is heard at a distant site of the chest in pneumothorax.

Coitus Sexual intercourse between male and female.

Coitus interruptus A method of birth control in which the erect penis is removed from the vagina before ejaculation occurs.

Colchicine A drug obtained from the seeds of *Colchicum autumnale.* Used in treating gout.

Cold 1. Of low temperature. 2. A viral infection affecting the membranes of the nose and throat and the bronchial tubes.

Cold agglutinin The agglutinin agglutinating RBCs at 4°C, commonly seen in viral and mycoplasma infections.

Cold common *SYN* – nasal catarrh, acute catarrhal inflammation of mucous membrane of nasal cavity, sinuses and pharynx caused by rhinovirus.

Cold pack Wrapping patient in cold water soaked clothing to reduce fever, for relief of pain and diminution of swelling in bruise.

Cold sore Herpes simplex *(See Herpes).*

Colectomy The excision of a portion or all of the colon.

Colestipol Ion exchange resin akin to cholestyramine.

Colic Acute paroxysmal abdominal pain.

Biliary colic Pain due to the presence of a gallstone in a bile duct.

Infantile colic Excessive crying due to pain and distress. Most common in the first 3 months of life. The infant may pull-up its legs and expel gas from the anus or "belch". Maybe due to air swallowing, milk intolerance or natural hyperactivity.

Intestinal colic Severe griping spasmodic abdominal pain which maybe a symptom of food poisoning or of intestinal obstruction.

Renal colic Pain due to the presence of a stone in the ureter.

Uterine colic Spasmodic pain originating in the uterus, as in dysmenorrhea.

Coliform Resembling the bacillus *Escherichia coli.*

Colistin An antibiotic produced from *Bacillus polymyxa.* Used to treat gastrointestinal and other bacterial infections.

Colitis Inflammation of the colon. It maybe due to a specific organism, as in dysentery, but the term *ulcerative colitis* Denotes a chronic disease, often of unknown cause, in which there are attacks of diarrhea, with the passage of blood and mucus.

Collagen A fibrous structural protein that constitutes the protein of the white (collagenous) fibers of skin, tendon, bone, cartilage and all other connective tissues. It also occurs dispersed in a gel to provide stiffening, as in the vitreous humor of the eye.

Collagen diseases A group of diseases having in common certain clinical and histological features that are manifestations of involvement of connective tissues *(See Connective tissues).*

Collapse 1. A state of extreme prostration due to detective action of the heart, severe shock or hemorrhage. 2. Falling in of a structure.

Collapse therapy Unilateral pneumothorax induced to promote healing/ stop bleeding of Koch's lesion.

Collapsing pulse Pulse of aortic regurgitation.

Collar bone The clavicle.

Collarbone The clavicle.

Collateral Accessory to.

Collateral circulation (See Circulation).

Colles' fascia Inner layer of superficial fascia of perineum.

Colles' fracture *A. Colles, Irish surgeon, 1773–1843.* Fracture of the lower end of the radius at the wrist following a fall on the outstretched hand. Typically, it produces the 'dinner fork' deformity.

Collecting tubule Small ducts in renal medulla that receive urine from several renal tubules. These ducts form papillary ducts of Bellini that open into renal papillae.

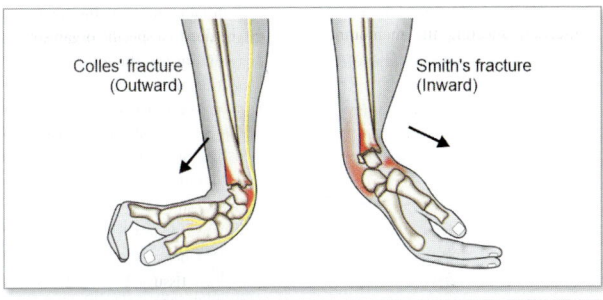

Colles' & Smith's Fracture

Collimator A shield, or cone device used in radiotherapy machines to help in determining the limits of the treatment field.

Colloid l. Glue-like. 2. The translucent, yellowish, gelatinous substance resulting from colloid degeneration. 3. A chemical system composed of a continuous medium of small particles which do not settle out under the influence of gravity and will not pass through a semipermeable membrane, as in dialysis.

Coloboma A congenital fissure of the eye affecting the choroid coat and the retina.

Colon The large intestine, from the cecum to the rectum.

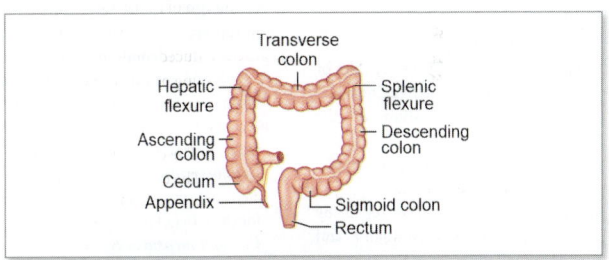

Parts of Colon

Ascending colon That part rising up to the right of the abdomen to in front of the liver.

Descending colon That part running down from in front of the spleen to the sigmoid colon.

Giant colon Megacolon.

Irritable colon (See *Irritable bowel syndrome*).

Pelvic colon, sigmoid colon That part lying in the pelvis and connecting the descending colon with the rectum.

Transverse colon That part lying across the upper abdomen connecting the ascending and descending portions.

Colonic Pertaining to the colon.

Colonic irrigation Colonic lavage.

Colonoscope A fibreoptic instrument, passed through the anus, for examining the interior of the colon.

Colony A mass of bacteria formed by multiplication of cells when bacteria are incubated under favorable conditions.

Coloprocetectomy Surgical removal of colon and rectum.

Colorimeter Instrument for measuring intensity of color.

Colostomy An artificial opening (stoma) in the large intestine brought to the surface of the abdomen for the purpose of evacuating the bowel.

Colostrum The fluid secreted by the breasts in the last few weeks of pregnancy and for the first 3 or 4 days after delivery, until lactation begins. Colostrum is high in protein and initially low in lactose; its fat content is equivalent to breast milk. It is an important source of passive antibody.

Colour blindness Achromatopsia.

Colour index An index of the amount of hemoglobin in red blood cells *(See Blood)*.

Colpitis Inflammation of the vagina.

Colpocele A hernia of either bladder or rectum into the vagina. Vaginocele.

Colpocystitis Inflammation of the bladder and vagina.

Colpohysterectomy Removal of the uterus through the vagina.

Colpoperineorrhaphy The repair by suturing of an injured vagina and torn perineum.

Colpopexy Suture of a prolapsed vagina to the abdominal wall.

Colpoplasty A plastic operation on the vagina.

Colpoptosis This is a condition associated with the prolapsed of vagina.

Colporrhaphy Repair of the vagina.
> *Anterior colporrhaphy* Repair for cystocele.
> *Posterior colporrhaphy* Repair for retrocele.

Colporrhexis A tearing or laceration of the vaginal vault.

Colposcope A speculum for examining the vagina and cervix by means of a magnifying lens; used for the early detection of malignant changes.

Colpostenosis Narrowing of vagina.

Colpotomy Also known as vaginotomy. This is a surgical procedure involving making an incision over the vagina. Anterior colpotomy is performed either to visualize the pelvic structure or to perform surgery on the fallopian tubes or ovaries. Posterior colpotomy is usually performed to drain an abscess in the pouch of Douglas.

Column A cylindrical supporting structure.

Coma A state of unconsciousness from which the patient cannot be aroused. Characterized by an absence of both spontaneous eye movements and response to painful stimuli *(See Glasgow coma scale)*.

Coma vigil Coma with open eyes and vacant look as in severe systemic infections.

Comatose In the condition of coma.

Comedo A blackhead. A plug of keratin of a hair follicle.

Comfort To provide relief of or freedom from pain, depression or anxiety.
> *Comfort eating* Eating at inappropriate times or eating unusual amounts for the relief of distress or anxiety.
> *Comfort measures* A specific action taken to promote the comfort of the patient, e.g., rearranging pillows or providing a change of position.

Comforter A baby's dummy or pacifier.

Comma bacillus Vibrio comma, organism of cholera.

Comma tract of Schultze The fasciculus interfascicularis, a tract of descending fibers located between the fasciculus cuneatus and fasciculus gracilis in the posterior funiculus of spinal cord.

Commensal Living on or within another organism and deriving benefit without harming or benefiting the host individual.

Comminuted Broken into small pieces, as in a comminuted fracture.

Commission on Human Medicines Established in 2005 to advice ministers and the licensing authority about the safety, quality and efficacy of human medicines; promotes the collection and investigation of information about adverse drug reactions; and considers representation from applicants or licence holders.

Commissioning The process by which health needs of the population are delivered and priorities determined. It is a strategic, long-term activity that frames service development within the NHS. Commissioning is a cyclical process involving: assessment of health needs, auditing of current service provision, setting priorities, service and practice development, with contracting and the evaluation of services. The commissioning process is undertaking in partnership with other agencies and is led in England by clinical commissioning groups (CCGs).

Commissure A site of union of corresponding parts, as the angle of the lips or eyelids.

Commode A bedside chair with a cutaway seat that allows a receptacle to be fitted underneath for the collection of urine and feces. Used by a patient who is unable to reach the nearest lavatory.

Commissurotomy Surgical incision of any commissure. Commonly refers to mitral commissurotomy in mitral stenosis.

Communication disease A disease, the causative agents of which may pass or be carried from a person, animal or the environment to a susceptible person either directly or indirectly.

Communicable disease A disease that maybe transmitted directly or indirectly from one person to another.

Communication skills In the broadest sense involve listening, speaking, writing and reading. In the context of health care, they generally focus on listening and giving information to patients. Communication skills cover both verbal and nonverbal forms of communication. Communication skills may extend to communicating with other clinicians, communicating at conferences or formal meetings, and presenting material in class settings.

Community A group of individuals living in an area, having a common interest, or belonging to the same organization.

Community care The care of individuals within the community, as an alternative to institutional or long-stay residential care.

Community Health Council An organization that enables the consumer's interests to be represented to those responsible for national health services at a local level.

Community nurse A nurse who is based within the community with a responsibility for providing nursing services within the patient's own home or ill health.

Therapeutic community Any treatment setting (usually psychiatric) which provides a living-learning situation through group processes emphasizing social,environmental and personal interactions.

Compartment syndrome A painful and potentially serious condition caused by a bleeding or swelling within an enclosed bundle of muscles known as a muscle compartment causing damage to the muscles and nearby nerves

Compatibility Mutual suitability. The mixing together of two substances without chemical change or loss of power *(See Blood group).*

Compensation 1. Making good a functional or structural defect. 2. Mental mechanism (unconscious) by which a person covers up a weakness by exaggerating a more desirable characteristic.

Compensatory techniques Assistance for patients/clients in developing new skills to compensate for a recognized disability or deficit.

Competence A set of professionally agreed deliverables, outputs and roles that the health care professional must be able to perform in a particular post.

Competency A set of behavior patterns, knowledge and skill that holder needs to bring to a position in order to perform the required role and functions with competence.

Complaint An act of expressing dissatisfaction with a service or individual; maybe written or verbal.

C. Management The policies and procedures in place within an NHS organization to respond to and learn from complaints received from patients, their families and members of the public regarding care, treatment and services.

Complement A substance present in normal serum which combines with the antigen-antibody complex (complement fixation) to destroy bacteria.

Complement fixation Test measurement of the amount of complement with antigen antibody complex. Complement fixation tests are widely used to detect antibodies for infectious diseases and include the Wassermann test for syphilis.

Compliance The property of altering size and shape in response to application of force, weight or release from such force, e.g., pulmonary compliance a measure of the force required to expand the lungs. Children have higher pulmonary compliance in comparison to adults. Compliance to drugs.

Complement system A series of small inactive plasma proteins that are an important part of the innate immune response to infection. When stimulated by the presence of either an antibody-antigen complex or certain microbial products or antigens, complement proteins act as a biochemical cascade, with one protein activating the next. This results in the formation of activated complement, which by various means, attacks and destroys pathogenic microorganisms, dissolves and removes immune complexes.

Complementary Pertaining to that which completes or makes perfect.

Complementary feed Feed given to infants to supplement breast-feeding when the mother has insufficient milk.

Complementary therapies A range of treatments, including yoga, reflexology, homeopathy, acupuncture and others, which maybe combined with traditional medicine.

Complete androgen insensitivity syndrome A condition that affects sexual development before birth and during puberty. People with this condition are genetically male but do not respond to male hormones and as a result have female external genitalia and breasts.

Complex A grouping of various things, as of signs and symptoms, forming a syndrome. In psychology, a grouping of ideas of emotional origin which are completely or partially represented in the unconscious mind.

Inferiority complex A compensation by assertiveness or aggression to cover a feeling of inadequacy *(See Electra complex and Oedipus complex).*

Complication An accident or second disease process arising during the course of or following the primary condition; maybe fatal.

Compos mentis [L.] Of sound mind.

Compound Composed of two or more parts or substances.

Compound astigmatism Myopia/hypermetropia of differing diopters in both longitudinal and vertical axes.

Compound fracture A fracture in which a wound through the skin has also occurred.

Comprehension Mental grasp of the meaning of a situation.

Compress Folded material, e.g., lint (wet or dry), applied to a part of the body for the relief of swelling and pain.

Compression 1. The act of pressing upon or together; the state of being pressed together. 2. In embryology, the shortening or omission of certain developmental stages.

Compression bandages Used in the treatment of leg ulcers to improve venous return and reduce venous hypertension. Following successful healing of the leg ulcer compression hose are worn to prevent reoccurrence.

Compression garments Tightly-fitted clothing used following burns or for a patient with lymphedema. They work by exerting pressure on the tissues thus preventing the build-up of fluid in the tissues.

Compulsion An overwhelming urge to perform an irrational act or ritual.

Compulsion neurosis Obsession that compels one to perform an absurd act.

Compulsive ideas An idea that continues to haunt against one's will.

Computed axial tomography Abbreviated CAT. The utilization of a computerized technique to examine a cross-section of the entire body. The CAT scanner produces an image of tissue density in a complete cross section of the part of the body being scanned.

Computed tomography (CT) The utilization of a computerized technique to examine a cross-section of the entire body. The CT scanner produces an image of tissue density in a complete cross-section of the part of the body being scanned.

Computer An electronic device for storing and retrieving numerical or textural information.

Computer-assisted design Computer use to assist in designing objects, e.g., reshape body parts in plastic surgery, artificial hip implant, crown preparation.

Computerized records Many health records are now held on computer systems which are required by law to be secure and to maintain confidentiality, usually achieved by limiting access. Most systems currently also provide a paper printout which is stored as a manual record *(See also Data Protection Act)*.

Conation A striving in a certain direction *(See Cognition)*.

Concanavalin A A lectin that stimulates proliferation of T lymphocytes but not B lymphocytes.

Concave Hollowed out. The opposite of convex.

Conceive To become pregnant, to form an idea, to form a mental image.

Concentration Strength of a substance solution, fixation of mind on one subject with exclusion of all other thoughts.

Concept An image or idea held in the mind.

Conception 1. The act of becoming pregnant, by the fertilization of an ovum. 2. A concept.

Conceptual framework A group of concepts that are broadly defined and organized to provide a rationale or structure for the interpretation of information.

Concha The outer ear or pinna; the turbinate inside nasal cavity.

Conchotomy Surgical incision of nasal concha.

Concoction Mixture of two medicinal substance aided by heating.

Concomitant Occurring at the same time.

Concretion A calculus or other hardened material present within an organ.

Concussion A violent jarring shock.

Concussion of the brain Temporary loss of consciousness produced by a fall or a blow on the head. There maybe amnesia, slow respiration and a weak pulse.

Conditioned response A response that does not occur naturally but maybe developed by regular association of some physiological function with an unrelated outside event, such as the ringing of a bell or flashing of a light. Soon the physiological function starts whenever the outside event occurs. Also called conditioned reflex.

Unconditioned response An unlearned response, i.e., one that occurs naturally.

Conditioning A form of learning in which a response is elicited by a neural stimulus that had previously been repeatedly presented in conjunction with the stimulus that originally elicited the response. Also called classical and respondent conditioning.

Conduction The transfer of electron, heat, ions or sound wave through a conducting medium or the process where by a state of excitation is transmitted.

Condom A contraceptive sheath worn during sexual intercourse and affording some protection for both partners against sexually transmitted diseases. Now available for both males and females.

Conductive deafness Deafness caused by the faulty conduction of sound from the outer to the inner ear.

Conductor 1. A substance through which electricity, light, beat or sound can pass. 2. Any part of the nervous system that conveys impulses.

Condyle A rounded eminence occurring at the end of some bones, and articulating with another bone.

Condyloma Pl. condylomata; an elevated wart-like lesion of the skin.

Condylomata acuminata Small, pointed papillomas of viral origin, usually occurring on the skin or mucous surfaces of the external genitalia or perianal region.

Condylomatalata Wide, flat, syphilitic condylomata occurring on most skin, especially about the genitals and anus.

Cone A solid figure with a rounded base, tapering upward to a point.

Cone biopsy The removal of a cone-shaped section from the cervix of the uterus. It is performed for confirmation of the diagnosis when a cervical smear test result suggests the presence of precancerous cells.

Retinal cone The cone shaped end of a light-sensitive cell in the retina, used for acute vision and for distinguishing colors.

Confabulation The production of fictitious memories, and the relating of experiences which have no relation to truth, to fill in the gaps due to loss of memory. A symptom of Korsakoff's syndrome.

Confidential enquiry A unique form of audit in which case notes are scrutinized by relevant professionals to identify substandard care and make recommendations for future practice. The triennial Confidential Enquiry into Maternal Deaths and the Confidential Enquiry into Stillbirths and Deaths in Infancy (CESDI) are directly related to maternity care, and midwives maybe involved in providing appropriate information. The Confidential

Enquiry into Perioperative Deaths is also available.

Confidentiality Spoken, written or given in confidence.

Cloaca 1. The common intestinal and urogenital opening present in vertebrates. 2. Opening through newly formed bone from a diseased area so that pus may escape *(See Involucrum)*.

Conflict A Mental state arising when two opposing wishes or impulses cause emotional tension and often cannot be resolved without repressing one of the impulses into the unconscious. Conflict situations maybe associated with an anxiety neurosis.

Confluent Running together.

Confusion Disturbed orientation with regard to time, place or person, sometimes accompanied by disordered consciousness.

Congener Two or more muscles with same function, or two substances with similar origin, function or structure.

Congenital Present at and existing from the time of birth.
Congenital dislocation of the hip Failure in position of the head of the femur and development of the acetabulum.
Congenital heart defect A Structural defect of the heart or great vessels or both.
Congenital infection An infection which takes place in utero. The most important congenital infections are rubella, cytomegalovirus, herpes simplex, human immune deficiency virus (HIV), syphilis and toxoplasmosis.

Congestion An abnormal accumulation of blood in any part.
Pulmonary congestion Congestion of the lung, as in pneumonia and congestive heart failure.

Coniology The study of dust and its effects.

Coniotomy Cricothyrotomy.

Conization Excision of a cone of tissue as in chronic cervicitis.

Conjugate Paired or joined.
Conjugate deviation Deviation of both eyes to either side.
Conjugate diagonal Distance measured from center of sacral promontory to the back of symphysis pubis. True conjugate is 1.5 to 2 cm less than diagonal conjugate.
Conjugate true It is anteriorposterior diameter of pelvic inlet; the distance between the midline superior point of the sacrum and the upper margin of symphysis pubis.

Conjugation A coupling together. In biology, the union of two unicellular organisms accompanied by an interchange of nuclear material.

Conjunctiva The mucous membrane covering the front of the eyeball and lining the eyelids.

Conjunctivitis Inflammation of the conjunctiva. "Pink eye" ophthalmia.
Catarrhal conjunctivitis A mild form, usually due to cold or irritation.
Granular conjunctivitis Trachoma.
Phlyctenular conjunctivitis Marked by small vesicles or ulcers on the membrane.
Purulent conjunctivitis Caused by virulent organisms, with discharge of pus.

Connective Joining together.
Connective tissues Those that develop from the mesenchyme and are formed of a matrix containing fibers and cells. Areolar tissue, cartilage and bone are examples.

Conn's syndrome Primary hyperaldosteronism with muscle weakness, polyuria, hypertension, hypokalemia and alkalosis.

Consanguinity Blood relationship.

Conscious The state of being awake or aware. Levels of consciousness are loosely defined states of awareness of and response to stimuli, essential for the assessment of an individual's neurological status. The level of consciousness is an accurate indicator of the degree of brain (dys) function.

Consensual Reflex stimulation of another or opposite part.

Consensual light reflex Contraction of opposite pupil from focusing of light on one side.

Consent In law, voluntary agreement with an action proposed by another. Consent is an act of reason; the person giving consent must be of sufficient mental capacity and in possession of all essential information in order to give valid and informed consent.

Consent forms In non-emergency situations, written informed consent is generally required before many clinical procedures, such as surgery (including biopsies), endoscopy and radiographic procedures involving catheterization.

The doctor must explain to the patient the diagnosis, the nature of the procedure, including the risks involved and the chances of success and the alternative methods of treatment that are available. It is recommended that consent forms should contain a signed declaration that the doctor has explained the nature of the procedure to the patient in non-technical words. Nurses or other members of the health care team maybe involved in filling out the consent form and witnessing the signature of the patient.

Conservative treatment The use of nonradical methods to restore health and preserve function.

Consolidation A state of becoming solid.

Consolidation of lung In pneumonia the infected lobe becomes solid with exudate.

Constipation Incomplete or infrequent action of the bowels, with consequent filling of the rectum with hard feces.

Atonic constipation Constipation due to lack of muscle tone in the bowel wall.

Spastic constipation A form of constipation where spasm of part of the bowel wall narrows the canal.

Consumer In health care, maybe the user, client, patient or carer, in terms of the services being provided.

Consumption 1. The act of consuming, or the process of being consumed. 2. A wasting away of the body; once applied to pulmonary tuberculosis.

Consummation 1. Giving oneself totally for a cause. 2. The completion of marriage by the first act of sexual intercourse.

Contact 1. A mutual touching of two bodies or persons. 2. An individual known to have been in association with an infected person or animal or a contaminated environment.

Contact dermatitis A skin rash marked by itching, swelling, blistering, oozing and scaling. It is caused by direct contact between the skin and a substance to which the person is allergic or sensitive.

Contact lens A glass or plastic lens worn under the eyelids in the front of the eye. It maybe worn for therapeutic or for cosmetic reasons.

Contact tracer A health care worker who visits people known to have an infectious disease, and their partners and family to encourage them to attend a clinic for health care in an attempt to prevent the spread of the infection in the community.

Contact tracing A public health measure taken to limit the spread of infectious disease, e.g., sexually transmitted diseases, tuberculosis.

Contagious Communicable; transmitted readily from one person to another either directly or indirectly.

Contagion 1. The communication of disease from one person to another by direct contact. 2. An infectious disease.

Containment A term used in communicable disease control, meaning prevention of spread of disease from a focus of infection.

Contamination 1. Introduction of disease germs or infectious materials into normally sterile objects. 2. Radiation in or on a place where it is not wanted.

Content analysis A research technique for the objective, systematic and quantitative description of communications and documentary evidence.

Continent 1. Able to control urination and defecation. 2. Exercising self-restraint, especially abstaining from sexual activity.

Continine Principal metabolite of nicotine excreted in urine.

Continuing care Ongoing care of the physically, mentally and emotionally handicapped, and those suffering from chronic incapacitating illness.

Continuing education Further study after the attainment of basic qualifications. This is vital for all professional practitioners so that they may keep up-to-date within their field and is accomplished in the form of organized study days or courses, or by individual reading.

Continuing healthcare Refers to a package of ongoing setting that has been assessed as primary health need, which might be a long-term condition or other chronic incapacitating illness.

Continuity of care The concept of a health care provider (general practitioner, health visitor or midwife, etc.) being continually involved with a patient throughout treatment over a period which may extend over years.

Continuous ambulatory peritoneal dialysis Abbreviated CAPD. The patient is ambulant while receiving peritoneal dialysis.

Continuous positive airway pressure Abbreviated CPAP. Medical gas is delivered to the patient at positive pressure to hold open alveoli that would normally close at the end of expiration, thereby increasing oxygenation and reducing the work of breathing.

Contortion A twisting into an unusual shape.

Contour Surface configuration of a part.

Contraception The prevention of conception and pregnancy.

Contraceptive An agent to prevent Conception, e.g., condom, cap that occludes the cervix, spermicidal pessary or cream, intrauterine device (IUD) and oral contraceptives (hormone pills).

Contract 1. To make or to enter into an agreement with a person, authority or company to deliver services or goods. 2. In health care, an agreement, usually written between two people with differing interests and concerns, who agree a course of action, behavior or treatment with defined goals. Consequences or penalties maybe included if the contract is not fulfilled.

Contraction A shortening or drawing together, especially applied to muscle action.

Uterine contractions Those occurring during labor.

Contraction isometric muscular exercise where muscles do not change its length.

Contraction isotonic Muscular contraction in which the muscle maintains constant tension by changing its length during contraction.

Contracture Fibrosis causing permanent contraction.

Dupuytren's contracture Contraction of the palmar fascia causing permanent bending and fixation of one or more fingers.

Volkmann's ischemic contracture Contraction resulting from impairment of the blood supply. May occur in upper or lower limbs.

Contraindication Any condition that makes a particular line of treatment impracticable or undesirable.

Contralateral Occurring on the opposite side.

Contrast In radiology, radiopaque material to provide a contrast in density between tissue or organ being X-rayed.

Contrast medium A substance used in radiography to make visible or more visible certain organs.

Contrecoup [Fr.] An injury occurring on the opposite side or at a distance from the site of the blow, e.g., brain damage on the opposite side of the skull to the blow.

Control 1. Restraint or command of objects or events. 2. A standard for testing where the procedure is identical in all respects to the experiment but the factor being studied is absent.

Birth control Contraception.

Control group A group of subjects who in the course of an experimental research project do not experience the factor under consideration. This enables the researcher to make a comparison with the effects produced on the experimental group.

Control of Substances Hazardous to Health (COSHH) Regulations that require the assessment of risk and action to be taken regarding the use of substances that maybe hazardous to health within the workplace.

Controlled drugs Preparations subject to the Misuse of Drugs Act (1971), Misuse of Drugs (Notification of and Supply to Addicts) Regulations (1973) and the Misuse of Drugs Regulations (1985), which regulate the prescribing and dispensing of psychoactive drugs, including narcotics, hallucinogens, depressants and stimulants.

Controlled trial A research method in which one group of subjects in a trial are not exposed to the experimental treatment or investigation, in an attempt to decrease the possibility of error and increase the possibility that the findings of the study are an accurate reflection of reality.

Controlled-dose transdermal absorption of drugs Application of a drug patch to the skin; gradual absorption gives a constant level in the blood. Examples of drugs used in this way include analgesics, some types of hormone and nicotine to assist a smoker to cease smoking.

Contusion A bruise.

Conus Shaped like cone.

Conus arteriosus The portion of right ventricle giving rise to pulmonary arteries.

Conus medularris Lower conical portion of spinal cord.

Convalescence Period of recovery following illness, injury or operation.

Convection A method of transmission of heat by the circulation of warmed molecules of a liquid or a gas.

Convergence The moving of two or more objects at same point.

Conversion 1. The act of changing into something of different form or properties. 2. The transformation of emotions into physical manifestations. 3. Manipulative correction of malposition of a fetal part during labor.

Conversion reaction Hysterical neuroses denoting a psychological conflict translated into physical ailment.

Convex Bowing outward. Having an outline like a segment of a sphere. The opposite of concave.

Convolution A fold or coil, e.g., of the cerebrum or renal tubules.

Convulsion Involuntary contractions of the voluntary muscles. Convulsive seizures are symptomatic of some neurological disorders; they are not in themselves a disease entity.

Clonic convulsion A convulsion marked by alternative contracting and relaxing of the muscles.

Febrile convulsion A convulsion occurring almost exclusively in children aged 6 months to 5 years of age, and associated with a fever of 40°C or higher.

Tonic convulsion Prolonged contraction of the muscles, as a result of an epileptic discharge *(See Epilepsy)*.

Cooley's anemia *TE Cooley, American pediatrician, 1871–1945.* Thalassemia.

Coombs' test *RRA Coombs., British immunologist, b. 1921.* A test to detect the presence of any antibody on the surface of the red blood cell. Used to detect rhesus incompatibility in maternal or fetal blood and in the diagnosis of hemolytic anemia.

Coordination Harmony of movement between several muscles or groups of muscle so that complicated maneuvers can be made.

Coping The process of contending with life difficulties in an effort to overcome or work through them.

Coping mechanisms Conscious or unconscious strategies or mechanisms that a person uses to cope with stress or anxiety.

Copolymer A polymer composed of two different kinds of monomers.

Copper Symbol Cu. A metallic element, traces of which are present in all human tissues.

Copper sulfate Deep blue crystals/granules, used as algicide/astringent.

Coprolalia The uncontrolled use of obscene speech.

Coprolith A mass of hard feces in the rectum or colon.

Coprophilia Unusual preoccupation with feces, a perversion in adults.

Coproporphyria Excessive coproporphyrin excretion in feces, as in inherited porphyrias.

Coproporphyrin A porphyrin present in urine and feces.

Copula Any connecting part.

Copulation Coitus. Sexual intercourse between male and female.

Coracoid Resembling in shape a crow's beak.

Coracoid process Process on anterior upper surface of scapula.

Cord A long cylindrical flexible structure.

Spermatic cord That which suspends the testicle in the scrotum, and contains the spermatic artery and vein and vas deferens.

Spinal cord The part of the central nervous system enclosed in the spinal column.

Umbilical cord The connection between the fetus and the placenta, through which the fetus receives nourishment.

Vocal cord's Folds of mucous membrane in the larynx, which vibrate to produce the voice.

Cordotomy Resectional of lateral spinothalamic tracts in the cord to relieve intractable pain.

Cori cycle In carbohydrate metabolism, the breakdown of muscle glycogen with formation of lactic acid which is converted to glycogen in liver. Liver glycogen is released as glucose which is taken up by muscles being then reconverted to muscle glycogen.

Corn A local hardening and thickening of the skin from pressure or friction, occurring usually on the feet.

Cornea The transparent portion of the anterior surface of the eyeball-continuous with the sclerotic coat.

Corical cornea Keratoconus.

Corneal Pertaining to the cornea.

Corneal graft A means of restoring sight by grafting healthy transparent cornea from a donor in place of diseased tissue. Keratoplasty.

Corneal reflex Closure of eye lid on touching the cornea: Afferent limb by trigeminal and efferent by facial nerves.

Corneoscleral Relating to both the cornea and sclera.

Corneoscleral junction The point where the edge of the cornea joins the sclera. The limbus.

Corneal transplant Either partial thickness of full thickness transfer of cornea from a healthy cadaver, donor to treat corneal opacity obstructing vision.

Corneoblelpharon Adhesion of eyelid to cornea.

Cornification Keratinization. The process whereby the skin becomes horny through the deposition of keratin.

Cornu A horn.

Cornu of the uterus One of the two horn-shaped projections where the uterine tubes join the uterus at the upper pole on either side.

Corona Any structure resembling a crown.

Corona radiata Ascending and descending fibers of internal capsule that above corpus collosum extend in all directions to reach cerebral cortex.

Coronal Relating to the crown of the head.

Coronal suture The junction of the frontal and parietal bones.

Coronal plane Plane dividing into front and back portions.

Coronary Encircling, crown-like.

Coronary angiography Opacification of coronary arteries by injection of iohexol or urograffin or any such contrast agent.

Coronary arteries The vessels that supply the heart.

Coronary artery bypass An operation carried out to bypass a coronary artery narrowed by atheroma using a graft from a healthy saphenous vein or internal mammary artery.

Coronary care unit A ward or unit within a hospital which provides for the monitoring and intensive care by a specialist team of staff of patients who have suffered an attack of coronary thrombosis and of those who are in the immediate postoperative period following heart surgery.

Coronary circulation (See *Circulation*).

Coronary thrombosis (See *Thrombosis*).

Coronary plexus A plexus of autonomic nerve fibers supplying the heart.

Coronary sinus The channel carrying venous drainage of heart into right atrium.

Coronavirus 1. A type of virus that can cause illness such as the common cold or serious diseases such as SARS and COVID-19.

Coronoid fossa An oval depression on anterior surface of distal end of humerus articulating with coronoid process of ulna.

Coronaviruses Members of a family (Coronaviridae) of large, enveloped, positive-stranded RNA viruses. Human coronaviruses (HCoVs) are a major cause of acute respiratory illnesses, e.g., the common cold (coryza). They can occasionally cause serious infections of the lower respiratory tract in children and adults and necrotizing enterocolitis in newborn.

Coroner A public official (e.g., a barrister, solicitor or doctor) who holds inquests concerning sudden, violent or suspicious deaths.

Corporate governance The accountability of an NHS Trust to meet standards in corporate management

155

working within the need to meet statutory financial objectives and targets.

Corporate working System in which managers and practitioners work within a team ethos, sharing a designated workload and providing equity of service.

Corpse A dead body; cadaver.

Corpulent Obese.

Corpulmanole Right heart failure secondary to pulmonary pathology.

Corpus A body.

Corpus albicans The scar tissue on the surface of the ovary which replaces the corpus luteum before the recommencement of menstruation.

Corpus callosum The mass of white matter that joins the two cerebral hemispheres together.

Corpus cavernosum Either of the two columns of the erectile tissue forming the body of the clitoris or the penis.

Corpus luteum The yellow body left on the surface of the ovary and formed from the remains of the graafian follicle after the discharge of the ovum. If it retrogresses, menstruation occurs, but it persists for several months if pregnancy supervenes.

Corpus striatum A mass of gray and white matter in the base of each cerebral hemisphere.

Corpuscle A small protoplasmic body or cell, as of blood or connective tissue.

Corrigan's pulse A full bounding pulse of aortic insufficiency.

Corrosive A substance that erodes and destroys.

Corrosive poisoning Poisoning by strong alkalies, acid, antiseptics, e.g., hydroxides of sodium, ammonium, potassium.

Corrugator The muscle of eye drawing eyebrow medially and inferiorly, arising from frontal bone and inserted on the skin of medial half of eyebrows.

Cortex [L.] An outer layer, as the bark of the trunk or root of a tree, or the outer layer of an organ or other structure, as distinguished from its inner substance.

Adrenal cortex The tissue surrounding the medulla or core of the adrenal gland.

Cerebral cortex The grey matter covering the two cerebral hemispheres.

Renal cortex The outer covering of the kidney.

Corticoid Steriod harmone secreted by adrenal cortex.

Corticospinal Relating to the cerebral cortex and the spinal cord.

Corticospinal tract The pyramidal tract. The nerve fibers making up the main pathway for rapid voluntary movement.

Corticosteroid Any of the hormones produced by the adrenal cortex or their synthetic substitutes. Glucocorticoids are responsible for carbohydrate, fat and protein metabolism. They have powerful anti-inflammatory properties. Mineralocorticoids, e.g., aldosterone, are responsible for salt and water regulation.

Corticosterone Hormone of adrenal cortex influencing carbohydrate metabolism. Na^+ and K^+ homeostasis.

Corticotrophin Adrenocorticotrophic hormone (ACTH).

Corticotrophin releasing factor The hypothalamic factor regulating secretion of corticotrophin.

Cortisol The naturally occurring hormone of the adrenal cortex. Hydrocortisone.

Cortisone A naturally occurring corticosteroid. Inactive in humans until converted into cortisol.

Cortisone acetate A synthetic preparation with anti-inflammatory and antiallergic properties.

Corynebacterium A genus of slender, rod-shaped, Gram-positive and non-motile bacteria.

Corynebacterium diptheriae Klebs-Loffler bacillus, the causative agent of diphtheria.

Coryza Acute infection of the upper respiratory tract, characterized by perfuse discharge from nasal mucous membranes, sneezing and watering of the eyes. The medical name for the common cold.

Cost-effectiveness A concept which relates cost to the effectiveness of a service and thus provides value for money, e.g., screening program to detect cervical cancer, rate of detection, and cost of the service and of treatment.

Cosmetic Agents or methods of improving physical appearance (appearance promoters).

Cosmetic surgery Commonly known as plastic surgery done to improve appearance, i.e., correction of ugly burns and scars, localized obesity, pendulous breast, facial wrinkles.

Cosmic Universe.

Costal Relating to the ribs.

Costal cartilages Those that connect the ribs to the sternum directly or indirectly.

Costen's syndrome Tempromandibular arthritis.

Costochondritis Inflammation of the cartilage that joins the ribs to the sternum. It will usually resolve after a few weeks.

Cot death *(See Sudden infant death syndrome)*.

Cotton p A round cotton ball having 1 cm diameter. It is used for applying medicines topically.

Cotton wool spots Soft wooly exudates in retina in hypertension and urermia, probably superficial infarcts.

Cotyledon A cup shaped depression. Applied to the subdivisions of the placenta.

Coughing Forcible downward displacement of lens caused to improve vision in cataract patients.

Cough Voluntary or reflex explosive expulsion of air from the lungs. Its purpose is usually to expel a foreign body or accumulations of mucus.

Drycough One where no expectoration occurs.

Wet cough One where expectoration of mucus or foreign body occurs.

Whooping cough Infectious disease caused by Bordetella pertussis.

Counseling A consultation and discussion in which one individual (the counselor) listens actively and offers guidance to another who is experiencing difficulties (the client). The counselor does not direct or make decisions for the client. The general aim is to solve problems and increase awareness. The emphasis is on clients finding their own solutions. *Disaster c.* Specialized counseling offered to victims of a major disaster, e.g., an aircraft crash or terrorist attack, or a natural event, e.g., an earthquake. The survivors of such disasters often experience psychological problems and post-traumatic stress disorder resulting in ill health.

Counter extension 1. The holding back of the upper fragment of a fractured bone while the lower is pulled into position. 2. The raising of the foot of the bed in such a way that the weight of the body counteracts the pull of the extension apparatus on the lower part of the limb. Used especially for fracture of the femur.

Counter Geiger Device for detection and counting of ionizing radiation.

Counter current exchanger The exchange of chemicals between two counter current streams separated by a membrane.

Counter immune-electrophoresis A process in which antigen and antibodies are placed in separate wells and an electric current is passed through diffusion medium. Antigens migrate to anode and antibodies to cathode. If the antigen and antibody correspond to each other, they upon meeting in the diffusion medium will precipitate and will form a precipit in band or line.

Counter incision A second incision made to facilitate drainage or to reduce tension on the stitches.

Counter irritant A substance that produces mild inflammation of the skin when applied to it, but relieves pain and congestion.

Counter shock An electric shock applied to heart to correct arrhythmia.

Counter traction The reduction of fractures by traction from two opposing directions at once.

Counterextension 1. The holding back of the upper fragment of a fractured bone while the lower is pulled into position. 2. The raising of the foot of the bed in such a way that the weight of the body counteracts the pull of the extension apparatus on the lower part of the limb. Used especially for fracture of the femur.

Counterirritant A substance that produces mild inflammation of the skin when applied to it, but relieves pain and congestion.

Countertraction The reduction of fractures by traction from two opposing directions at once.

Couple To join together, to have sexual union.

Coupling In cardiology, the frequent occurrence of a normal heart beat followed by an extraventricular one. Maybe found as a result of digitals overdose.

Couvade The experiencing of the symptoms of pregnancy and childbirth by the father. This psychosomatic phenomenon is common in many societies.

Courvoisier's law Sudden obstruction of bile duct by gallstone does not cause enlargement of gallbladder as opposed to gradual obstruction as in malignancy of pancreas/ampulla of Vater which consistently causes marked enlargement of gallbladder.

Couvelaire uterus Extravasation of blood into uterine musculature often demanding hysterectomy.

Covalent Sharing of electrons between two atoms.

Covid-19 Corona Virus Disease-19 (19 denotes year 2019 when the disease was first identified)

Cowden's disease Multiple hamartomas.

Cowling's rule Age of child on next birth day divided by 24 to give pediatric dose.

Cowper's gland A pair of compound tubular mucous glands beneath the bulb of male urethra, akin to Bartholin glands in female.

Coxa The hip joint.

Coxa valga A deformity of the hip in which there is an increase in the angle between the neck and the shaft of the femur.

Coxa vara A deformity in which the angle between the neck and the shaft of the femur is smaller than normal.

Coxalgia Pin in the hip.

Coxiella A genus of microorganisms of the order Rickettsiales.

Coxiella burnetii The causative agent of Q fever.

Coxsackie virus One of a group of enteroviruses that may give rise to a variety of illnesses, including meningitis, pleurodynia, acute myocarditis and acute pericarditis.

Crab louse *Phthirus pubis (See Louse).*

Crack Purified form of cocaine, produced by a technique known as 'freebasing' *(See Cocaine).*

Cracked pot sound Percussion note resembling cracked pot as in pulmonary cavity, hydrocephalus.

C

Cradle 1. A frame placed over the body or limb of a bed patient for protecting injured parts and preventing them from coming into contact with the bed clothes. 2. Infant's bed with protective sides and, in the past, often on rockers. 3. To support, hold, comfort in the arms.

Cradle cap An oily crust sometimes seen on the scalp of infants; also called milk crust (crusta lactea). Caused by excessive secretion of the sebaceous glands in the scalp.

Cramp A painful spasmodic muscular contraction which may result from fatigue.

Occupational cramp Occurs in miners and stokers; it is associated with intense heat and dehydration.

Cranial Relating to the cranium.

Cranial nerves The 12 pairs of nerves arising directly from the brain.

Cranioclast Instrument for crushing fetal skull to facilitate delivery of large head fetus.

Craniocleidodysostosis A congenital condition that involves defective ossification of bones of face, head, and clavicle.

Craniometry Measurement of skull bones.

Craniopharyngioma A cerebral tumor arising in the craniopharyngeal pouch just above the sella turcica.

Craniosacral therapy A form of osteopathic treatment in which very gentle manipulation of the cranium attempts to release tensions within the skull, which are thought to be the cause of various problems. The therapy has been successfully used to treat babies who become fractious after difficult forceps or vacuum extraction deliveries, or colic and hyperactivity in older infants.

Craniostenosis Premature closure of the suture lines of the skull in an infant. Surgery maybe required to relieve raised intracranial pressure.

Craniostosis Congenital ossification of cranial sutures.

Craniosynostosis Premature closure of the cranial sutures.

Craniotabes A patchy thinning of the bones of the vault of the skull of an infant; associated with rickets.

Craniotomy A surgical opening of the skull made to relieve pressure, arrest hemorrhage or remove a tumor.

Cranium 1. The skull. 2. The bony cavity that contains the brain.

Cravat bandage Triangular bandage folded to form a band around the injured part.

Crazybone Name for medial epicondyle of humerus, as slight trauma to it causes pain and tingling in fingers due to stimulation of ulnar nerve.

Crazybone reactive protien Acute phase reactant, a serum globulin whose concentration is increased in acute infections like rheumatic fever.

Creatine A nitrogenous compound present in muscle. It is also found in the urine in conditions in which muscle is rapidly broken down, e.g., acute fevers and starvation.

Creatine phosphate A high-energy phosphate store in muscle.

Creatine kinase Enzyme present in skeletal and cardiac muscles that acts in breakdown of ATP to ADP. Serum level is increased in myocardial infarction, skeletal muscle injury, and muscle dystrophy.

Creatinine A normal constituent of urine; a product of protein metabolism.

Creatinuria Increased concentration of creatine in the urine.

Crede's method Expulsion of placenta by putting downward pressure on the uterus through anterior abdominal wall and squeezing uterus but inversion is a danger.

Credentialing Review and examination of the credentials of health care professionals to ensure that they have training and the qualifications necessary to deliver care and support to the patient and the family.

Credibility A criterion for evaluating the data of qualitative research study, referring to the amount of confidence in the truth of the given information.

Credit Accumulation and Transfer System (CATS) Learning points or credits awarded by an academic institution to an individual for prior academic learning and/or evidence of the acquisition of professional expertise demonstrated, e.g., through a personal professional profile, contributing towards academic or professional awards, Originally developed to provide flexibility between academic institutions. *(See APEL and APL).*

Cremaster A fascia like muscle suspending and enveloping testicles and spermatic cord.

Cremasteric reflex Retraction of testes on stimulation of inner side of thigh, a superficial reflex mediated via L1, L2 segment.

Crepitation The grating sound caused by friction of the two ends of a fractured bone.

Crepitus 1. The discharge of flatus from the bowels. 2. Crepitation. 3. A crepitant rale.

Crescent Shaped like sickle e.g., menisci of knee joint, choroid atrophy in myopics (myopic crescent).

Cresol Coal tar derivative disinfectant containg 5% phenol.

Cresomania Hallucination of possession of great wealth.

Crest Ridge or elongated prominence. e.g., alveolar crest that surrounds teeth whose resorption can be delayed by flurbiprofen.

Crest Syndrome Calcinosis, Raynaud's phenomenon, esophageal dismotility, sclerodactily and telangiectasia, a variant of systemic sclerosis.

Cretin Hypothyroidism in babies manifesting as rough skin, mental subnormality, potbelly, coarse features, hypoactivity and delayed dentition.

Cretinism Congenital hypothyroidism. A condition caused by lack of thyroid secretion, characterized by arrested physical and mental development, dull facial expression with dry skin and lack of coordination.

Creutzfeldt-Jakob disease *HG Creutzfeldt, German physician, 1885–1964; A Jakob, German physician, 1884–1931.* Abbreviated CJD. A rapidly progressive disease of the nervous system affecting middle-aged and elderly people. The disease has been reported in younger people treated in the past with human pituitary extract for short stature, now no longer used. It is a spongi form encephalopathy similar to the bovine form (BSE) popularly known as 'mad cow disease', and is known to be associated with an abnormal protein or prion. There is no effective treatment. A new variant of CJD has recently been reported with a shorter incubation period.

Crevice A small fissure or crack e.g., gingival crevice, a fissure produced by the marginal gingival with tooth surface.

Crib A small bed with high legs and sides for infants and babies.

Cribriform Perforated like a sieve.
   Cribriform plate Part of the ethmoid bone *(See Ethmoid).*

Cricoid Ring-shaped.
   Cricoid cartilage The ring-shaped cartilage at the lower end of the larynx.

Cri-du-chat syndrome A chromosomal deletion disorder characterized by cry like a cat, microcephaly, mental retardation, dwarfism and laryngeal defect.

Crisis 1. A decisive point in acute disease; the turning point toward either recovery or death *(See Lysis)*. 2. A sudden paroxysmal intensification of symptoms in the course of a disease. 3. Life crisis; a period of disorganization that occurs when a person meets an obstacle to an important life goal such as the sudden death of a family member or a difficult family conflict.

Addisonian crisis. adrenal crisis Symptoms of fatigue, nausea and vomiting and collapse accompanying an acute attack of adrenal failure.

Blast crisis A sudden, severe change in the course of chronic myelocytic leukemia. The clinical picture resembles that seen in acute myelogenous leukemia, with an increase in the proportion of myeloblasts.

Crisis intervention Counseling or psychotherapy for patients in a life crisis that is directed at supporting the patient through the crisis and helping the patient to cope with the stressful event that precipitated it.

Identity crisis Usually occurring during adolescence, manifested by a loss of the sense of the sameness and historical continuity of one's self, and inability to accept the role the individual perceives as being expected by society.

Crista A crest or ridge, e.g., 1. Crysta ampularis, the localized thickening of membrane lining the ampulla of semicircular canals. 2. Crysta supraventricularis of heart.

Criterion The basis on which a decision is made, e.g., for drug dosage, treatment plans, research trials, etc.

Critical 1. Arising from a crisis. 2. Implying serious risk or uncertainty as to outcome.

C. appraisal An analysis of a research project using the parameters of research design, methodology, examination of results and relevance, e.g., relating the findings to practice.

C. care outreach team A team of specialist critical care practitioners based in hospital, whose main role is to share specialist skills and support ward staff in order to prevent admissions to the critical care facilities, and to facilitate appropriate discharges and transfers from the critical care unit.

C. care unit A unit within a hospital that supports and treats patients with critical disorders or diseases of the vital physiological systems. May also be called intensive care unit. *(See Intensive Care Unit)*.

C. path analysis In project management, tasks and actions are considered to be independent with the timing of each action crucial to the overall completion of the project. In clinical care, a schedule or pathway of procedures, or diagnostic tests for a patient is designed to ensure an efficient coordinated program of treatment.

C. thinking A purposeful, goal-directed approach based upon scientific evidence rather than assumption or memorization. Critical thinking is an organized approach to discovery that involves reflection and assimilation of information, which enables the nurse or health care provider to arrive at an informed decision or to make a judgment.

Crocodile tear Production of tear during mastication in patients with facial palsy due to abnormal regeneration, so named because crocodiles are said to weep after eating their victims.

Crohn's disease (Krohnz) *BB Crohn, American physician, 1884–1983.* Regional ileitis *(See Ileitis)*.

Crosby capsule *WH Crosby, American physician, b. 1914.* A capsule attached to the end of a flexible tube which is swallowed by the patient. When the capsule reaches the small intestine, as seen on radiological examination, a biopsy of the intestinal mucosa maybe taken.

Cromolyn sodium Disodium chromoglycate, useful in bronchial asthama, mast cell stabilizer.

Cross-fertilization Fusion of male and female gametes from different persons.

Cross-matching A test of the compatibility of donor blood to be transfused to a patient *(See Blood group)*.

Crossover Reciprocal exchange of genetic material between chromosomes.

Crotamiton A scabicide used as 2% ointment.

Croup A condition resulting from acute obstruction of the larynx caused by allergy, foreign body, infection or new growth; occurs chiefly in infants and children. There is spasmodic dyspnea, a harsh cough and stridor.

Crouzon's disease Congenital disease characterized by hypertelorism (wide spaced eyes) craniofacial dysostosis, exophthalmos, optic atrophy and divergent squint.

Crown Part of the tooth that appears above the gum.

Crowning The stage in labor when the top of the infant's head becomes visible at the vulva.

Crowing ligament (See Ligament).

Cruciate Cross shaped as in cruciate ligament of knee.

Crura Divergent bands resembling legs. For example, crura of diaphragm, connecting to spinal column, crura crebri; cerebral peduncles.

Crus [L.] 1. The leg, from knee to foot. 2. A leg-like part.

Crush syndrome The edema, oliguria and other symptoms of acute renal failure that follow crushing of a part, especially a large muscle mass, causing the release of myoglobin.

Crutch Appliance usually in the form of a light, tubular metal rod with hand grips and plastic loops for the forearms, to aid walking when the patient must not weight-bear (as in fractures of lower limbs) or when a lower limb is missing.

Crutch paralysis Crutch induces paralysis of brachial plexus/radial nerve.

Cryesthesia Abnormal sensitivity to cold.

Cryoanalgesia The relief of pain by application of cold by cryoprobe to peripheral nerves.

Cryobank A facility for freezing and preserving semen at low temperatures usually −196.5°C) for future use.

Cryocautery Cold application for therapeutic objective.

Cryoextractor An instrument in which intense cold coagulates the lens of the eye for removal in cataract extraction.

Cryoglobulin An abnormal globulin that precipitates when cooled but dissolves on heating, found in multiple myeloma, leukemia and mycoplasma pneumonia.

Cryoprecipitate Any precipitate that results from cooling. Of particular therapeutic value is the cryoprecipitate from fresh plasma, which is rich in factor VIII and is used to treat hemophilia.

Cryopreservation Maintenance of the viability of excised tissue or organs by storing at very low temperatures.

Cryosurgery The use of extreme cold to destroy tissue.

Cryotherapy Therapeutic use of cold.

Crypt Small cavity, i.e., anal cryps lying behind junction of anal skin and rectal mucosa, tonsillar crypts on tonsils surrounded by lymphnodules.

Cryptitis Inflammation of anal crypts.

Cryptococcosis Infection caused by the fungus *Cryptococcus neoformans*, having a predilection for the brain and meninges but also invading the skin, lungs and other parts. It particularly affects person's immunocompromised by disease or therapy.

Cryptorchidism Failure of the testicles to descend into the scrotum; cryptorchism.

Crypts of Lieberkühn *JN Lieberkühn, German anatomist, 1711–1756.* Glands, found in the mucous membrane of the small intestine, which secrete intestinal juice.

Cryptogenic of unknown or indeterminate origin.

Cryptomenorrhea Monthly subjective symptoms of menstruation without vaginal bleed usually due to unperforated hymen.

Cryptosporidiasis Acute diarrhea caused by protozoa cryptosporidium usually in immunocompromised.

Crystal Small particles with definite pattern and angles, e.g., apatite crystals of calcium phosphate with other elements; Charcot-Leyden crystals found in sputum of patients with asthma where in there is eosinophilia.

Crystallography Study of crystals pertains to study of renal and biliary calculi.

Crystalluria Appearance of crystals, in urine, commonly after administration of sulfa drugs.

Crystallography terminal The alpha carboxyl group of last amino acid.

Chemoreceptor trigger zone (CTZ) The area of medulla oblongata whose stimulation causes vomiting.

CT *(See Compound Axial Tomography)*.

Cu Symbol for copper.

Cubital fossa The hollow anterior to elbow bounded medially by pronater teres and laterally by brachioradialis.

Cubitus 1. The forearm. 2. The elbow.

Cubitus valgus Deformity of the elbow where the palm of the hand is abducted and thus faces outward.

Cubitus varus Deformity where there is adduction of the forearm.

Cue Something that gives a hint or idea of something else. A Cue is a verbal or non-verbal signal in communica-

tion from one person to another. It is a remembered item which connects with further information or meaning.

Cued recall Retrieval of information from memory with the help of cues, perhaps using the first letter of the word or name to be remembered.

Cuff Glove, structure encircling apart.

Cul-de-sac A blind pouch or cavity.

Culdocentesis Perforation of posterior upper vaginal wall for draining rectouterine pouch for diagnostic/therapeutic purposes.

Culdoscope An endoscope used in culdoscopy.

Culdoscopy Direct visual examination of the female viscera through an endoscope introduced into the pelvic cavity through the posterior vaginal fornix.

Culex Mosquito responsible for filariasis.

Culicide Agents that destroy gnats and mosquitoes.

Cullen's sign Bluish discoloration of periumbilical skin due to intraperitoneal hemorrhage, usually following pancreatitis, tubal pregnancy rupture.

Culmen Top or submit of a thing.

Cult People following an ideal or principle.

Culture 1. The propagation of microorganisms or of living tissue cells in special media conducive to their growth. 2. A collective noun for the symbolic and acquired aspects of human society, including convention, custom and language. 3. A singular noun for the customs and features of an ethnic (racial, religious or social) group.

Cumulative Adding to.

Cumulative action The toxic effects produced by prolonged use of a drug given in comparatively small doses. Usually occurs as a result of slow excretion of the drug.

Cumulative index to nursing and allied health literature (CINAHL) A computerized database of English language nursing and allied health literature.

Cumulus Small elevation.

Cupid's bow The normal bow shape of upper lip.

Cupola The dome at the apex of cochlea; the dome of pleura, covering apex of lung.

Cupping 1. The formation of a cup-shaped depression with the hand: (a) To produce a skin erythema, thereby improving local circulation; and (b) To loosen excessive secretions from air passages, and perhaps induce coughing. 2. The use of a cupping glass to stimulate skin blood flow.

Cuprous Monovalent copper Cu+.

CUPS Critical, unstable, potentially unstable, and stable. Priority classification of patients, used during the initial assessment of the patient.

Curare An extract from a South American plant used to poison the tips of arrows. Used in surgery to produce complete muscle relaxation, it is given intravenously as tubocurarine.

Curarization Anticonvulsant medication, by administration of agents negating effects of acetylcholine, i.e., suxamethonium.

Curative Anything which promotes healing by overcoming disease.

Curettage [Fr.] The scraping of a surface with a curette for therapeutic purposes or to obtain biopsy material.

Curette A spoon-shaped instrument used for the removal of unhealthy tissues by scraping.

Curie Unit of radiation equivalents to $10(10) \times 3.7$ disintegration per second.

Curietron An apparatus used for the treatment of cancer of the cervix and body of the uterus. The applicators are placed in the patient and the radioisotope is then moved in and out of the applicators by remote control.

Curling's ulcer An ulcer of the duodenum seen after severe burns of the body.

Current A flow, usually of electrical impulse.

Curriculum Course of study.

Curschmann's spirals Coiled spirals in sputum of asthmatic patients.

Cursor On the computer screen, a blinking character that indicates where the next character will appear.

Curvature The curving of a line, whether normal or abnormal.
    Spinal curavutre Abnormal deviation of the vertebral column.

Curvilinear Concerning or pertaining to a curved line.

Cushing's disease HW Cushing, American surgeon, 1869–1939. A condition of over-secretion by the adrenal cortex due to an adenoma of the pituitary gland. Symptoms include obesity, abnormal distribution of hair and atrophy of the genital organs.

Cushing's syndrome Symptoms arising out of hypercortisolism.

Cushingoid Referring to symptoms resembling those of Cushing's disease, e.g., the side effects of steroid therapy.

Cusp A pointed or rounded projection, such as on the crown of a tooth, or a segment of a cardiac valve.

Cutaneous Pertaining to the skin.

Cutdown An incision into a vein with insertion of a catheter for intravenous infusion. It is performed when an infusion cannot be started by venipuncture. Also used with hyper alimentation therapy when concentrated solutions need to be given into the superior vena cava.

Cuticle The narrow band of epidermis extending from the nail wall on to the nail surface; also called eponychium.

Cutis The skin.

Cyanemia Blue color blood.

C

Cyanhemoglobin Cyanide hemoglobin compound where blood appears cherry red as in cyanide poisoning.

Cyanocobalamin Vitamin B_{12} (anti anemic factor) found in liver, eggs and fish. It combines with the intrinsic factor secreted in gastric juice for absorption and is essential for erythrocyte maturation. Administered by injection in the treatment of pernicious anemia.

Cyanosis A bluish appearance of the skin and mucous membranes, caused by imperfect oxygenation of the blood. It indicates circulatory failure and is common in respiratory diseases. It is also seen in 'blue babies'.

Cyberstalking Internet harassment, for example, repetitive unsolicited and/or inappropriate emails, including hate, obscene or threatening mail or live chat harassment. *(See Bullying and Harassment)*.

Cyclamate A non-nutritive sweetener.

Cycle A series of recurring events.

Cardiac cycle The events occurring between one heartbeat and the next.

Menstrual cycle The changes that occur each month in the female reproductive system.

Cyclazocin Used in opioid addiction.

Cyclic Pertaining to or occurring in a cycle.

Cyclic AMP Adenosine 3'5' cyclic monophosphate, an intracellular messenger of end organ stimulation.

Cyclitis Inflammation of ciliary body.

Cyclizine An antihistamine.

Cyclobarbitone A short-acting barbiturate drug administered orally in cases of insomnia. Prolonged use may lead to dependence.

Cyclodialysis An operation used in glaucoma to improve drainage from the anterior chamber of the eye at the corneoscleral junction.

Cyclodiathermy A treatment for glaucoma without penetration of the eyeball. Diathermy is applied to the sclera to cause fibrosis around the ciliary body, so allowing the aqueous humor to drain.

Cyclo-oxygenase Enzyme converting arachidonic acid to prostaglandin.

Cyclopenthiazide An oral diuretic.

Cyclopentolate Eyedrops that paralyse the ciliary muscles and dilate the pupils.

Cyclophosphamide A cytotoxic drug used in the treatment of lymphomas and leukemia.

Cycloplegia Paralysis of the ciliary muscle of the eye.

Cyclopropane A gas used for general anesthesia. It is not irritating to the respiratory tract but is highly inflammable and is, therefore, potentially dangerous.

Cycloserine An antibiotic drug used in the treatment of tuberculosis by resistant to first-line therapy.

Cyclosporine An immunosuppressive agent which does not suppress the production of antibodies. Used as prophylaxis in graft-versus-host (GVH) disease and for the prevention of graft rejection in the field of organ and tissue transplantation.

Cyclothymia The alteration of mood seen in manic-depressive psychosis.

Cyesis Pregnancy.

Pseudo cyesis Signs and symptoms suggestive of pregnancy arising when no fertilization has taken place. 'Phantom pregnancy'.

Cyclotron A particle accelerator in which the particle is rotated between the ends of the magnet, gaining speed with each rotation.

Cylindroma Malignant tumor congaing a collection of cells forming cylinders.

Cyproheptadine Antiserotonin drug used in allergy and dumping syndrome.

Cyproterone An antiandrogen used to treat male hypersexuality and prostatic carcinoma.

Cyst 1. A cavity or sac with epithelium, containing liquid or semisolid matter. 2. A stage in the life cycle of certain protozoan parasites when they acquire tough protective coat.

Branchial cyst One formed in the neck from non-closure of the branchial cleft during development.

Chocolate cyst An ovarian cyst occurring in endometriosis.

Daughter cyst A small cyst that develops from a large one.

Dermoid cyst A congenital type containing skin, hair, teeth, etc. It is due to abnormal development of embryonic tissue.

Hydatid cyst The larval cyst stage of the tapeworm, usually found in the liver.

Meibomian cyst A swelling of a Meibomian gland caused by obstruction of its duct.

Multilocular cyst A cyst that is divided into compartments or locules.

Ovarian cyst A cyst of the ovary, usually nonmalignant, but sometimes becoming very large and requiring surgical removal.

Retention cyst Any cyst caused by blockage of a duct.

Sebaceous cyst A retention cyst caused by the blockage of a duct from a sebaceous gland so that the sebum collects.

Sublingual cyst A ranula.

Thyroglossal cyst One in the thyroglossaltract near the hyoid bone at the base of the tongue.

Cystadenoma An adenoma containing cyst, maybe serious when filled with clear fluid or pseudomucinous when contains thick viscid fluid.

Cysthionine An intermediate compound in the metabolism of methionine to cystine.

Cystathioninuria A hereditary disorder of cystathionine metabolism, marked by increased concentrations in the urine. Maybe associated with learning difficulties.

Cystectomy Complete or partial removal of the urinary bladder. The ureters are diverted into an isolated ileal segment (ileal conduit) or into the sigmoid colon.

Cysteine A sulphur-containing amino acid formed by the ingestion of dietary proteins.

Cysticercosis Formation of cysts by encapsulation of larvae of tapework (Taenia).

Cystic fibrosis Generalized hereditary disorder associated with accumulation of excessively thick and tenacious mucus and abnormal secretion of sweat and saliva; called also cystic fibrosis of the pancreas, and mucoviscidosis. The disease is inherited as a recessive trait. The severity of cystic fibrosis varies widely. Although it is congenital, it may not manifest itself during the early weeks of life, or it may cause intestinal obstruction and perforation in the newborn. The chief cause of complications in cystic fibrosis is the extremely thick mucus predisposing to repeated infection, leading to chronic lung disease.

Cysticercosis A disease caused by infestation with the cysticercus of *Taenia solium* (pork tapeworm).

Cysticercus The cystic or larval form of the tapeworm.

Cystine An amino acid closely related to cysteine. Sometimes excreted in urine in the form of minute crystals (cystinuria).

Cystinosis An inherited metabolic disorder in which cystine is deposited in the tissues.

Cystitis Inflammation of the urinary bladder.

Cystocele A prolapse of the bladder into the vagina.

Cystodiathermy The application of a high-frequency electric current to the bladder mucosa, usually for the removal of papillomas.

Cystography Radiography of the urinary bladder after the introduction of a radiopaque contrast medium.

Micturating cystography Radiographic examination during the act of passing urine.

Cystolithiasis Stone or stones in the urinary bladder.

Cystopexy An operation for stress incontinence in which the bladder neck is fastened to the fascia at the back of the symphysis pubis.

Cystoscope An endoscope for examining the interior of the urinary bladder.

Cystoscopy Incision of the urinary bladder for removal of calculi, etc. Suprapubic cystoscopy Incision above the pubes.

Cystostomy The operation of making a temporary or permanent opening into the urinary bladder.

Cystotomy Incision of the urinary bladder for removal of calculi, etc.

Suprapubic cystotomy Incision above the pubes.

Cystourethrography Radiography of the urinary bladder and urethra.

Cystourethroscope An instrument for examining the urethra and bladder.

Cytarabine (See Cytosine).

Cytarabine Compound of cytosine and D ribose.

Cytochrome A pigment important for cellular respiration.

Cytochrome oxidase Enzyme responsible for electron transfer from cytochromes to oxygen thus activating oxygen to combine with hydrogen to form water.

Cytochrome P450 A protein similar to Hb in the microsomes of livercells, catalyzing metabolism of steroid hormones and detoxification of many chemicals.

Cytogenesis Origin and development of cell.

Cytogenetics The study of cells during mitosis in order to examine the chromosomes and the relationship between chromosome abnormality and disease.

Cytology The microscopic study of the form and functions of the cells of the body.

Exfoliative cytology An aid to the early diagnosis of malignant disease. Secretions or surface cells are examined for premalignant changes.

Cytolysin A substance that causes cytolysis *(See Bacteriolysin and Hemolysin).*

Cystolysis The destruction of cells.

Cytomegalic Inclusion disease an infection due to cytomegalovirus. In the congenital form, there is hepatosplenomegaly with cirrhosis, and microcephaly with learning difficulties and development delay. Acquired disease may cause a clinical state similar to infectious mononucleosis.

Cytomegalovirus A virus belonging to the herpes simplex group.

Cytopheresis A technique to remove specific cellular components from the blood, e.g., white blood cells or platelets needed to treat a patient, or to remove abnormal constituents.

Cytoplasm The protoplasmic part of the cell surrounding the nucleus.

Cytosine One of the pyrimidine bases found in deoxyribonucleic acid (DNA).

Cytosine arabinoside An anti metabolite used in the treatment of acute leukemia. Cytarabine.

Cytotoxic 1. Having a deleterious effect upon cells. 2. An agent or drug that damages or destroys cells. Used to treat various forms of cancer.

Cytotoxin A toxin having a specific toxic action on cells of special organs.

D Symbol for dioptre.

Dacarbazine An alkylating agent used in treatment of malignant melanoma, Hodgkin's disease.

Dacryocystitis Inflammation of lacrimal gland.

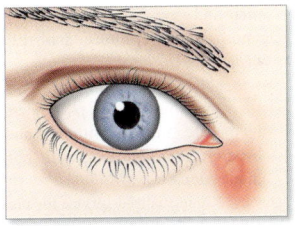

Dacryocystitis

Dacryostenosis Narrowing of lacrimal duct.

Dacryocystorhinostomy An operation to create a new opening between the lacrimal sac and the nasal cavity.

Dacryolith A calculus in a lacrimal duct.

Dacryoma A benign tumour which arises from the lacrimal epithelium.

Dactyl A finger or toe; a digit.

Dactylitis Chronic inflammation of phalanges and metatarsals.

Dactylology Communication between individuals by signs made with the fingers and hands.

Dactinomycin Anti tumor antibiotic.

Dalteparin A factor Xa inhibitor, anti-coagulant.

Dalton's law In a mixture of gases total pressure is equal to sum of partial pressure of each gas.

Daltonism Colour blindness; inability to distinguish red from green.

Danazol An anterior pituitary suppressant used in the treatment of endometriosis, associated infertility and benign breast disease.

Dance, Saint vitus *SYN* – chorea, i.e., involuntary quasipurposive nonrepetitive jerky movements.

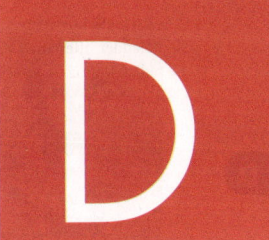

Dander Small scales from the hair or feathers of animals, which may be a cause of allergy in sensitive persons.

Dandruff White scales shed from the scalp. If moist from serous exudates they have a greasy appearance.

Dandy-Walker syndrome Congenital hydrocephalus due to blockage of foramen of Luschka and Magendie.

Dane Particle 42 nm sphere of hepatitis B virus.

Dantrolene A muscle relaxant.

Dapsone A sulphone drug used in the treatment of leprosy.

Daraprim Pyrimethamine, used in malaria.

Dariers disease (Keratosis follicularis) a congenital disorder characterized by verrucous papular growths that coalesce into plaques of various sizes on scalp, face, neck and trunk.

Darier's sign Burning and itching sensation in lesions of urticaria after stroking and it becomes red and raised.

Dark room Light tight room for processing X-ray films.

Dartos The subcutaneous muscle of scrotum.

Darwinism *C.R. Darwin, British Naturalist, 1809–1882.* The theory of the evolution of species through natural selection.

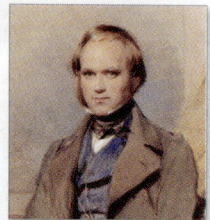

Charles Darwin

Data (s) datum; a collection of facts.

Continuous data Data that have a continuous set of values, e.g., for variables such as height, weight and antibody titres in response to vaccination.

Data processing The storage and analysis of data to produce statistical tabulations, often by computer.

Data Protection Act, 1984 This Act gives people the right to know what information is held about them on computers, including health related data. The Data Protection (Subject Access Modification) (Health) Order 1987 restricted access to health information which might cause serious physical or mental harm to an individual or reveal the identity of another person. The Act did not apply to manual records and in 1990 the access to Health Records Act was passed to enable people to have access to any computerized or manual health-related records made after 1991. Patients and clients must apply to gain access to their records; the same exceptions to access as in the original Data Protection Act remain.

Data set A collection of information made on a group and related to certain variables that are being investigated.

Discrete data Data with a single value or characteristic, e.g., colour of hair.

Database Information collected, stored, reviewed and updated, and used for evaluation and audit; e.g., a patient care database, in which information is gained at the initial interview, forms part of the care plan and is available for the evaluation of treatment and care.

Daunomycin A cytotoxic antibiotic; daunorubicin.

Daunorubicin Daunomycin.

Dawn phenomenon A phenomena in diabetes mellitus with morning hyperglycemia due to growth hormone release.

Day care A specialized service for preschool children, either as a substitute for or as an extension to family life. A similar service may be provided for the elderly needing care and support and to provide respite for family carers (*See Day center*).

Day center A specialized facility that offers care, treatment and a respite service for the elderly or the mentally ill.

Day nursery A center for the care, during the daytime, of children upto the age of 5 years; Provided by the social service department or by voluntary agencies. Priority is given to children from 'at risk' families and to those with a handicap.

Day patient care A service provided either in a specialized ward or in a hospital ward for treatment/investigation/minor surgery. The patient is admitted and discharged on the same day.

DB Symbol for decibel.

DBS Disclosure and Barring Service. The DBS provides criminal record checks for applicants to certain professions or roles in England and Wales. Different systems apply in Scotland and Northern Ireland.

D & C Dilatation and curettage.

DDT Dichlro Diphenyl Trichloroethane. A powerful insecticide

Deafness The inability to hear.

Conduction or middle ear deafness Deafness due to the sound wave failing to reach the cochlea.

Perceptive or nerve deafness Deafness due to damage to the cochlea or auditory nerve.

Deamination A process of hydrolysis, taking place in the liver, by which amino acids are broken down and urea is formed.

Death The cessation of all physical and chemical processes that occur in all living organisms or their cellular components.

Clinical death The absence of heart beat (no pulse can be felt) and cessation of breathing.

Cot death Sudden infant death syndrome (SIDS).

Death certificate Certificate issued by the registrar for deaths after receipt of a preliminary certificate completed and signed by an attending doctor, indicating the date and probable cause of death. Only after issue of this certificate, indicating that the death has been registered, can the body be disposed of.

Death instinct A concept, introduced by Freud, proposing a self destructive drive opposed by the sexual instinct, which perpetually seeks a renewal of life. May manifest itself as a repetition compulsion with the aim of annihilating one self.

Death rate The number of deaths per stated number of persons (100 or 10000 or 100000) in a certain region in a certain period.

Deathy rattle Rattle sound produced by passage of air through accumulated mucous in the bronchi in terminal patients due to want of cough reflex.

Debility A condition of weakness and lack of physical tone.

Debridement The removal of foreign substances and injured tissues from a traumatic wound. Part of the immediate treatment to promote healing.

Debrisan Trade name for a preparation of dextranomer beads used to assist wound-cleaning and the desloughing of ulcers.

Debrisoquin Antihypertensive agent.

Decadron Dexamethasone, a long acting corticosteroid.

Decadurabolin Nandrolone decanoate, an anabolic steroid.

Decalcification Removal of calcium-salts, e.g., from bone in disorders of calcium metabolism.

Decameter A measure of 10 meters.

Decannulation The removal of a cannula.

Decapitation Beheading.

Decapsulation Removal of a fibrous-capsule.

Decarboxylase Enzyme catalyzing release of carbondioxide from compounds like aminoacids.

Decay 1. The gradual decomposition of the dead organic matter. 2. The process or stage of ageing of living-matter.

Radioactive decay The process by which an unstable atom loses energy by the emission of gamma rays or beta or alpha particles and is transformed to a more stable atom.

Deceleration Decrease in velocity.

Decerebrate A person with brain damage whose neurological reactions are severely impaired and in whom cerebral functioning has ceased.

Decibel Symbol dB. A unit of intensity of sound, used particularly in estimating the degree of deafness.

Decidua The thickened lining of the uterus for the reception of the fertilized ovum to protect the developing embryo. It is shed when pregnancy terminates.

Deciduoma An intrauterine tumour containing decidual cells.

Deciduom amalignum Chorionepithelioma.

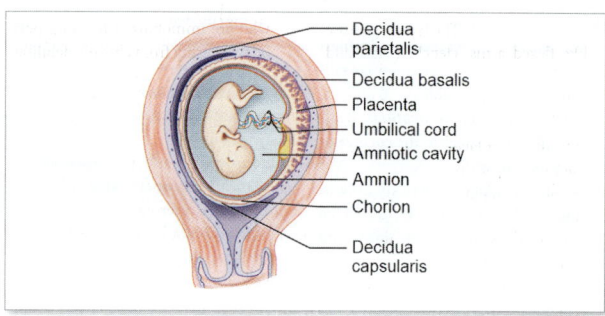

Decidua

Decidua parietalis
Decidua basalis
Placenta
Umbilical cord
Amniotic cavity
Amnion
Chorion
Decidua capsularis

Deciduous Falling off; subject to being shed, as deciduous teeth.

Deciliter 100 mL or 10 centiliter.

Decimeter 10 cm or 1/10 of meter.

Decision analysis A logically consistent approach to the common clinical problem of needing to make a decision when its consequences cannot be foretold with certainty. The biological variation, inconsistent drug response and poor clinical outcome data on many drug/therapeutic procedures make decision analysis a charter so that patient can be foretold in advance all about the possible outcome of treatment and he can choose the one he thinks best.

Decision making The process of using all the information available about a patient and arriving at a decision concerning therapeutic plan.

Declaration of Geneva The declaration adopted in 1948 by World Medical Association at Geneva.

Declaration of Hawaii The guidelines laid down by General Assembly of world psychiatric association for psychiatrists in 1976 at Hawaii.

Decline Progressively decrease.

Decoction A liquid medicinal preparation made by boiling vegetable substances with water.

Decompensation Failure to compensate. In particular, failure of the heart to overcome disability or increased workload.

Decomposition Decay, putrefaction.

Decompression Return to normal environmental pressure after exposure to greatly increased pressure.
Cerebral decompression Removal of a flap of the skull and incision of the dura mater for the purpose of relieving intracranial pressure.
Decompression sickness A disorder characterized by joint pains, respiratory manifestations, skin lesions and neurological signs, occurring as a result of rapid reduction in air pressure. Aviators flying at high altitudes and persons breathing compressed air in caissons and diving apparatus are particularly susceptible to this disorder.

Decongestant 1. Reducing congestionor swelling 2. An agent that reduces congestion or swelling, usually of the nasal membranes. Decongestants may be inhaled, taken as spray or nose drops, or used orally in liquid or tablet form.

Decontamination The freeing of a person or an object of some contaminating substance such as nerve gas, radioactive material, etc.

Decorticate posture The typical posture like flexed arms, clenched fists and extended legs in a comatose patient with lesion above upper brainstem.

Decortication An operation to strip the outer layer of an organ, e.g., the removal of the thickened pleura in the treatment of chronic empyema.

Decrudescence Diminution or abatement of the intensity of symptoms.

Decubitus The position assumed when lying down.

Decubitus projection A radiographic procedure that helps in the demonstration of air-fluid levels, using decubitus position and central ray of X-ray beam placed horizontally.

Decubitus ulcer An ulcer due to interference with the local circulation from prolonged or severe pressure on the surface body tissue resulting in tissue anoxia and cell death, also called bedsore and pressure sore.

Decussation A crossing, particularly of nerve fibres. A chiasma.

Pyramidal decussation The crossing of the pyramidal nerve fibres in the medulla oblongata.

Defecation Elimination of wastes and undigested food, as feces, from the rectum.

Dedifferentiation 1.The return of parts to a homogeneous state. 2. Process by which mature differentiated cells or tissues at sites of origin of immature elements of the same type, as in some cancers.

Deduction Reasoning from general to particular.

Deep reflex Reflexes influenced by higher cortical centers, e.g., ankle, knee, supination, biceps jerks.

Deep vein thrombosis Formation of thrombus in the deep-seated veins, especially of legs, characterized by pain and tenderness in the thighs or calves; occurs primarily in patients who are immobilized for long periods, suffering from chronic debilitating diseases, cancer, or after surgery.

Defecation Bowel evacuation.

Defecation syncope Syncope occurring during or immediately after defecation.

Defeminization Loss of female sexual characteristics.

Defence Behaviour directed to protection of the individual from injury.

Character defence Any character-trait, e.g., a mannerism, attitude or affectation, which serves as a defence mechanism.

Defence mechanism In psychology, an unconscious mental process or coping pattern that lessens the anxiety associated with a situation or internal conflict and protects the person from mental discomfort.

Insanity defence A legal concept that a person cannot be convicted of a crime if lacking criminal responsibility by reason of insanity at the time of commission of the crime.

Deferens Carrying away.

Deferroxamine Iron chelating agent used in thalassemia major, hemosiderosis.

Defervescence The period of abatement of fever.

Deferiprone Iron chelating agent.

Defibrillation The restoration of normal rhythm to the heart in ventricular or atrial fibrillation.

Defibrillator An instrument by which normal rhythm is restored in ventricular or atrial fibrillation by the application of a high voltage electric current.

Definition The precise.

Defibrination The removal of fibrin from blood plasma to prevent clotting. Used in the preparation of sera.

Diffinitive Clear and final without ambiguity.

Deficiency disease A condition caused by dietary or metabolic deficiency, including all diseases due to an insufficient supply of essential nutrients.

Deficit A deficiency or variation from that which is considered to be normal.

Deformity An alteration to the natural form or alignment of an organ.

Akerlund deformity X-ray deformity of duodenal cap in duodenal ulcer.

Boutonniere deformity flexion of PIP (proximal interphalangeal joint) and hyperextension of DIP (distal interphalangeal joint).

Madclung deformity radial deviation of hand due to overgrowth of distal ulna or shortening of radius.

Springel's deformity congenital elevation of scapula.

Swan-neck deformity hyperextension of PIP joint and flexion of DIP joint.

Degeneration Deterioration in organ structure or function.

Fatty degeneration Deposition of abnormal amounts of fat replacing normal cells.

Calcareous degeneration Deposition of calcium salts.

Cystic degeneration Degeneration with cyst formation.

Hyaline degeneration The degenerated tissues assume a homogeneous and glossy appearance.

Hydropic degeneration Appearance of water droplets in cytoplasm.

Pigmentary degeneration Degenerated cells change their colour.

Spongy degeneration Familial demyelination of deep cerebral cortex.

Subacute combined degeneration Degeneration of lateral and posterior columns of spinal cord as in Vit. B$_{12}$ deficiency.

Deglutition The act of swallowing.

Dehiscence Splitting open, as of a wound.

Dehydration Excessive loss of fluid from the body by persistent vomiting, diarrhea or sweating, or from the lack of intake. Severe dehydration is a serious condition that may lead to fatal shock, acidosis and the accumulation of waste products in the body, as in uremia.

Dehydrocholic acid A bile salt that stimulates the production of bile from the liver.

Dehydrocholesterol Precursor of Vit. D.

Dehydrocorticosterone Adrenal corticosteroid.

Dehydroepiandrosterone A 17 ketosteriod with androgenic activity.

Deinstitutionalization *(See Institutionalization)*.

Deiters' cells Supporting cells in organ of corti.

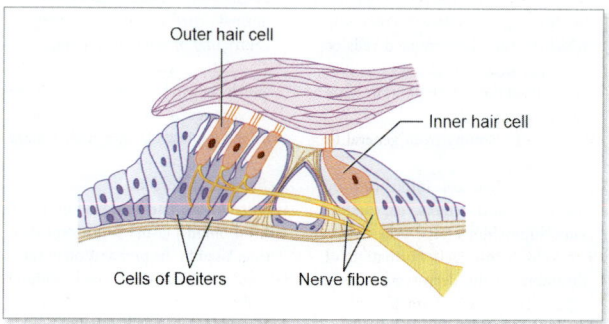

Outer hair cell

Inner hair cell

Cells of Deiters   Nerve fibres

Deiters' Cells

Deiter's nucleus Cell collection behind auditory nerve nucleus.

Deja entendu The illusion or experience of hearing a thing which he/she has previously heard.

Deja vu [Fr.] An illusion that a new experience is a repetition of a previous experience.

Deladelaphus Twins fused above thorax, but separated below.

Deleterious Harmful; injurious.

Deletion The loss of genetic material from one chromosome.

Delinquency Criminal or antisocial-conduct, especially among juveniles.

Delinquent One with antisocial/criminal behavior.

Delirium Mental excitement. A common condition in high fever. It is marked by an irregular expenditure of nervous energy, incoherent talk and delusions.

Delirium tremens An acute psychosis common in chronic alcoholism, usually following abstinence from alcohol.

Traumatic delirium A possible occurrence after severe head injury. There is much confusion and disorientation.

Delivery Childbirth; parturition.

Delouse To destroy or remove lice.

Delphi technique A long-range forecasting technique in which qualitative value judgements are made about information. Judgements are made independently and anonymously, pooled and summarized before being fed back to the contributors for another round of opinion.

Deltoid Triangular.

Deltoid ligament Internal lateral ligament of knee joint.

Deltoid muscle The triangular muscle of the shoulder arising from the clavicle and scapula, with insertion into the humerus.

Delusion A false idea or belief held by a person which cannot be corrected by reasoning.

Delusion of grandeur Erroneous belief in one's own greatness, wealth or position.

Delusion of persecution Paranoia.

Depressive delusion A sense of unworthiness or sinfulness.

Demeclocycline An antibiotic of tetracycline groups.

Dementia A global and progressive-deterioration of the mental faculties which is irreversible and affects memory, intellect, judgement, personality and emotional control. Dementia is the result of an organic brain syndrome. The term 'brain failure' is gradually replacing the term dementia because it conveys the fact that brain failure is a process,

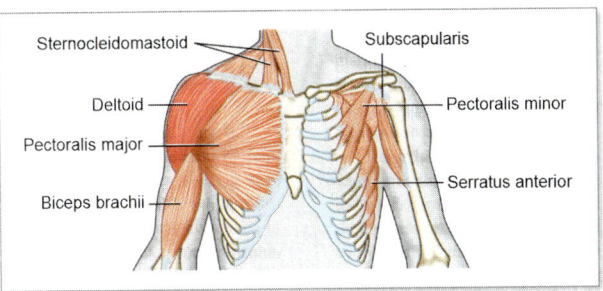

Sternocleidomastoid

Subscapularis

Deltoid

Pectoralis minor

Pectoralis major

Biceps brachii

Serratus anterior

Deltoid Muscle

while the term dementia simply suggests a state associated with nihilistic views on treatment and prognosis.

Arteriosclerotic dementia Dementia due to insufficient blood supply to the brain caused by arteriosclerosis.

Pre-senile dementia Occurring in people aged 40–60years, it is due to early degeneration of small cerebral blood vessels *(See Alzheimer's disease and Creutzfeldt-Jakob disease).*

Senile dementia Dementia occurring in old age as the result of cerebral atrophy.

Demerol Meperidine hydrochloride, opium derivative.

Demilune A crescent shaped group of serious cells forming a cap like structure over a mucous alveolus, commonly present in submandibular gland.

Demineralization Loss of minerals, calcium and phosphorus from bone.

Demodex A genus of mites parasitic in the hair follicles of the host.

Demography The social study of people viewed collectively with regard to race, occupation or conditions.

Demorphinization Gradual decrease in the dose of morphine in morphine addicts.

Demulcent An agent that soothes and allays irritation, especially of sensitive mucous membranes.

Demutization Overcoming mutism by teaching the patient to speak or use sign language.

Demyelination Destruction of the medullary or myelin sheaths of nerve fibres, such as occurs in disseminated sclerosis. Demyelinization.

Denaturation Addition of substances to ethyl alcohol to make it toxic and unfit for human consumption.

Denatured protein A protein that has lost some of its physical and chemical properties by treatment.

Dendrite One of the protoplasmic-filaments of a nerve cell by which impulses are transmitted from one neurone to another. Dendron.

Dendritic 1. Pertaining to a dendrite. 2. Branching.

Dendritic ulcer A corneal ulcer caused by the virus of herpes simplex. It has a branching appearance as it spreads.

Denervation Depriving a structure or organ from its nerve supply. Removal of the nerve supply to a part.

Dengue A painful viral disease that occurs in tropical countries throughout the world. The virus that causes the disease, one of four types of a group B arbovirus, is carried by *Aedes mosquitoes.* Because of the intense pain in the bones, dengue is also known as breakbone fever.

Denial A defence mechanism in which the existence of intolerable actions, ideas, changed circumstances, terminal illness, etc. is unconsciously denied.

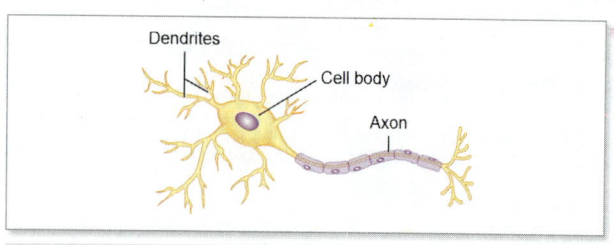

Dendrite

Densimeter An instrument for measuring optical density of a radiograph.

Densitometry Determining the amount of ionizing radiation to which a patient is being exposed.

Dental Relating to dentistry or to the teeth.

Dental arch The arch formed by cutting and chewing surfaces of teeth.

Dental consonant A consonant pronounced with the tongue at or near the front upper teeth.

Dental disk The disk with abrasive powder for cutting or polishing teeth.

Dental formula A brief method of expressing the dentition of mammals.

Dental hygienist A trained person carrying out dental procedures such as scaling of the teeth and oral cleansing, who works with the assistance of the dentist in providing preventive dental health care.

Dental plaque A gummy mass of microorganisms and minerals that grows on the crown and causes dissolution of enamel and tooth substance.

Dental pulp The embryonic connective tissue rich in vessels and nerves occupying the central space within the tooth and its roots.

Dental scalants Application of plastic films to the chewing surfaces of teeth to seal the pits and grooves where food and bacteria can be trapped.

Denticle A small tooth like projection, a calcified structure within pulp of tooth.

Dentifrice A powder or other substance used for cleaning the teeth.

Dentine The calcified substance forming the bulk of a tooth between the pulp and the enamel.

Dentinogenesis Formation of dentin in development of a tooth.

Dentist A person qualified to practice dentistry.

Dentistry The art and science of the teeth, mouth and associated tissues and bone. Dentistry also includes preventive dental care and education concerned with preserving the health of the teeth and gums as well as the supplying and fitting of dentures.

Dentition The process of teething.

Primary dentition Cutting of the temporary or milk teeth, beginning at the age of 6 or 7 months and continuing until the end of the second year. A full set consists of eight incisors, four canines and eight premolars: 20 in all. Deciduous dentition.

Secondary dentition Cutting of the permanent teeth, beginning in the 6th or 7th year, and being complete by the 12th to 15th year except for the posterior molars or 'wisdom teeth'. There are 32 permanent teeth; eight incisors, four canines, eight premolars or bicuspids and 12 molars. Permanent dentition.

Dentoid Tooth-like.

Dentulous Having one's natural teeth.

Denture A removable dental prosthesis, which may contain one artificial tooth, or several or a full set of teeth.

Denver development screening test widely used assessment for screening cognitive and behavioral problems in children up to the age of 6 years.

Deodorant A substance which destroys or masks an offensive odour.

Deontology Study of professional obligations and commitments.

Deoxycortone A naturally occurring adrenal steroid.

Deoxycortone acetate and deoxycortone pivalate Synthetic preparations used in the treatment of adrenocortical insufficiency.

Deoxycorticosterone A renal harmone with mineral corticoid activity.

Deoxygenated Deprived of oxygen.

Deoxygenated blood That which has lost much of its oxygen in the tissues

D

and is returning to the lungs for a fresh supply.

Deoxycholic acid A bile acid.

Deoxycoformycin Anti leukemic agent.

Deoxyribonuclease Enzyme causing hydrolysis in DNA.

Deoxyribonucleic acid Abbreviated DNA. A nucleic acid of complex molecular structure occurring in cell nuclei as the basic structure of the genes. It is responsible for the control and passing on of hereditary characteristics, and is present in all body cells of every species, including unicellular organisms and DNA viruses.

Department of health A central government department that is responsible for supporting the Secretary of State for Health and other health ministers in meeting their accountability to Parliament for all matters relating to the health of the nation.

Department of social security A central government department that is responsible for supporting the Secretary of State for Social Security and other social security ministers in meeting their accountability to Parliament for social security matters including the national insurance scheme, income support, child support, welfare benefits and social services.

Dependence 1. Addiction; the total psychophysical state of a drug user in which the usual or increasing doses of the drug are required to prevent the onset of withdrawal symptoms. 2. The level of reliance a person has on others for carrying out the activities of daily living.

Dependency A state of relying on another for love, affection, mothering, comfort, security, food, warmth, shelter, protection, etc.

Dependency studies The measurement of the need for care required by a patient based on the ability to carry out self-care. The main self-care activities measured are the ability to feed, the ability to carry out toilet requirements and the level of mobility, including dressing.

Dependency studies for staffing ratios Studies undertaken to determine the number of staff required to provide the appropriate skills to care for specific types and numbers of patient.

Depersonalization A condition in which patients feel that their personality has changed so that they become onlookers observing their own actions. It may occur in almost any mental illness.

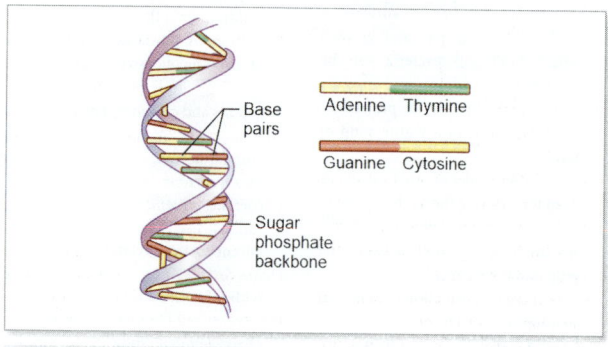

Deoxyribonucleic acid (DNA)

Depilation The process of hair removal.

Depletion Removal of substances like water, electrolyte, blood from the body.

Depilatory An agent that will remove hair.

Deplorization Electrical change in excitable cell in which inside of cell becomes positive.

Depolymerization The breakdown of polymers into monomers.

Depo medrone Methyl prednisone acetate.

Depot Storage, e.g., fat depot, contraceptive depot.

Depressant A drug that reduces functional activity of an organ. Anesthetics, sedatives, tranquillizers and alcohol are depressants.

Depression 1. A hollow or depressed area. 2. A lowering or decrease of functional activity. 3. In psychiatry, a morbid sadness, dejection or melancholy, distinguished from grief, which is realistic and proportionate to a personal loss. Profound depression may be symptomatic of a psychiatric disorder or it may constitute the principal manifestation of a neurosis or psychosis.

Endogenous depression Occurs sometimes without obvious cause in the course of manic depressive psychosis. The mood change is associated with slowing of thought and action and feelings of guilt.

Recessive depression Occurs as a result of some event, such as illness, loss of money, bereavement.

Deprivation Loss or absence of parts, organs, powers, or things that are needed.

Emotional deprivation Deprivation of adequate and appropriate inter personal or environmental experience in the early developmental years.

Maternal deprivation syndrome A group of symptoms, including stunted emotional and physical development, arising in infants who have been deprived of care and love provided by a mother or mothering figure. Deprivation of maternal care during the first 3 years of life is thought to be particularly critical as this is the optimal period for the forming of social attachments.

Sensory deprivation Deprivation of the usual external stimuli and the opportunity for perception.

Derbyshire Neck *(See Goitre)*.

Derealization Loss of a sense of reality. Surroundings and events seem unreal.

Dercum's Disease *SYN* – Adiposis dolorosa. Painful areas of fat accumulation in menopausal women.

Dereism Mental activity in which fantasy runs unhampered by logic and experience; describes autistic thinking.

Derivative Derived from another.

Dermal filler Injections used to fill out wrinkles and creases in skin used for cosmetic reasons.

Dermatillomania A compulsion to pick skin at the point where there are visible wounds. An impulse control disorder.

Dermatitis Inflammation of the skin.

Contact dermatitis That arising from touching a substance to which the person is sensitive.

Exfoliative dermatitis Widespread-scaling and itching of the skin, sometimes occurring as a reaction to treatment with certain drugs.

Industrial dermatitis, occupational dermatitis That caused by exposure to chemicals or other substances met with at work.

D

Sensitization dermatitis Dermatitis due to an allergic reaction.

Traumatic dermatitis Inflammation due to injury.

Varicose dermatitis Dermatitis, usually of the lower portion of the leg, due to varicosities of the smaller veins.

X-ray dermatitis Radiodermatitis; inflammatory reaction of the skin to radiotherapy.

Dermatoglyphics Study of the patterns of ridges of the skin of the fingers, palms, toes and soles. Of interest in anthropology and law enforcement as a means of establishing identity, and in medicine, both clinically and as a genetic indicator, particularly of chromosomal abnormalities.

Dermatographia A condition in which urticarial weals occur on the skin if a blunt instrument or fingernail is lightly drawn over it.

Dermatology The science of skin diseases.

Dermatome 1.Area of skin innervated by one segment of spinal cord. 2. Instrument to cut thin section of skin as in skin grafting. *(See Figure).*

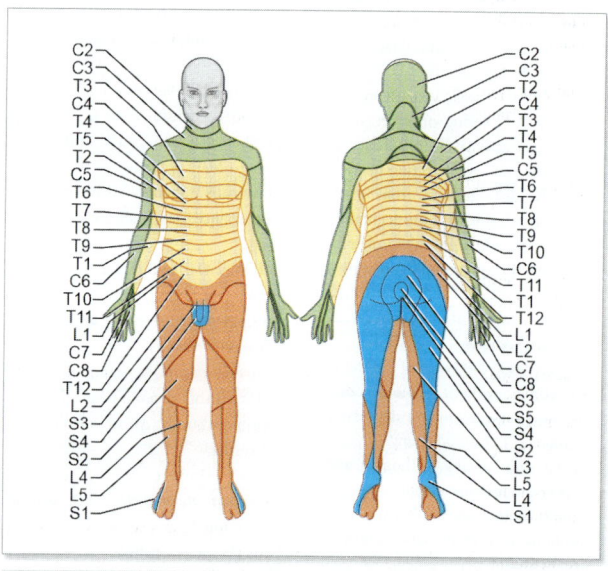

Dermatome

Dermatomycosis A fungal infection of the skin.

Dermatomyositis A collagen disease producing inflammation of the voluntary muscles with necrosis of the muscle fibres.

Dermatophobia Excessive fear about skin disease.

Dermatophyte A fungus that grows in skin or its appendage e.g., epidermophyton, trichophyton and microsoprum.

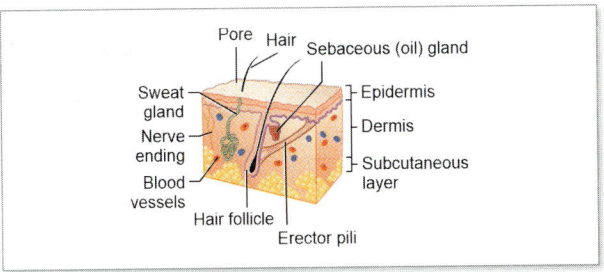

Dermis

Dermatophytosis Fungus infection of skin of hand and feet.

Dermatosis Any skin disease, especially one which does not produce inflammation.

Dermis The skin, especially the layer under the epidermis.

Dermoid Pertaining to the skin.

Dermoid cyst *(See Cyst)*.

Dermonosology The science of classification of skin disease.

Dermotropic Acting especially on the skin.

Dermodidymus A malformed fetus with two heads and neck but a single body and normal limbs.

Desalination Removal of salt, e.g., removal of salt from sea water to make the water drinkable.

Desaturation A process where by a saturated organic compound is converted into a unsaturated one.

Descemet's membrane Membrane between endothelial layer of cornea and substantia propria.

Desensitization 1. The prevention or reduction of immediate hypersensitivity reactions by the administration of graded doses of allergen; hyposensitization *(See also Immunotherapy)*. 2. In behaviour therapy, the treatment of phobias and related disorders by intentionally exposing the patient, in imagination or in real life, to emotionally distressing stimuli.

Designer drugs Drugs illicitly produced to suit the tastes of individuals but now used to describe synthetic variants (drug analogues) of potent controlled drugs (including narcotics and stimulants) but which are not themselves controlled. These substances currently circumvent existing drug legislation and many are relatively easy to synthesize from common industrial chemicals. Many designer drugs are extremely potent (some synthetic analogues of heroin are 1000 times as potent as heroin) and are consequently extremely dangerous.

Desert fever Coccidiodomycosis.

Desferrioxamine Iron chelating agent.

Desiccant Agent causing dryness.

Desipramine An antidepressant.

Desmitis Inflammation of a ligament.

Desmocyte A supporting tissue cell.

Desmoid Resembling a tendon.

Desmoplasia An abanormal tendency to form fibrous tissue or adhesive bands.

Desmopressin Synthetic vasopressin analogue.

Desonide A locally acting steroid.

Desquamation Peeling of the superficial layer of the skin, either in flakes or in powdery form.

Dessault's bandage Bandage for stabilizing fracture of clavicle.

Destructive Causing ruin, opposite to constructive.

Detachment Separation from or state of indifference to other people, one's surroundings or environment leading to social isolation.

Detachment of the retina Separation of the retina, or a part of it, from the choroid.

Detail In radiology, the sharpness with which an image is presented on a radiograph.

Detector An instrument for determining the presence of something.

Detector lie A polygraph, an instrument for determining minor physical changes assumed to occur under stress of lying or any other emotion.

Detergent A cleansing and antiseptic agent.

Deterioration Progressive impairment of function; worsening.

Determination Establishing the nature or precise identity of a substance, organism or event.

Detonation A violent noise caused by an explosive.

Detoxify To remove toxic quality of a substance. To treat toxic overdose of a drug/alcohol.

Detoxification The process of neutralizing toxic substances; detoxication.

Detritus Debris; material that has disintegrated.

Detrusor Muscle of the urinary bladder, the action of which is to push down.

Detumescence 1. The subsidence of a swelling. 2. The subsidence of an erect penis after ejaculation.

Deuteranopia Green colour blindness.

Deuterium Heavy hydrogen with two atoms.

Developer In radiology, the solution used to make the latent image visible on the radiograph.

Development The process of growth and differentiation.

Cognitive development The development of intelligence, conscious thought and problem-solving ability that begins in infancy.

Psychosexual development The development of the psychologial aspects of sexuality from birth to maturity.

Psychosocial development The development of the personality, including the acquisition of social attitudes and skills, from infancy through to maturity.

Developmental Pertaining to development.

Developmental anomaly Absence, deformity or excess of body parts as the result of faulty development of the embryo.

Developmental milestones Significant behaviours used to mark the process of development *(See Age (Achievement)*. Walking is a developmental milestone in locomotor development, conversation in cognitive development.

Deviance Generally any pattern of behaviour that violates prevailing standards of morality or behavior within a society. The term is usually qualified to indicate the specific form of deviance.

Deviant behavior Actions considered abnormal.

Deviation Variation from the normal. In ophthalmology, lack of coordination of the two eyes.

Device intrauterine contraceptive Devices placed in uterus to prevent contraception e.g., copper T.

Devitalization Loss of vitality; especially anesthetizing the pulp of a tooth.

Devitalized Devoid of vitality or life; dead.

Devolution Degradation or destructive process.

Dexamethasone A powerful anti-inflammatory glucocorticoid.

Dexchlorpheniramine Antihistaminic (polaramine).

Dexterity Motor skill.

Dextrality Right handedness.

Dextran A plasma volume expander, formed of large glucose molecules, which, given intravenously, increases the osmotic pressure of blood.

Dextrase Enzyme splitting dextrose into lactic acid.

Dextriferron Ferric hydroxide used in treating iron deficiency.

Dextrin A soluble carbohydrate that is the first product in the breakdown of starch and glycogen to sugar.

Dextroamphetamine An isomer of amphetamine, a CNS stimulant.

Dextrocardia Location of the heart in the right side of the thorax.

Dextrocardiogram Electrocardiogram representing right ventriclular forces.

Dextroduction Movement of visual axis to right.

Dextromethorphan A synthetic morphine derivative used as an antitussive.

Dextromoramide A narcotic used in the treatment of chronic pain in terminal disease.

Dextrophobia Abnormal aversion to objects on right side of body.

Dextropropoxyphene Analgesic with high addiction potency.

Dextroposition Displaced to right.

Dextrose An old chemical name for D glucose, an important energy source for all tissues and the sole energy source for the brain. The term dextrose continues to be used to refer to glucose solutions administered intravenously for fluid or nutrient replacement.

Diabetes A disease characterized by excessive excretion of urine (*See Polyuria*).

Bronze diabetes Hemochromatosis.

Diabetes insipidus Diabetes marked by an increased flow of urine of low specific gravity, accompanied by great thirst.

Diabetes mellitus A disturbance in the oxidation and utilization of glucose, which is secondary to a malfunction of the beta cells of the pancreas, whose function is the production and release of insulin. Because insulin is involved in the metabolism of carbohydrates, proteins and fats, diabetes is not limited to a disturbance of glucose metabolism. Polyuria, thirst and debility are common presenting symptoms. Type I diabetes results from the destruction of the insulin producing cells of the pancreas occurring most commonly in childhood or adolescence. Type II diabetes or maturity onset diabetes is due to an insufficiency of insulin and usually occurs after the age of 40 years. The goal of treatment is to maintain blood glucose and lipid levels within normal limits and to prevent complications. There is strong support for the concept that microvascular sequelae of the disease from retinopathy and kidney degeneration can be minimized by optimal control. In both types of diabetes treatment is aimed at promoting a sense of health and wellbeing. The diet must be controlled with adequate carbohydrate and the body weight stabilized. Type I is always treated with insulin. Type II may be treated with weight reduction, diet or the use of medications which promote the production of insulin by the pancreas. Insulin therapy has now been standardized at 100 units/mL. Combinations of soluble insulin with slower-acting preparations can be tailored to suit the individual patient in the 24-hrs control of blood sugar. All insulin has to be given by injection, usually subcutaneously. Pump systems to deliver continuous insulin under the skin are available.

D

Diabetic 1. Relating to diabetes. 2. A person affected with diabetes.

Diabetic gangrene, diabetic retinopathy and diabetic cataract Are complications of diabetes mellitus.

Diabetic tabes Diabetic neuropathy with neuritic leg pain and loss of knee jerk.

Diabetogenic Inducing diabetes. Some drugs or physical conditions, such as pregnancy or disease, precipitate the symptoms of diabetes in those prone to the disease.

Diabinese Chlorpropamide, an oral sulphonyl urea.

Diacele Third ventricle of brain.

Diacetic acid Acetoacetic acid, a ketone found in urine in diabetic ketoacidosis.

Diacerin Anti-inflammatory pain killer.

Diacetyl morphine Heroin, strong addictive potential.

Diadochokinesia Ability to make antagonistic movements like pronation and supination in quick succession.

Diagnosis Determination of the nature of a disease.

Clinical diagnosis Diagnosis made by the study of signs and symptoms.

Differential diagnosis There cognition of one disease among several presenting similar symptoms.

Nursing diagnosis A statement of a healthcare problem or the potential for one in the health status of the patient/client for which the nurse is competent to intervene and treat.

Dialysate The material passing through the membrane in dialysis.

Dialyser 1. The membrane used in dialysis. 2. The machine or 'artificial kidney' used to remove waste products from the blood in cases of renal failure.

Dialysis The process by which crystalline substances will pass through a semipermeable membrane, whereas colloids will not. In medicine, this process is usually employed to remove waste and toxic products from the blood in cases of renal insufficiency.

Peritoneal dialysis Use of the peritoneum as the semi permeable membrane. A dialyzing solution is infused into the abdominal cavity and allowed to run out again when sufficient time has elapsed for dialysis to have occurred. Waste products are thus removed from the blood *(See Haemodialysis)*.

Diameter A straight line passing through the center of a circle to opposite points on the circumference.

Cranial diameters Measurement of the skull, usually of the fetal head at term. If these are abnormal, delivery through the vagina may not be possible.

Pelvic diameters Measurements between the bones and joints of the pelvis made in women to determine whether the fetus can pass through at the time of childbirth.

Diamorphine hydrochloride a morphine derivative similar to heroin; a powerful analgesic and drug of addiction.

Diamox Acetazolamide, a carbonic anhydrase inhibitor.

Diapedesis The passage of white blood-cells through the walls of bloodcapillaries.

Diaphanometer A device for estimation of the amount of solids in a fluid by its transparency.

Diaphanoscope Device for transillumination of body cavities.

Diaphoresis Perspiration; particularly profuse perspiration.

Diaphoretic An agent that increases-perspiration, e.g., pilocarpine.

Diaphragm 1. The muscular dome shaped partition separating the thorax from the abdomen. 2. Any separating membrane or structure.

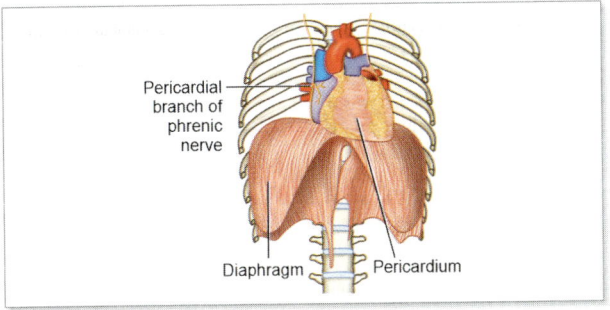

Pericardial branch of phrenic nerve

Diaphragm | Pericardium

Diaphragm

Contraceptive diaphragm A rubber cap which occludes the cervix.

Diaphragmatic hernia A protrusion of any or part of an abdominal organ through the diaphragm into the thoracic cavity.

Diaphysis The shaft of a long bone.

Diapophysis An upper articular surface of transverse process of vertebra.

Diarrhea Rapid movement of fecal matter through the intestine resulting in poor absorption of water, nutritive elements and electrolytes, and producing abnormally frequent evacuation of watery stools.

Summer diarrhea Gastroenteritis of infants, probably the result of a virus infection. It is highly contagious.

Tropical diarrhea Sprue.

Diarthrosis A freely moving articulation, e.g., ball and socket joint. A synovial joint.

Diascope A glass plate held against the skin for examining superficial lesions. Erythematous lesions blanch but not hemorrhagic lesions.

Diastage The enzyme converting starch to sugar.

Diastase 1. An enzyme, formed during germination of seeds, which converts starch into sugar. 2. One of the pancreatic enzymes excreted in the urine and the saliva.

Diastase test Used to estimate the excretion of diastase and therefore pancreatic function.

Diastasis The last part of diastole, of 0.2 second duration and is immediately followed by atrial contraction.

Diastole The phase of the cardiac cycle in which the heart relaxes between contractions; specifically, the period when the two ventricles are dilated by the blood flowing into them *(See Systole)*.

Diastolic pressure The period of least pressure in the arterial vascular system.

Diathermy Production of heat in a body tissue by a high frequency electric current.

Medical diathermy Sufficient heat is used to warm the tissues but not to harm them.

Short-wave diathermy Used in physiotherapy to relieve pain or treat infection.

Surgical diathermy Of very high frequency; used to coagulate blood vessels or to dissect tissues. Cautery.

Diathrosis A hinge joint.

Diatom One group of unicellular microscopic algae seen in lungs of patients with antemortem drowning.

Diatrizoate meglumine Radio-opaque dye for artereial use (gastrograffin).

Diatrizoate sodium Radiopaque dye for visualization of bladder, urinary tract, reproductive system.

Diaxon A neurone having two axons.

Diazepam A tranquillizer with muscle relaxant and anticonvulsive properties used to relieve anxiety and in the treatment of epilepsy.

Diazo reaction A deep red colour in urine produced by action of ammonia and *p*-diazobenzene- Sulfonic acid on aromatic substances of urine.

Diazoxide A vasodilator given by rapid intravenous injection in the treatment of hypertensive emergencies and orally in hypoglycemia due to a pancreatic tumour.

DIC Disseminated intravascular coagulation.

Dibasic Substance with two atoms of hydrogen in each molecule replaceable by a base.

Dibucaine hydrochloride Local anesthetic similar to cocaine.

Dicalcium Phosphate Dibasic calcium phosphate, used for calcium supplement.

Dichloralphenazone A hypnotic drug of the chloral group well suited for children and causing fewer gastrointestinal upsets.

Dichloramine A germicide, disinfectant containg chlorine.

Dichlorphenamide A diuretic used to reduce intraocular pressure inglaucoma.

Dichotomy Dividing into two parts.

Dichromation Ability to distinguish only two primary colours, i.e., red and green.

Dichromatic Pertaining to colourblindness when there is ability to see only two of the three primary colours.

Dick test A skin test for susceptibility to scarlet fever familiar to shick test for diphtheria.

Deiclofenac Analgesic-anti inflammatory agent.

Dicloxacillin sodium A semi-synthetic penicillin for treatment of penicillinase resistant staphylococci.

Dicophane Dichlorodiphenyltrichloroethane; chlorophenothane; DDT. An insecticide.

Dicrotic Having a double beat.

Dicrotic pulse A small wave of distension following the normal pulse beat; occurring at the closure of the aortic valve.

Dicumarol An anticoagulant that increases prothrombin time.

Dicyclomine An anticholinergic drug used in the treatment of peptic ulcer and spastic colon.

Didactic Pertains to teaching by lectures or texts as opposed to clinical or bedside teaching.

Didactylism Congenital condition in which there are only 2 digits on a hand or foot.

Didelphic Pertains to double uterus.

Didymitis Inflammation of testicle.

Didymodynia Pain in the testicle.

Dieldrin A chlorinated hydrocarbon used as insecticide.

Diencephalon The portion of brain encompassing epithalamus, thalamus, metathalamus and hypothalamus.

Dienestrol A synthetic oestrogen used to treat symptoms of atrophic vaginitis and kraurosis vulvae.

Dientamoeba fragilis Parasitic ameba inhabiting small instestine and causing diarrhea.

Diet The customary amount and kind of food and drink taken by a person from day to day; more narrowly, a diet planned to meet the specific requirements of the individual, including or excluding certain foods.

Bland diet One that is free from any irritating or stimulating foods.

Elimination diet One for diagnosis of food allergy, based on omission of foods that might cause symptoms in the patient.

High calorie diet One that furnishes more calories than needed to maintain weight, often more than 3500–4000 kcal/day.

High-fibre diet One relatively high in dietary fibre, which decreases bowel transit time and relieves constipation.

High-protein diet One containing large amounts of protein, consisting largely of meats, fish, milk, peas, beans and nuts.

Hospital diet A routine diet plan, provided in a hospital, that includes general, soft and liquid diets and modifications of them to suit the needs of specific patients.

Liquid diet A diet limited to liquids or to foods that can be changed to a liquid state *(See also Liquid (Diet)).*

Low calorie diet One containing fewer calories than needed to maintain weight, e.g., less than 1200 kcal/day for an adult.

Low-fat diet One containing limited amounts of fat.

Low-residue diet One with a minimum of cellulose and fibre and restriction of the connective tissue found in certain cuts of meat. It is prescribed for irritations of the intestinal tract after surgery of the large intestine, in partial intestinal obstruction, or when limited bowel movements are desirable, as in colostomy patients. Also called low-fibre diet.

Dietary chaos syndrome A syndrome in which patients believe that control of eating and body weight is the key to good health and wellbeing. A variety of approaches are used, which include bulimia and periods of abstinence from food, the use of laxatives or prolonged chewing of food without swallowing. *(See ANOREXIA and BULIMIA).*

Dietary reference values Abbreviated DRV. Published values (Department of Health) for most nutrients that provide for a range of intakes related to age gender and activity required to maintain health. These values are based upon the nutritional requirements of groups living in the UK.

Dietetics The science of applying the principles of nutrition to the feeding of individuals or groups.

Diethazine hydrochloride Anticholinergic used in treatment of Parkinsonism.

Diethyl carbamazine An anthelmintic drug used in the treatment of filariasis.

Diethylpropion An appetite suppressant in the treatment of obesity, similar in action to an amphetamine drug. Dependence can occur. Tradenames: Apisate and Tenuate Dospan.

Diethylstilbestrol Synthetic estrogen.

Diethytoluamide Insect repellant.

Diethyltryptamine Hallucinogenic agent.

Dietitian One who specializes in dietetics.

Dietl's crisis Renal colic from partial obstruction of ureter.

Dieulafoy's triad Tenderness, muscular rigidity and skin hyperesthesia at Mc Burney's point in acute appendicitis.

Differential Making a difference.

Differential blood count (See Blood count).

Differential diagnosis (See Diagnosis).

Differentiation 1. The distinguishing of one thing from another. 2. The actor process of acquiring completely individual characteristics, such as occurs in the progressive diversification of cells and tissues in the embryo. 3. Increase in morphological or chemical heterogeneity.

Diffraction The deflection that occurs when light rays are passed through crystals, prisms or other deflecting media.

Diffuse Scattered or widespread, as opposed to localized.

Diffusion 1. The spontaneous mixing of molecules of liquid or gas so that they become equally distributed.2. Dialysis.

Diflunisal A salicylic acid derivative that, like aspirin, has analgesic and anti-inflammatory properties. It has fewer side effects than aspirin, does not affect bleeding time or function, and has a long half-life that permits twice-daily dosage.

Digestion 1. The act or process of converting food into chemical substances that can be absorbed into the blood and utilized by the body tissues. 2. The subjection of substance to prolonged heat and moisture, so as to disintegrate and soften it.

Digit A finger or toe.

Accessory digit, supernumerary digit An additional digit occurring as a congenital abnormality.

Digital Coded in simple 'on-off' binary units such as in computers and the traditional view of the activation of neurones.

Digital radiography Radiography using computerized imaging instead of conventional film or screen imaging.

Digital reflex Sudden flexion of terminal phalanx when nail is suddenly tapped.

Digitalis A drug used to strengthen the heartbeat and slow down the conducting power of the atrioventricular bundle, thereby enabling the ventricles to beat more effectively. Particularly valuable in treating atrial fibrillation. Digoxin is the chief glycoside. The effects of digitalis are cumulative, indicated by a very slow pulse and coupling of the beats.

Digitalization The administration of digitalis in a dosage schedule designed to produce and then maintain optimal therapeutic concentrations of its cardio tonic glycosides.

Digitoxin Cardiotonic glycoside.

Digoxin *(See Digitalis).*

Dihydrocodeine A synthetic narcotic, analgesic and antitussive drug derived from codeine.

Dihydroergotamine A drug used in the treatment of migraine. Less effective than ergotamine, but with fewer side effects.

Dihydrosphingosine An amino alcohol present in sphingolipids.

Dihydrotachysterol A preparation closely related to vitamin D. Used in cases of vitamin D deficiency and in rickets.

Dihydroaluminium amino acetate A antacid.

Dihydroxycholecalciferol Sterols with hormonal properties akin to vit D. e.g., calcitrol.

Diiodohydropyquin Iodoquinol.

Diktyoma Tumour of ciliary epithelium.

Dilantin A derivative of glycerlyl urea (diphenylhydantoin sodium) used as antiepileptic, best for clonic/toxic clonic seizure.

Dilatation, dilation 1. The act of dilating or stretching. 2. The condition, as of an orifice or tubular structure, of being dilated or stretched beyond normal dimensions.

Dilatation and curettage Expanding of the opening of the womb to permit scraping of the walls of the uterus; also called D & C.

Dilation of the heart Compensatory enlargement of the cavities of the heart, with thinning of the walls.

Dilation and evacuation Cervical canal dilatation and evacuation of product of conception by suction/forcep.

Dilator 1. An instrument used for enlarging an opening or cavity such as the rectum, the male urethra or the cervix. 2. A muscle that causes dilatation. 3. A drug that causes dilatation, e.g., a vasodilator.

Hegar's dilator's A series of dilators used to widen the cervical canal before examination of the uterus under anesthesia.

Dilitiazem Calcium channel blocker useful for ischemic heart disease.

Diluent 1. Diluting. 2. An agent that dilutes or renders less potent or irritant.

Dimenhydrinate An antihistamine-drug, useful in preventing nausea and vomiting, particularly that associated with motion sickness.

Dimercaprol A drug which combines with heavy metals to form a stable compound, which is rapidly excreted. Used to treat poisoning by antimony, gold, mercury and other metals. Previously called British AntiLewisite or BAL.

Dimethicone A silicone oil used to protect the skin against water soluble irritants.

Dimethindene maleate Antihistamine.

Dimethisterone Progesterone compound.

Dimethyl phthalate Abbreviated DIMP. An insect repellent in liquid or ointment form that is effective for several hours when applied to the skin.

Dimethyl sulfoxide A solvent used to facilitate absorption of medicines through the skin.

Dimple sign A sign used to differentiate dermatofibroma from malignant nodular melanoma. Upon application of lateral pressure, the dermatofibroma will dimple or become indented, but melanoma protrudes above plane of skin.

Dinoprost tromethamine A drug causing uterine contraction hence used to induce abortion.

Dioctyl calcium, sodium/potassium/ sulfosuccinate A stool softner.

Diodone A contrast medium containing iodine which is similar to iodoxyl. Used in radiology of the urinary tract.

Diogenes syndrome Gross self-neglect, usually in the elderly.

Dioptre Symbol D. The unit used in measuring lenses for spectacles. When parallel light enters a lens and focuses at a distance of 1 m, the refractive power of the lens is 1 dioptre, and from this basis abnormalities are calculated.

Diosmin Antithrombotic, anticoagulant.

Dioxybenzone Chemical for protecting skin from sun.

Dipeptidase An enzyme that catalyzes the hydrolysis of dipeptides to amino acids.

Diphemanil methyl sulfate An anticholinergic agent used for treatment of peptic ulcer.

Diphenhydramine hydrochloride Antihistamine, (Benadryl).

Diphenoxylate Antidiarrheal agent smooth muscle relaxant (Lomotil).

Diphenylhydantioin sodium Anti convulsant.

Diphenylpyraline An antihistamine.

Diphonia Simultaneous production of two voice tones.

2-3 diphossphoglycerate An organic phosphate that effects affinity of hemoglobin for RBC and is depleted in stored blood.

Diphtheria A severe, notifiable, infectious disease, usually of children, characterized by the formation of membranes in the throat and nose and rarely the skin (in an open wound), and toxic neurological and cardiac complications; caused by the bacillus.
Corynebacterium diphtheriae. Primary prevention is provided by the routine immunization of the population in childhood *(See Appendices).*

Diphtheroid Resembling diphtheria. A general term applied to organisms or membranes similar to true diphtheria types.

Diphyllobothrium A genus of large tapeworm.

Diphyllobothrium latum The broad or fish tapeworm, grows up to 10 m long and may infest humans after the consumption of uncooked infected fish.

Dipipanone A potent analgesic used for the relief of severe pain.

Diplococcus 1. Any of the spherical, lanceolate or coffeebean-shapedbacteria occurring, usually in pairs, as a result of incomplete separation after cell division in a single plane. 2. Any organism of the genus *Diplococcus.*

Diplegia Paralysis of similar parts on either side of the body.

Diploe Spongy tissue between the two layers of compact bone.

Diploid 1. Having a pair of each chromosome characteristic of a species (in humans, 46). 2. A diploid individual or cell.

Diplomyelia Doubling of spinal cord due to a length wise fissure, often seen in patients of spina bifida.

Diplopia Double vision in which two images are seen in place of one, due to lack of coordination of the external muscles of the eye.

Dipole Two equal and opposite charges separated by a distance.

Diprophylline A theophylline derivative used in the treatment of bronchospasm or bronchial asthma associated with chronic bronchitis or asthma.

Dipsomania A morbid craving for alcohol, which occurs in bouts.

Dipstic A chemical impregnated paper strip used for analysis of chemical constituents in urine.

Direct current An electric current flowing continuously in one direction only.

Direct light reflex Contraction of pupil on focusing a light beam on it.

Directly observed therapy Strategy for ensuring a patient's compliance with a therapy in which there is oral administration of a drug to a patient and observing that each dose of prescribed drug is swallowed.

Dirofilaria A genus of microfilaria.

Disability Any restriction or lack (resulting from an impairment) of ability to perform an activity in the manner or within the range considered normal for a human being.

Developmental disability A substantial handicap of indefinite duration with onset before the age of 18 years and attributable to mental handicap, autism, cerebral palsy, epilepsy or other neuropathy.

Disaccharide Any of a class of sugars e.g., maltose, lactose, each molecule of which yields two molecules of monosaccharide on hydrolysis.

Disaccharide intolerance The inability to absorb disaccharides owing to an enzyme deficiency.

Disarticulation Amputation at a joint.

Disc A flattened circular structure.

Intervertebral disc A fibrocartilaginous pad that separates the bodies of two adjacent vertebrae.

Optic disc A white spot in the retina. It is the point of entrance of the optic nerve.

Discharge 1. A setting free or liberation; used for the release of a patient from hospital, clinic or therapy programme. 2. Material or force set free. 3. An excretion or substance evacuated.

Discharge planning The preparation required for the return of a patient to the usual life at home *(See Appendices).*

Disciplinary action Taken by the employer when member of staff has made a serious error, acted unprofessionally or negligently or has been convicted of a criminal offence. The process follows an agreed disciplinary procedure.

Discitis Inflammation of inter vertebral disk.

Disclosing solution A topically applied preparation which reveals plaque and other deposits on teeth by staining them.

Discography Radiographic examination after the injection of a radio-opaque contrast medium into an intervertebral disc.

Discoid eczema A long-term skin condition causing itchy, reddened, swollen and cracked patches on the skin.

Disconnection syndrome Disturbances of visual and language functions due to section of corpus collusum or occlusion of anterior cerebral artery, manifesting as inability to match an object held in one hand with that in the other when eyes are closed.

Discordance In genetics, the expression of a trait in only one of the twin pair.

Discrete Composed of separate parts that do not become blended.

Discrete Separate, distinct.

Discrimination The process of distinguishing or differentiating.

Disdiadochokinesia Inability to make quick alternating movements like pronation and supination common to cerebellar disease.

Disease Literally the lack of ease, or illness/suffering.

Autoimmune disease A state of immune aberration where body produces antibodies against healthy host tissues as in some cases of glomerulonephritis, hemolyticanemia, rheumatoid arthritis, myasthenia gravis, thyrotoxicosis, SLE, scleroederma etc.

Heavy chain disease Diseases in which heavy chain production of immunoglobulins is in excess. lgA chain excess manifests with abdominal lymphoma and malabsorption, lgM with repeated bacterial infections, lymphadenopathy and lgD chain with picture similar to multiple myeloma.

Hereditary disease Where Disease is transmitted from parent to offspring.

Motor neurone disease There is degeneration of anterior horn cells of spinal cord, cranial nerve nuclei in the brain stem, and pyramidal tracts, e.g., progressive muscular atrophy, amyotropic lateral sclerosis.

Psychosomatic disease Psychological factors contribute to initiation or exacerbation of the disease e.g., asthma, tension head-ache, neurodermatitis, peptic ulcer, etc.

Disengagement The emergence of fetal head from within the maternal pelvis.

Disintegration The falling apart of constituents of a substance.

Disimpaction Reduction of an impacted fracture.

Disinfect To destroy microorganisms, but not usually bacterial spores, reducing the number of micro organisms to a level which is not harmful to health.

Disinfectant An agent that destroys infection producing organisms. Heat and certain other physical agents, such as steam, can be disinfectants, but in common usage the term is reserved for chemical substances such as glutaraldehyde, sodium hypochlorite or phenol. Disinfectants are usually applied to inanimate objects because they are too strong to be used on living tissues. Chemical disinfectants are not always effective against spore\forming bacteria.

Disinfection The act of disinfecting.

Terminal disinfection Disinfection of a sick room and its contents at the termination of a disease.

Disinfestation Destruction of insects, rodents or pests present on the person or the clothes or in the surroundings, and which may transmit disease.

Dislocation The displacement of a bone from its natural position upon another at a joint; luxation.

Dismemberment The amputation of a limb or a part of it.

Disopyramide A drug given orally or by slow intravenous injection to treat ventricular arrhythmia.

Disodium edentate A chelating agent used to treat hypercalcemia.

Disopyramide phosphate Anti-arrhythmic agent of class II.

Disorientation The loss of proper bearings or a state of mental confusion as to time, place or identity.

Dispensary Any place where drugs or medicines are actually dispensed.

Disperate Suspension of finely divided particles in liquid.

Dispression Dissipation or disappearance of colloid in a fluid.

Dispersonalization Mental state in which individual denies presence of some of his body parts or personality.

Displacement Removal to an abnormal location or position.

Activity displacement In psychology unconscious transference of an emotion from its original object on to a more acceptable substitute.

Disposition A tendency to suffer from certain diseases.

Disproportion A part being different in size from that considered to be normal.

Dissect 1. To cut carefully in the study of anatomy. 2. During operation, to separate according to natural lines of structure.

Dissection The cutting of parts for purpose of separation and study.

Disseminated Widely scattered or dispersed.

Disseminated intravascular coagulation Abbreviated DIC. Widespread formation of thromboses in the capillaries. It is a secondary complication of a diverse group of obstetric, surgical hemolytic and neoplastic disorders.

Dissipation Dispersion of matter.

Dissociation Separation. 1. The splitting up of molecules of matter into their component parts, e.g., by heat or electrolysis. 2. In psychology, the separation of ideas, emotions or experiences from the rest of the mind, giving rise to a lack of unity of which the patient is not aware.

Dissociation AV Atria and ventricles beat independently as sinus node impulse does not reach the ventricle.

Dissociation of personality Split in consciousness resulting in two different phases of personality, neither being aware of words, acts or feelings of others.

Dissolution Breaking up the integrity of anatomical entity.

Dissolve Dispersion of a solid within a liquid.

Dissonance Disagreement.

Distal Situated away from the center of the body or point of origin. The opposite of proximal.

Distalgesic A proprietary analgesic composed of dextropropoxyphene and paracetamol.

Distance Space between two objects.

Focal distance Distance from the optical center of lens to focal point.

Distend To stretch; to inflate.

Distensibility The property of being stretchable.

Distension Enlargement.

Abdominal distension Enlargement of the abdomen by gas in the intestines or fluid in the abdominal cavity.

Distichia, distichiasis The presence of a double row of eyelashes, one or both of which are turned against the eyeball, causing irritation.

Distillate Substance obtained by distillation.

Distillation Condensation of vapor that has been obtained from a liquid heated to volatilization point.

Distome A fluke with two suckers.

Distomiasis Infestation with flukes.

Distortion Change from regular to irregular/altered shape.

Distractibility Inability to focus ones attention or mental wandering.

Distraction State of mental confusion.

Distraugh The mental state of being deeply troubled, having conflicting thoughts.

Distress Physical or mental agony.

Distribution 1. The sharing out or spreading of an agent, object or population within an area. 2. In research the relative frequencies with which scores of a different size occur.

Districhiasis Two hair growing from the same hair follicle.

Disulfiram A drug used in aversion therapy in alcoholism. Antabuse is a proprietary preparation.

Dithranol A synthetic preparation used in the treatment of psoriasis and eczema.

Diuresis Increased excretion of urine.

Diuretic 1. Increasing urine excretion or the amount of urine. 2. An agent that promotes urine secretion. Diuretic drugs are classified by chemical structure and pharmacological action, although a diuretic medication may contain drugs from one or more of groups, e.g., loop diuretics, osmotic and potassium sparing diuretics, and thiazides.

Diurnal Occurring during daytime or period of light. Diurnal animals have one period of rest and one of activity in 24 hours.

Divalent A molecule with two electric charges.

Divalproex Antiepileptic.

Divergence Separation from a common center.

Diverticulitis Inflammation of a diverticulum. It is most common in the colon; lower abdominal pain with colic and constipation may occur. Intestinal obstruction or abscesses may develop as a result of collections of bacteria and irritating agents being trapped in small blind pouches formed in the intestinal walls.

Diverticulosis The presence of diverticula in the colon without inflammation.

Diverticulum A pouch or pocket in the lining of a hollow organ, as in the bladder, esophagus or large intestine. *Meckel's diverticulum* A small sac occurring in the ileum as a congenital abnormality.

Diving reflex Emersion in cold water or sprinkling of cold water on body causes parasympathetic stimulation with reduced cardiac output and increasing A-V block. Hence used to treat paroxysmal supraventricular tachycardia.

Division Separation into parts.

Divulsion Forcibly pulling apart.

Dizygotic, Dizygous Pertaining to or derived from two separate zygotes (fertilized ova) said of twins.

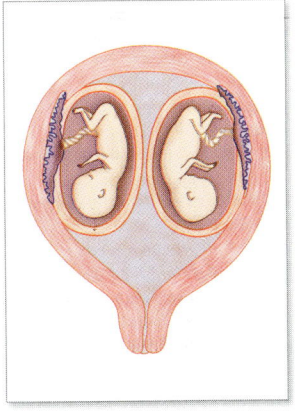

Dizygotic, Dizygous Twins

Dizziness A feeling of unsteadiness or haziness, accompanied by anxiety.

DNA Deoxyribonucleic acid.

Dobutamine A heart muscle stimulant administered parenterally in short-term treatment of adults with cardiac decompensation either from organic heart disease or from cardiac surgical procedures.

Doctor A person qualified to practice medicine.

Bare foot doctor A practitioner of traditional or native medicine in China who have not attended any medical school.

Doctrine The system of principles taught or advocated.

Docusate sodium A stool softner.

Doderlein's bacillus *A.S.G. Doderlein, German obstetrician and gynecologist, 1860–1941.* A lacto bacillus occurring normally in vaginal secretions.

Dohle bodies Inclusions in neutrophils as seen in burn, trauma, infection and neoplastic diseases.

Dolicocephalic Having a skull with long antero-posterior diameter.

Dolicomorphic A long and slender body (ectomorph).

Doll's headmaneuver A test to know brainstem damage in comatose patients. Normally eyes move together to the opposite side of head rotation.

Dolophine hydrochloride Methadone.

Dolor [L.] Pain.

Dolorimeter Device for measurement of degree of pain.

Domiciliary Within or at home.

Domicillary midwifery The confinement of a woman in her own home, attended by a midwife and possibly by the family doctor.

Domicillary services Health and social services provided within the home of the patient/client.

Dominant In genetics, capable of expression when carried by only one of a pair of homologous chromosomes. The opposite to recessive.

Dominant gene One which will produce its characteristics when it is present in either a hetero or homozygous state, i.e., it may be inherited from one parent only.

Domino' booking A plan of maternity care whereby a mother has her baby in a consultant unit, cared for by the community midwife. They return home following delivery after an interval of at least 6 hrs. The name derives from domiciliary midwife in and out.

Domperidone Antiemetic increases gastric motility, useful in dyspepsia.

Donath - Landsteiner phenomenon A test for paroxysmal cold hemoglobinuria where cold hemolysin combines to RBCs at 5°C and upon warming these red cells hemolyze.

Donnan's equilibrium A equilibrium is established between two solutions separated by a semipermeable membrane so that the sum of anions and cations on one side is equal to that on other side.

Donor 1. An organism that supplies living tissue to be used in another body, such as a person who furnishes blood for transfusion or an organ for transplantation. 2. A substance or compound that contributes part of itself to another substance (acceptor).

Universal donor A person with group O blood; such blood is some times used in emergency transfusion. Transfusion of blood cells rather than whole blood is preferred.

Donavan body Organism of granuloma inguinale, i.e., *Chlamydia trachomatis*.

Dopa The precursor of dopamine and an intermediate product in the biosynthesis of noradrenaline and adrenaline. It is used in Parkinson's disease and manganese poisoning. Also called L-dopa and levodopa.

Dopamine A substance allied to noradrenaline and used in the treatment of cardiogenic shock. Also occurs naturally in the adrenal medulla and the brain, where it functions as a transmitter of nervous impulses.

Dopamine hydrochloride A vasopressor catecholamine and neurotransmitter, also implicated in some forms of psychosis and abnormal movement disorder.

Doping In sports medicine, use of drugs to improve sports performance, commonly androgenic anabolic steroids.

Doppler A method to measure blood flow in arteries and veins.

Doppler effect The relationship of the apparent frequency of waves, as of sound, light and radio waves, to the relative motion of the source of the waves and the observer.

Doppler ultrasound flow meter A device for measuring blood flow that transmits sound at a frequency of several megahertz along a blood vessel. Rapid pulsatile changes in flow as well as steady flow can be recorded; hence, it is helpful in assessing intermittent claudication, thrombus obstruction of deep veins and other abnormalities of blood flow in the major arteries and veins.

Doraphobia Aversion to touching the hair or fur of animals.

Dorllo's canal A bony canal in the tip of temporal bone enclosing abducens nerve.

Dorsal Relating to the back or posterior part of an organ.

Dorsal nerves Branches of spinal nerves that pass dorsally to innervate structures near to vertebral column.

Dorsal slit A surgical method of making the foreskin of penis easily retractable. The foreskin is cut in dorsal midline but not far enough to extend to mucous membrane next to glans.

Dorsiflexion Bending backwards of the fingers or toes, i.e., upwards.

Dorsum 1. The back. 2. The upper or posterior surface.

Dosage Pertains to quantity, frequency and number of doses of a drug/radiation.

Dose Amount of medicine/radiation to be given to a tissue or target.

Absorbed dose Dose of ionizing radiation imparted to a tissue or target.

Cumulative dose Total dose of radiation resulting from repeated exposures.

Maximum permissible dose The maximum amount of radiation exposure permitted to person whose occupation requires working with radioactive agents.

Therapeutic dose Dose required to produce therapeutic effect.

Dose calculation for children Young's formula

$$\frac{\text{Age of years.}}{\text{Age} + 12} \times \text{adult dose or Body}$$

surface area of child/1.7 adult dose.

Dose response curve A graph showing the degree of effect of a drug in relation to its doses.

Dosimeter One of various devices used to detect and measure exposure to radiation; worn by personnel near to radiation sources.

Dothiepin A tricyclic antidepressant and sedative drug.

Double-blind trial A test for the real effect of a new drug or treatment in clinical practice. Neither the patient nor the staff administering the treatment knows which of two apparently identical treatments is the new one being tested.

Double contrast examination Radiographic examination in which both a radiopaque and a radioluscent contrast medium are used simultaneously to visualize internal anatomy.

Double personality Dual personality seen in hysteria and schizophrenia.

Douche A stream of fluid directed to flush out a cavity of the body.

Douglas fold The arcuate line of the sheath of rectus muscle.

Douglas's pouch *Douglas. British anatomist, 1675–1742.* Peritoneal space lying between uterus and front of rectum. Rectouterine pouch.

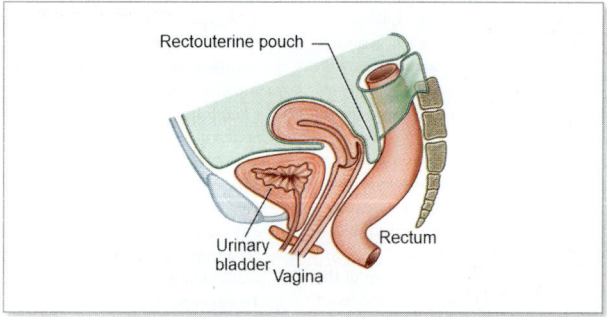

Douglas's Pouch

Doula From the Greek word, meaning 'woman who serves other women'. In maternity terms, one who provides emotional and practical support throughout pregnancy, and labour and postnatally.

Down's syndrome *J.L.H. Down, British physician, 1828–1896.* A congenital condition characterized by physical malformations and some degree of mental handicap. The disorder was formerly known as mongolism. It is also called trisomy 21 syndrome because the disorder is concerned with a defect in chromosome 21. There is a relatively high incidence in children of mothers who are in the older childbearing age. A particular type of Down's syndrome that occurs in children of younger mothers tends to occur in certain families. The term trisomy refers to the presence of three representative chromosomes in a cell instead of the usual pair. In Down's syndrome the 21st chromosome pair fails to separate when the germ cell (usually the ovum) is being formed. Thus the ovum contains 24 chromo-

somes, and when it is fertilized by a normal sperm carrying 23 chromosomes, the child is born with an extra chromosome (or total of 47) per cell.

Doxapram A respiratory stimulant used in carbon monoxide poisoning.

Doxepin A tricyclic antidepressant.

Doxorubicin Anthracycline, antitumor antibiotic.

Doxycycline Broad spectrum tetracycline.

Doxylamine A sedative.

Dracontiasis A tropical disease caused by infestation with the guinea worm; acquired by drinking contaminated water.

Dracunculus A genus of roundworms; includes the guinea worm.

Drain 1. To withdraw liquid generally. 2. Any device by which a channel or open area may be established for exit of fluids or purulent material from a cavity, wound or infected area.

Drainage The free flow of fluid from a wound/cavity.

Closed drainage Drainage without access of air into drained site via the tube.

Negative pressure drainage Drainage where negative pressure is maintained within the tube, e.g., pneumothorax drainage.

Open drainage Drainage without exclusion of air.

Postural drainage Drainage of sinuses and bronchi by gravity.

Dramamine Diphenhydramine, an agent for vertigo.

Dramatism Dramatic behavior and lofty speech as in lunatics.

Drama therapy The therapeutic use of drama, in which clients are encouraged to act out their feelings in order to overcome problems.

Drastic Acting strongly.

Draught A liquid medicinal dose to be gulped at once; drink.

Draw sheet The rubber cloth spread on the bed to protect the mattress and linen from drainage and soilage.

Drawer sign Sign of cruciate ligament rupture of knee.

Dream Mental activity that occurs during deep (see REM) sleep, usually in the form of vivid images, emotions and imagined events. Often rapidly forgotten on waking.

Dreaming The activity of engaging in fantasies or speculation during quiescent waking periods. Also called day dreaming. Some research suggests that this activity helps to promote mental health for the individual concerned.

Drepanocyte Resembling sickle cell.

Dressing Material applied to cover a wound or a diseased surface of the body.

Drift Movement due to an external force, in an aimless fashion.

Drill (*SYN*-burr) Device for rotating sharp cutting instrument e.g., cavity preparation in dentistry.

Drip A colloquial term used to denote intravenous infusion of fluid (blood, saline, glucose) into the body.

Drive (driev) In psychology, an urge or motivating force.

Dromostanolone An antineoplastic agent.

Dromotropic Fibers in cardiac nerves influencing conduction.

Dronabinol Synthetic tetrahydrocanabinol, a psychoactive substance.

Droperidol A major tranquillizer used to control behavioural disturbances.

Droplet infection Infection due to inhalation of respiratory pathogens suspended in liquid particles exhaled from someone already infected.

Dropsy An old-fashioned term used to describe excess fluid in the tissues (edema).

Drotaverine Antispasmodic drug.

Drowning Asphyxiation due to immersion in liquid.

Drowsiness The state of almost falling asleep.

Drug 1. Any medicinal substance. 2. A narcotic.

Drug abuse The use of drugs for purposes other than those for which they are prescribed or recommended. The major groups of drugs and medicines generally considered to be most commonly misused are stimulants ('uppers'), depressants ('downers'), psychedelics and narcotics.

Drug addiction A state of periodic or chronic intoxication produced by the repeated consumption of a drug, characterized by (a) An overwhelming desire or need (compulsion) to continue use of the drug and to obtain it by any means; (b) A tendency to increase the dosage; (c) A psychological and usually a physical dependence on its effects; and (d) A detrimental effect on the individual and on society.

Drug dependence A psychic and often physical dependence upon a drug.

Drug fever Fever caused by drugs.

Drug idiosyncrasy An individual response to a drug that is unique to that person and quite different from what is expected.

Drug interaction Modification of the potency of one drug by another (or others) taken concurrently or sequentially. Some drug interactions are harmful and some may have therapeutic benefits. Present knowledge of drug interactions is limited. Drugs may also interact with various foods. In general, these interactions fall into three categories: (a) Food malabsorption; (b) Nutritional status; and (c) Alteration of drug response by nutrients. In teaching patients self care in the taking of prescribed medications, one should explain the need for meticulously following directions related to the intake of food and drink while the medication regimen is being followed.

Drug rash Rash produced by intake or application of drugs.

Drug reaction Adverse and undesired reactions in some individuals to a substance.

Drug receptors The protein molecules on cell surface that bind to a particular drug and then activate a series of reactions through which the drug produces the desired pharmacological effect.

Drug tolerance A progressive reduction in the effect of a drug following repeated use. To achieve the desired effect increasingly larger doses of the medication are needed.

Drunkness Alcoholic intoxication with blood ethyl alcohol level exceeding 0.3-0.4%.

Drusen Small hyaline, globular pathological growths formed on Descemet's membrane.

Dry eye syndrome A common condition in which the eyes do not make sufficient tears. Also known as keratoconjunctivitis sicca or dry eyes.

Dry socket Infection of the soft tissues of a tooth socket, occurring 2 or 3 days after tooth extraction, often a lower molar. It is a painful condition requiring dental treatment with socket irrigation and local and/or systemic antibiotics.

DSH Deliberate self-harm. *(See PARASUICIDE).*

Duazomycin Glutamine antagonist, anticancer drug.

Dubowitz score A method used to assess gestational age in a low-birth-weight infant.

Duchenne dystrophy *G. B. A. Duchenne, French neurologist, 1806–1875.* Progressive muscular dystrophy occurring in childhood, due to repeated consumption of a drug.

Ducrey's bacillus Small rod shaped organism found in pairs, causative agent of soft sore.

Duct A tube or channel for the passage of fluid, particularly one conveying the secretion of gland.

Ductless Without an excretory duct.
Ductless glands Endocrine glands.

Ductus A duct.
Ductus arteriosus A passage connecting the pulmonary artery and aorta in intrauterine life, which normally closes at birth. When it remains open it is called persistent ductus arteriosus *(See also Patent ductus arteriosus).*
Ductus Venosus The duct through which the umbilical vein drains into inferior venacava in fetus.

Duffy system A blood grouping system.

Duloxetine Antidepressant.

Dumping A rapid evacuation of the contents of an organ.
Dumping syndrome A feeling of fullness, weakness, sweating and dizziness which may occur after meals following a partial gastrectomy.

Duodenal Pertaining to the duodenum.
Duodenal bulb First part of duodenum beyond pylorus.

Duodenal intubation The use of a special tube which is passed via the mouth and stomach into the duodenum. Used for withdrawal of duodenal contents for pathological examination.

Duodenal ulcer A peptic ulcer occurring in the duodenum near the pylorus.

Duodenostomy The formation of an artificial opening into the duodenum, through the abdominal wall, for purposes of feeding in cases of gastric disease.

Duodenum The first 20–25 cm of the small intestine, from the pyloric opening of the stomach to the jejunum. The pancreatic and common bile ducts open into it.

Dupuytren's contraction or contracture *Baron G. Dupuytren, French surgeon, 1777–1835.* Contracture of the palmar fascia, causing permanent bending and fixation of one or more fingers.

Dura mater A strong fibrous membrane forming the outer covering of the brain and spinal cord.

Duritis *SYN* – pachymeningitis, inflammation of dura.

Duroziez murmur Systolic and diastolic murmur heard over an artery when pressure is applied just distal to stethoscope.

Dust Minute fine particles of earth.

Ear dust Fine calcareous bodies found in gelatinous substance of otolith membrane of ear.

House dust Matters included in house dust are mites, hairs, pollen, and smoke particles.

Dutasteride Antiandrogen for prostatic hypertrophy.

Duty of candour A contractual duty imposed on all providers of care to NHS patients to provide to the service user and any other relevant person all necessary support and all relevant information in the event of a reportable patient safety incident.

Duty of care 1. The legal responsibility in the law of negligence that a person must take reasonable care to avoid causing harm. 2. A nurse, midwife or medical practitioner has an accepted duty to a patient or client irrespective of any contractual agreement existing between the parties. The law has developed a set of rules on the expected standard of care to assist in determining whether or not a professional has neglected their duty of care, based on the standards prevailing at the time of any case questioning the issue.

Duty of partnership Duty placed on NHS bodies and local government to develop joint local delivery plans involving other parts of the NHS, local Voluntary organizations and businesses.

Dwarfism The state of being short in stature. Arrest of growth and development, e.g., due to renal rickets, cretinism or deficient pituitary function.

Dyclonine hydrochlorides A topical anesthetic.

Dye Any colored or colouring agent, employed for staining slides for histopathological examination or manufacturing test reagents.

Dynamic Pertains to vital force or inherent power; opposite of static.

Dynamograph Device for recording muscular strength.

Dynamometer An instrument for measuring the force of muscular contracture.

Dyne Force needed for imparting acceleration of 1 cm. per second to a 1 gm mass.

Dynorphins An endogenous opioid peptide.

Dysacusis Difficulty in hearing, discomfort caused by loud noise.

Dysarthria Difficulty in articulation or speech.

D

Dysarthrosis A deformed, dislocated or false joint.

Dysautonomia A hereditary disease involving autonomic nervous system characterized by motor in coordination, fluctuating blood pressure, mental retardation, etc.

Dysbasia Difficulty in walking.

Dyscalculia Inability to solve mathematical problems.

Dyschondroplasia A condition in which cartilage is deposited in the shaft or some bones. The affected bones become shortened and deformed.

Dyscrasia A morbid condition, usually referring to an imbalance of component elements *(See also Blood dyscrasia)*.

Dysdiadochokinesia A sign of cerebellar disease in which the ability to perform rapid alternating movements, such as rotating the hands, is lost.

Dysentery Inflammation of the intestine, especially of the colon, with abdominal pain, tenesmus and frequent stools, often containing blood and mucus. The causative agent may be chemical irritants, bacteria, protozoa, viruses or parasitic worms.

Amebic dysentery Common in tropical countries; caused by the protozoon.

Entamoeba histolytica Spread is decreased in places with high standards of hygiene and sanitation. Also called amoebiasis.

Bacillary dysentery The most common and acute form of the disease, caused by bacteria of the genus.

Shigella. Also called shigellosis.

Dysesthesia Abnormal sensation on the skin with tingling, numbness, burning, etc.

Dysfunction Impairment of function.

Dysgammaglobulinemia An immunological deficiency state marked by selective deficiencies of one or more but not all, classes of immunoglobulin, resulting in heightened susceptibility to infectious diseases.

Dysgenesis Defective development.

Dysgerminoma A malignant tumour derived from germinal cells that have not been differentiated to either sex, occurring in either the ovary or the testicle.

Dysgeusia Impairment or perversion of gustatory sense so that normal taste is interpreted as being unpleasant.

Dysgraphia Difficulty in writing.

Dyshidrosis A disturbance of the sweat mechanism in which an itching vesicular rash may be present.

Dyskeratosis Altered keratinization of epithelial cells of epidermis, characteristic of many skin disorders.

Dyskinesia Impairment of voluntary movement.

Dyslalia Impairment of speech, caused by a physical disorder.

Dyslexia Difficulty in reading or learning to read; accompanied by difficulty in writing and spelling correctly.

Dyslogia difficulty in expression of ideas or impairment of the ability to reason or think logically. This is usually due to a lesion of central nervous system.

Dysmaturity The condition of being small or immature for gestational age; said of fetuses that are the product of a pregnancy involving placental insufficiency or dysfunction. Also called small for dates, or light for gestational age.

Dysmyelia This refers to a group of disorders associated with congenital malformation of the upper and lower extremities. These disorders are usually characterized by hypoplasia or partial and total aplasia of the tubular bones of the extremities or complete loss of an extremity.

Dysmenorrhea Painful menstruation.

Primary (spasmodic) dysmenorrhea Painful menstruation

occurring without apparent cause. The onset is usually shortly after puberty and occurs with each subsequent period. May be helped by hormonal therapy.

Secondary (congestive) dysmenorrhea Painful menstruation occurring in a woman who has previously had normal periods for some years. Often due to endometritis. The condition tends to worsen as the local congestion increases.

Dysmorphia A deformity or an abnormality in shape.

Dysostosis Abnormal development of bone.

Dysoxia Inability of mitochondria to utilize oxygen properly.

Dyspareunia Painful or difficult coitus in women.

Dyspepsia Indigestion. There may be abdominal discomfort, flatulence, nausea and sometimes vomiting.

Nervous dyspepsia Dyspepsia in which anxiety and tension aggravate the symptoms.

Dysphagia Difficulty in swallowing.

Dysphasia Difficulty in speaking as the result of a brain lesion. There is a lack of coordination and an inability to arrange words in their correct order.

Dysplasia Abnormal development of tissue.

Dyspnea Difficult or laboured breathing.

Expiratory dyspnea Difficulty inexpelling air.

Inspiratory dyspnea Difficulty in taking in air.

Dysphria Excessive depression feeling without apparent cause.

Dyspraxia Partial loss of ability to perform coordinated movements.

Dysrhythmia Disturbance of a regularly occurring pattern. Often applied to an abnormality of rhythm of the brainwaves as shown in an electroencephalogram.

Dystaxia Difficulty in controlling voluntary movements.

Dystonia A lack of tonicity in a tissue, often referring to the muscles.

Dystrophia Dystrophy.

D myotonica A rare hereditary disease of early adult life in which there is progressive muscle wasting and gonadal atrophy.

Dystrophy A disorder of an organ or tissue caused by faulty nutrition of the affected part.

Muscular d A group of hereditary diseases in which there is progressive muscular weakness and wasting.

Dysuria Difficult or painful micturition.

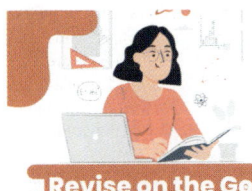

To access

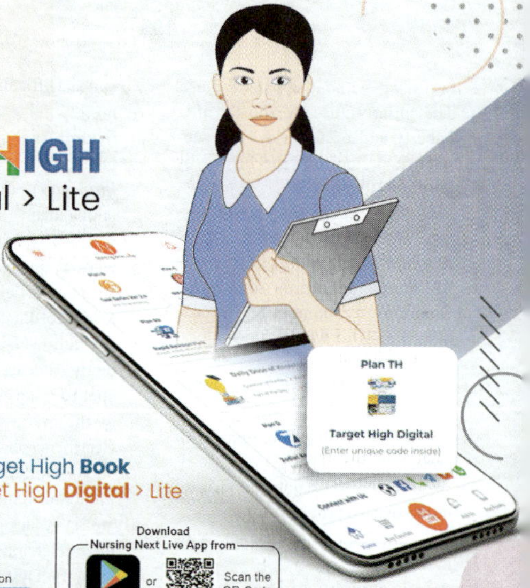

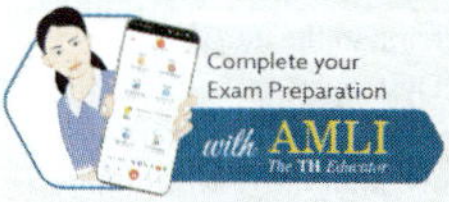

TARGET HIGH
Digital › Lite

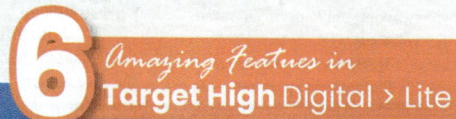

6 Amazing Features in
Target High Digital › Lite

Eales' disease Retinal vein thrombophlebits with recurrent hemorrhages into retina and vitreous.

Ear The organ of hearing and of equilibrium. It consists of three parts: (a) The *external ear*, made up of the expanded portion, or pinna, and the auditory canal, separated from the middle ear by the drum, or tympanum; (b) The *middle ear*, an irregular cavity containing three small bones (incus, malleus and stapes) that link the tympanic membrane to the internal ear; it also communicates with the pharyngotympanic tube and the mastoid cells; (c) The *internal ear*, which consists of a bony and a membranous labyrinth (the cochlea and semicircular canals).

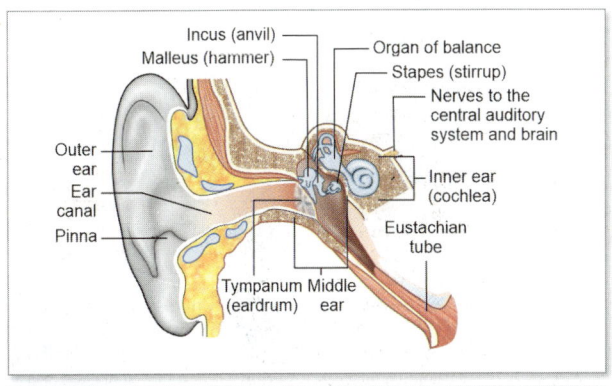

Incus (anvil)
Malleus (hammer)
Organ of balance
Stapes (stirrup)
Nerves to the central auditory system and brain
Outer ear
Ear canal
Pinna
Inner ear (cochlea)
Eustachian tube
Tympanum (eardrum)
Middle ear

Structure of Ear

EB virus Epstein-Barr virus.

EBM Expressed breast milk *(See Expression)*.

Ear dust Calcareous concretions in the membranous labyrinth.

Ear plug Device for plugging the external auditory canal, thereby preventing access of sound to internal ear.

Earwax Sticky honey colored cerumen secreted by glands at outer one-third of ear canal mixed with dust.

Eaton agent Mycoplasma pneumonia.

Ebastine Antiallergic agent.

Ebola Hemorrhagic Fever (EHF) A severe and acute, fatal, hemorrhagic viral disease, also known as Ebola virus disease, principally seen in central and west African countries, caused by the Ebola virus, of the family Filoviridae. Death occurs in up to 90% of cases. Ebola virus can be transmitted in several ways, the most significant being person-to-person through direct contact with body fluids (e.g., blood, semen, vaginal fluid) of an infected person.

Ebola virus disease A central African viral hemorrhagic fever with acute onset and characteristic morbilli-form rash. The incubation period is 2–21 days. Outbreaks have been reported in Sudan and Zaire. It has no known source, although it is probably zoonosis. Person-to-person spread in hospitals and laboratories by accidental inoculation of blood and tissue fluids has occurred.

Ebstein's anomaly Downward displacement of septal leaflet of tricuspid valve with gross tricuspid regurgitation.

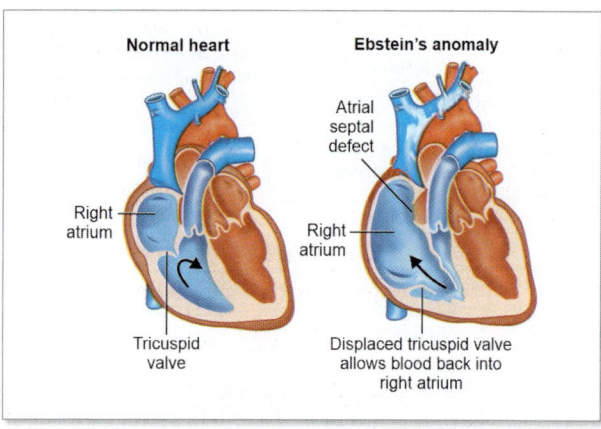

Normal heart / **Ebstein's anomaly**

Atrial septal defect

Right atrium

Right atrium

Tricuspid valve

Displaced tricuspid valve allows blood back into right atrium

Ebstein's Anomaly

Eclampsia A severe condition in which convulsions may occur as a result of an acute toxemia of pregnancy.

Ecchymosis A bruise; an effusion of blood under the skin causing discoloration.

Eccrine Secreting externally. Applied particularly to the sweat glands, which are generally distributed over the body *(See Apocrine)*.

ECG Electrocardiogram.

Echeosis Mental disturbance caused by noise.

Echinococcosis Infestation with *T. echinococcus*.

Echinococcus A genus of tapeworm. *Echinococus granulosus* infests dogs and may also infect humans. The larval form develops into cysts (hydatids), which occur in the liver, lung, brain and other organs.

Echinocyte Abnormal erythrocyte with multiple spiny projections from surface.

Echinostoma A genus of fluke found in aquatic birds.

Echo A reverberating sound produced when sound waves are reflected back to their source.

Echocardiography A method to examine the movements of the heart by the use of ultrasound.

Echoencephalography A method of brain investigation by ultrasonic echoes.

Echokinesis Involuntary repetition of another's gestures.

Echolalia The pathological involuntary repetition of phrases or words spoken by another person.

Echopraxia The automatic repetition of the movements of others.

Echovirus A group of viruses (enteroviruses), the name of which was derived from the first letters of the description "enteric cytopathogenic human orphan". At the time of the isolation of the viruses the diseases they caused were not known, hence the term "orphan". It is now known that these viruses produce many types of human disease, especially aseptic meningitis, diarrhea and respiratory diseases.

E-cigarette A handheld electronic device that mimics the effects of smoking tobacco cigarettes by heating a liquid to generate an aerosol, called a vapour that is inhaled. Also known as vaping.

Eclampsia A severe condition in which convulsions may occur as a result of an acute toxemia of pregnancy.

Eclecticism An old system of medicine where treatment is dependent upon individual signs and symptoms rather than the disease as a whole.

Ecmnesia Forgetfulness of recent events with remembrance of more remote ones.

Ecology The study of the relationship between living organisms and the environment.

Econazole A topical antifungal agent.

Economo's disease Encephalitis lethargica.

Economy The management of money or domestic affairs.

Token economy In behavior therapy, a programme of treatment in which the patient earns tokens, exchangeable for tangible rewards, by engaging in appropriate personal and social behavior, and loses tokens for antisocial behavior.

Ectasia Dilatation of any tubular structure.

Ecstasy 1. A feeling of exaltation. It maybe accompanied by sensory impairment and lack of activity but with an expression of rapture. 2. An illegal drug that has become extremely popular since the late 1980s. It is particularly widely used as an accompaniment to modern dance music. Has resulted in several fatalities in young people. Causes intense thirst leading to the drinking of large quantities of water resulting in fatal damage of the body's fluid balance, kidney failure and coma. Also known as 'MDMA', 'E' or 'ecky'.

Ecthyma A shallow skin lesion with crusting, often followed by pigmentation and scarring.

Ectocervix The portion of cervical canal outlined by squamous epithelium.

ECT Electroconvulsive therapy.

Ectoderm The outer germinal layer of the developing embryo from which the skin and nervous system are derived.

Ectogenous Produced outside an organism *(See Endogenous).*

Ectomorph Linear slender body build with poor musculature.

Ectoparasite A parasite that spends all or part of its life on the external surface of its host, e.g., a louse.

Ectopia Displacement or abnormal position of any part.

Ectopiacordis Congenital malposition of the heart outside the thoracic cavity.

Ectopiavesicae A defect of the abdominal wall in which the bladder is exposed.

Ectopic 1. Pertaining to or characterized by ectopy. 2. Located away from the normal position. 3. Arising or produced at an abnormal site or in at issue where it is not normally found.

Ectopic pregnancy Pregnancy in which the fertilized ovum becomes implanted outside the uterus instead of in the wall of the uterus. Also called extrauterine pregnancy.

Ectopic rhythm Any abnormal or irregular cardiac rhythm.

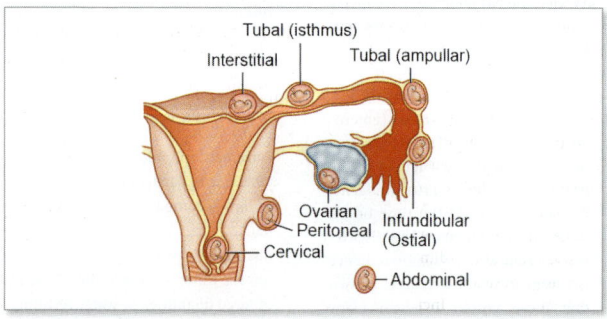

Ectopic Pregnancy

Ectoplasm The outer most layer of cell protoplasm.

Ectostosis Formation of bone beneath periosteum.

Ectothrix Fungus growing on hair shafts.

Ectotrichophyton Fungi causing hair and skin infection.

Ectozoon Parasite living on another animal.

Ectomelia Hypoplasia of long bones of limbs.

Ectopy Displacement or malposition, especially if congenital.

Ectropion Eversion of an eyelid, often due to contraction of the skin or to paralysis. It causes a persistent overflow of tears and hypertrophy of exposed conjunctiva.

Eczema 1. A general term for any superficial inflammatory process involving primarily the epidermis, marked early by redness, itching, minute papules and vesicles, weeping, oozing and crusting, and later by scaling, lichenification and often pigmentation. 2. Atopic dermatitis. Eczema is a common allergic reaction in children but it also occurs in adults. Childhood eczema often begins in infancy, the rash appearing on the face, neck and folds of elbows and knees. It may disappear by itself when an offending food is removed from the diet, or it may become more extensive and in some instances cover the entire surface of the body. Severe eczema can be complicated by skin infections. The cause of eczema can be either exogenous (due to external or traumatic factors) or endogenous (due to internal or constitutional factors).

Edema Excessive tissue accumulation water, either localized or generalized, can be due to poor venous drainage, lymphatic obstruction, increased venous pressure (CHF), hypoalbuminemia, or increased water retention.

Angioneurotic edema Local edema due to hypersensitivity to drugs, food, physical agents (cold) or idiopathic.

Brain edema Brain swelling due to water accumulation as following injury, toxemia or infection.

Cardiac edema Dependent edema of congestive heart failure.

Edema of glottis Usually follows infections with cough, hoarseness and dyspnea.

High altitude edema Pulmonary edema of mountaineers related to low partial pressure of oxygen.

Laryngeal edema Usually of allergic origin but life-threatening.

Non-pitting edema Myxomatous tissue accumulation appearing as edema without any dimple or pressure, e.g., myxedema.

Pulmonary edema Increased fluid accumulation in lungs following left heart failure, toxic gas inhalation, or ARDS.

Edentulous Without natural teeth.

EDTA Ethylenediaminetetraacetic acid.

Edge A margin or border.

Edrophonium chloride A cholinergic drug (anticholinesterage).

Edwards' syndrome Also known as trisomy 18, a serious genetic condition caused by an additional copy of chromosome 18. Babies born with Edwards' syndrome tend to be very small and have serious complications. They rarely live for more than few weeks and if they survive are likely to have severe physical and learning disabilities.

EEG Electroencephalogram.

Efavirenz Anti-HIV agent.

Effacement Taking up of the cervix. The process by which the internal os dilates, so opening out the cervical canal and leaving only a circular orifice, the external os. This process precedes cervical dilatation, particularly in a primigravida, while both occur simultaneously in a multigravida during labor.

Effect Result of an action or force.

Cumulative effect Drug effect on repeated administration of a drug.

Effective 1. The extent to which something succeeds. 2. A result produced by agent, action or force, e.g., resources to achieve desired outcomes. Cost effectiveness.

E dose The amount of a drug given to a patient to achieve the required treatment result.

Effector A motor or sensory nerve ending in a muscle, gland or organ.

Effeminate A male having physical characteristic or mannerism of a female.

Efferent Conveying from the center to the periphery *(See also Afferent)*.

Efferent nerves Nerves coming from the brain to supply the muscles and glands.

Effervescence Formation of bubbles of gas rising to surface of fluids.

Effleurage [Fr.] Stroking movement in massage. In natural childbirth, a light circular stroke of the lower abdomen, done in rhythm to control breathing, to aid in relaxation of the abdominal muscles, and to increase concentration during a uterine contraction. The stroking is accomplished by moving the wrist only. Also used in back massage.

Effort syndrome A condition characterized by breathlessness, palpitations, chest pain and fatigue, caused by an abnormal anxiety; often found in soldiers but may also occur in other individuals.

Effluent Fluid discharged from sewage treatment or industrial plant.

Effusion The escape of blood, serum or other fluid into surrounding tissues or cavities.

Ego In psychoanalytical theory, that part of the mind which the individual experiences as self. The ego is concerned with satisfying the unconscious primitive demands of the 'id' in a socially acceptable form.

Egocentrism A type of thinking in which a person has difficulty in seeing another's point of view. This self-centring is normal in young children but in adults may indicate delayed cognitive development.

Egoism An inflated estimate of one's value or effectiveness.

Egophony A nasal sound like bleating of a goat, present on lung tissue above effusion.

Ehlers-Danlos syndrome An inherited disorder of elastic connective tissue characterized by fragile hyperelastic skin, hyper mobile joints.

Eicosanoids Metabolites of arachidonic acid metabolism like prostaglandins, thromboxane and leukotrienes.

Eidetic Having the ability to visualize exactly objects or events which have previously been seen. Having a photographic memory.

Eisenmenger's complex *V Eisenmenger, German physician 1864–1932.* A congenital heart defect in which a ventricular septal defect is associated with increased pulmonary vascular resistance.

Ejaculation The act of ejecting semen, a reflex action that occurs as the result of sexual stimulation.

Ejaculatory duct The terminal portion of seminal duct formed by the union of the ductus deferens and excretory duct of the seminal vesicle.

Ejection fraction The percentage of blood ejected from left ventricle into aorta with each cardiac contraction.

Elastase Proteolytic pancreatic enzyme.

Elastic Capable of stretching.

Elastic bandage One that will stretch and will exert continuous pressure on the part bandaged.

Elastic cartilage Yellow cartilage of epiglottis, pharynx, external ear, auditory tubes.

Elastic stocking A woven rubber stocking sometimes worn for varicose veins.

Elastic tissue Connective tissue containing yellow elastic fibers.

Elastin The protein of elastic tissue.

Elation In psychiatry, a feeling of well-being or a state of excitement. It occurs to a marked degree in hypomania and to an intense degree in mania *(See Euphoria)*.

Elastometry The measurement of elasticity of tissues.

Elbow The joint between the upper arm and the forearm. It is formed by the humerus above and the radius and ulna below.

Tennis elbow Tendinitis of lateral forearm muscles near their origin from lateral epicondyle of humerus (lateral epicondylitis).

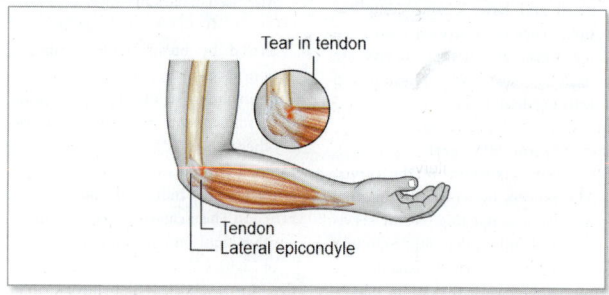

Tear in tendon

Tendon
Lateral epicondyle

Tennis Elbow

Elective Usually pertaining to a surgical procedure that is performed by choice, as opposed to an emergency life-saving procedure. Timing of the procedure may also be arranged to be mutually convenient for the patient and surgeon.

Elder abuse *(See abuse)*

Elective therapy A planned convenient therapy/operation.

Electra complex Libidinous fixation of a daughter toward her father. The female version of the Oedipus complex.

Electric shock Tissue injury from passage of electricity.

Electricity A form of kinetic energy having magnetic, chemical, mechanical and thermal effects; formed from interaction of positive and negative charges.

Electroanalgesia Pain relief by use of low intensity electric currents.

Electro-oculography *(See Electro-retinography).*

Electrocardiogram Abbreviated ECG. A tracing made of the various phases of the heart's action by means of an electrocardiograph. The normal electrocardiogram is composed of a P wave, Q, R and S waves (known as the QRS complex, or QRS wave), and a T wave. The P wave occurs at the beginning of each contraction of the atria. The QRS wave occurs at the beginning of each contraction of the ventricles. The T wave seen in a normal electrocardiogram occurs as the ventricles recover electrically and prepare for the next contraction. There is a refractory period between these waves.

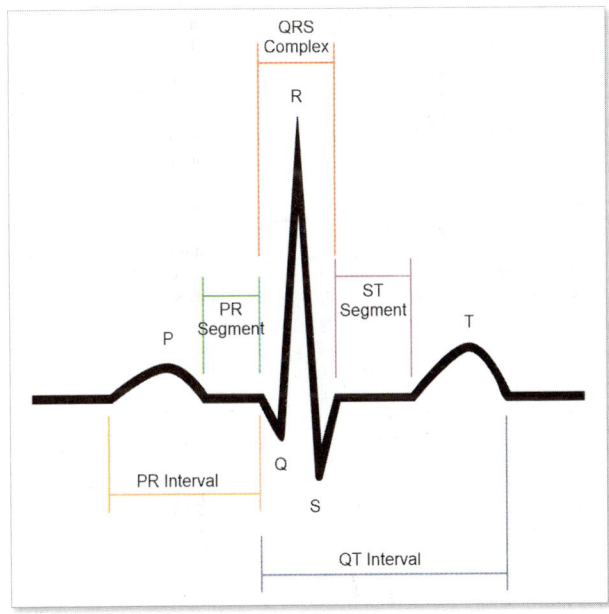

Electrocardiogram

Electrocardiograph A machine that records the electrical potential of the heart from electrodes on the chest and limbs.

Electrocautery An instrument for the destruction of tissue by means of an electrically heated needle or wire loop.

Electrocoagulation A method of coagulation using a high-frequency current. A form of surgical diathermy.

Electroconvulsive therapy Abbreviated ECT. Electroplexy. The passage of an electric current through the frontal lobes of the brain, which causes a convulsion. It is used in the treatment of depression and sometimes of schizophrenia. A general anesthetic and muscle relaxant are given before treatment.

Electrocution Death by electric current.

Electrocorticography Electroencephalography with the electrodes applied directly to the cortex of the brain during surgery to locate a small lesion, e.g., a scar.

Electrode The terminal of a conducting system or cell of a battery, through which electricity enters or leaves the body.

Electrodesiccation Drying of cells or tissues by means of high frequency electric spark used for achieving hemostasis following bleeding from small capillaries and veins during surgery.

Electrodialysis A method of separating electrolytes from colloids by passing current through the solution.

Electrodynamometer Instrument used to measure strength of current.

Electroejaculation Production of ejaculation by electrical stimulation from a probe placed in rectum, e.g., in paraplegics for artificial insemination.

Electroencephalogram Abbreviated EEG. A tracing of the electrical activity of the brain. Abnormal rhythm is an aid to diagnosis in epilepsy and cerebral tumor.

Electroencephalograph A machine for recording the electrical activity of the cortex of the brain. The electrodes are applied to the scalp.

Electrogoniometer Electrical device for measuring angles of joints and their range of motion.

Electrology The branch of science dealing with properties of electricity.

Electrolysis 1. Chemical decomposition by means of electricity, e.g., an electric current passed through water decomposes it into oxygen and hydrogen. 2. The destruction of tissue by means of electricity, e.g., the removal of surplus hair.

Electrolyte A compound which, when dissolved in a solution, will dissociate into ions. These ions are electrically charged particles and will thus conduct electricity.

Electrolyte balance The maintenance of the correct balance between the different elements in the body tissues and fluids.

Electrometer An instrument for measuring difference in electric potential.

Electromotive force (EMF) The difference in potential that causes the flow of electricity. It is measured in volts.

Electromyography Preparation, study and interpretation of electromyograms.

Electromyogram A graphic record of the contraction of muscle on electric stimulation.

Electron A negatively charged particle revolving round the nucleus of an atom.

Electron microscope A type of microscope employing a beam of electrons rather than a beam of light, which allows very small particles such as viruses, to be identified.

Electronic health record Abbreviate EHR. Longitudinal record of a patient's health and **health** care which combines information from primary health care with periodic care from other institutions.

Electronic patient record abbreviated ERP. A computerized record of the care provided for a patient both in primary and secondary settings.

Electronics The science of all systems involving use of electric devices, e.g., communication, data control and processing.

Electronystagmography A method of recording nystagmus from electrical activity of extraocular muscles.

Electrooculogram Recording of electric currents produced by eye movements.

Electrophoresis A method of analyzing the different proteins in blood serum by passing an electric current through the serum to separate the electrically charged particles. The particles gradually separate into bands as a result of the difference in rate of movement according to the electrical charge on the particles.

Electroplexy Electroconvulsive therapy.

Electrophysiology Branch of physiology dealing with relationships of body functions to electrical phenomena.

Electroretinography A method of examining the retina of the eye by means of electrodes and light stimulation for assessment of retinal damage.

Element 1. Any of the primary parts or constituents of a compound. 2. In chemistry, a simple substance that cannot be decomposed by ordinary chemical means; the basic 'stuff' of which all matter is composed.

Elephantiasis A chronic disease of the lymphatics producing excessive thickening of the skin and swelling of the parts affected, usually the lower limbs. It may be due to filariasis in tropical and subtropical climates.

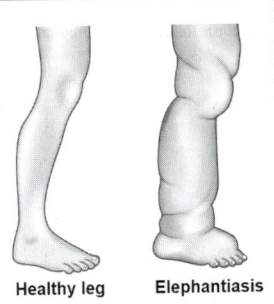

Healthy leg   Elephantiasis

Elephantiasis

Elevator An instrument used as a lever for raising bone, etc.

Periosteal elevator Instrument that strips the periosteum in bone surgery.

Elimination The removal of waste matter, particularly from the body. Excretion.

Elimination diet A diet regime used to determine which foods cause allergic response. Offending food then is discovered when one by one food is gradually introduced into diet.

ELISA Abbreviation for enzyme-linked immunosorbent assay, a blood test first used for the detection of antibodies to the human immunodeficiency virus (HIV) but which may be used to detect the presence of other antibodies in the blood. It may give a false-negative or false-positive result: a follow-up test should always be offered after a positive result.

Elixir A sweetened spirituous liquid, used largely as a flavoring agent to hide the unpleasant taste of some drugs.

Ellipsoid Spindle shaped.

Elliptocyte Oval shaped red blood cell. Normally, 15% of human RBC are oval and bird and reptiles have normally all RBC in elliptocytic form.

Elliptocytosis Benign hereditary disease, causing hemolytic anemia.

Ellis-van Creveld syndrome Congenital syndrome consisting of polydactyly, chondrodysplasia and congenital heart defects (ASD).

Emaciation Excessive wasting of body tissues. Extreme thinness.

Email An electronic method of exchanging digital messages between people using digital devices such as computers and mobile phones.

Emasculation The removal of the penis or testicles; castration.

Embalming Use of antiseptics and preservatives to prevent premature biodegradation of dead body.

Embarrass To interfere with or compromise function.

Embden-Meyerh of pathway Anaerobic metabolism of glucose to lactic acid in humans.

Embolectomy Surgical removal of an embolus, frequently arterial emboli that are cutting off the blood supply to the limbs.

Embolism Obstruction of a blood vessel by a traveling blood clot or particle of matter.

Air embolism The presence of gas or air bubbles, usually sucked into the large veins from a wound in the neck or chest.

Cerebral embolism Obstruction of a vessel in the brain.

Coronary embolism The blockage of a coronary vessel with a clot.

Fat embolism Globules of fat released into the blood from a fractured bone.

Infective embolism Detached particles of infected blood clot from an area of inflammation which, obstructing small vessels, result in abscess formation, i.e., pyemia.

Pulmonary embolism Blocking of the pulmonary artery or one of its branches by a detached clot, usually due to thrombosis in the femoral or iliac veins.

Retinal embolism Blockage, due to air or a blood clot, of the central retinal artery, resulting in loss of vision.

Embolus A substance carried by the bloodstream until it causes obstruction by blocking a blood vessel *(See Embolism).*

Embrocation A liquid applied to the body by rubbing to treat strains. A liniment.

Embramine Antiallergic agent.

Embryo The fertilized ovum in its earliest stages, i.e., until it shows human characteristics during the second month. After this it is termed as fetus.

Embryogeny The growth and development of embryo.

Embryology The study of the growth and development of the embryo from the unicellular stage until birth.

Emergency A sudden crisis requiring urgent intervention.

Emergency cardiac care (ECC) Care necessary to deal with an acute cardiopulmonary event like infarction, arrhythmia, pulmonary embolism.

Emergency obstetric unit An emergency team from a consultant obstetric unit which goes out to obstetric emergencies in the community or, in general practitioner units, taking the appropriate equipment, including A-negative blood for transfusion.

Emergency protection order A court order whereby a child is arbitrarily removed from the care of the parents in the interests of the child's safety.

Emesis Vomiting.

Emetic An agent that can induce vomiting.

Emic Perspectives that are shared and understood by members of a group, community or culture; 'the insiders'. These views may contrast to those of 'outsiders' *(see ETIC).* Used in ethnographic and qualitative research.

Emigration Passage of WBC through walls of capillaries.

Eminence A projection, usually rounded, from a surface, e.g., of a bone.

Emissary An outlet.

Emission Involuntary ejection (of semen).

EMLA A cream for local application to a skin site, containing a mixture of local anesthetics. Particularly useful for children as it allows for painful tests and biopsies to be performed with minimal pain and discomfort.

Emmetropia When the eyes are at rest parallel rays are focused exactly on retina; i.e., normal refraction.

Emmetropic Normal vision.

Emollient Any substance used to soothe or soften the skin.

Emotion Feeling or affect; a state of arousal characterized by alteration of feeling, tone and by physiological and behavioral changes. The physical form of emotion may be outward and evident to others, as in crying, laughing, blushing or a variety of facial expressions; however, emotion is not always reflected in the appearance and actions even though psychic changes are taking place. Joy, grief, fear and anger are examples of emotions.

Empathy The power of projecting oneself into the feelings of another person or into a situation.

Emphysema The abnormal presence of air in tissues or cavities of the body. *Pulmonary emphysema* A chronic disease of the lungs. Distension of alveoli causes intervening walls to be broken down and bullae to form on the lung surface. It also causes distension of the bronchioles and eventual loss of elasticity so that inspired air cannot be expired, making breathing difficult. *Surgical emphysema* The presence of air or any other gas in the subcutaneous tissues, introduced through a wound and evidenced by crepitation on pressure.

Empirical Based on experience and not on scientific reasoning.

Empowerment The capacity to empower, to give power or authority, e.g., to patients through the mechanism of the "Patient's Charter" or the "Changing Childbirth Report" for pregnant women, to take control over their own care and to work in partnership with care providers.

Emprosthotonos A form of spasm in which body is flexed forward, opposite to opisthotonus.

Empyema A collection of pus in a cavity, most commonly referring to the pleural cavity.

Empyesis Any pustular skin lesion.

Empyocele Suppurating hydrocele.

Emulsification Breaking down of large fat globules into smaller ones by bile acid that lower surface tension.

Emulsion A mixture in which an oil is suspended in water by the addition of an emulsifying agent.

En face [Fr.] A position in which the mother's face and that of her infant are on the same plane and approximately 20 cm apart; a position usually held during breastfeeding.

Enable 1. To provide a person with the authority, power, means or the opportunity to develop and achieve what is important to them as an individual or as a member of a community or organization. 2. To make possible or easy.

Enalapril Converting enzyme inhibitor, used in heart failure, hypertension.

Enamel The hard outer covering of the crown of a tooth.

Enamel organ A cup-shaped structure that forms on the dental lamaina of an embryo.

Enantiopathy Treatment of one disease by using another disease that produces symptoms antagonistic to former.

Enarthrosis A freely moving joint, e.g., ball and socket joint.

Enathem Eruption on mucous membrane.

Encanthis A small fleshy growth at the inner canthus of the eye, which may form an abscess.

Encapsulated Enclosed in a capsule.

Encephalagia Deep-seated headache.

Encephalin An opiate-like substance produced by the pituitary which has analgesic effects. This substance may also be produced synthetically *(See Endorphin)*.

Encephalitis Inflammation of the brain. There are many types of encephalitis, depending on the causative agent and the structures involved. The symptoms may be mild, with headache, general malaise and muscle ache similar to that associated with influenza. The more acute and serious symptoms may include fever, delirium, convulsions and coma, and in a significant number of patients result in death.

Encephalocele Herniation of the brain through the skull.

Encephalogram (air) X-ray of brain with air injected into ventricular system.

Encephalography Radiographic examination of the ventricles of the brain after the insertion of air or a gas through a lumbar or cisternal puncture.

Encephalomalacia Softening of the brain.

Encephalomyelitis Inflammation of the brain and spinal cord.

Encephalon The brain with the spinal cord, constituting the central nervous system.

Encephalopathy Cerebral dysfunction with diffuse disease or damage of the brain.

Dialysis encephalopathy Associated with long-term use of hemodialysis; marked by speech disorders and myoclonic fits progressing to global dementia.

Hepatic encephalopathy A condition caused by liver failure, leading to dementia and then coma.

Hypertensive encephalopathy A transient disturbance of function associated with hypertension. Disorientation, excitability and abnormal behavior occur, which may be reversed if the pressure is reduced.

Wernicke's encephalopathy A complication associated with chronic alcoholism; characterized by paralysis of the eye muscles, diplopia, nystagmus, ataxia and mental changes.

Encephalo trigeminal angiomatosis *(See Sturge-Weber Syndrome)*

Enchondroma A benign cartilaginous tumor occurring within a bone and expanding the diaphysis.

Encopresis Incontinence of feces not due to organic defect or illness.

Endarterectomy The surgical removal of the lining of an artery, usually because of narrowing of the vessel by atheromatous plaques.

Thrombo endarterectomy Removal of a clot with the lining.

Endarteritis Inflammation of the innermost coat of an artery.

Endarteritis obliterans A type that causes collapse and obstruction in small arteries.

Endemic Pertaining to a disease prevalent in a particular locality.

Endemiology The study of all the factors pertaining to endemic disease.

Endocarditis Inflammation of the endocardium characterized by vegetations on the endocardium and heart valves due to infection by microorganisms, fungi or rickettsia, or to rheumatic fever.

Endocardium The membrane lining the heart.

Endocervicitis Inflammation of the membrane lining the uterine cervix.

Endocrine Secreting within. Applied to those glands whose secretions (hormones) flow directly into the blood and not outward through a duct. The chief endocrine glands are the thyroid, parathyroids, suprarenals and pituitary. The pancreas, stomach, liver, ovaries and testes also produce internal secretions *(See Exocrine)*.

Endocrinology The science of the endocrine glands and their secretions.

Endocytosis A method of ingestion of a foreign substance by a cell.

Endoderm The innermost of the three germ layers of the embryo along with the mesoderm (intermediate) and ectoderm (outer) layers. It gives rise to the lining of most of the respiratory tract and to the intestinal tract and its glands.

Endodontis A branch of dentistry concerned with diagnosis, treatment and prevention of diseases of dental pulp and its surrounding tissue.

Endogenous Produced within the organism; *(See Exogenous)*.

Endogenous depression One in which the disease derives from internal causes.

Endolymph The fluid inside the membranous labyrinth of the ear.

Endometer Electronic device used to determine the length of tooth root canal.

Endometriosis The presence of endometrium in an abnormal situation, e.g., in the ovaries, the intestines or the urinary bladder. The ectopic tissue undergoes the same hormonal changes as normal endometrium. As there is no outlet for bleeding when menstruation occurs, the woman suffers severe pain.

Endometritis Inflammation of the endometrium.

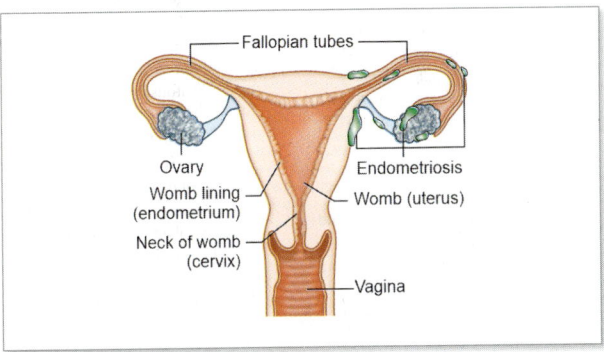

Endometriosis

Endometrium The mucous membrane lining the uterus.

Endomorph Body build characterized by predominance of tissues derived from endoderm.

Endomyocarditis Inflammation of the lining membrane and muscles of the heart.

Endomysium A thin layer of connective tissue that surrounds each striated muscle fiber.

Endoneurium A delicate connective tissue sheath that surrounds nerve fibers.

Endonuclease Enzyme that clears ends of polynucleotides.

Endoparasite A parasite that lives within the body of its host.

Endopelvic fascia The downward continuation of the parietal peritoneum of abdomen that supports pelvic viscera.

Endopeptidase Proteolytic enzyme that cleaves peptides.

Endophthalmitis Inflammation of the ocular cavity and adjacent structures.

Endorgan The expanded end of a nerve fiber in a peripheral tissue.

Endorphin One of a group of opiate like peptides produced naturally by the body at neural synapses at various points in the central nervous system, where they modulate the transmission of pain perceptions. Endorphins raise the pain threshold and produce sedation and euphoria; the effects are blocked by naloxone, a narcotic antagonist.

Endosalpingitis Inflammation of lining of fallopian tubes.

Endoscope An instrument used for direct visual inspection of a hollow organ or cavity.

Endosome The vacuole formed when material is absorbed in the cell by process of endocytosis. The vacuole fuses with lysosome.

Endospore *(See Spore)*

Endosteitis Inflammation of the endosteum.

Endosteoma A neoplasm in the medullary cavity of a bone.

Endosteum The lining membrane of bone cavities.

Endothelioma A malignant growth originating in the endothelium.

Endotheliosis Increased growth of endothelial cells.

Endothelium The membranous lining of serous, synovial and other internal surfaces.

Endothrix Fungus growth within hair.

Endotoxemia Toxemia due to presence of endotoxin in blood.

Endotoxin A poison produced by and retained within a bacterium, which is released only after the destruction of the bacterial cell *(See Exotoxin)*.

Endotracheal Within the trachea.

Endotracheal tube An airway catheter which is inserted into the trachea when a patient requires ventilator support. It also allows for the removal of secretions by suction.

Endplate The terminal end of nerve fiber to a muscle.

End of life care Care pathway for people nearing the end of life. Also incorporates planning for future care, making wishes and preferences known in advance.

End product The final product of a chemical/metabolic process.

Enema 1. Introduction of fluid into the rectum. 2. A solution introduced into the rectum to promote evacuation of feces or as a means of administering nutrient or medicinal substances. 3. Introduction of a radiopaque material in a radiological examination of the colon *(barium enema),* or via a tube inserted into the jejunum in a radiological examination of the small bowel *(small bowel enema)*.

Energy The capacity of a system in doing work.

Energy expenditure basal (BEE) Harris Benedict equation.
For women $6.55 + (9.6 \times W) + (1.8 \times H) - (4.7 \times A)$.
For men $66 + (13.7 \times W) + (5 \times H) - (6.8 \times A)$.
Where A = Age in years, H = Height in cm and W = Weight in kg.
Energy expenditure is increased by 13% over basal needs for each °C rise in temperature than normal. Stress, burn, trauma increase the need of calories to the extent of 40 – 100%.

Enflurane Anesthetic agent (volatile).

Enervation 1. General weakness and loss of strength. 2. Removal of a nerve.

Engagement The entry of the presenting part of the fetus, normally the head, into the true pelvis. Occurs in the last stage of pregnancy.

Engorgement Vascular congestion.

Enkephalins Polypeptides produced in brain that bind to opioid receptors to produce analgesia.

Enolase An enzyme present in muscle tissue that converts phosphoglyceric acid to phosphopyruvic acid.

Enophthalmos A condition in which the eyeball is abnormally sunken into its socket.

Enoxaparin Factor Xa inhibitor, anticoagulant.

Enriched Addition of something extra.

Ensiform Xiphoid; sword-shaped.
Ensiform cartilage The lowest portion of the sternum.

Entamoeba A genus of protozoa, some of which are parasitic in man.
Entamoeba histolytica The cause of amebic dysentery.

Enteral Within the gastrointestinal tract.
Enteral diets or enteral feeding Diets taken by mouth or through a nasogastric tube.

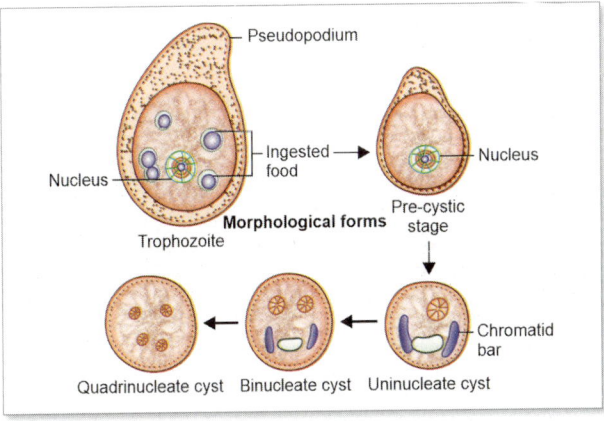

Entamoeba Histolytica

Enterectomy Excision of a portion of the intestine.

Enteric Pertaining to the intestine.
Enteric coated A special coating applied to tablets or capsules which prevents release and absorption of their contents until they reach the intestine.

Enteritis Inflammation of the small intestine.

Enterobacteriaceae A family of Gram-negative, rod-shaped bacteria, many of which are normally found in the human intestine.

Enterobiasis Infestation by thread worms.

Enterobius A genus of nematode worms.
Enterobius vermicularis The thread worm or pin worm, a small white worm parasitic in the upper part of the large intestine. Gravid females migrate to the anal region to deposit their eggs, sometimes causing severe itching. Infection is frequent in children.

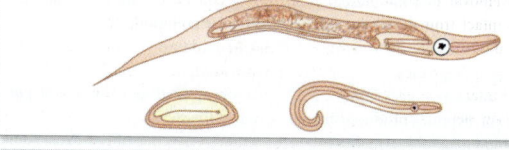

Enterobius Vermicularis

Enterococcus Any streptococcus of the human intestine. An example is *Streptococcus faecalis,* only harmful out of its normal habitat, when it may cause a urinary infection or endocarditis.

Enterocolostomy Inflammation of both the large and the small intestine.

Enterocolitis Inflammation of both the large and the small intestine.

Enterocoloctomy Surgical joining of small intestine to colon.

Enterocystoplasty Use of a portion of small intestine to enlarge the bladder.

Enteroenterostomy Establishing communication between two intestinal segments that are not continuous.

Enterogastrone A hormone secreted by intestinal mucosa but decreases gastric emptying. Fat stimulates its secretion.

Enterokinase An intestinal enzyme that converts trypsinogen into trypsin; enteropeptidase.

Enterolith Concretions in intestine.

Enteromyiasis Disease caused by maggots (larva of flies) in the intestine.

Enteron The elementary canal.

Enteropathogen Microorganism that causes intestinal infection.

Enteropeptidase Enzyme of duodenal mucosa that helps conversion of trypsinogen to trypsin.

Enteropexy Fixation of intestine to abdominal wall.

Enterostomy The formation of an external opening into the small intestine.

It may be (a) Temporary, to relieve obstruction, or (b) Permanent in the form of an ileostomy in cases of total colectomy.

Enterotomy Any incision of the intestine.

Enterotoxin A toxin that is produced by one of the many organisms that cause food poisoning. Such toxins frequently prove more resistant to destruction than the bacteria themselves.

Enterovirus A virus that infects the gastrointestinal tract and then attacks the central nervous system. This subgroup includes Coxsackie, polio and echoviruses, and are now known, together with rhinoviruses, as picornaviruses.

Enterozoon An animal parasite infesting the intestines.

Enthesis The use of metallic or other inert substances to substitute or replace lost tissue.

Enthesitis Inflammation at site of attachment of a tendon to bone.

Entomology Study of insects and their relationship to disease.

Entonox Trade name for a mixture of nitrous oxide and oxygen, 50% of each, premixed in one cylinder and used as an analgesic.

Entopic phenomena Visual phenomena like seeing floating bodies, circles of light, black spots, transient flashes of light.

Entropion Inversion of an eyelid, so that the lashes rub against the eyeball.

Enucleation Removal of an organ or other mass intact from its supporting tissues, as of the eyeball from the orbit.

Enuresis Involuntary passing of urine, usually during sleep at night (bedwetting).

Envenomation Introduction of poisonous venum into body by bite or sting.

Environment The surroundings of an organism which influence its development and behavior.

Environmental Health Officer The person employed by the local authority to improve and regulate the environment and to enforce statutory regulations. Responsibilities include housing, food hygiene, refuse collection, infestation, and air and noise pollution, etc.

Enzootic Endemic disease confined to animals.

Enzyme A protein that will catalyse a biological reaction *(See Catalyst)*.

Enzyme induction Increase in enzyme level due to its increased production or decrease degradation. Drugs commonly causing hepatic enzyme induction are barbiturates.

Enzyme-linked immunosorbent assay *(See Elisa)*.

Eosin A red dye used to stain biological specimens. A derivative of bromine and fluorescein.

Eosinophil Cell having an affinity for eosin. A type of white blood cell containing eosin-staining granules.

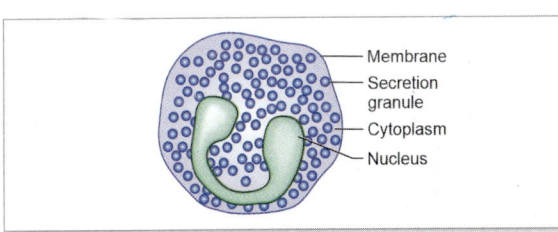

Eosinophil

Eosinophilia Excessive numbers of eosinophils present in the blood.

Ependyma The membrane lining the cerebral ventricles and the central canal of the spinal cord.

Ependymitis Inflammation of ependyma.

Ependymoma A neoplasm arising from the lining cells of the ventricles or central canal of the spinal cord. It gives rise to signs of hydrocephalus and is treated by surgery and radiotherapy.

Ephebiatrics Adolescent medicine.

Ephebology Study of puberty and its changes.

Ephedrine Sympathomimetic agent used locally as decongestant and systemically for bronchodilation and raising blood pressure.

Epiandrosterone Androgenic hormone normally present in urine.

Epiblast *SYN-* Ectoderm; outer layer of cells of blastoderm.

Ephidrosis Profuse sweating; hyperhidrosis.

Epiblepharon A congenital condition in which an excess of skin of the eyelid folds over the lid margin so that the eyelashes are pressed against the eyeball.

Epicanthus A vertical fold of skin on either side of the nose, sometimes covering the inner canthus; a normal characteristic in persons of certain races, but anomalous in others.

Epicardium The visceral layer of the pericardium.

Epichondal Dorsal to notochord.

Epichorion The portion of decidua of placenta that covers the ovum.

Epicondyle A protuberance on a long bone above its condyle.

Epicondylitis Also known as tennis elbow caused by strenuous overuse of the muscles and tendons of the forearm.

Epicritic Pertaining to sensory nerve fibers in the skin which give the appreciation of touch and temperature.

Epicyte An epithelial cell.

Epidemic The presence in a population of disease or infection in excess of that usually expected.

Epidemiology The study of the distribution of diseases in populations. It includes the attack rate (incidence) and the numbers affected at any particular time (prevalence).

Epidermis The nonvascular outer layer or cuticle of the skin. It consists of layers of cells which protect the dermis.

Epidermization Conversion of deeper germinative layers of cells into outer layers of epidermis.

Epidermoid Pertaining to certain tumors which have the appearance of epidermal tissue.

Epidermophyton A genus of fungi that attack skin and nails, but not hair. The cause of ringworm and athlete's foot.

Epididymis [Gr.] An elongated, cord like structure along the posterior border of the testis, whose coiled duct provides for the storage, transport and maturation of spermatozoa.

Epididymitis Inflammation of the epididymis.

Epididymography Radiographic examination of epididymis after introduction of contrast.

Epididymo-orchitis Inflammation of the epididymis and the testis.

Epidural Outside the dura mater.

Epidural analgesia Also known as extradural or peridural anesthesia. A form of pain relief for childbirth and chronic pain, obtained by the injection of a local analgesic into the epidural space in order to block the spinal nerves. It may be approached by two routes: (1) Caudal, through the sacrococcygeal membrane covering the sacral hiatus; or (2) Lumbar, through the intervertebral space and ligamentum flavum.

Epigastric reflex Contraction of upper portion of rectus abdomen is when skin of epigastric region is scratched.

Epigastrium Region of the abdomensituated over the stomach.

Epiglottis A cartilaginous structurewhich covers the opening from the pharynx into the larynx during swallowing and prevents food from passing into the trachea.

Epiglottitis Inflammation of epiglottis, usually bacterial often threatens airway obstruction of treatment is delayed.

Epilate To extract hair by the roots.

Epilation Removal of hairs with their roots. It may be effected by pulling out the hairs or by electrolysis.

Epilemma Neurilemma of small branches of nerve filament.

Epilatory An agent that produces epilation.

Epilepsy Convulsive attacks due to disordered electrical activity of the brain cells. In a major attack of "grand mal" the patient falls to the ground unconscious, following an aura or unpleasant sensation. There are first tonic and then clonic contractions, from which stage the patient passes into a deep sleep. A minor attack of "petit mal" is a momentary loss of consciousness only. Both these types of epilepsy are idiopathic and are not caused by any damage to the brain.

Focal or Jacksonian epilepsy A symptom of a cerebral lesion. The convulsive movements are often localized and close observation of the onset and course of the attack may greatly assist diagnosis.

Temporal lobe epilepsy Characterized by hallucinations of sight, hearing, taste and smell, paroxysmal disorders of memory and automatism. Caused by temporal or parietal lobe disease.

Epileptic Concerning epilepsy.

Epileptiform Resembling an epileptic fit.

Epiloia Tuberous sclerosis. A congenital disorder with areas of hardening in the cerebral cortex and other organs, characterized clinically by mental handicap and epilepsy.

Epimoephosis Regeneration of a part of organism by growth from cut surface.

Epimysium Outermost sheath of connective tissue surrounding a skeletal muscle.

Epinephrine Adrenaline.

Epinephritis Inflammation of adrenal gland.

Epinephroma Lipomatoid tumor of kidney.

Epineurium The sheath of tissue surrounding a nerve.

Epiphora Persistent overflow of tears, often due to obstruction in the lacrimal passages or to ectropion.

Epilphylaxis Increase in defensive power of body.

Epiphysiolysis Separation of an epiphysis.

Epiphysis The end of a long bone, developed separately from but attached by cartilage to the diaphysis (the shaft), with which it eventually unites. Growth in length takes place from the line of junction.

Epiphysitis Inflammation of an epiphysis especially that of knee, hip, shoulder in infants.

Epiplocele Hernia containing omentum.

Epiploic Pertains to omentum.

Epipygus A developmental anomaly where accessory limb is attached to the buttocks.

Epirubicin Antitumor antibiotic.

Episcleral Overlying sclera of eye.

Episcleritis Inflammation of the outer coat of the eyeball. It is seen as a slightly raised bluish nodule under the conjunctiva.

Episiotomy An incision made in the perineum when it will not stretch sufficiently during the second stage of labor.

Epispadias A malformation in which there is an abnormal opening of the urethra on to the dorsal surface of the penis *(See Hypospadias)*.

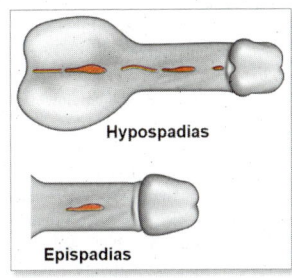

Epispadias

Episplenitis Inflammation of splenic capsule.

Epistais Suppression of any discharge.

Epistaxis Bleeding from the nose.

Epitendon The connective tissue holding a tendon with its sheath.

Epithelial cells Cells irregular in shape, having a single nucleus.

Epithelial tissue Those tissues covering outer surface of body and lining the internal passages or cavities.

The cells lie in close proximity of each other with little intercellular substance.

Epithelioid Resembling epithelium.

Epithelioma Any tumor originating in the epithelium.

Epithelium The surface layer of cells of the skin or lining tissues.

Epithelization Development of epithelium. The final stage in the healing of a surface wound. Epithelialization.

Epsilon-aminocaproic acid Synthetic substance, antifibrinolytic, used to check bleeding.

Epsom Salt = $MgSO_4$, a cathartic.

Epizoon Any external animal parasite.

Epstein-Barr virus *MA Epstein, British pathologist, b. 1921. Y Barr Canadian pathologist, b. 1932.* A herpes virus that causes infectious mononucleosis, it has been isolated from cells cultured from Burkitt's lymphoma, and has been found in certain cases of nasopharyngeal cancer. Also called EB virus.

Epulis Complete elimination of disease.

Erben's reflex Slowing of pulse when head and trunk are forcibly bent forward.

Equality and Human Rights Commission (EHRC) Launched in 2007, the Commission is an independent statutory body established under the Equality Act 2006 and 2010. The EHRC has statutory remit to promote and monitor human rights; and to protect, enforce and promote equality across the nine 'protected grounds: age, disability, gender, race, religion and belief, pregnancy and maternity, marriage and civil partnership, sexual orientation and gender reassignment.

Erb's palsy *WH Erb, German physician, 1840–1921.* Paralysis of the arm, often due to birth injury causing pressure on the brachial plexus or lower cervical nerve roots.

Erectile Having the power of becoming erect.

   Erectile tissue Vascular tissue which, under stimulus, becomes congested and swollen, causing erection of that part. The penis consists largely of erectile tissue.

Erection The enlarged and rigid state of the sexually aroused penis. Erection can also occur in the clitoris and the nipples of the female.

Erector spinae reflex Irrigation of skin of back causes hardening due to contraction of erector spinae.

Erepsin The enzyme of succus entericus, secreted by the intestinal glands, which splits peptones into aminoacids.

Erg In physics, the amount of work done when a force of 1 dyne acts through a distance 1 cm.

Ergasthenia Weakness due to overwork.

Ergocalciferol Vitamin D_2.

Ergocristine An ergot alkaloid.

Ergograph An apparatus for recording contractions of muscles and measuring the amount of work done.

Ergometer An apparatus for measuring amount of work performed.

Ergometrine An alkaloid of ergot which stimulates contraction of the uterine muscle.

Ergonomics The scientific study of human beings in relation to their work and the effective use of human energy.

Ergonovine maleate An ergot derivative used in treatment of migraine. It also stimulates contraction of uterus.

Ergosterol A sterol occurring in animal and plant tissues which, on ultraviolet irradiation, becomes a potent antirachitic substance, vitamin D_2 (ergocalciferol).

Ergot A drug from a fungus that grows on rye. Used chiefly to contract the uterus and check hemorrhage at child birth.

Ergotamine tartarate An alkaloid of ergot used in the treatment of migraine or to enhance uterine contraction.

Ergotism The effects of poisoning from ergot, which may lead to gangrene of the fingers and toes.

Erode To wear away.

Erogenous Arousing erotic feelings.

Erogenous zones Areas of the body, stimulation of which produces erotic desire, e.g., the oral, anal and genital orifices and the nipples.

Erosion The breaking down of tissue, usually by ulceration.

Cervical erosion A covering of columnar epithelium on the vaginal part of the uterine cervix, arising from erosion of the squamous epithelium, which normally covers it.

Erotic Pertaining to sexual love or lust.

Eroticism, erotism A sexual instinct or desire; the expression of one's instinctual energy or drive, especially the sex drive.

Erotology The study of love and its manifestations.

Erotomania Pathological exaggeration of sexual behavior.

Erotophobia Aversion to sexual love or its manifestations.

Erratic Fluctuating, unpredictable.

Error Mistake, miscalculation.

Eructation Belching; the escape of gas from the stomach through the mouth.

Eruption A breaking out, e.g., of a skin lesion or the cutting of teeth.

Erysipelas A febrile disease characterized by inflammation and redness of the skin and subcutaneous tissues, and caused by group A hemolytic streptococci.

Erysipeloid An infective dermatitis or cellulitis due to infection with *Erysipelothrixinsidiosa;* it usually begins in a wound (often the result of a prick by a fish bone) and remains localized, rarely becoming generalized and septicemic.

Erythema Redness of the skin caused by congestion of the capillaries in its lower layers. It occurs with any skin injury, infection or inflammation.

Erythema induratum A manifestation of vasculitis.

Erythema multiforme An acute eruption of the skin, which may be due to an allergy or to drug sensitivity.

Erythema nodosum A painful disease in which bright-red, tender nodes occur below the knee or on the forearm; it may be associated with tuberculosis.

Erythematous Characterized by erythema.

Erythrasma A skin disease due to infection by *Corynebacterium minitissimum,* attacking the armpits or groins. It causes no irritation but is contagious.

Erythritylte tranitrate Anti anginal agent.

Erythroblast Originally, any nucleated erythrocyte, but now more generally used to designate the nucleated precursor from which an erythrocyte develops.

Erythroblastosis The presence of erythroblasts in the blood.

Erythroblastosis fetalis A severe hemolytic anemia with an excess of erythroblasts in the newly born. It is due to rhesus incompatibility between the child's and the mother's blood.

Erythrocyanosis Swelling and blueness of the legs and thighs occurring mainly in young women and during cold weather.

Erythrocyte A mature red blood cell. The cells contain hemoglobin and serve to transport oxygen. They are developed in the red bone marrow found in the cancellous tissue of all bones. The hemopoietic factor

E

vitamin B$_{12}$ is essential for the change from proerythroblast to normoblast, and iron, thyroxine and vitamin C are also necessary for its perfect structure.

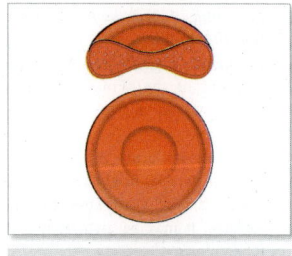

Erythrocyte

Erythrocyte sedimentation rate Abbreviated ESR. The rate at which the cells of citrated blood form a deposit in a graduated 200 mm tube (Westergren method). The normal is less than 10 mm of clear plasma in 1 hour. This is much increased in severe infection and acute rheumatism.

Erythrocythemia Increase in numbers of red blood cells due to overactivity of the bone marrow; Vaquez's disease; polycythemia vera.

Erythrocytopenia Erythropenia; deficiency in numbers of red blood cells.

Erythrocytosis Ethrocythemia.

Erythrodema An infantile disease characterized by itchy lesions of hands and feet, and polyarthritis.

Erythroderma Abnormal redness of the skin, usually over a large area.

Erythredema polyneuropathy A disease of infancy and early childhood. Marked by pain, swelling and ink coloration of the fingers and toes, and by listlessness, irritability, failure to thrive, profuse perspiration and sometimes scarlet coloration of the cheeks and tip of the nose. Called also acrodynia, pink disease.

Erythrodontia Reddish-brown staining of teeth.

Erythroid Concerning red blood cells.

Erythroleukemia A variant of acute myeloid leukemia with anemia, bizarre red cell morphology, erythroid hyperplasia in bone marrow.

Erythromelia Painless erythema of extensor surface of arm.

Erythromelalgia Burning and throbbing in feet that come and go.

Erythromycin A broad-spectrum antibiotic produced by a strain of *Streptomyces erythreus*. It is effective against a wide variety of organisms, including Gram-negative and Gram-positive bacteria.

Erythropoiesis The manufacture of red blood corpuscles.

Erythropoietin A hormone, produced by the kidney, which stimulates the production of red blood cells in the bone marrow.

Erythropoietin therapy The use of erythropoietin to promote new blood formation as an alternative to blood transfusion.

Erythropsia A defect of vision in which all objects appear red. Often occurs after a cataract operation.

Esculent Suitable for use as food.

Eschar A slough or scab which forms after the destruction of living tissue by gangrene, infection or burning.

Escherichia A genus of *Enterobacteriaceae*.

Escherichia coli An organism normally present in the intestines of humans and other vertebrates. Although not generally pathogenic, it may set up infections of the gallbladder, bile ducts, and urinary and intestinal tracts.

Esmarch's tourniquet *JFA von Esmarch, German surgeon, 1823–1908.* A rubber bandage used in surgery to express blood from a limb and render it less vascular.

Esophagoenterostomy Making communication between esophagus and intestine following resection of stomach as in gastric malignancy.

Esophagomyotomy Incision of muscular coat of esophagus as in achalasia cardia.

Esophagoplication Reduction of dilatation of esophagus by taking tucks in its walls.

Esophagotomy Surgical incision into the esophagus as in achalasia cardia.

Esophagus The musculo-membranous tube extending from pharynx to stomach.

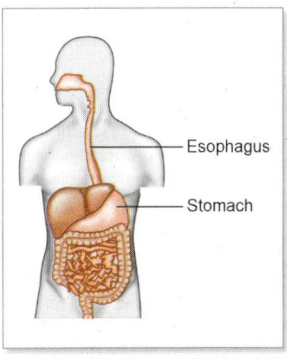

Esophagus — Stomach

Esophagus

Esophoria Latent convergent strabismus. The eyes turn inwards only when one is covered up.

Esotropia Convergent strabismus. One or other eye turns inwards, resulting in double vision.

ESP Extrasensory perception.

ESR Erythrocyte sedimentation rate.

ESRD End-stage renal disease *(See Renal)*.

Essence 1. An indispensable part of anything. 2. A volatile oil dissolved in alcohol.

Essential Indispensable.

Essential amino acids Those amino acids that must be obtained in the diet and are necessary for the maintenance of tissue growth and repair *(See Amino acid)*.

Essential fatty acids Unsaturated fatty acids that are necessary for body growth.

Essential oils Specially prepared aromatic oils which are obtained from the different parts of plants including flowers, leaves, seeds, wood, roots and balk. Used in aromatherapy.

Ester A compound formed by the combination of an acid and an alcohol with the elimination of water.

Esterase An enzyme that causes the hydrolysis of esters into acids and alcohol.

Esthesia Perception, feeling, sensation.

Esthesiometer Device for measuring tactile sensibility.

Estradiol Steroid hormone of ovary with estrogenic properties.

Estriol Metabolic product of estrone and estradiol.

Estrogen Substance having estrogenic activity, i.e., development of female sex characteristics, cyclic changes in endometrium and vaginal epithelium, breast changes.

Estrone Natural estrogenic hormone less active than estradiol but more active than estriol.

Estrus The cyclic period of sexual activity in mammals; during estrus animal is said to be "in heat".

Etching Application of corrosives material to a glass/metal to create a pattern or design.

Ethambutol A drug used in combination with other drugs in the treatment of tuberculosis.

Ethanol Alcohol.

Ethanolamine An intravenous sclerosing agent used to inject varicose veins.

Ethaverine hydrochloride Mild coronary artery dilator.

Ethchlorvynol Hypnotic agent.

E

Ether A volatile inflammable liquid formerly used as a general anesthetic agent.

Ether diethyl Inflammable anesthetic agent.

Ethics A code of moral principles.

Nursing ethics The code governing a nurse's behavior with patients and their relatives, and with colleagues.

Ethmoidectomy Surgical removal of a portion of the ethmoid bone.

Ethinamate Mild sedative – hypnotic agent.

Ethinyl estradiol An estrogenic hormone.

Ethionamide Bacteriostatic second line antitubercular drug.

Ethionine Progestational agent used in contraceptive.

Ethoheptazine Analgesic agent.

Ethmoid A sieve-like bone separating the cavity of the nose from the cranium. The olfactory nerves pass through its perforations.

Ethmoiditis Inflammation of ethmoidal air cells causing pain in between eyes, headache and nasal discharge.

Ethnic Pertaining to a social group, members of which share cultural bonds or physical (racial) characteristics.

Ethnic minority A social grouping of people who share cultural or racial factors but who constitute a minority within the greater culture or society.

Ethnocentrism The belief that one's own group, community, society or even way of doing things is superior to those of others, leading to mistrust or doubt about others' values and beliefs.

Ethnography A qualitative research approach developed by anthropologists with the purpose of describing an aspect of a culture, but also aimed at learning about the culture or factor being studied.

Ethnology The science dealing with the human races, their descent, relationship, etc.

Ethoheptazine An analgesic related to pethidine. It relieves pain and muscle spasm.

Ethopropazine Anticholinergic used in parkinsonism.

Ethosuximide An anticonvulsant used in the treatment of "petit mal" epilepsy.

Ethotoin Sparingly used anticonvulsant.

Ethylchloride A volatile liquid used as a local anesthetic. When sprayed on intact skin it causes local insensitivity, through freezing.

Ethyl cellulose Ether of cellulose, used for drug preparation.

Ethylene glycol Antifreeze, poisonous.

Ethylene oxide A gas that is sporicidal and viricidal and capable of penetrating relatively inaccessible parts of an apparatus during sterilization. It is used for equipment, which is too delicate to be sterilized by other methods.

Ethylenediamine Solvent for theophyline.

Ethylenediaminetetraacetic acid Abbreviated EDTA. A chelating agent used in the treatment of lead-poisoning.

Ethylmorphine Used as cough suppressant.

Ethylnorepinephrine Adrenergic drug used in asthma.

Ethylestrenol An anabolic steroid that may be used to treat severe weight loss, debility and osteoporosis.

Etic The perspectives of a group, community or culture held by observers who are 'outsiders' or non-participants.

Etidronate Drug used in Paget's disease.

Etiolation Paleness of the skin due to lack of exposure to sunlight.

Etiology *(See Aetiology).*

Etofamide An intraluminal amebicide.

Etoposide Podophylotoxin for malignant diseases.

Etoricoxib Anti-inflammatory, analgesic.

Etretinate Retinoid used for acne.

Eucalyptus oil An oil derived from the leaves of the eucalyptus tree; it has mild antiseptic properties and is used in the treatment of nasal catarrh.

Eucapnia Normal CO_2 concentration in blood.

Eudiometer Instrument for testing purity of air and making analysis of gases.

Eugenics The study of measures that maybe taken to improve future generations, both physically and mentally.

Eugenol A local anesthetic and antiseptic, derived from oil of cloves and cinnamon, used in dentistry.

Eugeria The state of a high quality of life in old age. Eugeria should be the normal state for the elderly but maybe affected by physical or mental illness.

Eugynon E. 30, E. 50 Proprietary preparations of contraceptive tablets containing estrogen and progesterone.

Eunuch A castrated male.

Eunuchoidism Deficient male sexual characteristics.

Euphoria An exaggerated feeling of well-being, often not justified by circumstances. Less than elation.

Euplastic Capable of being transformed into healthy tissue. The term may be applied to a wound that is healing well.

Euploidy In genetics, a state of having complete sets of chromosomes.

Eurhythmics Gentle body exercises performed to music.

European Health Insurance Card (EHIC) Gives access to health care across the European Economic Area and Switzerland.

European Medicines Agency Authorizes the use of medicinal products in the European Union. Works with national medicines regulatory bodies and aims to protect and promote the health of the citizens of European Member States (see also Medicines And Healthcare Products Regulatory Agency).

European Pressure Ulcer Advisory Panel (EPUAP) Set up to find best evidence to prevent and treat pressure ulcers. Guidelines from EPUAP includes an international pressure ulcer classification system.

European Union Nursing Directives The EU directives seek to ensure that nurses and midwives from the member states of the EU receive similar educational programs, which meet defined standards to facilitate free movement of nursing personnel between the member states.

Eustachian tube B Eustachio, Italian anatomist, 1520–1574. The pharyngotympanic tube.

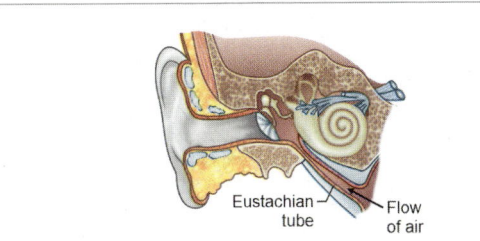

Eustachian Tube

Eustachian valve Valve at the entrance of inferior venacava.

Eustachitis Inflammation of the Eustachian tube.

Euthanasia 1. An easy or good death. 2. The deliberate ending of life of a person suffering from an incurable disease; this can be voluntary or involuntary.

Euthenics The science of improvement of population through modification of environment.

Euthyroid Having a normally functioning thyroid gland.

Evacuate To discharge especially bladder and bowel; to transfer patient from one site to another.

Evacuant 1. Promoting evacuation. 2. An agent that promotes evacuation.

Evacuation 1. An emptying or removal, especially the removal of any material from the body by discharge through a natural or artificial passage. 2. Material discharged from the body, especially the discharge from the bowels.

Evacuator An instrument that produces evacuation, e.g., one designed to wash out small particles of stone from the bladder after lithotripsy.

Evaluation A critical appraisal or assessment; a judgment of the value, worth, character or effectiveness of that which is being assessed. In the health-care field this includes assessment of the patient's position on the health/illness continuum, and of the effectiveness of patient care activities in bringing about a change in the patient's position. Accepted as the fourth phase of the nursing process.

Evanescescent Not permanent, brief duration.

Evans blue A dye used for as diagnostic agent.

Evaporation Change from liquid to gaseous state.

Evenomation Removal of venom from biting site.

Eventration 1. The protrusion of the intestines through the abdominal wall. 2. Removal of abdominal viscera.

Eversion Turning outwards.

Eversion of the Eyelid Ectropion. The upper eyelid may be everted for examination of the eye or for the removal of a foreign body.

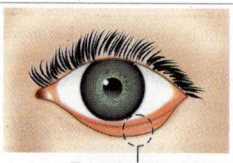

Turned out eyelid
from muscle laxity

Ectropion

Evidence-based practice Systematically appraising clinical situations and then using up-to-date research findings as a basis for the nursing or medical decisions. An approach to clinical practice first developed at Mc Master University (Canada) which is based on the following four principles: (a) Clinical and other health-care decisions should be *based on the best evidence* available from patients and populations as well as from the laboratory; (b) The patient's problem determines the nature and source of evidence to be sought, rather than habit, protocolor tradition; (c) Identifying the best evidence calls for the integration of epidemiological and biostatistic always of thinking with those derived from pathophysiology and clinical experience; (d) The conclusions of this search and critical appraisal of evidence are worthwhile only if they are translated into actions that affect patients.

Evisceration Removal of internal organs.

Evisceration of the eye Removal of the contents of the eyeball, but not the sclera.

Evoked response Study of function of sense organs even though patient is unconscious by giving sensory stimuli and recording the electric response along the propagation pathway to brain.

Evolution The development of living organisms which change their characteristics during succeeding generations.

Evulsion Extraction by force.

Ewing's tumour *J. Ewing. American pathologist, 1866–1943.* A form of sarcoma usually affecting the shaft of a long bone in young adults.

Exacerbation An increase in the severity of the symptoms of a disease.

Exanthem An infectious disease characterized by a skin rash.

Exanthematous Pertaining to any disease associated with a skin eruption.

Excavation Scooping out.

Dental excavation The removal of decay from a tooth before inserting a filling.

Exception In health care the justification for clinical variance made by a practitioner and usually peer reviewed by others.

Exchange transfusion Transfusion and withdrawal of small amounts of blood until blood volume is entirely replaced; used in autoimmune hemolytic anemia, hyperbilirubinemia.

Excipient The vehicle for the drug.

Excise Removal by surgery.

Excision The cutting out of a part.

Excitation The act of stimulating.

Excitation wave The wave of irritability originating in sino-atrial node and conduction system to ventricular muscles.

Excitement A physiological and emotional response to a stimulus.

Excoriation An abrasion of the skin.

Excrement Fecal matter; waste matter from the body.

Excrescence Abnormal outgrowth of tissue, e.g., a wart.

Excreta The natural discharges of the excretory system: feces, urine and sweat.

Excretion The discharge of waste from the body.

Exenteration Evisceration.

Exercise Performance of physical exertion for improvement of health or correction of physical deformity.

Active exercise Motion imparted to a part by voluntary contraction and relaxation of its controlling muscles.

Isometric exercise Active exercise performed against stable resistance, without change in the length of the muscle. No movement occurs at any joints over which the muscle passes.

Passive exercise Motion imparted to a segment of the body by another individual, or a machine or other outside force, or produced by voluntary effort of another segment of the patient's own body.

Range of movement (ROM) exercises Exercises that move each joint through its full range of movement, that is, to the highest degree of movement of which each joint is normally capable.

Exercise electrocardiogram *SYN* – Stress test.

Exercise tolerance test A test to determine the efficiency of cardio respiratory system, e.g., treadmill testing.

Exflagellation The formation of microgametes (flagellated bodies) from micro gametocytes. Occurs in plasmodia in the stomach of mosquitos.

Exfoliation The splitting off from the surface of dead tissue in thin flaky layers.

Exhalation 1. The giving off of a vapor. 2. The act of breathing out.

Exhibitionism 1. Showing off; a desire to attract attention. 2. Exposing the genitals to persons of the opposite sex in socially unacceptable circumstances.

Exhumation Removal of a dead body from grave.

Exner's nerve Nerve from pharyngeal plexus to cricothyroid membrane.

Exocrine Pertaining to those glands that discharge their secretion by means of a duct, e.g., salivary glands *(See Endocrine).*

Exodontology Branch of dentistry dealing with dental extraction.

Exoerythrocytic Occuring outside RBC.

Exogenous Of external origin.

Exomphalos 1. Hernia of the abdominal viscera into the umbilical cord. 2. Congenital umbilical hernia.

Exophthalmometer An instrument for measuring the extent of protrusion of the eyeball.

Experiential learning Learning from experiencing a situation. May also be facilitated with the use of role play or of a simulated situation and reflecting upon the experience.

Exphoria Tendency of visual axes to diverge outwards.

Exophthalmos Abnormal protrusion of the eyeball which results in a marked stare. May be due to injury or disease and is often associated with thyrotoxicosis.

Exoplasm Outer protoplasm of a cell.

Exostosis A bony outgrowth from the surface of a bone.

Exotic Not native.

Exotoxin A poison produced by a bacterial cell and released into the tissues surrounding it *(See Endotoxin).*

Exotropia Divergent strabismus; the eyes turn outward.

Expanded role The opportunity for nurses, midwives and health visitors to undertake an expanded role in relation to patient care beyond that traditionally recognized.

Expected or estimated date of delivery abbreviated EDD. Used in midwifery and obstetrics to calculate the date of delivery of a baby. This is calculated by counting forward 9 months and adding 7 days from the first day of the last normal menstrual period of counting back 3 months and adding 7 days.

Expected outcome In a nursing care plan the rationale for a statement regarding a nursing intervention and what it is expected to achieve.

Expectorant A remedy that promote and facilitates expectoration.

Expectoration Sputum, secretions coughed up from the air passages. Its characteristics are a valuable aid in diagnosis and note should be taken of the quantity ejected, its color and the amount of effort required. Frothiness denotes that it comes from an air-containing cavity, fluidity indicates edema of the lung.

Expiration 1. The act of breathing out. 2. Termination or death.

Explode To burst.

Exploration The operation of surgically investigating any part of the body.

Exponent The mathematical method of indicating the power.

Exposure The amount of radiation delivered/received.

Expression 1. The aspect or appearance of the face as determined by the physical or emotional state. 2. The act of squeezing out or evacuating by pressure, e.g., the removal of breast milk by hand or breast pump. 3. The manifestation of a heritable trait in an individual carrying the gene or genes that determine it.

Exsanguination Extensive blood loss due to internal or external hemorrhage.

Extension 1. The straightening out of a flexed joint, such as the knee or elbow, 2. The application of traction to a fractured or dislocated limb by means of a weight.

Extensor A muscle that extends or straightens a limb.

Exterior On the outside.

Exteriorize 1. To bring an organ or part of one to the outside of the body by surgery. 2. In psychiatry, to turn one's interests outward.

Extinction The process of extinguishing or putting out.

Extirpation Excision of a part.

Extorsion Rotation of a part outward.

Extra Prefix denoting outside, additional or beyond.

Etracapsular Outside the capsule. May refer to a fracture occurring at the end of the bone but outside the joint capsule, or to cataract extraction.

Extracellular Outside the cell.

Extracellular fluid Tissue fluid that surrounds the cells.

Extracorporeal Outside the body.

Extracorporeal membrane oxygenator (ECMO) A device for oxygenation of blood used for patients of acute respiratory failure.

Extracorporeal shock wave lithotripsy (ECSWL) Shock wave dissolution of renal and gallstones.

Extract A concentrated preparation of a drug made by extracting its soluble principles by steeping in water or alcohol and then evaporating the fluid.

Extraction 1. The process or act of pulling or drawing out. 2. The preparation of an extract.

Breech extraction Extraction of an infant from the uterus in cases of breech presentation.

Vacuum extraction Removal of the uterine contents by application of a vacuum. An alternative to the forceps method of delivering a baby.

Extradural Outside dura matter.

Extramural Outside the wall of an organ or vessel.

Extracular eye muscles Muscles attached to the capsule of eye controlling its movements.

Extrapyramidal Outside the pyramidal (cerebrospinal) tract.

Extrapyramidal system The nerve tracts and pathways which are not within the pyramidal tracts.

Extrasensory Outside or beyond any of the known senses.

Extrasensory perception Abbreviated ESP. Appreciation of the thoughts of others or of current or future events without any normal means of communication.

Extrasystole Premature contraction of the atria or ventricles *(See Systole).*

Extrauterine Occurring outside the uterus.

Extrauterine pregnancy Ectopic gestation; development of a fetus outside the uterus.

Extravasation Effusion or escape of fluid from its normal course into surrounding tissues.

Extravasation of blood A bruise.

Extremity Distal part; a hand or foot.

Extrinsic Originating externally.

Extrinsic factor A substance present in meat and other food stuffs. Also called cyanobalamin (vitamin B_{12}), it is necessary for the manufacture of red blood cells. The intrinsic factor produced in the stomach is necessary for the absorption of vitamin B_{12}.

E

Extrinsic muscle A muscle originating away from the part that it controls, such as those controlling the movements of the eye.

Extrophy Congenital turning inside out of an organ.

Extroversion Turning inside out, e.g., of the uterus, as sometimes occurs after labor.

Extrovert A person who is sociable, a good mixer, outgoing and interested in what is going on in the social environment. A personality type first described by Jung *(See Introvert)*.

Extubation Removal of a tube used in intubation.

Exuberant Excessive growth of tissue, joyful, happy.

Exudate A protein-rich fluid, high in cell count can be pus, catarrhal, hemorrhagic, fibrinous.

Exudation The slow discharge of serous fluid through the walls of the blood cells and its deposition in or on the tissues.

Exude To pass out slowly through the tissues.

Eye The organ of sight. A globular structure with three coats. The nerve tissue of the retina receives impressions of images via the pupil and lens. From this the optic nerve conveys the impressions to the visual area of the cerebrum.

Eye tooth An upper canine tooth.

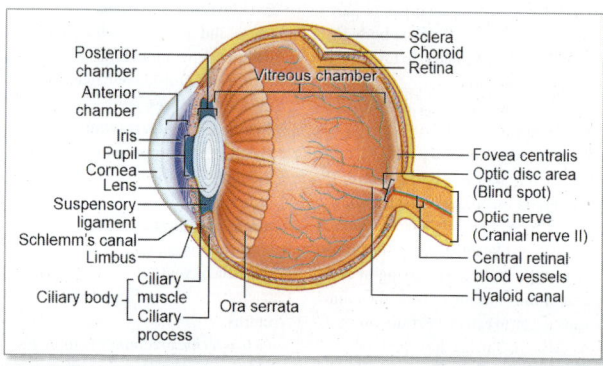

Structure of Eye

Eye bank An organization that collects corneas and stores them for transplantation.

Eyelid A protective covering of the eye, composed of muscle and dense connective tissue covered with skin, lined with conjunctiva and fringed with eyelashes.

Eyelids Contain the meibomian glands.

Eye muscle imbalance Incoordinate action of extraocular muscles causing esophoria or exophoria.

Eyetooth An upper canine tooth.

Eyestrain Tiredness of eye due to errors of refraction, overuse, debility, anemia.

Ezetimibe A lipid lowering agent.

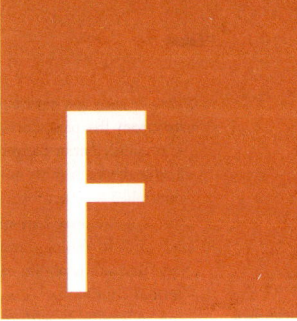

F Symbol for Fahrenheit and fluorine.

Fabere test *Flexion, abduction, external rotation, and extension of hip* test for the identification of hip arthritis.

Fabricated or induced illness *(see Munchausen syndrome and Munchausen syndrome by Proxy)*

Fabrication Deliberately false statement told as if it were true, present in Korsakoff's syndrome.

Fabry's disease An inherited disorder of metabolism with accumulations of glycolipid in tissues.

Face The front of the head from the forehead to the chin.

   Face presentation The appearance of the face of the fetus first at the cervix during labor.

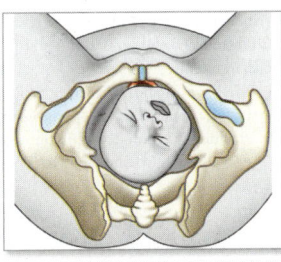

Face Presentation

Facet A small flat area on the surface of a bone.

   Facet syndrome A slight dislocation of the small facet joints of the vertebrae giving rise to pain and muscle spasm.

Facetectomy Excision of anticular facet of vertebra.

Facial Pertaining to the face or lower anterior portion of the head.

   Facial center Brain center responsible for facial movements.

   Facial nerve The seventh cranial nerve, which supplies the salivary glands and superficial face muscles.

   Facial paralysis (See Paralysis).

   Facial reflex Contraction of facial muscles following pressure on eyeball.

   Facial spasm Involuntary contraction of muscles supplied by facial nerve.

Facies Facial expression; it often gives some indication of the patient's condition.

   Adenoid facies The open mouth and vacant expression associated with mouth breathing and nasal obstruction.

   Aortica facies Seen in aortic insufficiency; with bluish sclera, sunken cheeks and shallow face.

   Parkinson facies Fixed expression, due to paucity of movement of facial muscles, characteristic of Parkinsonism.

   Hepatica facies Sunken eyes, yellow conjunctiva.

Facilitation Hastening of an action.

Factitious False, not natural, artificial.

Factitious disorder Disease not genuine, produced voluntarily for gain, etc. Munchausen syndrome.

Factor 1. Any of several substances necessary to produce a result. 2. A coefficient or conversion factor. 3. One of two or more quantities that multiplied together form a product.

Factor V Leiden *(see Thrombophilia)*

Facultative In biology and bacteriology, having the ability to live under certain conditions. Thus, a bacteria can be facultative with respect to O_2 and be able to live with or without O_2.

Faculty A normal mental attribute or sense; teaching staff.

Faeces Waste matter excreted by the bowel, consisting of indigestible cellulose, food which has escaped digestion, bacteria (living and dead) and water.

Faecalith A hard stony mass of Fecal material. A coprolith.

Faget's sign A slower pulse than expected for the rise in temperature, a feature of enteric fever and viral infections.

Fahrenheit scale *GD Fahrenheit, German physicist, 1686–1736.* A scale of heat measurement. It registers the freezing point of water at 32°, the normal heat of the humanbody at 98.4° and the boiling point of water at 212° *(See Celsius).*

Failure Inability to perform or to function properly.

Failure to thrive Retardation of normal growth and development in an infant. Causes are numerous but malnutrition or difficulty in absorbing essential nutrients is a main factor, as well as those that are psychosocial in origin, e.g., maternal deprivation syndrome.

Heart failure Inability of the heart to maintain a circulation sufficient to meet the body's needs.

Hepatic failure Liver failure with cholemia due to cirrhosis, acute hepatic necrosis, etc.

Kidney failure, renal failure Inability of the kidney to excrete metabolites at normal plasma levels under normal loading, or inability to retain electrolytes when intake is normal; in the acute form, marked by uremia and usually by oliguria, with hyperkalemia and pulmonary edema.

Respiratory failure, ventilatory failure A life-threatening condition in which respiratory function is inadequate to maintain the body's needs for oxygen supply and carbon dioxide removal while at rest.

Fainting *(See Syncope).*

Faith healing An attempt to cure disease or disability with the use of spiritual powers or by the influence of the personality of the healer.

Falciform Sickle shaped.

Falciform ligament A fold of peritoneum which separates the two main lobes of the liver and connects it with the anterior abdominal wall and the diaphragm.

Faliciform ligament of liver Sickle-shaped reflection of peritoneum attaching liver to diaphragm and separating right lobe from left lobe *(see Figure).*

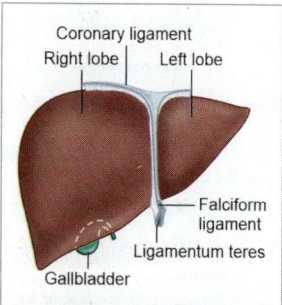

Faliciform Ligament

Falciform process That portion of falciform ligament along the inner margin of ramus of ischium.

Fall Moving downwards quickly and without control. The tendency to fall to the ground increases with age when reflex actions are slower. Various conditions of the elderly, e.g., poor sight or walking disorders, increase risk of falls as does the taking of sleeping pills or tranquilizer drugs. Broken bones are a common complication, most usually in women, who are more prone to osteoporosis. A fall or the fear of falling can have an adverse psychological effect on an elderly person, who may become reluctant to leave the home. Community care staff as falls specialist nurses or other practitioners can provide practical advice and support to prevent or minimize further falls, e.g., ensuring that floor coverings and wiring are made safe, suitable footwear is worn, good lighting is available and hand rails are secure and safe.

Fallopian tube *G Fallopio, Italian anatomist, 1523–1563.* Uterine tube. One of a pair of tubes, about 10–14 cm long, arising out of the upper part of the uterus. The distal end of each tube is fimbriated and lies near an ovary. The tubes function is to conduct the ova from the ovaries to the interior of the uterus. An oviduct.

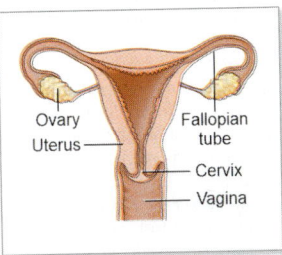

Fallopian Tube

Fallot's tetralogy *ELA Fallot, French physician, 1850–1911.* A congenital heart disease with four characteristic defects: (a) Pulmonary stenosis; (b) Interventricular defect of the septum; (c) Overriding of the aorta, i.e., opening into both right and left ventricles; (d) Hypertrophy of the right ventricle.

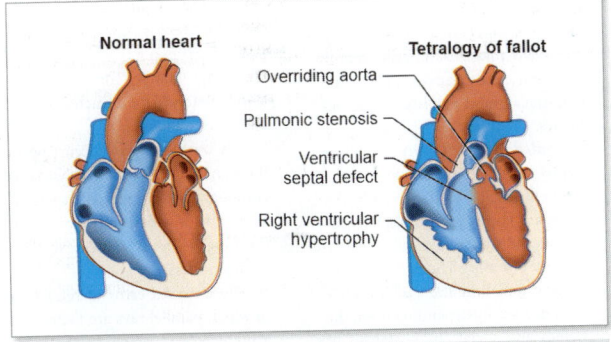

Fallot's Tetralogy

Fallout Settling of radioactive fission products from atmosphere after nuclear explosion.

False-positive A test indicating that the disease is present when in fact it is not.

False-negative A test indicating the disease is not present when actually it is present.

False ribs The lower five pairs of ribs that do not unite directly with the sternum.

Falx A sickle-shaped structure. *Falx-cerebri* The fold of duramater that separates the two cerebral hemispheres.

Famciclovir Antiviral agent for herpes.

Familial Occurring in or affecting members of a family more than would be expected by chance.

Familial Mediterranean fever Inherited autosomal recessive disorder in person of Irish or Italian descent manifesting with periodic fever, chest/abdominal pain and a propensity for amyloidosis.

Familial periodic paralysis Paralysis occurring at awakening with hypokalemia or even normokalemia.

Family 1. A group of people related by blood or marriage, especially husband, wife and their children. 2. A taxonomic category below an order and above a genus.

Blended family A family unit composed of a married couple and their offspring, including some from previous marriages.

Extended family A nuclear family and their close relatives, such as the children's grand parents, aunts and uncles.

Extended nuclear family A nuclear family who never the less make frequent social contacts with the extended family group despite geographical distance.

Family planning The arrangement, spacing and limitation of the children in a family depending upon the wishes and social circumstances of the parents.

Family therapy A therapeutic process whereby the psycho therapist treats several members of the family simultaneously.

Nuclear family A couple and their children, by birth or adoption, who are living together and are more or less isolated from their extended family.

Single parent family A lone parent and offspring living together as a family unit.

Famotidine H_2 receptor blocker, used for peptic ulcer disease.

Fanconi's syndrome F Fanconi, Swiss *pediatrician, 1892–1979.* A rare inherited disorder of metabolism in which reabsorption of phosphate, amino acids and sugar by the renal tubules is impaired. The kidneys fail to produce acid urine, and resulting features are thirst, polyuria and rickets, leading to chronic renal failure.

Fang The root of a tooth.

Fantasy An imagined sequence of events or mental images that serves to satisfy unconscious wishes or to express unconscious conflicts.

Farad A unit of electrical capacity. The capacity of a condenser that charged with 1 coulomb, gives a difference of potential of 1 volt.

Faradism Therapeutic use of an interrupted current to stimulate muscles and nerves.

Farinaceous Starchy or containing starch. Refers to foods such as wheat, oats, barley and rice.

Farmer's lung A disease occurring in those in contact with mouldy hay. It is thought to be due to a hypersensitivity, with widespread reaction in the lung tissue. It causes excessive breathlessness.

Farsightedness An error of refraction in which parallel rays are focused at a point behind retina, so that near objects are not seen clearly.

FAS Fetal alcohol syndrome.

Fascia A sheath of connective tissue enclosing muscles or other organs.

Fascicle A fasciculus.

Fasciculation Isolated fine muscle twitching which gives a flickering appearance.

Fasciculus A small bundle of nerve or muscle fibers; a fascicle.

Fasciectomy Excision of portion of fascia.

Fasciolopsis buski A fluke infesting intestinal tract of certain mammals including man.

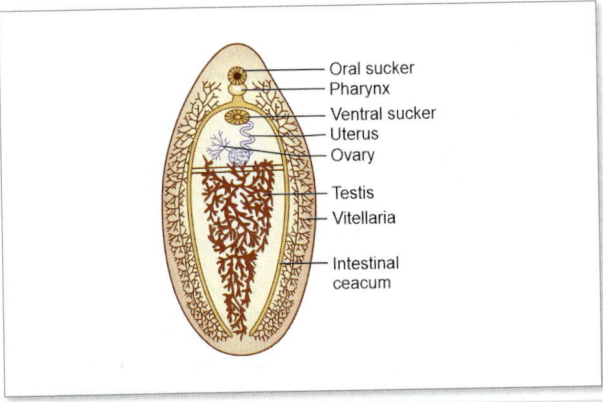

Fasciolopsis buski

Fascitis Inflammation of fascia.

Fastigium The highest point; The most posterior portion of fourth ventricle in brain.

Fasting Accepting no food.

Fat 1. The adipose or fatty tissue of the body. 2. Neutral fat; a triglyceride which is an ester of fatty acids and glycerol.

Wool-fat Lanolin *(See also Brown fat).*

Fatigue A state of weariness which may range from mental disinclination for effort to profound exhaustion after great physical and mental effort.

Muscle fat May occur during prolonged effort owing to oxygen lack and accumulation of waste products.

Fatty Containing or similar to fat.

Fatty acid (See Essential).

Fatty change Abnormal accumulation of fat within the cell.

Fatty degeneration A degenerative change in tissue cells due to the invasion of fat and consequent weakening of the organ. The change occurs as a result of incorrect diet, shortage of oxygen in the tissues or excessive consumption of alcohol.

Fauces The opening from the mouth into the pharynx.

Pillars of the fauces The twofolds of muscle covered with mucous membrane that pass from the soft palate on either side of the fauces. One fold passes into the tongue, the other into the pharynx, and between them is situated the tonsil.

Faucial reflex Sensation of vomiting resulting from irritation of fauces.

Favism An acute hemolytic anemia caused by ingestion of fava beans or inhalation of the pollen of the plant, usually occurring in certain individuals as a result of a genetic abnormality with a deficiency in an enzyme, glucose 6-phosphatede-hydrogenase, in the erythrocytes. Called also fabism.

Favus A type of ringworm infection with formation of scabs, in appearance like a honeycomb. It usually affects the scalp and is due to a fungus infection *(Trichophyton schoenleinii).*

Fc Fragment A part of antibody.

Fc Receptor A receptor on phagocyte that binds to Fc fragment of IgG and IgE.

Fe Symbol for iron (L. ferrum).

Fear A normal emotional response, in contrast to anxiety and phobia, to consciously recognized external sources of danger; it is manifested by alarm, apprehension or disquiet.

Obsessional fear A recurring irrational fear that is not amenable to ordinary reassurance; a phobia.

Febrile Characterized by or relating to fever.

Febrile convulsion A convulsion which occurs in childhood and is associated with pyrexia.

Feces Excreta, stool

Feculent Having sediment.

Fecundation Fertilization.

Fecundity The ability to produce offspring frequently and in large numbers. In demography, the physiological ability to reproduce, as opposed to fertility.

Federations Groups of general practices that formally work together to provide services for their practice populations.

Feedback A method of control where some of the output is returned as input for monitoring purposes. Feedback mechanisms are important in the regulation of such physiological processes as hormone and enzyme reactions.

Negative feedback A rise in the output of a substance is detected and further output is thus inhibited.

Positive feedback A rise in output causes either a direct or indirect rise in the output of another substance.

Feeder A device permitting independent eating by severe neurologically disabled person.

Feeder artificial Tube feeding, the tube passed through esophagus or rectum.

Feeling The conscious phase of nervous activity. Emotions are centrally stimulated feelings.

Fehling's solution A solution for testing urine sugar, prepared by dissolving 34.66 g of copper sulfate in 500 ml of water to make solution A and 173 g potassium iodide and 50 g. of sodium hydroxide in 500 mL of water to make solution B. When urine containing sugar is boiled after addition of both the solutions, a red precipitative of cuprous oxide is formed.

Felbamate A newer antiepileptic agent.

Felodipine A calcium-channel blocker used in hypertension.

Felon An abscess of the distal phalanx of a finger; a whitlow.

Felty's syndrome *AR Felty, American physician, 1895–1963.* The triad of rheumatoid arthritis, splenomegaly and leukopenia. Often associated with anemia, lymphadenopathy and vasculitic cutaneous ulceration.

Female Woman, sex that produces ova.

Female genital mutilation Female circumcision involving excision of the labia majora, labia minora and clitoris and in some cases, partial closure of the introitus. It is prevalent in African countries such as Sudan. Prior to pregnancy it may cause problems with micturition and intercourse. Special care will be required during labor and delivery, and excision and separation of the tissues may be carried out; cesarean section may be necessary.

Feminism Male developing secondary sexual characteristic of female.

Feminization 1. The normal induction or development of female sexual characteristics. 2. The induction or development of female secondary sexual characteristics in the male.

Testicular feminization A condition in which the subject is pheno typically female, but lacks nuclear sex chromatin and is of XY chromosomal sex.

Femoral Pertaining to the femur. *Femoral artery* That of the thigh from groin to knee.

Femoral canal The opening below the inguinal ligament through which the femoral artery passes from the abdomen to the thigh.

Femur The thigh bone.

Fenbufen A nonsteroidal antiinflammatory drug (NSAID) that acts as a pro drug. It is associated with a lower incidence of gastro intestinal hemorrhage but a higher incidence of skin rashes than other NSAIDs.

Fenestra A window-like opening. *Fenestra ovalis* The oval opening between the middle and the internal ear.

Fenfluramine An adrenergic agent.

Fenofibrate Lipid-lowering agent.

Fenoprofen An anti-inflammatory drug used in the treatment of arthritic conditions.

Fenoterol Beta-adrenergic agonist used in bronchial asthma.

Fenoverine Antispasmodic agent.

Fentanyl A short-acting narcotic analgesic, widely used during anesthesia, especially for children and the elderly.

Ferment To decompose.

Fern A flowerless plant, whose extracts are used as anthelmintic.

Fern pattern Palm leaf (arborization) pattern of cervical mucus when allowed to dry on a glass slide; dependent on salt concentration in mucus which is further dependent upon amount of estrogen in the mucus. This test is only positive in midcycle. If positive in late cycle, indicates lack of progesterone.

Ferritin A complex formed of an iron and protein molecule; one of the forms in which iron is stored in the body.

Ferrokinetics Study of absorption, utilizatiion, storage and excretion of iron.

Ferroprotein Important oxygen transferring enzyme.

Ferrous Containing iron. *Ferrous fumarate, ferrous gluconate, ferroussuccinate and ferrous sulfate* Are iron salts which are given orally to treat iron-deficiency anemia.

Ferric Trivalent iron, oxidized form.

Ferrule A rubber cap used on the end of walking sticks, frames and crutches to prevent slipping.

Fertilization The impregnation of the female sex cell, the ovum, by a male sex cell, a spermatozoon.

In vitro fertilization Artificial fertilization of the ovum in laboratory conditions. The timing and conditions for implantation into a uterus have to be perfect if successful pregnancy is to ensure.

Fester To become superficially inflamed and to suppurate.

Fervescence Increase of fever.

Festination An involuntary tendency to take short accelerating steps in walking; seen in conditions such as Parkinson's disease.

Fetal Pertaining to the fetus. *Fetal alcohol syndrome* Abbreviated FAS. Physical and mental abnormalities due to maternal alcohol intake during pregnancy. Abnormalities may include microcephaly, growth deficiencies, mental handicap, hyperactivity, heart murmurs and skeletal malformation. The exact amount of alcohol consumption that will produce fetal damage is unknown, but

F

the periods of gestation during which the alcohol is most likely to result in fetal damage are 3–4. 5 months after conception and during the last trimester.

Fetal assessment Determination of the well-being of the fetus. Assessment techniques and procedures include: (a) Medical and family histories and physical examination of the mother; (b) Ultrasonography; (c) Assessment of fetal activity using the Cardiff kick chart; (d) Chemical assessment of placental function; (e) Assays of amniotic fluid obtained by Amniocentesis; and (f) Electronic and ultrasonic fetal heart rate monitoring.

Fetal distress The clinical manifestation of fetal hypoxia which may be due to maternal or fetal causes.

Fetal position A position resembling that of the fetus in the womb, sometimes adopted by a child or adult in a state of distress or depression.

Feticide Killing of the fetus.

Fetishism A state in which an object is regarded with an irrational fear, or an erotic attraction which may be so strong that the object is necessary for achieving sexual excitement.

Fetor An offensive smell.

Fetoprotein A fetal antigen often present in adults. Amniotic fluid fetoprotein level can indicate about fetal well-being and maturity. Level is increased in defects of neuroaxis. Increased level in adults indicates hepatoma.

Fetoscope An endoscope for viewing the fetus in utero.

Fetotoxic Materials toxic to developing fetus, e.g., alcohol, sedatives tetracycline, tobacco.

Fetus The developing baby between the eighth week and the end of pregnancy.

Fetus amorphous Shapeless fetus, barely recognizable as fetus.

Fetus calcified Fetus dyeing in utero with calcification.

Fetus in fetu A small imperfect fetus is developed within body of another fetus (e.g., desmoids).

Fetus mummified A dead fetus that has assumed mummified form.

Fetus papyraceus In twin pregnancy, the dead fetus is pressed flat by living fetus.

FEV1 Forced expiratory volume in 1 second. After full inspiration patient exhales as hard and as fast as possible into spirometer and the amount of air exhaled in 1 second is recorded. FEV1 is reduced in obstructive lung disease.

Fever 1. An abnormally high body temperature; pyrexia. 2. Any disease characterized by marked increase of body temperature.

Fexofenadine H_1 receptor, blocker, antiallergic.

Fibre A thread-like structure.

Fibril A small fiber, often the component of a cell or a fiber, can be myofibril or neurofibril.

Fibreoptics The transmission of light rays along flexible tubes by means of very fine glass or plastic fibers. Use is made of this in endoscopic instruments such as the gastroscope.

Fibrescope An endoscope in which fiberoptics are used.

Fibrillation A quivering, vibratory movement of muscle fibers.

Atrial fibrillation Rapid contractions of the atrium causing irregular contraction of the ventricles in both rhythm and force.

Ventricular fibrillation Fine rapid twitching of the ventricles leading to circulatory arrest. Rapidly fatal unless it can be controlled.

Fibrin An insoluble protein that is essential to clotting of blood formed from fibrinogen by action of thrombin.

Fibrinogen A soluble protein which is present in blood plasma and is converted into fibrin by the action of thrombin when the blood clots.

Fibrinogenolysis Dissolution of fibrin.

Fibrinogenopenia Reduction in blood fibrinogen.

Fibrinolysin A proteolytic enzyme that dissolves fibrin.

Fibrinolysis The dissolution of fibrin by the action of fibrinolysin. The process by which clots are removed from the circulation after healing has taken place.

Fibrinoid Resembling fibrin.

Fibrinoid change Change in connective tissue with immunologic injury, the tissue becoming homogeneous, swollen and band like.

Fibrinopenia A deficiency of fibrinogen in the blood. There is a tendency to bleed as the coagulation time is increased.

Fibrinokinase Enzyme of animal tissue that activates plasiminogen.

Fibrinopeptide The substance removed from fibrinogen during blood coagulation; fibrin degradation product.

Fibrinosis Excess fibrin in blood.

Fibroadenoma A benign tumor of glandular and fibrous tissue *(See Adenoma)*.

Fibroangioma A benign tumor of glandular and fibrous tissue *(See Adenoma)*.

Fibroblast A connective tissue cell.

Fibrocartilage Cartilage with fibrous tissue in it.

Fibrochondritis Inflammation of fibrocartilage.

Fibrocystic Fibrous and cystic. *Fibrocystic disease of breast* Painful lump in breast, the pain and size fluctuating with menstrual cycle; 50% of women in reproductive age have this problem and carry a 2–5% greater risk of developing breast cancer.

Fibrocystic disease of the pancreas An inherited disease affecting the mucus-secreting glands, the sweat glands and the pancreas. It is characterized by fatty stools and repeated lung infections. Mucoviscidosis; cystic fibrosis.

Fibroid 1. Having a fibrous structure. 2. A fibroma or a fibromyoma, usually one occurring in the uterus.

Fibroma A benign tumor of connective tissue.

Fibromatosis Simultaneous development of multiple fibromas.

Fibromatosis gingivae An inherited condition in which there is hypertrophy of gums prior to eruption of teeth.

Fibromyoma A tumor consisting of fibrous and muscle tissue; frequently found in or on the uterus.

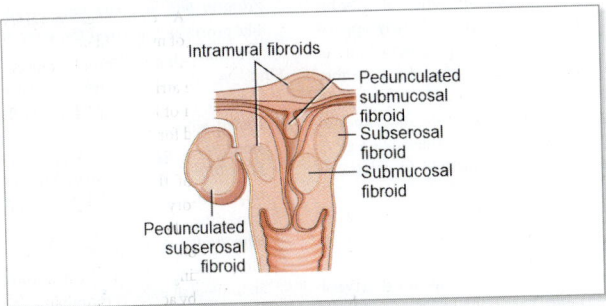

Intramural fibroids

Pedunculated submucosal fibroid

Subserosal fibroid

Submucosal fibroid

Pedunculated subserosal fibroid

Fibromyoma

Fibromyositis Inflammation of muscle in surrounding connective tissue, a non-specific illness characterized by pain, tenderness, stiffness of joint capsule.

Fibromyxoma A fibroma that has undergone partial myxomatous degeneration.

Fibromyxosarcoma A sarcoma containing fibrous and myxoid tissue or sarcoma that has undergone mucoid degeneration.

Fibronectin A group of proteins whose presence in cervical secretion may act as marker for preterm labor.

Fibropapilloma Mixed fibroma and papilloma seen in bladder.

Fibroplasia The formation of fibrous tissue when a wound heals.

Retrolental fibroplasia A condition characterized by the presence of fibrous tissue behind the lens, leading to detachment of the retina and blindness, attributed to use of oxygen in the care of preterm infants.

Fibrosarcoma A malignant tumor arising in fibrous tissue.

Fibrosis Fibrous tissue formation, such as occurs in scar tissue or as the result of inflammation. It is the cause of adhesions of the peritoneum or other serious membranes.

Fibrosis of the lung Condition that may precede bronchiectasis and emphysema.

Fibrositis Inflammation of fibrous tissue. The term is loosely applied to pain and stiffness, particularly of the back muscles, for which no other cause can be found.

Fibula The slender bone from knee to ankle, on the outer side of the leg.

Fick method A method to determine cardiac output.

Field of vision The area within view, as for the fixed eye or a camera, or in an operation.

Fifth cranial nerve Trigeminal nerve, a mixed nerve with its sensory – motor nuclei in Pons-medulla.

Fifth disease Parvovirus infection with rash mimicking rubella.

FIGO staging system Staging system for gyneocological cancers developed by International Federation of Gynecology and Obstetrics.

FIGLU excretion test Test for folic acid deficiency. When histidine is administered to a patient with folic acid deficiency form iminoglutamic acid excretion in urine is increased.

Fight or flight response Activation of the sympathetic nervous system in response to danger or stress.

Filament A small thread-like structure.

Filaria A genus of nematode worms which may be found in the connective tissues and lymphatics, having been transmitted to humans by mosquitoes. Found mainly in the tropics and subtropics.

Filariasis An infection by filaria, particularly by *Wuchereria bancrofti,* resulting in blockage of the lymphatics, which causes swelling of the surrounding tissues. Elephantiasis may occur.

Filarioidea A genus of nematode worms, which may be found in the connective tissues and lymphatics, transmitted to humans by mosquitoes. Found mainly in the tropics and subtropics.

Filiform Thread like.

Filiform papillae The fine thread-like processes that cover the anterior two-thirds of the tongue.

Film A thin membrane/covering; photographic film usually cellulose coated with a light-sensitive emulsion.

Film bitewing Technique used for taking film of several teeth at the same time.

Film badge A badge containing a film to calculate the total exposure of an individual to X-rays.

Filter A device for eliminating certain elements, such as (a) Particles of certain size from a solution, or (b) Rays of a certain wavelength from a stream of radiant energy.

Millipore filter Trade name for a device used to filter nutrient solutions as they are administered intravenously.

Filtrate The fluid that passes through a filter.

Filtration 1. The removal of precipitate from a liquid by means of a filter. 2. The removal of rays of a certain wavelength from an electromagnetic beam.

Angle filtration The angle of the anterior chamber of the eye through which the aqueous humor drains; blockage of this channel give rise to glaucoma.

Glomerular filtration The protein free plasma filtered while passage of blood through glomeruli.

Filum A thread-like structure.

Filum coronaria A fibrous band extending from the base of the median cusp of tricuspid valve to the aortic annulus.

Filum terminale A long slender filament at the terminal end of cord terminating in coccyx.

Fimbria A fringe.

Fimbriae of the uterine tube The thread-like projections that surround the pelvic opening of the uterine tube.

Finasteride Anti-androgen used for prostatic hypertrophy.

Fine motor skills Skills pertaining to synergy of small muscles of hand.

Finger A digit of the hand.

Clubbed finger One with enlargement of the terminal phalanx with constant osseous changes; occurs in many heart and lung diseases.

Hammer finger, mallet finger Permanent flexion of the distal phalanx of a finger due to avulsion of the extensor tendon.

Trigger finger Temporary flexion of a finger which is overcome in a sudden jerk by active or passive extension of the finger. It is caused by thickening of the flexor tendon in a narrowed tendon sheath.

Webbed fingers Fingers more or less united by strands of tissue; syndactyly.

Finger print An imprint made by the cutaneous ridges of fingers, used for the purpose of identification.

Fingerprint The impression left upon a surface of the ridged pattern of the skin of the fingertips. Loops, whorls, arches and combinations of these form distinct patterns for each human individual and not even identical twins have the same fingerprint pattern.

Firm A medical or surgical hospital team, usually comprising two house officers, a senior house officer (SHO), a registrar and a senior registrar, directed by a consultant physician or surgeon.

First aid Emergency assistance to injured/sick individuals prior to physicians' care or transportation to hospital. Common situations necessitating first aid are; foreign body, coma, convulsion, burn, poisoning, etc.

First cranial nerve Nerve carrying smell sensation from olfactory mucosa.

First degree A-V block Partial block of conduction in A-V node characterized by prolonged P-R interval. When occurring independently does not need treatment but if with anterior myocardial infarction or bundle branch block, it may progress to complete heart block and hence needs permanent pacemaker.

Fish skin disease A disease of skin characterized by increase of the horny layer and deficiency of the skin secretion.

F

Fission A form of asexual reproduction by dividing into two equal parts, as in bacteria.

Binary fission The splitting in two of the nucleus and the protoplasm of a cell, as in protozoa.

Nuclear fission The splitting of the nucleus of an atom, with the release of a great quantity of energy.

Fissiparous Reproducing by fission.

Fissure A narrow slit or cleft.

Anal fissure A painful crack in the mucous membrane of the anus.

Auricular fissure Fissure of petrous part of temporal bone.

Broca fissure Fissure encircling the third left frontal convolution of the brain.

Inferior orbital fissure Fissure at the apex of orbit, through which pass the infraorbital blood vessels and maxillary branch of trigeminal nerve.

Fissure of Rolando A furrow in the cortex of each cerebral hemisphere, dividing the sensory from the motor area; the central sulcus.

Fissure of Sylvius Fissure separating frontal and parietal lobes from temporal lobe.

Fissure transverse 1. Fissure between cerebrum and cerebellum of brain. 2. Fissure on the lower surface of liver serving as the hilum for entrance of hepatic vessels and exit of ducts.

Fistula An abnormal passage between two epithelial surfaces, usually connecting the cavity of one organ with another or a cavity with the surface of the body.

Anal fistula The result of an ischiorectal abscess where the channel is from the anus to the skin.

Biliary fistula A leakage of bile to the exterior, following operation on the gallbladder or ducts.

Blind fistula One which is open at only one end.

Fecal fistula One in which the channel is from the intestine through the wound caused by an operation on the intestines when sepsis is present.

Rectovaginal fistula Fistula from the rectum to the vagina which may result from a severe perineal tear during childbirth.

Tracheo-esophageal fistula An opening from the trachea into the esophagus; a congenital deformity.

Vesicovaginal fistula An opening from the bladder to the vagina, either from error during operation or from ulceration, as may occur in carcinoma of the cervix.

Fit A commonly used term for paroxysmal motor discharges leading to sudden convulsive movements, as in epilepsy, eclampsia and hysteria. The term is sometimes applied to apoplexy.

Fitness Associated with a sense of well-being, and the ability to undertake sustained physical exertion without undue breathlessness. Fitness needs to be maintained on a regular basis by the person taking regular physical exertion or exercise.

Fixation 1. The process of rendering something immovable, such as a joint or a fractured bone. 2. In psychology, a term used to describe a failure to progress wholly or in part through the normal stages of psychological development to a fully developed personality. 3. In ophthalmology, directing the sight straight at an object.

Flaccid Soft, flabby.

Flaccid paralysis (See Paralysis).

Flagellate A protozoon with one or more flagella.

Flagellation Whipping, massage by strokes, a form of sexual aberration in which sexual urge is brought about by being whipped or whipping the partner.

Flagellin Protein of Flagella resembling myosin.

Flagellum A hair like motile process on a protozoon.

Flagyl Trade name for a preparation of metronidazole, an antibacterial and antiprotozoal.

Flail Exhibiting abnormal or pathological mobility, as in flail chest or flail joint.

Flail chest A loss of stability of the chest wall due to multiple rib fractures or detachment of the sternum from the ribs as a result of a severe crushing chest injury. The loose chest segment moves in a direction that is the reverse of normal.

Flail joint An unusually movable joint.

Flange In dentistry, the part of an artificial denture that extends from embedded teeth to the border of denture.

Flank The part of body between ribs and upper border of ilium.

Flap A mass of tissue, used for grafting in plastic surgery, which is left attached to its blood supply and used to repair defects either adjacent to it or at some distance from it.

Pedicle flap Flap made by suturing the edges to form a tube. Then one end of the tube is severed and sutured to another site. By use of this jump flap technique, such a flap may be moved in several stages, a great distance.

Periodontal flap Gingival flap removed or re-positioned to eliminate periodontal pockets or to correct mucogingival defects.

Flare The response of the skin to an allergic or hypersensitivity reaction. Reddening of the skin that spreads outward.

Flashbacks The return of imagery and hallucinations after the immediate effect of hallucinogens is worn off.

Flash point The temperature at which substance will burst into flames spontaneously.

Flatfoot A condition due to absence or sinking of the medial longitudinal arch of the foot, caused by weakening of the ligaments and tendons. Pes planus.

Flatness Resonance heard on percussion over solid organs or when there is fluid in the thoracic cavity.

Flatulence Excessive formation of gases in the stomach or intestine.

Flatulent Suffering from flatulence.

Flatulent distension Swelling due to gas in the stomach or intestines. It is a common complication after abdominal operations and is caused by intestinal stasis.

Flatus Gas in the stomach or intestine.

Flatus tube A rectal tube which is pushed to facilitate expulsion of gas.

Flavi virus Previously called group B arbo virus responsible for yellow fever, dengue fever and encephalitis.

Flavin One of a group of natural water soluble pigments occurring in milk, yeast, bacteria and some plants.

Flavism Having a yellow tinge.

Flavobacterium A group of bacteria producing orange-yellow pigments in culture. Flavobacterium meningosepticum causes virulent meningitis in prematures.

Flavoprotein A group of conjugated proteins that constitute yellow enzyme for cellular respiration.

Flavour The quality that affects the sense of taste.

Flavoxate Urinary antispasmodic.

Flbroangioma A benign tumor of glandular and fibrous tissue. *(See ADENOMA)*

Flea A small, wingless blood-sucking insect parasite. The common human flea, *Pulexirritans,* rarely transmits disease. Cat and dog fleas, *Ctenocephalides,* are also relatively harmless. The rat fleas *Xenopsylla* and *Nosopsyllus* are the vectors of bubonic plague.

Flecainide acetate Antiarrhythmic agent.

Fleece of Stilling Mesh work of white fibers that surrounds the dentate nucleus of cerebellum.

Fleming Alexander Scottish physician who in 1945 was awarded Nobel prize for discovering penicillin.

Flesh Soft tissues of animal body, especially the muscles.

Fletcher factor A blood clotting factor, prekallikrein.

Flexibility Adaptibility, quality of being bent without breaking.

Flexibilitas cerea Waxy flexibility; a cataleptic state in which the limbs retain any position in which they are placed. A symptom of some forms of schizophrenia; also occurs occasionally in hysteria.

Flexion Bending; moving a joint so that the two or more bones forming it draw toward each other.

Plantar flexion Bending the fingers or toes downwards.

Flexner's bacillus *S Flexner, American bacteriologist, 1863–1946.* One of the groups of pathogenic bacteria which cause bacillary dysentery; *Shigella flexneri.*

Flexor Any muscle causing flexion of a limb or other part of the body.

Left colic flexor Bend in colon where transverse colon continues as descending colon *SYN* – splenic flexure.

Rightcolic flexor Bend in colon where ascending colon becomes the transverse colon *SYN* – hepatic flexure.

Flexure A bend or curve.

Flicker The visual sensation of alternating intervals of brightness caused by rhythmically interrupting light stimuli.

Flight of ideas The rapid movement of ideas and speech from one fragmentary topic to another that occurs in mania.

Floaters Wisps or strands within the eye that are visible to the patient.

Usually caused by detachment and collapse of the vitreous humor and the normal ageing process.

Flocculation The gathering together of fine dispersed particles in a solution into larger visible particles.

Flocculus 1. A small tuft of wool like fibers. 2. Lobes of cerebellum behind the middle cerebral peduncle.

Flooding 1. Excessive loss of blood from the uterus. 2. A form of desensitization for the treatment of phobias and related disorders. The patient is repeatedly exposed, in imagination or real life, to emotionally distressing aversive stimuli of high intensity. Also called implosion.

Floppy–valves syndrome Mitral valve prolapsed.

Florid Having a flushed facial appearance.

Floss To use dental floss or tape to remove plaque or calculus.

Flour Ground wheat powder.

Flow meter An instrument used to measure the flow of liquids or gases.

Flow state An altered state of consciousness in which the mind functions at the peak, time may seem to be distorted and a sense of happiness seems to pervade that period.

Flowmeter An instrument used to measure the flow of liquids or gases.

Floxuridine An antimetabolite used in cancer treatment.

Flucloxacillin An antibiotic drug used in the treatment of infection by penicillin resistant bacteria.

Fluconazole Benzimidazole antifungal for candidiasis, cryptococcosis.

Fluctuation A wave-like motion felt on palpation of the abdomen.

Flucytosine Antifungal agent.

Fludrocortisone A synthetic corticosteroid used in the treatment of adrenal disorders.

Flufenamic acid Nonsteroidal anti-inflammatory agent.

Flufenazine enanthate A phenothiazine type antipsychotic drug.

Fluid 1. A liquid or gas; any liquid of the body. 2. Composed of molecules which freely change their relative positions without separation of the mass.

Amniotic fluid The fluid within the amnion that bathes the developing fetus and protects it from mechanical injury.

Body fluids The fluids within the body, composed of water, electrolytes and nonelectrolytes. The volume and distribution of body fluids vary with age, sex and amount of adipose tissue.

Cerebrospinal fluid The fluid contained within the ventricles of the brain, the subarachnoid space and the central canal of the spinal cord.

Interstitial fluid The extra cellular-fluid bathing most tissues, excluding the fluid within the lymph and blood vessels.

Fluid balance A state in which the volume of body water and its solutes (electrolytes and non-electrolytes) is within normal limits and there is normal distribution of fluids within the intracellular and extra cellular compartments. The total volume of body fluids should be about 60% of the body weight.

Fluke One of a groups of parasitic flat worms (Trematoda). Different varieties may affect the blood, the intestines, the liver or the lungs.

Flumethasone Synthetic corticosteroid.

Flunarizine Calcium-channel blocker for migrane.

Fluocinolone acetonide Synthetic corticosteroid.

Fluorescein A dye used to detect corneal ulceration. When it is dropped on the eye the ulcer stains green.

Fluorescence The property of reflecting back light waves, usually of a lower frequency than those absorbed so that invisible light (e.g., ultraviolet) may become visible.

Fluorescent Capable of producing fluorescence.

Fluorescent screen A screen that becomes fluorescent when exposed to X-rays.

Fluorescent treponemal antibody test A serological test for syphilis; the first to become positive after infection.

Fluoridation The adding of fluorine to water, in those areas where it is lacking, in order to reduce the incidence of dental caries.

Fluorine Symbol F. Any binary compound of fluorine.

Fluorapatite A compound formed when the enamel of teeth is treated with appropriate concentration of fluoride to form hydroxyapatite which is less acid soluble, hence resistant to caries.

Fluorometer Device for determining amount of radiation produced by X-rays.

Fluoroscope An instrument for the study of moving internal organs and contrast medium using X-rays.

Fluoroscopy Patient examination by fluoroscope.

Fluorosis Chronic fluorine poisoning causing mottling of tooth enamel, and hyperluscency of bone.

Fluorouracil An antimetabolite cytotoxic drug used particularly in the treatment of solid tumors.

Fluoxetine Antidepressant.

Fluoxymesterone An anabolic and androgenic hormone.

Fluphenazine A major tranquillizer.

Flupenthixol Antipsychotic agent.

Flurandrenolide A corticosteroid.

Flurandrenolone A topical steroid used for eczema and other inflammatory skin conditions that have not responded to weaker steroids.

Flurazepam Sedative–hypnotic agent.

Flurbiprofen A nonsteroidal anti-inflammatory drug.

Flurogestone A progestational drug.

Fluroxene An anesthetic agent administered by inhalation.

Flush A redness of the face and neck.

Hectic flush One occurring in conditions such as septic poisoning and pulmonary tuberculosis.

Hot flush One occurring during the menopause, accompanied by a feeling of heat.

Flutamide Antiandrogen used for BPH.

Fluticasone Steroid inhaler for asthma.

Flutter An irregularity of the heartbeat.

Atrial flutter Rapid atrial contraction (200–400/min.) but with a regular heart beat due to 1:2/1:3 AV block.

Diaphragmatic flutter Rapid diaphragmatic contraction.

Mediastinum flutter Abnormal side to side motion of diaphragm.

Fluvoxamine Anti- depressant.

Flux An excessive flow or discharge from an organ or cavity of body.

Foam Production of gas bubble interspersed with fluid.

Foam solubility test Procedure for determining the presence or absence of surfactant active material in amniotic fluid. Surfactant deficit is diagnostic of respiratory distress syndrome.

Focus 1. The point of convergence of light or sound waves. 2. The local seat of a disease.

Focusing The ability of the eye to alter its lens power to focus correctly at different distances.

Fog Water droplets in air.

Fogging 1. A method of testing vision used particularly in testing astigmatism and in postcycloplegic examination. 2. Unwanted density on the radiographic film resulting from exposure to secondary radiation, light, chemicals, heat, etc.

Foil A thin pliable sheet of metal. Gold foils are used in dental restoration work.

Fold A doubling back.

Aryepiglottic fold The ridge like lateral walls of the entrance to larynx.

Gastric fold Gastric mucosal folds; mostly longitudinal.

Rectum fold Transverse mucosal folds of rectum, *SYN*-valves of Houston.

Foley's catheter A urinary tract catheter with balloon attachment at the end.

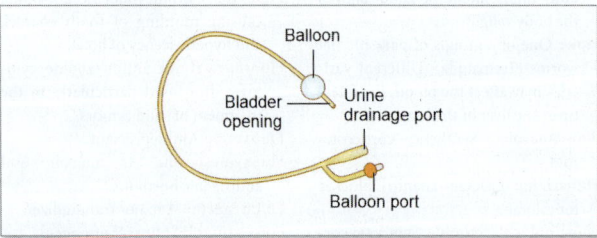

Foley's Catheter

Foliaceous Resembling leaf.

Folic acid One of the vitamins of the B complex. Folic acid is involved in the synthesis of amino acids and DNA; its deficiency causes megaloblastic anemia. Green vegetables, liver and yeast are major sources.

Folic acid antagonist Any anti-metabolite cytotoxic drug that inhibits the action of the folic acid enzyme.

Folinic acid The active form of folic acid.

Folie à deux [Fr.] The occurrence of identical psychoses simultaneously in two closely associated persons.

Follicle A very small sac or gland.

Hair follicle The sheath in which a hair grows.

Follicle stimulating hormone Abbreviated FSH. A hormone, produced by the anterior pituitary gland, which controls the maturation of the Graafian follicles in the ovary.

Follicular Pertaining to a follicle.

Follicular conjunctivitis Inflammation occurring in the lower conjunctival fornix.

Follicular tonsillitis Tonsillitis arising from infection of the tonsillar follicles.

Folliculitis barbae Ring work of beard.

Fulliculoma A tumor of ovary originating in Graffian follicle in which cells resemble the cells of stratum granulosum.

Folliculosis An abnormal increase in the number of lymph follicles.

Conjunctival folliculosis A benign non-inflammatory over growth of follicles of the conjunctiva of the eyelids.

Follow-up The continued care or monitoring of a patient after the initial visit or examination.

Fomentation Treatment by warm, moist applications; also, the substance thus applied.

Fomes *(See Fomites).*

Fomites [L.] Sing. fomes; inanimate objects or material on which disease producing agents may be conveyed.

Fontana's spaces Spaces between the processes of ligamentum pectinatum of iris, conveying aqueous humor.

Fontanelle A soft membranous space between the cranial bones of an infant.

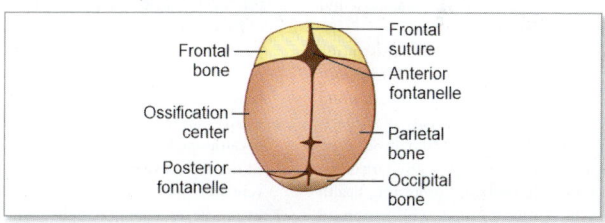

Fontanelle

Anterior fontanelle That between the parietal and frontal bones, which closes at about the age of 18 months. Rickets causes delay in this process.

Posterior fontanelle The junction of the occipital and parietal bones, at the sagittal suture, which closes within 3 months of birth.

Fartan's procedure Palliative surgical procedure in children with single effective ventricle either because

of heart valve defects, abnormality of pumping of the heart, or a complex congenital heart disease where it is not possible or advisable to do bi-ventricular repair.

Food Anything which, when taken into the body, serves to nourish or build up the tissues or to supply body heat.

Food additives Substances other than basic food stuffs that are present in

F

food during production, processing, storage or packaging.

Food adulterants Substances making food impure or toxic like organisms, pesticide residues, poisonous substance or substances added to increase weight or bulk of food.

Food allergy Sensitivity to one or more of the components of a normal diet, e.g., peanut allergy, which is rare but may be dangerous.

Food poisoning A group of notifiable acute illnesses caused by ingestion of contaminated food. It may result from toxemia from foods, such as those inherently poisonous or those contaminated by poisons, foods containing poisons formed by bacteria, or food-borne infections. Food-poisoning usually causes inflammation of the gastrointestinal tract (gastroenteritis). This may occur quite suddenly, soon after the food has been eaten. The symptoms are acute, and include tenderness, pain or cramps in the abdomen, nausea, vomiting, diarrhea, weakness and dizziness *(See Botulism).*

Food and Drug Administration (FDA) In USA, an official regulatory body for food, drugs, cosmetics, and medical devices, a part of Department of Health and Human Services.

Food Standards Agency Organization charged with protecting health in relation to food, with powers to act throughout the food chain to develop policies. Advises consumers, ministers and the food industry on all aspects of food safety and standards. In Scotland, this function is carried out by Food Standards Scotland.

Foodball Gastric stone made up of fruit and vegetable skins, seeds and fibers. *SYN* – phytobezoar.

Food chain Sequential transfer of food energy from green plants to herbivorous animals and then to man through animal flesh. Interruption of this chain can result in ecological disaster.

Food poisoning Illness resulting from ingestion of foods, containing poisonous substances, e.g., mushroom poisoning, insecticides contaminating food, milk from cows that have eaten some poisonous plants, ingestion of putrefied or decomposed food.

Food requirement Requirement of calorie and protein depending upon age, muscular work and environment. Average active healthy (70 kg) man requires 2,700 cal/day and average healthy woman 2000 cal/day. Persons in sedentary work require less calories. Protein requirement of adult is 1 g/kg of their ideal weight. Pregnancy and lactation demand 15–25% extra calories. In growing children protein requirement is 2–3 g/kg/day.

Foot The terminal part of the lower limb.

Athlete's foot Ringworm of the foot; tinea pedis.

Foot drop Inability to keep the foot at the correct angle owing to paralysis of the flexors of the ankle.

Foot presentation The presentation of one or both legs instead of the head during labor.

Foot and mouth disease A viral disease of cattle and horses.

Foot board A device that helps to prevent foot drop.

Foot candle An amount of light equivalent to one lumen per square foot.

Foot plate The flat part of stapes, the bone of middle ear.

Foot print An impression of foot used for identification of infants.

Forage Creating a channel through enlarged prostate by use of an electric cautery.

Foramen An opening or hole, especially in a bone.

Foramen magnum The hole in the occipital bone through which the spinal cord passes.

Foramen ovale The hole between the left and right atria in the fetus.

Obturator foramen The large hole in the innominate bone.

Optic foramen The opening in the posterior part of the orbit through which the optic nerve and the ophthalmic artery passes.

Forbe's disease Type III glycogen storage disease.

Force A push or pull exerted upon an object, measured in newtons. 1 newton is equivalent to 0.225 pound force.

Electromotive force Energy that causes flow of electricity in a conductor.

Forceps Surgical instruments used for lifting or compressing an object.

Forceps alligator Toothed forceps with a double clamp.

Artery (Spencer Wells forceps) Compress bleeding points during an operation.

Forceps clamp Any forceps with automatic lock.

Forceps dental Forceps of varying shapes for grasping teeth during extraction.

Cheatle forceps Long forceps for lifting utensils.

Obstetric forceps Various patterns are used in difficult labor to facilitate delivery.

Forceps towel/tissue Forceps for clipping towels to operation site or grasping delicate tissue

Vulsellum forceps Have claw-like ends for exerting traction *(see Figure)*.

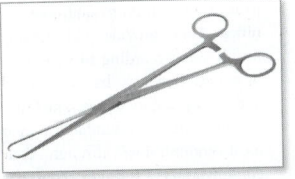

Vulsellum Forceps

Fordyce's disease Enlarged ectopic sebaceous glands in mucosa of mouth and genitals.

Fordyce-Fox disease A disease similar to prickly heat in which itchy follicular papules are present in axilla, areola of breast, labia, etc.

Forensic Pertaining to or applied in legal proceedings.

Forensic medicine The branch that is concerned with the law and has a bearing on legal problems. It includes the investigation of unexplained death or injury.

Forensic dentistry Application of science of dentistry for the purposes of law, e.g., establishing identity.

Forensic medicine Medicine in relation to law, legal aspects of medical ethics and standards.

Foreskin The prepuce.

Fore waters Mucus discharge from vagina during pregnancy.

Forgetfulness The inability to remember or recall events, appointments, objects, etc. of daily life. Failure to retrieve memories may occur as a normal result of inattention although it is a common difficulty that develops with increasing age. In the elderly, worsening forgetfulness may be associated with the development of dementia.

Fork turning An elongated instrument that bifurcates at one end, used for testing hearing, bone conduction and vibration.

Formaldehyde A gaseous compound with strongly disinfectant properties. It is used in solution for disinfection of excreta and utensils and also in the preparation of toxoids from toxins.

Formalin Aqueous solution of 37% formaldehyde.

Formation A structure, shape or figure.

Reticular formation Found in medulla oblongata between the pyramids and floor of the fourth ventricle, supposed to be the activating or arousal system for consciousness.

Forme fruste An aborted or incomplete form of disease arrested before running its course.

Formestane Antiestrogen.

Formic acid A clear pungent acid obtained from oxidation of formaldehyde or wood alcohol, responsible for pain and swelling following stings and bites.

Formication Sensation of insects creeping upon the body.

Formiminoglutanic acid (FIGLU) A chemical intermediate in the metabolism of histidine to glutamic acid. In folic acid deficiency states FIGLU excretion is increased in urine.

Formoterol Inhaled steroid.

Formula [L.] 1. An expression, using numbers or symbols, of the composition of, or of directions for preparing, a compound, such as a medicine; or of a procedure to follow to obtain a desired result; or of a single concept. 2. A mixture for feeding an infant, composed of milk and/or other ingredients.

Formulary A prescriber's handbook of drugs.

Fornication Sexual intercourse between unmarried partners.

Fornix An arch.

Conjunctival fornix The reflection of the conjunctiva from the eyelids on to the eyeball.

Fornix cerebri An arched structure at the back and base of the brain.

Fornix of the vagina The recesses at the top of the vagina in front (anterior fornix), back (posterior fornix) and sides (lateral fornix) of the cervix uteri.

Forskolin Cardiac stimulant for congestive failure.

Fortification spectrum Appearance of dark patch with zigzag outline in the visual field causing temporary blindness in that portion of eye.

Fossa A small depression or pit. Usually applied to fossae in bones.

Cubital fossa The triangular depression at the front of the elbow.

Iliac fossa The depression on the inner surface of the iliac bone.

Pituitary fossa The depression in the sphenoid bone *(See Sellaturcica)*.

Foster children Children under the care of foster parents.

Foster parents persons who undertake for reward the care of children who are not related to them within the meaning of the Children Act (1989).

Fothergill's operation *WE Fothergill, British gynaecologist, 1865–1926.* Amputation of the cervix, with anterior and posterior colporrhaphy for prolapse of the uterus.

Foundation doctor Junior doctors in their first two years following graduation from medical school. Abbreviated to F1 for first-year foundation doctors and F2 for second-year doctors.

Foundation NHS Trusts Foundation Trusts are subject to the same standards, performance ratings and systems of inspection as other NHS organizations, although they are free from the direction of the Secretary of State for Health. NHS foundation trusts are not-for-profit, public benefit corporations. They are part of the NHS and currently provide over half of all NHS hospital, mental health and ambulance services in England and Wales. NHS foundation trusts were created to devolve decision making from central government to local organizations and communities. They provide and develop health care according to core NHS principles-free care based on need and not the ability to pay. The foundation trusts are accountable to their local communities through their commissioners through contracts and also to Parliament and the Care

Quality Commission through the legal requirement to register and to meet the required standards of the care provided. Monitor, now part of NHS IMPROVEMENT, is the independent regulator. Anyone who lives in the area which the foundation trust serves or who works for a foundation trust, or has been a patient or service user can become a member of the trust.

Fourchette [Fr.] The fold of membrane at the perineal end of the vulva.

Fourth cranial nerve Trochlear nerve emerging from dorsal surface of midbrain, supplying superior oblique.

Fovea A fossa; a small depression, particularly that of the retina which contains a large number of cones, giving form and color, and is, therefore, the area of most accurate vision.

Fowler's position Semi-sitting position with angulation of upper portion of body at 45°–60°; knees may or may not be bent.

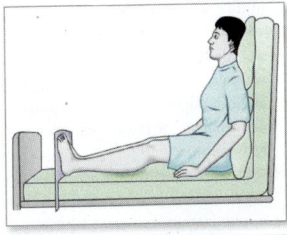

Fowler's Position

Foxglove Common name for plant digitalis purpurea.

Fraction of inspired oxygen (FiO₂) The concentraction of O_2 in the inspired air.

Fractional test meal Fractional examination of stomach contents for free and total hydrochloric acid.

Fracture 1. To break a part, especially a bone. 2. A break in the continuity of bone. The signs and symptoms are pain, swelling, deformity, shortening of the limb, loss of power, abnormal mobility, and crepitus. Fractures are generally caused by trauma, either by a direct or an indirect force on the bone. Fractures may also be caused by muscle spasm or by disease that results in decalcification of the bone. The different types and classification of fractures are shown in the Figure.

March fracture A hairline crack in the long bone of the foot caused by repeated trauma associated with long marches and with jogging.

Pathological fracture One due to weakening of the bone structure by pathological processes, such as neoplasia, osteomalacia or osteomyelitis.

Pott's fracture A fracture dislocation of the ankle involving the lower end of the fibula and sometimes the internal malleolus of the tibia.

Spontaneous fracture One that occurs as a result of little or no violence, usually of a bone weakened by disease.

Fragile – X syndrome Mutation in X-chromosome manifesting with mental retardation and greatly enlarged testicles after puberty.

Fragilitas Brittleness as of the hair.

Fragility State of brittleness.

Fragility erythrocyte Rupture of RBC in various strengths of salt solution. Normal blood starts hemolyzing at about 0. 44% and complete at 0.35%.

Frailty A distinctive health state related to the aging process in which multiple body systems gradually become diminished.

F. score The assessment of people who are frail or quantify their level of frailty in order to provide a consistent approach to management.

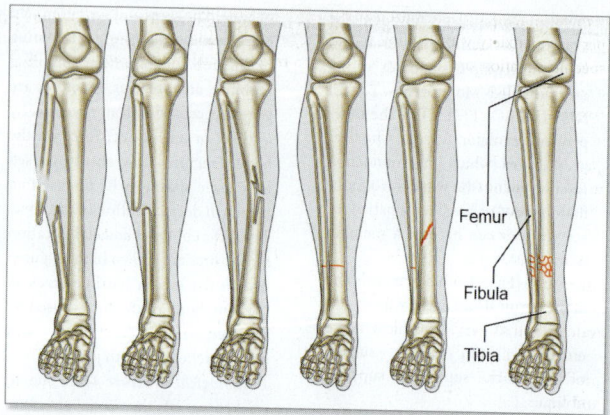

Types of Fracture

Frambesia Infectious disease caused by a spirochete.

Frambesioma Primary lesion of yaws in the form of a protruding nodule.

Frame A rigid supporting structure or a structure for immobilizing a part.

Braun frame A metal frame used to elevate the lower limb in fractures of the tibia and fibula.

Quadriplegic standing frame A device for supporting in the upright position a patient whose four limbs are paralyzed.

Stryker frame One consisting of canvas stretched on anterior and posterior frames, on which the patient can be rotated around the longitudinal axis.

Walking frame A walking aid with three or four legs.

Framycetin An aminoglycoside antibiotic, very similar to neomycin. Used for topical application.

Franceschetti's syndrome Mandibulo-facial dysostosis *SYN* – Trecher – Collin's syndrome.

Francisellatularensis Non-motile, encapsulated Gram-negative organism causing plague.

Fratricide Murder of one's brother or sister.

Freckle A brown pigmented spot on the skin.

Hutchinson's melanotic freckle A non-invasive malignant melanoma which occurs mainly on the face of middle-aged women.

Free association In psychoanalysis a spontaneous mental process whereby words used in a nonlogical chain suggest ideas, thoughts or feelings without selection or repression.

Freedom of Information Act All NHS organizations are required to have a publication scheme, which sets out the type of information that it publishes or intends to publish, the form in which the information is published and details of any changes. NHS organizations must answer requests for information within the terms of the individual right of access given by the Act. This applies to all types of recorded information held by the organization regardless of its date, although the Act does include some specific exemptions.

Free-floating anxiety Generalized and pervasive anxiety with no link to a specific situation or object creating a feeling of unease and dread for the patient.

Frei's test *WS Frei, German dermatologist; 1885–1943.* An intradermal test to aid the diagnosis of lymphogranuloma venereum.

Freiberg's disease *AH Freiberg, American surgeon, 1868–1940.* Osteochondritis of the second metatarsal bone, in which there is pain on walking and standing.

Fremitus A thrill or vibration, e.g., that produced in the chest by speaking and felt on palpation.

French scale A system indicating outer catheter diameters. Each unit of scale is equivalent to 1/3 mm.

Frenkel exercise These exercise involve teaching patient muscle and joint sensation in order to restore the lost coordination. Especially useful in cases of tabes dorsalis and other ataxic conditions.

Frenotomy The cutting of the frenulum of the tongue to cure tongue-tie.

Frenulum A fold of mucous membrane which limits the movement of an organ.

Frenulum of the tongue The fold under the tongue.

Frenzy A state of violent mental agitation or excitement. Frenzy response in electrodiagnostic study of spinal reflexes, the time required for a stimulus applied to a motor nerve to travel in the opposite direction up the nerve to the spinal cord and return.

Fretum A constriction.

Freudian *S Freud, Austrian psychiatrist 1856–1939.* Relating to the theories of Freud who was the originator of psychoanalysis and the psychoanalytical theory of the cause of neurosis.

Frey's syndrome A rare condition affecting young children characterized by facial flushing and sweating after eating.

Freudian Freud's theories of unconscious or repressed libido on past experiences or desires as the cause of various neuroses, and cure for which is the restoration of such conditions to consciousness through psychoanalysis.

Friable Easily crumbled or torn.

Friction The act of rubbing one object against another.

Friction massage A circular or transverse pressure applied by fingertip or thumb to a localized area. Used for the relief of pain.

Friction murmur The grating sound heard in auscultation when two rough surfaces rub together, as in dry pleurisy.

Friedlander's bacillus *K Friedlander, German pathologist, 1847–1887.* The cause of rare form of pneumonia. Klebsiella friedlanderi.

Friedreich's ataxia or disease *N Friedreich, German physician, 1825–1882.* A rare form of hereditary ataxia.

Friends and family test Gives patients the opportunity through the completion of a short questionnaire to provide feedback on services they have used. Services receive this feedback and can take actions in real-time to address feedback.

Fright Extreme sudden fear.

Frigid Cold, irresponsive to emotions or lack of sexual desire in women.

Frigidity an absence of normal sexual desire; usually refers to women.

Frogbelly Flaccid atonic abdomen of children with rickets.

Frog face Facies of chronic sinusitis.

Frolich's syndrome *A Frolich, Austrian neurologist, 1871–1953.* A group of symptoms associated with disease of the pituitary body; increased adiposy, atrophy of the genital organs and development of feminine characteristics.

Fröhlich's syndrome A. Frohlich, Austrian neurologist, 1871-1953. A group of symptoms associated with disease of the pituitary body, increased adiposity, atrophy of the genital organs, and development of feminine characteristics. Also known as Adiposogenital Dystrophy.

Froin's syndrome High CSF protein content that rapidly coagulates and is yellow caused by spinal canal obstruction.

Froment's sign Flexion of distal phalanx of thumb when a sheet of paper is held between thumb and index finger, a feature of ulnar nerve palsy.

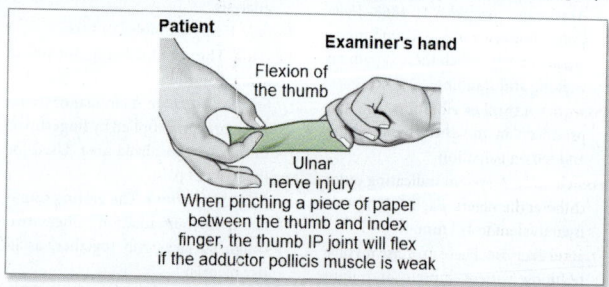

Froment's Sign

Frontal 1. Relating to the forehead. 2. Relating to the front or anterior aspect of a structure.

Frontal lobe Four main convolutions infront of central sulcus of cerebrum.

Frontal plane Plane parallel with the long axis of body and at right angles to the median sagittal plane.

Frontal sinus A pair of hollow asymmetrical spaces in the frontal bone above the orbits, filled with air and lined by mucus membrane.

Front tap reflex Contraction of gastrocnemius muscles when stretched muscles of extended legs are percussed.

Frostbite Impairment of circulation, chiefly affecting the fingers, the toes, the nose and the ears, due to exposure to severe cold. The first stage is represented by chilblains. Advanced cases show thrombosis and dry gangrene.

Frost uremic Deposit of urea crystals on skin in uremia patient.

Frottage [Fr.] 1. A rubbing movement in massage. 2. Sexual gratification by rubbing against another person's body.

Frozen section A technique of examining and reporting on pathological tissue cut from a patient while on surgical table, thus deciding future course of action in the theatre itself.

Frozen shoulder A stiff and painful shoulder; capsulitis. Treatment may include stretching under anesthesia, combined with exercises. The case is unknown.

Frozen watchfulness The state of young child who is unresponsive to its surroundings, but is clearly aware of them. The state of frozen watchfulness is usually a marker of child abuse.

Fructokinase Enzyme that transfers high energy phosphate from a donor to fructose.

Fructose Fruit sugar, a monosaccharide.

Fructose intolerance Inability to metabolize fructose in absence of enzyme aldolase thus producing nausea, vomiting, sweating, tremor, hypoglycemia on fructose consumption.

Frustration Disappointment.

Frusemide A diuretic with a rapid and powerful action used in the treatment of edema and of acute renal failure.

FSH Follicle-stimulating hormone.

Fucose A mucopolysaccharide present in blood group substances and in human milk.

Fucosidosis Hereditary disease with thick skin, heart disease, hyperhydrosis and poor neural growth resulting from improper metabolism of fucose.

Fugitive Inconstant symptoms, transient, wandering

Fugue A period of altered awareness during which a person may wander for hours or days and perform purposive actions although memory for the period may be lost. It may follow an epileptic fit or occur in hysteria or schizophrenia.

Fulguration The destruction by diathermy of papillomata (warts), particularly inside the urinary bladder.

Full term In obstetric child born between 38 and 41 weeks of gestation.

Fulminating Sudden in onset and rapid in course.

Fumaric acid One of the organic acids in the citric acid cycle.

Fumigation Disinfection by exposure to the fumes of a vaporized germicide.

Function 1. The natural action or intended purpose of a person, or structure. 2. To perform special work or an action.

Functional disease Emotional response to physical disease, taking the form of conversion or hysterical response.

Fundoplication Surgical reduction in size of opening into fundus of stomach, used in treating reflux esophagitis.

Fundoscopy Visual examination of fundus of eye.

Fundus The base of an organ or the part farthest removed from the opening.

Fundus of the eye The posterior part of the inside of the eye as shown by the ophthalmoscope.

Fundus of the stomach Part above the cardiac orifice.

Fundus of the uterus The top of the uterus, the part farthest from the cervix.

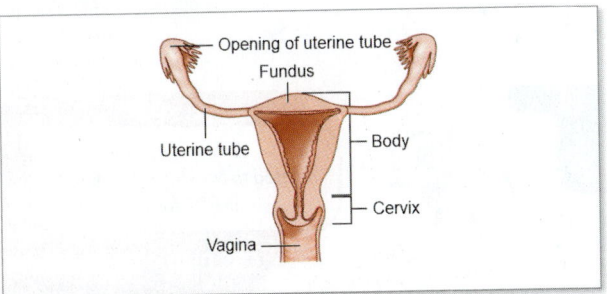

Fundus of the Uterus

Fungal nail infection Infection affecting the finger nail, toe nail or nail bed. It is not usually serious but can be difficult to treat and nails can become thickened and unsightly. Also known as Onychomycosis.

Fungate To grow rapidly and produce, fungus-like growths. Often occurs in the late stages of malignant tumors.

Fungicide A preparation that destroys fungal infection.

Fungiform Shaped like a fungus or mushroom.

Fungus A low form of vegetable life which includes mushrooms and moulds. Some varieties cause disease, such as actionomycosis and ringworm.

Funis The umbilical cord.

Funnel chest A developmental deformity in which there is a depression in the sternum and an inward curvature of the ribs and costal cartilage.

Furor A state of intense excitement during which violent acts may be performed. This may occur often in epileptic fit.

Furuncle A boil.

Furunculoid Resembling boil.

Furunculosis A staphylococcal infection represented by many, or crops of boils.

Furunculus A furuncle.

Furunculus orientalis A protozoal infection, mainly of the tropics, which causes a chronic ulceration. Cutaneous leishmaniasis.

Fuscin A dark-brown pigment present in pigment epithelium of retina.

Fusidic acid An antibiotic used to treat penicillin-resistant staphylococci. It is usually used in combination with another antibiotic effective against staphylococci.

Fusiform Shaped like a spindle.

Fusion 1. The union between two adjacent structures. 2. The coordination of separate images of the same object in the two eyes into one image.

Fusobacterium A genus of anaerobic Gram-negative bacteria found as normal flora in the mouth and large-bowel, and often in necrotic tissue, probably as secondary invaders.

Fusobacterium waves Flutter waves in atrial fibrillation.

Fybogel Trade name for preparations of ispaghula husk, a laxative.

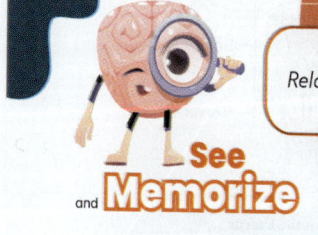

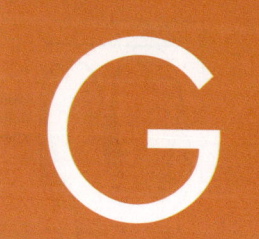

G Symbol for gram and guanine

Ga Symbol for gallium.

GABA Gamma amino butyric acid, a neurotransmitter.

Gabapentin An antiepileptic agent.

Gadolinium A rare element used as NMR contrast agent.

Gag 1. An instrument placed between the teeth to keep the mouth open. 2. The reflex action that occurs when the back of the throat is stimulated.

Gail score An indicator for assessing the risk of a woman to develop breast cancer in the next 5 years.

Gait Manner of walking.

Ataxic gait The foot is raised high, descends suddenly, and the whole sole strikes the ground. Staggering, unsteady gait.

Cerebellar gait A staggering walk indicative of cerebellar disease.

Double step gait Gait in which alternate steps are of a different length or at a different rate.

Equine gait High stepping gait of peroneal nerve palsy.

Four-point gait A method which maybe adopted when using sticks or crutches, which allows maximum stability.

Hemiplegic gait The parlayzed limb abducts and makes a circle to come to front to touch the ground.

Scissor gait Gait in which legs cross while walking.

Slapping gait High stepping ataxic gait due to loss of proprioception as in tabesdorsalis.

Spastic gait Stiff, shuffling walk, the legs being kept together.

Waddling gait Walk resembling that of a duck as in muscular dystrophy.

Galactan A complex carbohydrate that forms galactose on hydrolysis.

Galactase A proteolytic ferment of milk.

Galactocele A tumor caused by occlusion of a milk duct; hydrocele containing milk-like fluid.

Galactogogue Agent promoting secretion of milk.

Galactokinase Enzyme transferring high energy phosphate groups from a donor to D-Galactose.

Galactometer Device for measuring specific gravity of milk.

Galactorrhea 1. An excessive flow of milk. 2. Secretion of milk after breast-feeding has ceased.

Galactosemia An inborn error of metabolism in which there is inability to convert galactose to glucose. The disorder becomes manifest soon after birth and is characterized by feeding problems, vomiting, diarrhea, abdominal distension, enlargement of the liver and mental handicap. Treatment consists of exclusion from the diet of milk and all foods containing galactose or lactose.

Galactose A monosaccharide derived from lactose. D-Galactose is found in lactose or milk sugar and cerebrosides of the brain.

Galactose tolerance test A laboratory test to determine the liver's ability to convert the sugar galactose into glycogen.

Galactosuria Excretion of galactose in urine.

Galeazzi's sign A clinical test for determining the presence of congenital hip dislocation in infants and toddlers; with the child lying supine,

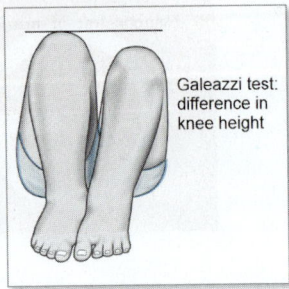

Galeazzi test: difference in knee height

Galeazzi's Sign

knees and hips flexed to 90; dislocation is evidenced if one knee is higher than other.

Galen's veins These veins run through the telachorodiae formed by the joining of the terminal and choroid veins. They form venacerebra magna, that empties into straight sinus.

Gall Bile, a digestive fluid secreted by the liver and stored in the gallbladder.

Gallamine A synthetic muscle relaxant, chemically related to curare but less potent and shorter-acting.

Gallbladder The sac under the lower surface of the liver, which acts as a reservoir for bile.

Gallipot A small receptacle for lotions.

Gallium Symbol Ga. A radioisotope used in detecting some soft-tissue disorders.

Gallium scan A radioactive isotope of gallium maybe administered intravenously in a total body scan to detect metastatic spread, lymphomas, or a focus of infection.

Gallon Measure of liquid equivalent to 4.55 liters.

Gallop rhythm Heart rhythm that may occur when there is ventricular over load.

Gallstone A concretion formed in the gallbladder or bile ducts. Gallstones are often multiple and faceted.

Gallstone colic (See Biliary (Colic)).

Galvanic current Direct electric current from battery.

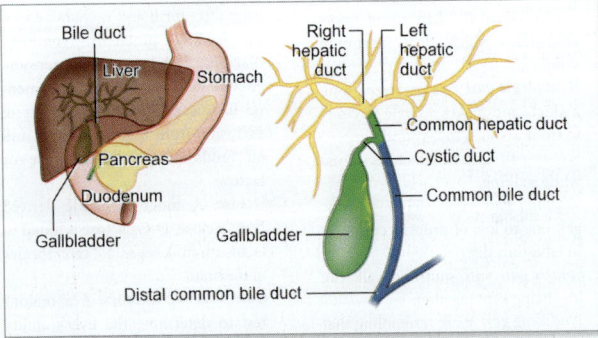

Gallbladder

Galvanometer An instrument for detecting or measuring the strength of a current of electricity.

Galvanoscope An instrument that shows presence and direction of galvanic current.

Gamete A sex cell which combines with another to form a zygote, from which a complete organism develops; A spermatozoon or an ovum.

Gamete intrafallopian transfer (GIFT) Obtaining ova through laparoscope and fusing it with sperm and placing it in fallopian tube for completion of fertilization and transfer to uterus.

Gametocide Agent that destroys malaria gametocytes.

Gametocyte A cell that is undergoing gametogenesis.

Gametogenesis The production of the gametes by the gonads.

Gamma The third letter in the Greek alphabet, γ.

Gamma-benzene hexachloride A drug used as a cream, lotion or as a shampoo to treat head lice.

Gamma camera An apparatus for depicting a part of the body into which radioactive isotopes emitting gamma rays have been introduced.

Gamma encephalography A method of localizing a brain tumor by using radioactive isotopes emitting gamma rays.

Gamma globulin A class of plasma proteins composed almost entirely of IgG, an immunoglobulin protein that contains most antibody activity.

Gamma knife surgery A modality of treatment of brain tumor, where radiation beam is focused on tumor tissue with stereotaxic precision.

Gamma rays Electromagnetic rays, of shorter wavelength and with greater penetration than X-rays, which are given off by certain radioactive substances and which are used in radiotherapy. Also used in the sterilization of articles that would be destroyed by the heat and moisture required in autoclaving.

Gammopathy Diseases with high gammaglobulin, e.g, multiple myeloma.

Gamna's disease This is a form of chronic splenomegaly characterized by thickening of the splenic capsule and presence of multiple, small, dense, rust like densities containing iron. These bodies are known as Gamna-Gandy bodies.

Gamophobia Neurotic fear of marriage.

Gangliocyte A ganglion cell.

Ganglioma Tumor of lymphatic gland.

Ganglion 1. A collection of nerve cells and fibers, forming an independent nerve centre, as is found in the sympathetic nervous system. 2. A cystic swelling on a tendon.

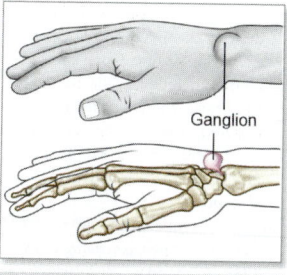

Ganglion

Ganglionectomy Excision of a ganglion.

Ganglioneuroma A nerve cell tumor containing ganglion cells.

Ganglionic blockade Blockage of neurotransmission in autonomic ganglia by drugs that occupy receptor sites for acetylcholine or stabilize post-synaptic membrane against action of acetylcholine liberated in presynoptic nerve endings.

Ganglioside A particular class of glycosphingolipid present in nerve tissue and in the spleen.

Gangrene Death of body tissue, generally in considerable mass, due to either loss of blood supply or the effects of certain infections.

Dry gangrene Occurs gradually and results from slow reduction of the blood flow in the arteries. There is no subsequent bacterial decomposition; the tissues become dry and shrivelled. It occurs only in the extremities, and can occur with arteriosclerosis and diabetes (mellitus).

G

Gas gangrene Results from dirty lacerated wounds infected by anaerobic bacteria, especially species of *Clostridium.* It is an acute, severe, painful condition in which muscles and subcutaneous tissues become filled with gas and a serosanguinous exudate.

Moist gangrene Caused by sudden stoppage of blood, resulting from burning by heat or acid, severe freezing, physical accident that destroys the tissue, or a clot or other embolism. At first, tissue affected by moist gangrene has the colour of a bad bruise, and is swollen and often blistered. The gangrene is likely to spread with great speed. Toxins are formed in the affected tissues and absorbed.

Ganser's syndrome (state) *S.J.M. Ganser, German psychiatrist, 1853–1931.* Amnesia, disturbance of consciousness and hallucinations, associated with senseless answers to questions, and absurd acts. Usually a transient response to a troublesome situation, e.g., prisoners on remand (prison psychosis).

Gardnerella vaginalis A bacteria causing vaginitis.

Gardener's syndrome Familial polyposis of colon, an autosomal dominant condition with propensity or development of carcinoma.

Gargle 1. A solution for rinsing the mouth and throat. 2. To rinse the mouth and throat by holding a solution in the open mouth and agitating it by expulsion of air from the lungs.

Gargoylism A congenital condition characterized by dwarfism, kyphosis and skeletal abnormalities with mental retardation.(Hurler's syndrome).

Garlic An edible strongly flavored bulb containing chemical allicin, possessing antithrombotic properties.

Garment (pneumatic-anti-shock) An inflatable garment used to combat shock, stabilize fracture, promote hemostasis, increase peripheral vascular resistance.

Garre's disease Chronic sclerosing osteomyelitis.

Gartner's bacillus Another name for *Salmonella enteritidis* bacillus, which is responsible for causing gastroenteritis in human beings and animals.

Gartner's duct A vestigial structure representing the persistent mesonephric duct.

Gas Molecules of a substance very loosely combined; a vapor.

Gas and air analgesia An authorized form of analgesia using nitrous oxide and air, by which the pains of labor are lessened without affecting uterine contractions.

Laughing gas Nitrous oxide.

Marsh gas Methane.

Sternutatory gas One which causes sneezing.

Tear gas One that is irritating to the eyes and causes excessive lacrimation.

Gas mustard Dichloroethyl sulfide, a poisonous gas used in warfare.

Gasoline A distillation product of petroleum often containing toxic additives like tetraethyl lead or tricresyl phosphate.

Gasser's ganglion *J.L. Gasser, Austrian anatomist, 1723–1765.* The trigeminal ganglion. The ganglion of the sensory root of the fifth cranial nerve.

Gastrectomy Excision of part or whole of the stomach.

Billroth gastrectomy Removal of most of the lesser curvature and pyloric portion and joining of the duodenum to the refashioned stomach. This cuts down the production of secretin and acid.

Partial gastrectomy Removal of a part, usually the distal portion, of the stomach. Commonly performed in the surgical treatment of peptic ulcer.

Polya gastrectomy Removal of the first part of the duodenum and the greater part of the stomach, and anastomosis of the stomach to the jejunum. The blind portion of the duodenum supplies the bile and pancreatic and duodenal secretions.

Gastric Pertaining to the stomach.

Gastric analysis Analysis of the stomach contents by microscopy and tests to determine the amount of acid present.

Gastric bypass Surgical creation of a small gastric pouch that empties directly into the jejunum through a gastrojejunostomy, thereby causing food to bypass the duodenum; performed for the treatment of gross obesity.

Gastric digestion Pepsin secreted in the stomach hydrolyzes proteins to proteoses and peptones. HCl is essential for activity of pepsin.

Gastric flu A popular term for what maybe any of several disorders of the stomach and intestinal tract. The symptoms are nausea, diarrhea, abdominal cramps and fever.

Gastric glands Tubular glands lying in gastric mucosa that contain peptic cells secreting pepsinogen, oxyntic cells secreting HCl and mucus cells lying at the neck of gland secreting cytoprotective gastric mucin.

Gastric juice The clear fluid secreted by the glands of the stomach to assist digestion. It contains an enzyme called pepsin, which acts upon proteins in the presence of weak hydrochloric acid.

Gastric lavage A treatment for some types of poisoning where the stomach contents are washed out through a stomach tube.

Gastric ulcer Ulceration of the gastric mucosa, associated with hyperacidity and often precipitated by *Helicobacter pylori* organisms. The condition is often aggravated by stress.

Gastrin A hormone, secreted by the walls of the stomach, which excites continued secretion of digestive juice while food is in the stomach.

Gastrinoma Tumor of gastrin secreting cells causing Zollinger–Ellison syndrome.

Gastritis Inflammation of the lining of the stomach characterized by epigastric pain, vomiting and dyspepsia.

Gastrocnemius Larger superficial muscle in the back of lower leg that helps to plantar flex the foot and flex the knee upon the thigh.

Gastrocolic Pertaining to the stomach and colon.

Gastrocolic reflex After a meal, increased peristalsis causes the colon to empty into the rectum. This gives rise to a desire to defecate.

Gastroduodenoscopy Visual examination of stomach and duodenum by endoscope.

Gastroduodenostomy A surgical anastomosis between the stomach and the duodenum.

Gastroesophagostomy A surgical anastomosis between the stomach and the esophagus.

Gastroenteritis Inflammation of the lining of the stomach and intestine. Psychological causes of gastroenteritis include fear, anger and other forms of emotional upset. Allergic reactions to certain foods can cause gastroenteritis, e.g., irritation by excessive use of alcohol. Severe gastroenteritis, with such symptoms as headache, nausea, vomiting, weakness, diarrhea and gas pains, may result from various viral and bacterial infections, such as influenza.

Gastroenterology The study of diseases of the gastrointestinal tract.

Gastroenterostomy A surgical anastomosis between the stomach and small intestine.

Gastroepiploic Pertains to stomach and greater omentum.

G

Gastroesophageal reflux Reflux of acid contents of stomach into lower esophagus due to obesity, hiatus hernia, anticholinergic use, pregnancy etc.

Gastrografin A proprietary oral diagnostic radiopaque contrast medium.

Gastro-esophagostomy A surgical anastomosis between the stomach and the esophagus.

Gastroileac Pertaining to the stomach and ileum.

G. reflex Food entering the stomach sets up powerful peristalsis in the ileum and opening of the ileocecal valve.

Gastroileal Pertaining to the stomach and ileum.

Gastroileal reflex Food entering the stomach sets up powerful peristalsis in the ileum and opening of the ileocecal valve.

Gastrointestinal Pertaining to the stomach and intestine.

GI tract The alimentary tract.

Gastrointestinal decompression Removal of gas and fluids from GI tract through Ryle's tube.

Gastrojejunostomy A surgical anastomosis between the stomach and the jejunum.

Gastrolysis Surgical breaking of adhesions between the stomach and adjoining structures.

Gastroptosis Downward displacement of stomach.

Gastroscope An endoscope specially designed for passage into the stomach to permit examination of its interior. The gastroscope is a hollow, cylindrical tube, fitted with special lenses and lights, which acts by reflecting light and creating a mirror effect, making it possible to 'go around corners', and facilitating visualization of the curvature of the stomach.

Gastrostomy The creation of an opening into the stomach. This procedure is done to provide for the administration of food and liquids when stricture of the esophagus or other conditions make swallowing impossible *(See Artificial (Feeding))*.

Gastrotomy A surgical incision of the stomach.

Gastrula An early stage in the development of the fertilized ovum.

Gate control theory of pain Theory proposing that a neural mechanism in the dorsal horns of the spinal cord acts like a gate, which can increase or decrease the flow of nerve impulses from peripheral fibers to the central nervous system. It is the position of the gate that determines how much information is transmitted to the brain and therefore the amount of pain generated. Influences such as anxiety and anticipation cause the gate to open and therefore increase the level of pain experienced, whereas other factors may cause the gate to close, thereby reducing the pain.

Gate theory The hypothesis that painful stimuli can be prevented from reaching higher centers for recognition by stimulation of sensory nerves, a key mechanism explaining acupuncture analgesia.

Gatekeepers The individuals or groups in an organization who regulate access to goods and services.

Gateway drug Generic name for alcohol, cocaine or cannabis referring to their supposed roles as conduits leading on to the taking of harder drugs.

Gaucher's disease *P.C.E. Gaucher, French physician, 1854–1918.* A rare familial disease in which fat is deposited in the reticuloendothelial cells, causing an enlarged spleen and anemia.

Gault's reflex Blinking of eye following a loud noise close to ear, a test helpful in people malingering deafness.

Gauss sign Unusual mobility of uterus in early pregnancy.

Gauze A thin open-meshed material used for dressing wounds.

Gavage [Fr.] Forced feeding; the giving of fluids and nourishment by esophageal or other type of tube directly into the stomach.

Gay Popular term for a homosexual, usually male.

Gay bowel syndrome The damaging effects of male homosexual practices on the lower bowel; also includes anal fissures, anal fistulas, hemorrhoids and ulcers.

Gay's glands Large sebaceous circumanal glands.

Geigel reflex Contraction of muscles of lower abdomen on stimulation of inner aspect of thigh in females. It corresponds to cremasteric reflex.

Geiger counter *H. Geiger, German physicist, 1882–1945.* An instrument for detecting and registering radioactivity. The apparatus is sensitive to the rays emitted.

Gel Jelly like semisolid state.

Gelasmus Spasmodic laughter of insane.

Gelatin An albuminoid, obtained from connective tissue or bone. Used in pharmacy for suppositories and capsules, and in bacteriology as a culture medium. In absorbable film and sponge, it is used in surgical procedures.

Gelatinase An enzyme present in bacteria, molds and yeasts that liquefies gelatin.

Gelatinous Having consistency of gelatin.

Gelfoam Absorbable gelatin foam, a hemostatic.

Gemcitabine Anticancer agent.

Gemfibrozil Lipid lowering agent (mainly triglycerides).

Gemifloxacin Quinolone antibiotic.

Gemination Development of two teeth or two crowns within a single root.

Gemistocyte Swollen astrocyte with eccentric nucleus seen adjacent to areas of infarct/edema.

Gemmation Cell reproduction by budding.

Gender Sex; the category to which an individual is assigned on the basis of sex.

Gender identity disorder A psychiatric label for those disorders marked by a sense of inappropriateness and feel discomfort concerning one's sexual anatomy and sex role. This category usually includes transvestism, trans-sexual and gender identity disorders in childhood.

Gene One of the biological units of heredity, self-reproducing and located at a definite position (locus) on a particular chromosome.

Allelic gene Pairs of genes located at same site on chromosome pair.

Dominant gene One that is capable of transmitting its characteristics irrespective of the genes from the other parent.

Histocompatible gene Gene that controls the specificity of antigenic expression by tissues.

Recessive gene One that can pass on its characteristics only if it is present with a similar recessive gene from the other parent *(See Mendel's theory).*

Gene amplification The duplication of regions of DNA to form multiple copies of a specific portion of the original region.

Gene map A map of the human genome i.e., a map of each chromosome.

Gene therapy The use of 'healthy' genes to cure/treat a hereditary disease.

General household survey (GHS) Started in 1971, now under the auspices of the Office for National Statistics; initially for use by all government departments but also provides a secondary data source for the social sciences. It is a continuous

G

survey and includes five main areas of investigation: family data, employment, housing, education and health.

General adaptation syndrome (GAS) An organism's nonspecific response to stress occurring in 3 stages. 1. Alarm reaction with pituitary adrenal hyperactivity to face the stress by fight or flight. 2. Stage of adaptation when the physical symptoms diminish and 3. Stage of exhaustion when body can no longer respond to stress related emotional disturbances, cardiovascular problems, etc.

General medical council (GMC) The regulating body of all medical practitioners within the UK. It licenses doctors to practice and is charged with: (a) keeping the register of practicing doctors up to date; (b) fostering good medical practice; (c) promoting high standards in medical education; and (d) dealing firmly and fairly with doctors worse fitness for practice is in doubt.

General practitioner (GP) The role of the general practitioner or primary care physician is unique. Besides being the first point of contact for most patients, GPs must offer the first treatment or referral for all problems which are presented to them. In addition, GPs give personal and continuing care to their patients, often over the course of many years.

Generalized anxiety disorder (GAD) A long term condition causing anxiety to a range of situations and issues. Feelings of anxiety are constant and can affect daily living.

Generation 1. The act of forming a new organism 2. Period of time between birth of parents and birth of their children.

Generator pulse Device producing stimuli intermittently, e.g., cardiac pacemaker.

Generic Distinctive, general.

Genesiology The science of reproduction.

Genesis Act of reproducing, generation, origin of anything.

Genetic 1. Pertaining to reproduction or to birth or origin. 2. Inherited.

Genetic code The arrangement of genetic material stored in the DNA molecule of the chromosome.

Genetic counseling Supportive service for prospective parents who can receive advice as to the likelihood of their children being born with a genetically transmitted disorder.

Genetic engineering The synthesis, modification or repair of genetic DNA by synthetic means.

Genetics The study of heredity and natural development.

Gene transfer Transfer gene from one person to another for repair of inherited defect in the recipient.

Geneva convention Declaration in Geneva that the sick and wounded victims of war including persons involved in their care like doctors, nurses, ambulance drivers, stretcher bearers are neutral and would not therefore be target of military action.

Genioplasty Plastic surgery of cheek or chin.

Genital herpes Caused by the herpes simplex virus (HSV types 1 or 2) and presents with painful blisters on or around the genitalia and transmitted through sexual contact.

Genital warts Small fleshy lumps appearing on the genitalia caused by strains of the human papillovirus (HPV) and transmitted through sexual contact.

Genitalia The organs of reproduction.

Genitourinary Referring to both the reproductive organs and the urinary tract.

Genius An individual with exceptional mental or creative capability.

Genome The total amount of genetic information in the chromosomes of an organism, including genes and DNA sequences.

Genotype The genetic characteristics of an individual.

Gentamicin An antibiotic effective against many Gram-negative bacteria, especially *Pseudomonas* species, as well as certain gram-positive bacteria, especially *Staphylococcus aureus*.

Gentian Dried rhizome roots of plant gentian lutea.

Gentian violet A dye derived from coaltar. Widely used as a stain in histology, cytology and bacteriology. Also is anti-infective and antifungal.

Genu [L.] The knee.

Genu valgum Knockknee. A condition in which knees are close to each other and ankles are wide apart (>5 cm).

Genu varum Bowleg Curving out of the legs.

Genu recurvatum Hyperextension at the knee joint.

Genu pectoral Relating to the knee and chest.

Genu pectoral position The knee-chest position *(See Position)*.

G

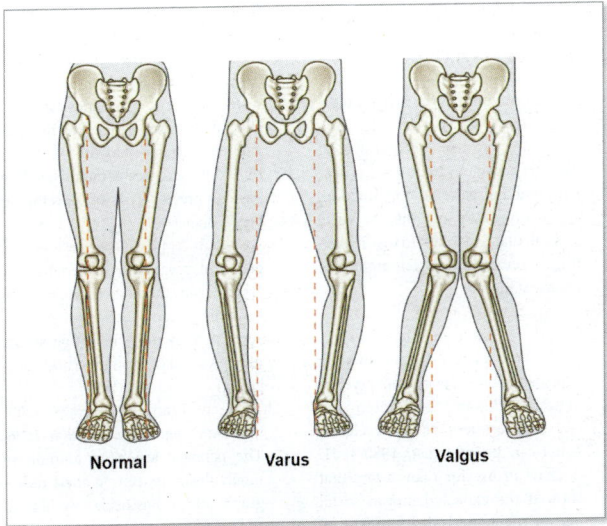

| Normal | Varus | Valgus |

Genu Varus & Genu Valgus

Genupectoral Relating to the knees and chest.

G. position The knee – chest position. *(See Position)*

Genus In biology, taxonomic division between species and family.

Gerdy's fibers Superficial transverse ligament of palm.

Geriatrics The branch of medicine covering old age and the disorders arising from it.

Gerlach's valve Inconstant valve at the opening of appendix into the cecum.

Germ 1. A microbe. 2. That from which something may develop; a seed.

German measles *(See Rubella)*.

Germicide An agent capable of destroying pathogenic micro organisms.

Germinal center A light area of lymphocytopoietic cells that occupies the center of lymphatic nodules, of spleen, tonsils and lymph nodes.

Germinal epithelium The epithelium that covers the surface of the genital ridge of an embryo.

Germination Development of impregnated ovum into an embryo or sprouting of spore.

Germinoma A neoplasm of the testis or ovum.

Geroderma Appearance of senility brought about by premature loss of hair, wrinkling of skin, general body atrophy.

Gerontology The study of old age and the ageing processes.

Gerotophilia Fondness or love for old.

Gerota's capsule The perirenal fascia.

Gerstmann's syndrome Neurological disorder caused by brain lesions near temporal and parietal lobe junction, characterized by inability to write and calculate, inability to distinguish fingers on hand, and left-right side disorientation.

Gessel's developmental chart *A. Gessell, American psychologist, 1880–1961.* A chart which shows the expected motor, social and psychological development of children.

Gesell's developmental chart A. Gesell, American psychologist, 1880-1961. A chart in use for many years that showed the expected motor, social and psychological development of children. Use has fallen over the years.

Gestaltism A theory of holism in psychology, which claims that ideas come as a whole and are not subdivisible.

Gestation The period of development of the young in mammals, from the time of fertilization of the ovum to birth *(See also Pregnancy).*

Ectopic gestation Fetal development in some part other than the uterus, usually the uterine tube.

Interstitial gestation Tubal gestation in which ovum develops in a portion of fallopian tube.

Secondary gestation Gestation in which the ovum becomes dislodged from the original seat of implantation and continues to develop at new site.

Gestation period The duration of pregnancy; in the human female about 280 days when measured from the first day of the last menstrual period.

Gestation assessment Assessment of fetal age and maturity by ultrasound.

Gestational diabetes High blood sugar occurring in non-diabetic women during pregnancy. It usually disappears after birth but women who have has the condition should be screened annually as they have a greater risk of developing type 2 diabetes.

Gestational trophoblastic disease A group of pregnancy-related tumors arising from the tissue that grows to form the placenta during pregnancy.

Gesture A body movement that assists in expression of thoughts (body language).

Ghon focus (gon) *A. Ghon, Czechoslovakian pathologist, 1866–1936.* The primary lesion of pulmonary tuberculosis, as seen on chest radiograph, after it has healed by fibrosis and calcification.

Ghrelin A 28-amino acid hormone produced by stomach cells and responsible for fat storage and stimulation of hunger.

Giant cell A large cell with several nuclei.

Giant cell tumour 1. A connective tissue tumor of bone marrow 2. Tumor of tendon sheath 3. Chondroblastoma.

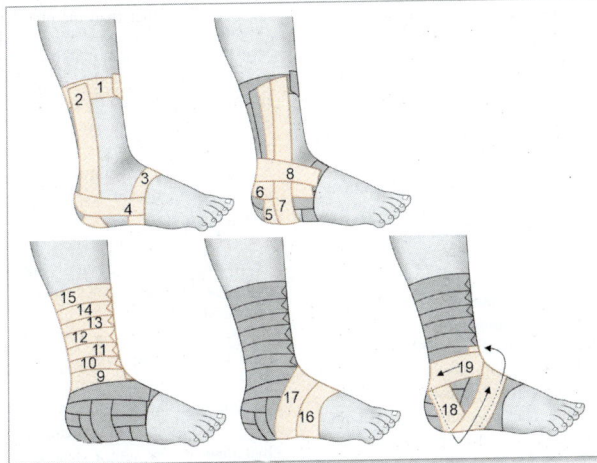

Gibney's Bandage

Gibney's bandage Used to treat sprain in the ankle or support ankle.

Giardiasis *A. Giard, French biologist, 1846–1908.* An infection with *Giardia lamblia,* a pear-shaped protozoon that causes a persistent protracted diarrhea, often resulting in intestinal malabsorption.

Gibbus Humped back, commonly due to compression fracture, collapse.

Gibson's murmur Murmur of patent ductus arteriosus.

Giddiness Light headed sensation.

Giemsa's stain A stain for staining blood smears for differential count and detection of parasitic microorganisms.

Gigantism Abnormal growth of the body, often due to over activity of the anterior lobe of the pituitary gland.

Gilbert's syndrome Hereditary deficiency of glucuronyl transferase with unconjugated hyperbilirubinemia.

Gilles de la Tourette's syndrome (disease) *G.E.A.B. Gilles de la Tourette, French neurologist, 1857–1904.* Multiple tics, especially of the upper part of the body, often associated with involuntary obscene utterances. The condition usually has its onset in childhood and often becomes chronic. The cause is unknown.

Gilliam's operation *D.T. Gilliam, American gynecologist, 1844–1923.* The correction of retroversion of the uterus by shortening the round ligaments; ventrosuspension.

Gimbernat's ligament The lateral portion of inguinal ligament forming medial portion of femoral ring.

Gingiva The gum; connective tissue surrounding the necks of the teeth.

Gingivectomy The surgical removal of the gum margins to get rid of pockets and improve the shape of the gums.

Gingivitis Inflammation of the gums characterized by redness, swelling and tendency to bleed.

Ginkgo Extract from the maidenhair tree, used by herbalists and naturopaths and claimed to be helpful in circulatory disorders, reduced circulation in the brain, senility, depression and premenstrual syndrome.

Ginseng Used widely in Chinese medicine; reputed to have the power to cure many diseases and to have properties to improve sexual health and impotence.

Giralde's organ A remnant of Wolffian body at posterior side of testicle.

Girdle Structure that resembles a circular belt or band.

Girdle symptoms Feeling of constriction in the chest, as in tabesdorsalis, or cord compression.

Gitter cell A honeycombed cell packed with lipid granules.

Gitalin A cardiac glycoside.

Glabella That portion of frontal bone lying between the superciliary arches just above root of nose.

Glacial Resembling ice.

Gland An organ composed of cells which secrete fluid prepared from the blood, either for use in the body, or for excretion as waste material.

Ductless (endocrine) gland One that produces an internal secretion but has no canal (duct) to carry the secretion away, e.g., the thyroid gland.

Exocrine gland One that discharges its secretion through a duct, e.g., the parotid gland.

Lymph gland (See Lymph (Nodes).

Mucous gland One that secretes mucus.

Glanders A disease of horses communicable to humans, and caused by the glanders bacillus, *Pseudomonas-mallei.*

Glandular Pertaining to a gland.

Glandular fever (See Infectious mononucleosis).

Glans An acorn-shaped body, such as the rounded end of the penis or the clitoris.

Glanzmann's thrombasthenia Congenital abnormality of platelets with easy bruising, prolonged bleeding time and poor clot retraction.

Glasgow coma scale A standardized system for quickly evaluating the level of consciousness in the critically ill. Measures include: eye opening according to four criteria, verbal response against five criteria, and motor response using six criteria. Scores of 7 or less qualify as 'coma'. Coma is defined as no response and no eye opening.

Glass photochromatic The glass becoming dark on exposure to light and regaining transparency on being away from light.

Bifocal glass Glasses in which the refractory power of lower portion of glass is for near vision and the upper portion for distant vision.

Glass test A simple test for meningitis that involves pressing a clear glass against a rash. If the rash remains visible it may indicate purpura, which occurs in meningitis. *(See Meningitis).*

Glaucoma Raised intraocular pressure.

Closed-angle glaucoma One that occurs when there is a mechanical defect in the drainage angle; maybe primary or secondary. It maybe acute, when there is pain and blurring of vision, or chronic, when there maybe no pain, but a gradual loss of vision.

Open angle glaucoma Chronic primary glaucoma in which the angle remains open but drainage becomes gradually diminished.

Primary glaucoma One that occurs without any previous disease. It is a common cause of blindness, partial or complete, in the elderly.

Secondary glaucoma One that occurs when some ocular disease is complicated by an increase in intra-ocular pressure.

Gleet Chronic gonococcal urethritis marked by a transparent mucous discharge.

Glenoid Resembling a hollow.

Glenoid cavity The socket of the shoulder joint.

Glenoid fossa The fossa of temporal bone that receives the condyle or capitulum of the mandible.

Glia Neuroglia; the connective tissue of the brain and spinal cord.

Gliadin A water insoluble protein present in the gluten of wheat.

Glibenclamide An oral hypoglycemic agent of the sulphonylurea group used in the treatment of maturity onset diabetes mellitus (Type II).

Glioblastoma A malignant glioma arising in the cerebral hemispheres.

Glioma A malignant tumor composed of neuroglial cells affecting the brain and spinal cord; seldom metastasizes.

Gliomatosis Formation of glioma.

Glipizide Sulphonyl urea compound for diabetes.

Globin A protein used in the formation of hemoglobin.

Globulins A protein group, forming constituents of the blood (serum g.) and cerebrospinal fluid.

Antihemophilic globulin A clotting component of plasma, deficient in hemophiliacs.

Gamma globulin That fration of globulin responsible for body immunity.

Antilymphocyte globulin Globulin from a person who has become immunized to lymphocytes; used as immunosuppressants.

Globus A ball or globe.

Globus hystericus A symptom of hysteria when a patient feels unable to swallow because there is a lump in the throat.

Globus pallidus The pale medial part of the lentiform nucleus of the brain.

Glomangioma A benign tumor developing from an arteriovenous glomus of skin.

Glomerular disease A group of disorders mostly autoimmune or due to some secondary cause that involve the glomerulus manifesting with proteinuria, hematuria and hypertension.

Glomeruli Cluster of capillary vessels enveloped in Bowman's capsule in cortex of kidney.

Glomerulitis Inflammation of the glomeruli of the kidney.

Glomerulonephritis A bilateral, non-infectious inflammation of the kidneys. The cause is unknown but the condition is associated with immunological disturbance. It maybe acute, presenting rapidly but reversibly, or it maybe chronic, presenting slowly and irreversibly.

Glomerulopathy Any disease of glomeruli.

Glomerulosclerosis Degenerative changes in the glomerular capillaries of the renal tubule, leading to renal failure.

Glomerulus The tuft of capillaries within the nephron, which filters urine from the blood.

Glomoid Similar appearance of glomeruli.

Glomus A small round mass made up of tiny blood vessels and found in stroma containing many nerve fibers.

Glossal Relating to the tongue.

Glossina A genus of biting flies, the tsetse flies.

Glossitis Inflammation of the tongue.

Glossodynamometer Device for measuring contractile power of tongue muscles.

Glossograph An instrument for measuring tongue movement during speech.

Glossolalia 'Speaking in tongues' unintelligible speech. The patient speaks in an imaginary language.

Glossopharyngeal Pertaining to the tongue and pharynx.

G

Glossopharyngeal nerve The ninth cranial nerve carrying taste sensation.

Glossoplegia Paralysis of the tongue.

Glottis The space between the vocal cords. The term is sometimes used for that part of the larynx which is associated with voice production.

Glucagon A polypeptide produced by the pancreas. It aids in glycogen breakdown in the liver and raises the blood sugar level.

Glucagonoma A malignant tumor of alpha cells of pancreas.

Glucocerebroside A cerebroside with glucose in the molecule, present in tissues in patients of Gaucher's disease.

Glucocorticoid Any corticoid substance that raises the concentration of liver glycogen and blood sugar, i.e., cortisol (hydrocortisone), cortisone and corticosterone.

Glucogenesis Formation of glucose from glycogen.

Glucokinase An enzyme in liver that converts glucose to glucose 6 phosphate.

Gluconeogenesis The production of glucose from the non-nitrogen portion of the amino acids after deamination. It occurs in the liver and kidneys.

Glucosamine An aminosaccharide present in chitin and mucus.

Glucose Dextrose or grape-sugar; a simple sugar, a monosaccharide in certain food stuffs, especially fruit, and in normal blood; the chief source of energy for living organisms *(See Dextrose).*

Glucose-6-phosphate dehydrogenase A red-cell enzyme. Inherited deficiency causes a tendency to hemolytic anemia *(See Favism).*

Glucose tolerance test Test in which a quantity of glucose is given and the concentration of glucose in the blood is estimated at intervals afterwards.

Used mainly when diabetes mellitus is suspected.

Glucoside A glycoside that upon hydrolysis yields glucose and additional products. e.g., digitalin, present in digitalis.

Glucosuria Abnormal amount of sugar in urine.

Glucoronic acid An acid that possess detoxifying action.

Glucuronide Combination of glucoronic acid with phenol, alcohol, etc.

Glue ear The accumulation of sticky material in the middle ear resulting in impaired hearing, most common in young school children.

Glue sniffing Solvent abuse.

Glutamic acid One of the 22 amino-acids formed by the digestion of dietary protein.

Glutamic-oxaloacetic transaminase An enzyme found in cardiac muscle and the liver. Raised serum levels (SGOT) may indicate an acute myocardial infarction or the presence of liver disease.

Glutamic-pyruvic transaminase An enzyme found in the liver. Measurement of serum levels (SGPT) is used in the study and diagnosis of liver diseases

Glutamine The monoamide of amino-glutaric acid, essential for hydrolysis of proteins.

Glutaraldehyde A disinfectant active against all viruses, fungi, vegetative bacteria and spores. Used in aqueous solution for sterilization of non-heat resistant equipment.

Glutaric aciduria type 1 A rare inherited condition characterized by an inability to process certain amino acids. Babies are tested for the condition as part of Newborn Blood Spot Screening. The condition can be treated with diet and medication.

Gluteal Relating to the buttocks.

Gluteal muscles Three muscles which form the fleshy part of the buttocks.

Gluten The protein of wheat and other grains.

Gluten free diet Elimination of gluten from the diet by exclusion of all products prepared from wheat, rye, barley and oats.

Gluten-induced enteropathy Coeliac disease manifesting with malabsorption and diarrhea.

Gluburide Sulphonyl urea compound for diabetes mellitus.

Glybenclamide Sulphonyl urea for Non Insulin Dependent Diabetes Mellitus (NIDDM).

Glycemic index (GI) The classification of carbohydrate foods based on their overall effects on blood glucose levels. Carbohydrates are ranked 1 to 100. Foods with a low GI factor, e.g., wholegrain cereals, raise blood glucose levels a little and are absorbed more slowly and evenly, whereas those with a high GI factor, e.g., refined flours and sugars, raise blood glucose levels sharply and considerably. Low level GI diets have been shown to improve blood glucose and lipid levels in people with type 1 and type 2 diabetes.

Glyceride An ester of glycerin compounded with an acid.

Glycerin A colorless syrupy substance obtained from fats and fixed oils. It has a hygroscopic action. As an emollient, it is an ingredient of many skin preparations.

Glycerin suppository One composed of glycerin and gelatin, used as an evacuant.

Glycerin of thymol An antiseptic mouthwash and gargle.

Glyceryl A trivalent radical of glycerol.

Glycerylmonostearate An emulsifying agent used in preparing creams and ointments.

Glyceryltrinitrate Nitroglycerin. It is a vasodilator used to relieve certain types of pain, especially in the prophylaxis and treatment of angina pectoris. It is administered sublingually or by transdermal patch or gel.

Glycine A non-essential amino acid.

Glycocholic acid Bile acid present in bile, a conjugate of cholic acid and glysine.

Glycogen The form in which carbohydrate is stored in the liver and muscles. Animal starch.

Glycogen storage disease Inherited disease in which there is a deficiency in the synthesis of glycogen. This accumulates in the liver, causing enlargement.

Glycogenesis The process of glycogen formation from the blood glucose.

Glycogenolysis The breakdown of glycogen in the body so that it maybe utilized.

Glycoside A crystalline body in plants which, when acted on by acids or ferments, produces sugar. If the sugar is glucose it maybe termed a glucoside *(See Digitalis)*.

Glycosuria An excess of glucose in the urine, a symptom of diabetes mellitus.

Renal glycosuria Sugar in the urine, in an otherwise healthy person, due to an inherited inability to reabsorb glucose normally.

Glymidine A drug of the sulphonylurea group used in the treatment of diabetes mellitus.

Gnathic Pertaining to the jaw.

Gnathoplasty A plastic operation on the jaw.

Gnathostoma A genus of nematodes that inhabit alimentary tract, that secretes mucus by rupture of cell wall.

Goal A statement of what a nursing intervention is expected to achieve in either the short or long term. May also be referred to as an outcome. *(See Nursing)*.

G

Goblet cell A goblet-shaped cell, found in the intestinal epithelium, which produces mucus.

Godfrey's test Test for identifying tearing of posterior cruciate ligament.

Goiter Enlargement of the thyroid gland, causing a swelling in the front part of the neck.

Adenomatous goiter Thyroid enlargement due to adenoma.

Colloid goiter An enlarged but soft thyroid gland with no signs of hyperthyroidism.

Diffuse goiter Diffused increase in thyroid tissue in contrast to its nodular form as in adenomatous goiter.

Endemic goiter Sometimes referred to as Derbyshire neck, is usually caused by lack of iodine in the diet.

Exophthalmic goiter Hyperthyroidism with marked protrusion of the eye balls (exophthalmos). Graves' disease.

Intrathoracic goiter Enlargement of the gland mainly in the thorax, so the swelling may not be easily visible.

Sporadic goiter A simple non-toxic enlargement.

Substernal goiter Enlargement of the gland behind the sternum so that swelling in the neck may not be apparent.

Toxic goiter Signs of excess of thyroxine in the blood where the gland has not been previously enlarged. The patient complains of weight loss and is generally nervous. Exophthalmos maybe present.

Gold Symbol Au. A metallic element used in treating rheumatoid arthritis. Gold salts are among the most toxic of therapeutic agents. Toxic reactions may vary from mild to severe kidney or liver damage and blood dyscrasias.

Radioactive gold An isotope which gives off beta and gamma rays. Used in the form of small grains or seeds, it maybe implanted into malignant tissues. In colloidal form it maybe instilled into a serous cavity to treat malignant effusions.

Golden hour The initial 60 minutes after a major traumatic injury during which the definitive care and surgical intervention must be given to the patient for counter-acting long term and irreversible damage to vital organs.

Gold standard A standard with which other tests or procedures are compared.

Golgi apparatus *C. Golgi, Italian histologist, 1844–1926.* Specialized structures seen near the nucleus of a cell during microscopic examination.

Golgi cells Multipolar nerve cells in the cerebral cortex and posterior bones of spinal cord.

Golgi corpuscle A sensory nerve ending or receptor found in tendons and aponeuroses.

Golgi's organ The sensory end-organs in muscle tendons that are sensitive to stretch.

Goll's tract *SYN* – fasciculus gracilis, posterior white column of spinal cord.

Gonad A reproductive gland; the testicle or ovary.

Gonadal dysgenesis Congenital disorder with failure of ovaries to respond to pituitary gonadotrophin stimulation resulting in amenorrhea, failure of sexual maturation and short stature. Webbing of neck, cubitus valgus maybe present. Genetic pattern is 45XO (*SYN* – Turners' syndrome).

Gonadotropin Any hormone having a stimulating effect on the gonads. Two such hormones are secreted by the anterior pituitary: follicle stimulating hormone (FSH) and luteinizing hormone (LH), both of which are active, but with differing effects, in the two sexes.

Gonadotropic hormones (See Gonadotrophin).

Chorionic gonadotrophin A gonad-stimulating hormone produced by cytotrophoblastic cells of the placenta; used in the treatment of underdevelopment of the gonads and to induce ovulation in infertile women.

Gonadotropin releasing hormone Produced in hypothalamus, it acts on pituitary to cause release of Gonadotropic hormones.

Gonadotropic Having influence on the gonads.

Goniometer Apparatus to measure joint movement and angles.

Gonion [Gr.] The mid-point of the mandible (lower jaw).

Gonioscope An apparatus for examining the angle of the anterior chamber of the eye.

Goniotomy An operation for glaucoma; it consists in opening Schlemm's canal under direct vision.

Gonococcus *Neisseria gonorrhoeae,* a diplococcus which causes gonorrhea.

Gonorrhea A common venereal disease caused by *Neisseria gonorrhoeae* infecting the genital tract of either sex, causing a discharge and pain on micturition, although the disease is often asymptomatic in females. Spread by the bloodstream, it may give rise to iritis or arthritis. Scar tissue formation may bring about urethral stricture or infertility owing to occlusion of the uterine tubes. The eyes of babies maybe infected at birth during passage through the birth canal of an infected mother. The condition is called ophthalmia neonatorum (notifiable disease). In the past, it was a major cause of blindness in babies.

Gonorrheal Relating to gonorrhea.

Gonorrhael arthritis Intractable infection of joints, causing great pain and disability.

Goodell's sign Softening of the cervix during pregnancy.

Good Pasture's syndrome IgA nephropathy with hemoptysis and hemosiderosis.

Good Samaritan law Legal stipulation for protection of those who give first aid in emergency situation.

Goose flesh Transcient roughness of skin with contraction of arrector-pili muscles, as a reaction to cold or shock.

Goren's reflex Extension of great toe on pressure to calf muscles, a sign of pyramidal tract disease.

Gorget An instrument grooved to protect soft tissues from injury as pointed instrument is inserted in a body cavity.

Gossypol A toxic chemical of cotton seed.

Gouge A curved chisel used for scooping out diseased bone or other hard substances.

Goundou Bilateral hyperostosis of nasal bones.

Gout A hereditary form of arthritis with an excess of uric acid in the blood. It is characterized by painful inflammation and swelling of the smaller joints, especially those of the big toe and thumb. Inflammation is accompanied by the deposit of urates around the joints.

Gower's sign Clinical sign of muscular dystrophy in childhood. Affected children use their arms to push themselves by moving their hands up their thighs.

Gower's tract Spinocerebellar tract.

GPI General paralysis of the insane; dementia paralytica *(See Paralysis).*

Graafian follicle *R. de Graaf, Dutch physician and anatomist, 1641–1673.* A follicle which is formed in the ovary and contains an ovum. A follicle matures during each menstrual cycle, ruptures and releases the ovum (ovulation), which is then picked up by the fimbriated end of the uterine tube.

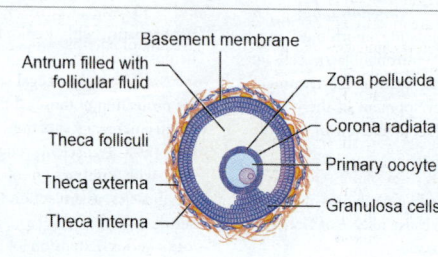

Basement membrane
Antrum filled with follicular fluid
Theca folliculi
Theca externa
Theca interna
Zona pellucida
Corona radiata
Primary oocyte
Granulosa cells

Graafian Follicle

G

Gracile nucleus Nucleus in medulla oblongata where fasciculus gracilis ends.

Gracilis A long slender muscle on the medial aspect of thigh.

Gradenigo's syndrome Suppurative otitis media with abducens nerve palsy.

Graft 1. Any tissue or organ for implantation or transplantation. 2. To implant or transplant such tissue.
Autogenous graft A graft taken from and given to the same individual.
Bone graft A portion of bone transplanted to repair another bone.
Corneal graft A portion of cornea, usually from a recently dead person, used to repair a diseased cornea.
Homologous graft Tissue obtained from the body of another animal of the same species but with a genotype differing from that of the recipient; a homo graft or allograft.
Pedicle graft A skin graft, one end of which attached to its original site until the grafting has become established.

Graft-versus-host disease (reaction) Abbreviated GVH disease. A condition that occurs when immunologically competent cells or their precursors are transplanted into an immunologically incompetent recipient (host) that is not histocompatible with the donor. Characteristic signs include skin lesions, ulceration, alopecia, painful joints and hemolytic anemia. GVH disease is a frequent complication of bone marrow transplants. Human leukocyte antigen (HLA) matching of the donor and recipient reduces the possibility of GVH disease.

Gram Symbol g. The fundamental SI unit of weight, equal to one thousandth of a kilogram.

Gram's stain *H. Gram, Danish physician, 1853–1938.* A method of staining bacteria which is used to classify them into gram-negative and gram-positive.

Grande multipara A woman who has given birth four or more children. Increasing parity can lead to an increased risk of problems in pregnancy, labor and the puerperium.

Grandiose In psychiatry, unrealistic and exaggerated concept of self worth, importance, ability, power and wealth.

Grand mal (Fr.) Major epilepsy *(See Epilepsy).*

Granular Containing small particles.
Granular casts The degenerated cells from the lining of renal tubules excreted in the urine in certain kidney disorders.

Granulation 1. The division of a hard solid substance into small particles. 2. The growth of new tissue by which ulcers and wounds heal when the edges are not in apposition. It consists of new capillaries and fibroblasts which fill in the space and later form fibrous tissue. The resulting scar is often unsightly.

Granule 1. A small particle or grain. 2. A small pill made of sucrose.

Granulocyte Any cell containing granules in its cytoplasm, especially polymorphonuclear leukocytes which contain neutrophilic, basophilic and eosinophilic granules in their cytoplasm.

Granulocytopenia A marked reduction in the number of granulocytes in the blood. The condition may precede agranulocytosis.

Granuloma A tumor composed of granulation tissue, usually due to chronic infection or invasion by a foreign body.

Granulomatosis An infection producing granulomata.

Lipoid granulocytosis Xanthomatosis; Hand-Schuller-Christian disease.

Malignant granulocytosis Lymphadenoma; Hodgkin's disease.

Granulopoiesis Formation of blood granulocytes.

Granulosa cell tumour Tumor of ovary secreting estrogens, hence feminizing in nature.

Graphesthesia The ability by which outlines, numbers, words, symbols traced or written upon skin are recognized.

Grasp to hold.

Grattage Removal of morbid growth by rubbing with a brush.

Grunt Abnormal sound heard during labored exhalation.

Gravel Small 'sandy' calculi formed in the kidneys and bladder and sometimes excreted with the urine. They can also form in the gallbladder where they can accumulate or cause low-grade cholecystitis.

Graves' disease *R.J. Graves, Irish physician, 1796–1853.* Exophthalmicgoitre; thyrotoxicosis.

Gravid Pregnant.

Gravity Weight.

Specific gravity The weight of a substance compared with that of an equal volume of water.

Gray matter Nervous tissue lying peripherally in brain and somewhat centrally in spinal cord where myelinated fibers do not predominate.

Gray (symbol Gy.) The SI unit used to denote the absorbed dose in radiation therapy.

Gray syndrome occusin new born Ashen gray colour, vomiting, cyanosis and flaccidity of newborn when treated with chloramphenicol.

Grey-scale display A method to show the texture of tissue on ultrasound display. The amplitude of each echo is represented by varying shades of grey. A bright white outline is seen from specular surfaces, a mottled grey from various tissue areas, and black from collections of fluid, such as the bladder and amniotic sac.

Grid A chart with horizontal and vertical lines on which curves maybe plotted.

Grief *(See Bereavement).*

Grinder's disease Chronic lung disease due to dust inhalation (*SYN*-Pneumoconiosis).

Gripes Spasmodic bowel pain, intestinal colic.

Griseofulvin An oral antifungal antibiotic that is used in the treatment of infections of the skin, hair and nails.

Grits Coarsely ground corn.

Groin The junction of the upper thigh with the abdomen. The groins slope outwards and upwards from the pubic region.

Grommet Ventilation tube placed across the tympanic membrane for

G

equalization of pressure in treatment of retracted tympanic membrane secondary to eustachian block/catarrh.

Groove Long narrow channel.

Ground itch Skin inflammation in foot due to invasion by larva of hookworm.

Grounded theory A qualitative research approach, which emphasizes the process of theory generation from systematically collected and stored data, the concept being that the theory remains 'grounded in' the data, demonstrating the fit between the theory and the supporting empirical evidence.

Group therapy A form of psychotherapy in which a group of patients meet regularly with the therapist in order to discuss and share problems, anxieties and fears in a psychotherapeutic setting. The group also provides emotional support for self-revelation and a structured environment for trying out new ways of relating to people.

Growing pains Recurrent quasi rheumatic limb pains peculiar to early youth, once believed to be caused by the growing process. It is now recognized that growth does not cause pain and that these pains can be a symptom of many different disorders.

Growth 1. The progressive development of a living thing, especially the process by which the body reaches its point of complete physical development. 2. An abnormal formation of tissue, such as a tumor.

Growth hormone A substance that stimulates growth, especially a secretion of the pituitary gland that directly influences protein, carbohydrate and lipid metabolism, and controls the rate of skeletal and visceral growth *(See Creutzfeldt-Jakob disease (CJD))*.

Guanethidine It is an adrenergic blocking agent. A drug used in treatment of hypertension.

Guanine A purine base, one of the constituents of all nucleic acids.

Guardian ad litem A person usually from the local authority social service department, who is appointed by a court to look after the interests of a child before its full Adoption Order is granted. Meanwhile the prospective adoptive parents have continuous possession of the child, and are visited and interviewed by the guardian *ad litem* to ensure that the home will be satisfactory.

Guardian Caldicott A named member of an NHS Trust who is responsible for agreeing and reviewing internal protocols governing the protection and use of patient identified information by staff within the health care system. This nominated person is also responsible for ensuring that these protocols meet the requirements of relevant national guidance and/or policies and that all systems in place are regularly monitored.

Gudden's law In division of a nerve, degeneration on the proximal portion is towards nerve cell.

Gugu lipid Lipid lowering agent.

Guided imagery A complementary therapy that uses pleasant mental images of events, feelings or sensations as a distraction method in coping with pain.

Guillain-Barre syndrome *G. Guillain, French neurologist, 1876–1961; A. Barre, French neurologist, 1880–1967.* Acute infective polyneuritis. After an infection, usually respiratory, there is a general weakness or paralysis which frequently affects the respiratory muscles as well as the peripheral ones.

Guillotine A surgical instrument used for excising tonsils.

Guilt Feeling grief for doing what is thought to be wrong.

Guinea pig A small rodent used in laboratory research.

Guinea worm A nematode worm, *Dracunculus medinensis*, which burrows into human tissues, particularly into the legs or feet.

Gulf War syndrome Also known as Gulf War illness, experienced by military personnel during the Gulf War and later wars. Has a variety of symptoms including chronic fatigue, muscle and joint pains, headaches, memory loss, depression and irritability. Possibly due to chemical exposure (e.g., to insecticides or nerve gas) or the interaction of multiple vaccinations and drugs given to protect personnel from the perceived threat of chemical or biological warfare combined with prolonged fatigue and stress.

Gum The fleshy tissue covering the alveolar process of jaw.

Gumboil The opening on the gum of an abscess at the root of a tooth.

Gumma A soft, degenerating tumor characteristic of the tertiary stage of syphilis. It may occur in any organ or tissue.

Gustatory Relating to taste.

Gustometry Measurement of sense of acuteness of taste.

Gut The intestine.

Guttering Groove in bone.

Guyon's canal A space at wrist between flexor retinaculum and palmar carpal ligament through which ulnar artery and ulnar nerve enter into the hand.

Guyon's sign Ballotment of kidney.

Guthrie test A blood test carried out on a neonate between the 6th and 14th days of life to diagnose phenylketonuria.

Gutta A drop.

    Guttapercha The juice of a tropical tree which, when dried, forms an elastic semisolid substance. Used in dentistry as a root filler.

GVH disease Graft-versus-host disease.

Gy Symbol for gray.

Gymnophobia Abnormal aversion to seeing a naked body.

Gynecoid Resembling female.

Gynecologist One who specializes in the diseases of the female genital tract.

Gynecology The science of those diseases that are peculiar to the female genital tract.

Gynecomastia Excessive growth of the male breast.

Gynndroid Individual having hermaphroditic sexual characteristics to be mistaken for a person of opposite sex.

Gypsum Plaster of Paris (calcium sulfate).

Gyrus A convolution, as of the cerebral cortex.

○●○

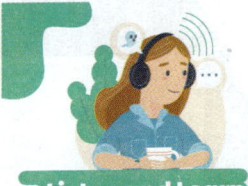

CBS Digital Dictionary *for Nurses*

Learn to Pronounce Correctly
(Audio Pronunciation of Difficult Words)

Listen and Learn

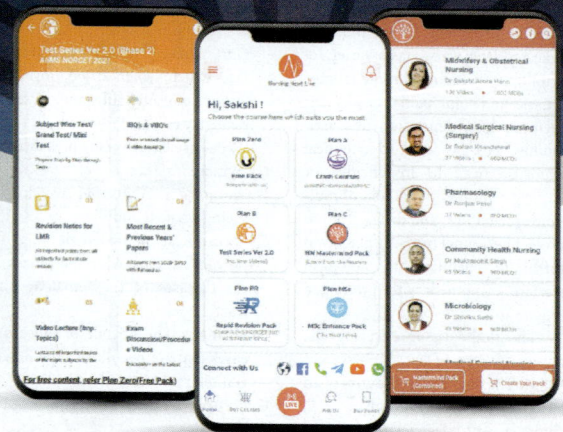

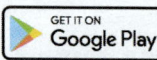
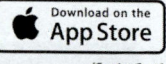
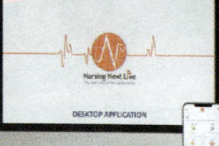

H Symbol for hydrogen.

HAART Highly active antiretroviral therapy involving a combination of various antiretroviral drugs which aim to treat patients of HIV.

Habenula A whip like structure; A stalk attached to pineal body of brain; a narrow band like structure.

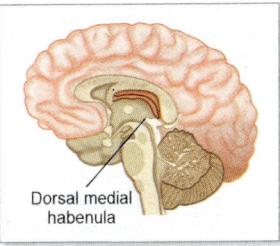

Dorsal medial habenula

Habenula

Habenular commissure A transverse band of fibers connecting the two habenular areas.

Habenular trigone A depressed triangular area located on the lateral aspect of the posterior third ventricle.

Habilitation The process of education and training person with disability both physical and mental to improve their ability to function in society.

Habit Automatic response to a specific situation acquired as a result of repetition and learning.

Drug habit Drug addiction.

Habit training A method used in psychiatric nursing whereby deteriorated patients can be rehabilitated and taught personal hygiene by constant repetition and encouragement.

Habituation The gradual adaptation to a stimulus or to the environment. The acquisition of a habit. e.g., a condition resulting from the repeated consumption of a drug, but with little or no tendency to increase the dose; there maybe psychic but no physical dependence on the drug.

Habitus A physical appearance that indicates a tendency to certain diseases or positioning of internal organs in certain planes.

Hacking cough Recurrent nonproductive cough.

Haemangioblastoma A tumor of the brain or spinal cord consisting of proliferated blood vessel cells.

Haemangioma A benign tumor formed by dilated blood vessels. *Strawberry Hemangioma* A birthmark, which maybecome very large, but frequently disappears in a few years.

Haemarthrosis An effusion of blood into a joint.

Haematemesis Vomiting of blood. If it has been in the stomach for some time and become partially digested by gastric juice, it is of a dark color and contains particles resembling coffee grounds.

Haematin The iron-containing part of hemoglobin.

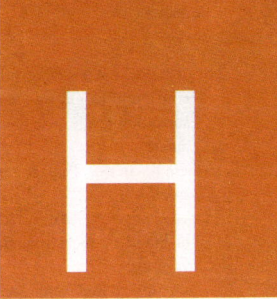

Haematocele A swelling produced by effusion of blood, e.g., in the sheath surrounding a testicle or a broad ligament.

Haematochezia Passage of bloody stool.

Haematocolpos An accumulation of blood or menstrual fluid in the vagina.

Haematocrit Red blood cells volume in blood.

Haematoidin A yellow-brown or red pigment formed from hemoglobin under reduced oxygen tension.

Haematology The science dealing with the nature, functions and diseases of blood.

Haematoma A swelling containing clotted blood.

Haematometra An accumulation of blood or menstrual fluid in the uterus.

Haematuria Passage of blood in urine.

Haematomyelia An effusion of blood into the spinal cord.

Haematosalpinx An accumulation of blood in the uterine tubes; haemosalpinx.

Haematuria The presence of blood in the urine, due to injury or disease of any of the urinary organs.

Haeme A protoporphyrin with 4 pyrrole groups that binds to oxygen for its carriage to tissues.

Haemocoagulation Clumping of RBC.

Haemoagglutinin An agglutinin that clumps RBC.

Haemobilia Blood in bile duct.

Haemochromatosis A congenital disorder of iron metabolism leading to excess iron accumulation in liver pancreas, and heart, SYN-bronze diabetes.

Haemoconcentration A loss of circulating fluid from the blood resulting in an increase in the proportion of red blood cells to plasma. The viscosity of the blood is increased.

Haemocyanin An oxygen carrying blue pigment in the plasma of arthropods and moluscus.

Haemocytoblast The primitive reticuloendothelial stem cell of bone marrow differentiating into various blood components.

Haemocytogenesis Formation of blood cells.

Haemocytology The study of the cellular contents of blood.

Haemocytometer An apparatus for counting the blood corpuscles in a specific volume of blood.

Haemodialysis The removal of waste material from the blood of a patient with acute or chronic renal failure by means of a dialyser or artificial kidney. The apparatus is coupled with an artery and dialysis is achieved by the blood and rinsing fluid (dialysate) passing through a semipermeable membrane. Blood is returned through a vein.

Haemodialyzer Device used in performing hemodialysis.

Haemodilution Reduction in relative concentration of RBC due to plasma volume expansion.

Haemodynamics Study of blood circulation.

Haemoflagellate Any flagellate protozoan of the blood, e.g., *Trypanosome, Leishmania.*

Haemofuscin A brown pigment derived from hemoglobins.

Haemoglobin (Hb) The complex protein molecule contained within the red blood cells which gives them their color and by which oxygen is transported.

Haemoglobinemia The presence of hemoglobin in the blood plasma.

Haemoglobinometer An instrument for estimating the hemoglobin content of the blood.

Haemoglobinuria Presence of hemoglobin in urine.

Haemoglobinopathy Anyone of a group of hereditary disorders, including sickle-cell anemia and thalassemia, in which there is an abnormality in the production of hemoglobin.

Haemogram Differential blood count.

Haemolysin A substance that destroys red blood cells. It maybe an antibody, a bacterial toxin or a component of a virus.

Haemolysis The disintegration of red blood cells. Excessive haemolysis, which may produce anemia, maybe caused by poisoning or by bacterial infection.

Haemolytic Having the power to destroy red blood cells.

Haemolytic disease of the new born A condition associated with rhesus incompatibility *(See Rhesus factor).*

Haemolytic uremic syndrome Characterized by microangiopathic haemolytic anemia, acute nephropathy and thrombocytopenia in children usually preceded by upper respiratory illness of GI upset.

Haemoperfusion Perfusioin of blood through substances, such as activated charcoal or ion exchange resins, to remove toxic material. The blood is not separated from the chemical or solution by semipermeable dialysis membrane unlike hemodialysis.

Haemopericardium Accumulation of blood in the pericardial sac.

Haemoperitoneum Accumulation of blood in peritoneal cavity.

Haemopexin A glycoprotein of beta-globulin that binds to hemin but not hemoglobin.

Haemophilia A condition characterized by impaired coagulability of the blood, and a strong tendency to bleed. Over 80% of all patients with haemophilia have haemophilia A (classic haemophilia), which is characterized by a deficiency of clotting factor VIII. Haemophilia B (Christ-mas disease), which affects about 15% of all haemophiliac patients, results from a deficiency of factor IX. Inherited as an X-linked recessive trait, it is transmitted by females only, to their male offsprings.

In order to avoid the debilitating and crippling effects of haemophilia, treatment must raise the level of the deficient clotting factor and maintain it in order to stop local bleeding. The patient must learn to avoid trauma and to obtain prompt treatment for bleeding episodes. Before surgery or dental treatment the patient must be given an infusion of the appropriate clotting factor.

Haemophilus A genus of Gram-negative rod-like bacteria.

Haemophilus ducreyi The cause of soft chancre.

Haemophilus influenza A species once thought to be the cause of epidemic influenza; it produces a highly fatal form of meningitis, especially in infants.

Haemophilus pertussis The cause of whooping cough; Bordet- Gengou bacillus.

Haemophthalmia Bleeding into the vitreous of the eye, usually the result of trauma; haemophthalmos.

Haemopneumothorax The presence of blood and air in the pleural cavity, usually the result of injury.

Haemopoiesis The formation of red blood cells, which normally takes place in the bone marrow and continues throughout life.

Extramedullary haemopoiesis The formation of blood cells other than in the bone marrow, e.g., in the liver or spleen.

Haemopoietic Relating to red blood cell formation.

Haemopoietic factors Those necessary for the development of red blood cells, e.g., vitamin B_{12} and folic acid.

H

H

Haemoptysis The coughing up of blood from the lungs or bronchi. Being aerated, it is bright-red and frothy.

Haemorrhage An escape of blood from a ruptured blood vessel, externally or internally. Arterial haemorrhage involves bright-red blood which escapes in rhythmic spurts, corresponding to the beats of the heart. Venous haemorrhage involves dark-red blood which escapes in an even flow. Haemorrhage may also be: primary, at the time of operation or injury; reactionary or recurrent, occurring later when the blood pressure rises and a ligature slips or a vessel opens up; secondary, as a rule about 10 days after injury, and usually due to sepsis. Special types are as follows:

Antepartum haemorrhage Which occurs before labor starts *(See Placenta (Praevia)).*

Cerebral haemorrhage An episode of bleeding into the cerebrum; one of the three main forms of stroke.

Concealed haemorrhage Collection of the blood in a cavity of the body.

Intracranial haemorrhage Bleeding within the cranium, which maybe extradural, subdural, subarachnoid or cerebral.

Intradural haemorrhage Bleeding beneath the dura mater. It maybe due to injury and causes signs of compression. The cerebrospinal fluid will be bloodstained.

Postpartum haemorrhage That which occurs within 12–24 hours of delivery, from the genital tract, and which either measures 500 mL or more, or which adversely affects the woman's condition. Secondary postpartum haemorrhage is excessive bleeding more than 24 hours after delivery.

Haemorrhagic Pertaining to or characterized by haemorrhage.

Haemorrhagic disease of the newborn A self-limited haemorrhagic disorder of the first days of life caused by deficiency of vitamin K-dependent blood clotting factors II, VII, IX and X. It should be prevented by the prophylactic administration of vitamin K to all newborn babies.

Viral haemorrhagic fevers A group of notifiable virus diseases of diverse etiology but with similar characteristics of fever, headache, myalgia, prostration and haemorrhagic symptoms. They include dengue haemorrhagic fever, Marburg disease, Ebola virus disease, Lassa fever and yellow fever.

Haemorrhoid A "pile" or locally dilated rectal vein. Piles maybe either external or internal to the anal sphincter. Pain is caused on defecation, and bleeding may occur.

Haemorrhoidectomy The surgical removal of haemorrhoids.

Haemosiderosis Iron deposits in the tissues resulting from excessive haemolysis of red blood cells.

Haemostasis The arrest of bleeding or the slowing up of blood flow in a vessel.

Haemostatic A drug or remedy for arresting haemorrhage; a styptic.

Haemothorax Blood in the thoracic cavity, e.g., from injury to soft tissues as a result of fracture of a rib.

HAI Hospital-acquired infection.

Hageman factor Blood coagulation factor, helps in kinin synthesis.

Hair A delicate keratinized epidermal filament growing out of the skin. The root of the hair is enclosed beneath the skin in a tubular follicle.

Hair ball (See Bezoar).

Hair analysis Investigation for chemical composition of hair to exclude toxic chemical intoxication, state of nutrition and monitoring course of certain diseases.

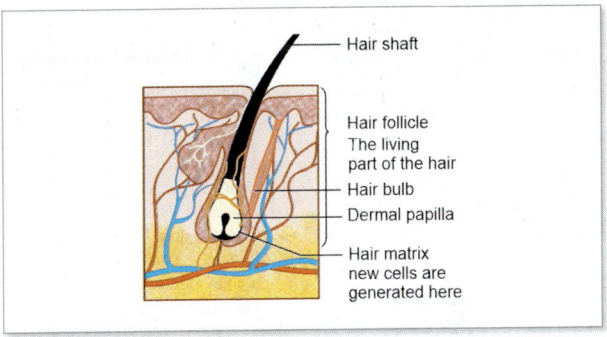

- Hair shaft
- Hair follicle
  The living
  part of the hair
- Hair bulb
- Dermal papilla
- Hair matrix
  new cells are
  generated here

Structure of Hair

H

Hair bulb The lower expanded portion of a hair.

Hair follicle An invagination of the epidermis that forms a cylindrical depression extending into subepidermal layer. Sebaceous glands and arrectores pili muscles are attached to these hair follicles.

Hair papilla A projection of dermis extending into hair bulb at the bottom of hair follicle. It contains capillaries through which hair receives its nourishment.

Hair transplantation Technique of transferring skin containing hair follicles from one place to another; done to treat alopecia.

Hailey-Hailey disease Benign familial pemphigus.

Hairy tongue Tongue covered with hair-like papilla with threads of aspergillus or candida.

Halal Meat from an animal that has been killed according to Islamic law and is therefore awful to be eaten by Muslims.

Halazone A chloramines water disinfectant.

Halcinonide A corticosteroid.

Haldol Trade name for a preparation of haloperidol, an antipsychotic agent.

Half-life 1. Time required for radioactive substance to reduce to one-half its energy due to metabolism or excretion. 2. Time required for radioactive nuclei undergoing decay to lose half their radioactivity 3. Time taken by body to inactivate half of the administered drug/chemical (biological half-life).

Halfway house A facility to house mental patients who do not need hospitalization but who are not ready for independent living.

Halibut oil A vitamin (A and D)- rich oil derived from the liver of halibut.

Halide Compound containing a halogen, i.e., bromine, chlorine, fluorine or iodine.

Halitosis Foul-smelling breath.

Hallervorden-Spatz disease An inherited progressive degenerative disease beginning in childhood manifesting with rigidity, athetotic movements and mental retardation.

Hallucination A sensory impression (sight, touch, sound, smell or taste) that has no basis in external stimulation. Hallucinations can have psychological causes, as in mental illness, or they can result from drugs, alcohol, organic illnesses, such as brain tumor or senility, or exhaustion.

Hallucinations rating scale Abbreviated HRS. It is a scale that uses 11 items to determine auditory hallucinations in patients. It also assesses the way in which the hallucinations are experienced and controlled by the patient.

Hallucinogen An agent that causes hallucinations, e.g., LSD and cannabis.

Hallucinosis The state of having hallucinations.

Hallux The big toe.

Hallux valgus A deformity in which the big toe is bent toward the other toes.

Hallux varus A deformity in which the big toe is bent outward away from the other toes.

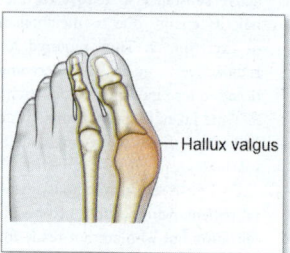

Hallux Valgus

Halo A circular structure, such as a luminous circle seen surrounding an object or light.

Halo glaucomatous A narrow light zone surrounding the optic disk in glaucoma.

Halo effect A beneficial effect noted after a health care intervention, visit or research project. The halo effect cannot be attributed to the content of the interview, visit or project but is the outcome of indefinable factors as a result of the intervention.

Halo splint An orthopedic device used to immobilize the head and neck to assist in the healing of cervical injuries and postoperatively after cervical surgery.

Halofantrine Antimalarial agent.

Halogen One of the nonmetallic elements (others are chlorine, iodine, bromine and fluorine).

Haloperidol A sedative and tranquilizer used in the treatment of schizophrenia and other psychiatric disorders, particularly mania.

Haloprogin Halogenated phenolic ether, fungicidal.

Halothane A widely used anesthetic; used as an inhalation to induce and maintain anesthesia.

Halsted's operation Operation done for radical correction of inguinal hernia.

Halsted's suture Suture placed through the subcuticular fascia that is used for exact skin approximation.

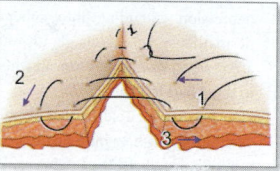

Halsted's Suture

Hamamelis A soothing agent prepared from witch hazel and used in suppository form in the treatment of hemorrhoids.

Hamartoma A benign nodule which is an overgrowth of mature tissue.

Hamate bone The medial bone in the distal row of carpal bones of wrist.

Hammer The malleus.

Hammer toe A deformity in which the first phalanx is bent upwards, with plantar flexion of the second and third phalanx.

Hammer finger Flexion deformity of the distal joint of a finger, caused by avulsion of extensor tendon.

Hamstring The flexors of the knee joint that are situated at the back of the thigh.

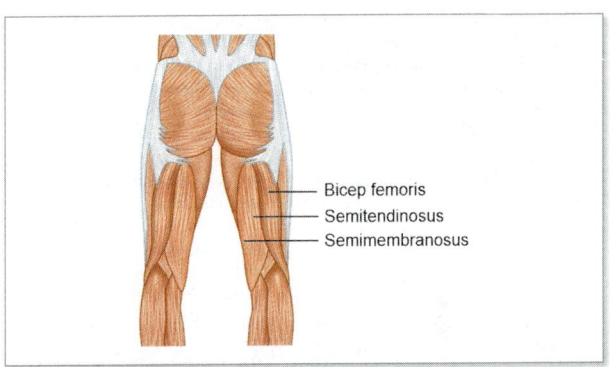

Hamstring Muscles

Ham test Test for diagnosis of paroxysmal nocturnal hemoglobinuria. The red cells lyse in acidic medium.

Hand drugs An imprecise term used in relation to drugs that are highly addictive, e.g., heroin or cocaine, and therefore prone to misuse.

Hand The terminal part of the arm below the wrist.

Claw hand A paralytic condition in which the hand is flexed and the fingers contracted, caused by injury to nerves or muscles.

Cleft hand A congenital deformity in which the cleft between the third and fourth fingers extends into the palm.

Hand, foot and mouth disease A mild infectious disease in children, caused by coxsackievirus, which results in vesicle formation on all three sites. Not the same as foot and mouth disease.

Hand washing *(See Annexure 11).*

Hand-arm vibration syndrome Pain and numbness with blanching in the hand and arm due to the use of vibrating tools, usually in the workplace. The syndrome tends to develop slowly over time and gangrene may develop. Exposure to cold tends to aggravate the condition.

Hand-Schüller-Christian disease *A. Hand, American pediatrician, 1868–1949; A. Schüller Austrian neurologist, 1874–1958; HA Christian, American physician, 1876–1951.* A disease of the reticuloendothelial system in which granulomata-containing cholesterol are formed, chiefly in the skull.

Handicap A disadvantage for a given individual, resulting from an impairment or a disability that limits or prevents the fulfilment of a role that is normal (depending on age, sex, and social and cultural factors) for that individual.

Hangman's fracture Fracture dislocation of upper cervical spine due to judicial hanging.

Hang nail Partly detached piece of skin at root or lateral edge of finger or toe nail.

Hangover Headache, depression, fatigue and irritability present some times after consumption of alcohol or CNS depressant.

Hansen's bacillus Lepra bacillus.

Hansen's disease *GHA Hansen, Norwegian physician, 1841–1912.* Leprosy, caused by Hansen's bacillus, *Mycobacterium leprae*.

Haploid Having one set of chromosomes after division instead of two.

Hapten That portion of an antigen determining its immunological specificity.

Haptephobia Aversion of being touched by another person.

Haptoglobin Mucoprotein accepting hemoglobin in plasma on release in hemolytic conditions. Hence hepatoglobin is decreased in hemolytic disorders and increased in certain inflammatory conditions.

Harassment Any repetitive physical or verbal conduct that causes distress in another person, including physically threatening, humiliating, offensive or derogatory acts or utterances. Harassment is unlawful and examples include bullying, workplace violence, sexual harassment, racial, age or gender discrimination and cyberstalking. Harassment can occur in health care settings and this may take many forms, but an example is when a consultant, manager or senior professional repeatedly makes derisory or critical comments to another member of staff in front of patients or colleagues, it leads to loss of confidence and feeling of incapability in the workplace in that person.

Hardness Water with less cleansing action due to presence of soluble salts of calcium and magnesium. These compounds precipitate with soap.

Harelip A cleft in the upper lip due to faulty fusion of median nasal process and the lateral maxillary processes.

Harelip suture A twisted figure-of- eight suture used in surgical correction of harelip.

Harlequin fetus Newborn with skin features of ichthyosis with deep red fissures.

Harpoon A device with a hook on the end for obtaining small pieces of tissue.

Harrison's groove or sulcus *E. Harrison, British physician, 1789-1838.* A horizontal groove along the lower border of the thorax corresponding to the costal insertion of the diaphragm; seen in rickets.

Harris-Benedict equation Equation for calculating basal body energy expenditure.

Hartman's solution A solution of 0.6 g NaCl, 0.03 g KCl, 0.02 g $CaCl_2$ and 0.31 g sodium lactate in 100 mL of water used for fluid and electrolyte replacement.

Hartmann's solution A saline solution containing sodium lactate used intravenously in treating acidosis.

Hartnup disease A hereditary defect in amino acid metabolism which may produce learning difficulties (named after the first person found to suffer from it).

Harvey, William British physician who described circulation of blood.

Hashimoto's disease *H Hashimoto, Japanese surgeon, 1881–1934.* A lymphoadenoid goitre caused by the formation of antibodies to thyroglobulin. It is an autoimmune condition giving rise to hypothyroidism.

Hashish Indian hemp *(See Cannabis).*

Hassal's corpuscle Spherical bodies with central area of degeneration with surrounding flattened cells, seen in thymus gland.

Haunch The hips and buttocks.

Haustration A haustrum, or the process of forming one.

Haustrum Anyone of the pouches formed by the sacculations of the colon.

Haversian canal *C Havers, British physician and anatomist, 1650–1702.* One of the minute canals that permeate compact bone, containing blood and lymph vessels to maintain its nutrition *(See Bone).*

Haversian gland Minute projections from the surface of synovial tissue into the joint space.

Haversian system Architectural unit of bone consisting of haversian canals, with alternate layers of intercellular matrix surrounding it in concentric cylinders.

Hawthorne effect The term given to the usual beneficial effect of a study on the persons participating in the study. It was named after an industrial management study in the USA, where the effect was first identified.

Hay fever An atopic allergy characterized by sneezing, itching and watery eyes, running nose and a burning sensation of the palate and throat. It is a localized anaphylactic reaction to an extrinsic allergen, most commonly pollens and the spores of molds. When the allergen comes in contact with mast cell bound IgE immunoglobulin in the tissues of the conjunctiva, nasal mucosa and bronchial tree, the cells release mediators of anaphylaxis and heal/produce the characteristic symptoms of hay fever. Atopy.

hCG Human chorionic gonadotropin *(See Gonadotropin).*

HCl Hydrochloric acid

He Symbol for helium.

HEA Health education authority. A special health authority responsible for giving authoritative advice both nationally and locally on a wide range of health education issues through campaigns and publications (formerly the Health Education Council). Now an integral part of the health service and thus participates with other health authorities in planning health service policies and priorities.

Head The anterior or superior part of a structure or organism, in vertebrates containing the brain and the organs of special sense.

Head injury Traumatic injury to the head resulting from a fall or violent blow. Such an injury maybe open or closed and may involve a brain concussion, skull fracture, or contusions of the brain. All head injuries are potentially dangerous because there maybe a slow leakage of blood from damaged blood vessels into the brain, or the formation of a blood clot which gradually increases pressure against brain tissue. Long-term effects of head injury may include chronic headache, disturbances in mental and motor function, and a host of other symptoms that may or may not be psychogenic. Organic brain damage and post-traumatic epilepsy resulting from scar formation are possible sequels to head injury.

Headache A pain or ache in the head. A symptom rather than a disorder. It accompanies many diseases and conditions, including emotional distress *(See also Migraine).*

Heaf test *FGR Heaf, British physician, 1894–1973.* A form of tuberculin testing. A drop of tuberculin solution on the skin is injected by means of a number of very short needles mounted on a spring-loaded device (Heaf's gun).

Healing The process of return to normal function after a period of disease or injury.

Healing by first intention Union of the edges of a clean incised wound without visible granulations, and leaving only a faint linear scar.

Healing by second intention Union of the edges of an open wound by the formation of granulations from the bottom and sides.

Healing by third intention Union of a wound that is closed surgically several days after the injury.

Health and Care Professions Council (HCPC) Previously the Health Professions Council, is a UK independent body created in 2001 to protect the public by setting and maintaining

H

standards for proficiency and conduct for the professions it regulates. It currently regulates several professions including: arts therapists; biomedical scientists; chiropodists/podiatrists; clinical scientists; dietitians; hearing aid dispenser; occupational therapists; operating department practitioners; orthoptists; paramedics; physiotherapists; practitioner psychologists; prosthetists/orthotists; radiographers; social workers (in England); speech and language therapists. Health Protection Agency (HPA) became part of Public Health England in 2013.

Health and Safety at Work Act 1974 Comprehensive legislation that came into force in 1975. It deals with the welfare, health and safety of all employers and employees, except domestic workers in a private house. The Health and Safety Executive (HSE) enforces health and safety law in the UK. The HSE is the independent watchdog for work-related health, safety and illness. It acts in the public interest to reduce work-related deaths and serious injury. It is an executive non-departmental body sponsored by the Department for Work and Pensions.

The Health and Safety Commission (HSC) Merged into the HSE in 2008.

Health record Is any record information relating to someone's physical or mental health that has been made by (or on behalf of) a health professional. This could be anything from the notes made by a GP in a local surgery to results of an MRI scan or X-rays. Health records contain personal, sensitive and confidential information. They are usually held electronically or occasionally as paper files by a range of health professionals both in the NHS and the private sector. For the purpose of the Data Protection Act, a registered professional can be one of the following people; registered medical practitioner, dentist, dispensing optician or optometrist, pharmacist or pharmacy technician, child psychotherapist, a scientist employed in a hospital as head of department, registered nurse or midwife, osteopath or chiropractor, any person registered as a member of a profession to which the health and social work professions order extends.

Health Service Ombudsman UK Appointed to protect the interests of patients in relation to the administration and provision of health care delivered in the NHS. The Commissioner is responsible to Parliament and can investigate complaints and allegations of maladministration by a health authority, NHS Trusts and the clinical practice of medical practitioners. See Ombudsman.

Health The World Health Organization (WHO, 1998) states that "Health is a dynamic state of complete physical, mental social and spiritual wellbeing and not merely the absence of disease or infirmity".

Health assessment An evaluation made by a health-care professional of an individual's health status, which takes account of the health history and lifestyle together with the findings of a physical examination.

Health authority A body through which the National Health Service is administered at district level.

Health center A community health organization for providing ambulatory health care and coordinating the efforts of all health agencies, commonly focused around the general practitioner's services.

Health culture A system that attempts to explain and treat health problems and illness and to maintain health. Part of the wider culture to which people belong, it maybe a traditional or a biomedical system.

Health education officer An officer appointed to make health education resources available to the community.

Health services The term is usually employed to connote the system or program by which health care is made available to the population and financed by government or private enterprise, or both.

Health statistics Summative data on any aspect of the health of populations; for example, mortality, morbidity, use of health services, treatment outcome, costs of health care.

Holistic health A system of preventive medicine that takes into account the whole individual, and that person's own responsibility for well-being, with the total influences (social, psychological, environmental) that affect health, including nutrition, exercise and mental relaxation.

Public health The field of medicine that is concerned with safeguarding and improving the health of the community as a whole.

Health care-associated infection (HCAI; sometimes abbreviated as HAI); Also known as nosocomial infections. An infection acquired during an episode of health care in either acute (hospital) or non-acute settings, usually as a result of a clinical intervention, such as urinary catheterization or the insertion of a vascular access device. *(See Annexure 11).*

Health certificate An official statement signed by a physician attesting to state of health.

Health care assistant Abbreviated HCA. A support worker in the clinical area who works under the supervision of a registered practitioner responsible for the quality of care delivered by the HCA. An HCA should receive training for their role

including accessing a clinical health-care apprenticeship.

Health care system An organized plan of health services. The term is usually employed to denote the system or program by which health care is made available to the population and financed by government or private enterprise or both.

Health education Various methods of education aimed at the prevention of disease. All nurses, midwives and health visitors have particular responsibilities and opportunities to promote good health.

Health hazard Any substance, condition or circumstances not conducive to good health.

Health visitor A registered nurse who may also be a midwife and who has completed a 52-week full-time course in social and preventive medicine leading to a health visiting certificate. The main area of responsibility of health visitors is health education and preventive care of mothers and children under 5 years old, although some specialize in school health and preventive care of the elderly.

Hearing The reception of sound waves and their transmission onward to the brain in the form of nerve impulses.

Hearing aid An apparatus, usually electronic, to amplify sounds before they reach the inner ear.

Heart A hollow, muscular organ which pumps the blood throughout the body, situated behind the sternum slightly toward the left side of the thorax.

Heart attack Myocardial infarction.

Heart block Impairment of conduction in heart excitation; often applied specifically to atrioventricular heart block.

Heart failure Maybe acute, as in coronary thrombosis, or chronic.

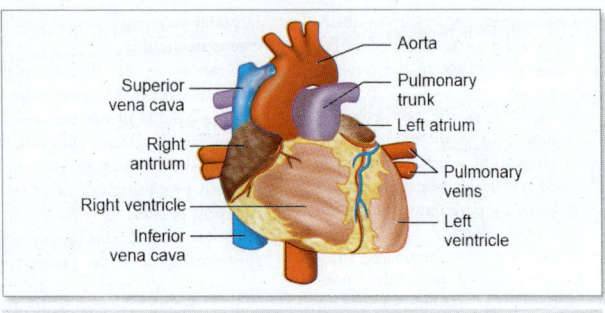

Labels on the diagram: Superior vena cava, Right antrium, Right ventricle, Inferior vena cava, Aorta, Pulmonary trunk, Left atrium, Pulmonary veins, Left veintricle

Heart

H

Heart-lung machine An apparatus used to perform the functions of both the heart and the lungs during heart surgery.

Heart murmur An abnormal sound heard in the heart, frequently caused by disease of the valves. Occurs when the blood flow through the heart exceeds a certain velocity.

Heart sounds The sound heard when listening to the heartbeat. They are caused by the closure of the valves.

Heartburn Indigestion marked by a burning sensation in the oesophagus, often with regurgitation of acid fluid. Pyrosis.

Heat Warmth. A form of energy, which may cause an increase in temperature or a change of state, e.g., the conversion of water into steam.

Heat exhaustion A rapid pulse, anorexia, dizziness, and cramps in arms, legs or abdomen, sometimes followed by sudden collapse, caused by loss of body fluids and salts under very hot conditions.

Prickly heat Miliaria; heat rash. Acute itching caused by blocking of the ducts of the sweat glands following profuse sweating.

Heat stroke A severe life-threatening condition resulting from prolonged exposure to heat *(See Sunstroke).*

Hebephrenia A form of schizophrenia characterized by thought disorder and emotional incongruity. Delusions and hallucinations are common.

Heberden's nodes *W Heberden, British physician, 1710–1801.* Bony or cartilaginous outgrowths causing deformity of the terminal finger joints in osteoarthritis.

Hebetude Emotional dullness. A common symptom in dementia and schizophrenia.

Hectic Occurring regularly.

Hectic fever A regularly occurring increase in temperature; it is frequently observed in pulmonary tuberculosis.

Hectic flush A redness of the face accompanying a sudden rise in temperature.

Hedonism Excessive devotion to pleasure.

Hegar's dilators *A Hegar, German gynecologist, 1830-1914.* A series of graduate dilators used to dilate the uterine cervix.

Heimlich maneuver *HJ Heimlich, American physician, b. 1920.* A technique for removing foreign matter from the trachea of a choking person. Wrap the arms around the victim and allow that person's torso to hang forward. Make a fist with one hand and grasp it with the other, then with both hands against the victim's abdomen (above the navel and below the rib cage), forcefully press into the abdomen with a sharp upward thrust. The manoeuvre maybe repeated several times if necessary to clear the air passages. If the victim is unconscious or prone, turn that person on to the back, kneel astride the torso and with both hands use the manoeuvre as described.

Heinz bodies Inclusions in erythrocytes consisting of damaged aggregated hemoglobin and is associated with some forms of hemolytic anemia.

Helicobacter A genus of spiral and flagellated Gram-negative bacteria.

Helicobacter pylori A species found in the stomach. May cause damage to the prostaglandins protecting the mucosal cells in the stomach wall, leading to progressive gastritis and ulceration.

Heliotherapy Treatment of disease by exposure of the body to sunlight.

Helium Symbol He. An inert gas sometimes used in conjunction with oxygen to facilitate respiration in obstructional types of dyspnea and for decompressing deep-sea divers.

Helix 1. A spiral twist. Used to describe the configuration of certain molecules, e.g., deoxyribonucleic acid (DNA). 2. The outer rim of the auricle of the ear.

HELLP syndrome Life-threatening complication of pregnancy characterized by hemolysis, elevated liver enzymes, and low platelet count and considered to be a variant of preeclampsia.

Hellin's law One in about 89 pregnancies ends in the birth of twins; one in 892, or 7921, in the birth of triplets; one in 893, or 704, 969, in the birth of quadruplets. Infertility treatments have raised the rate of multiple pregnancies.

Helminthiasis An infestation with worms.

Hemeralopia Day blindness. The vision is poor in a bright light but is comparatively good when the light is dim *(See Nyctalopia).*

Hemianesthesia Anesthesia (loss of sensation) of one-half of body due to lesion in internal capsule.

Hemianopia Partial blindness, in which the patient can see only half of the normal field of vision. It arises from disorders of the optic tract and of the occipital lobe.

Hemiballismus Involuntary chorea-like movements only on one side of the body.

Hemicolectomy The removal of the ascending part of the transverse colon with an ileotransverse colostomy.

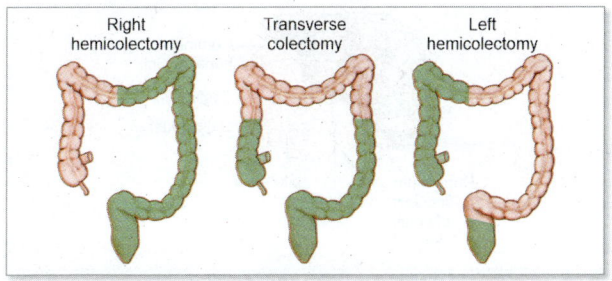

Hemicolectomy

Hemiparesis Paralysis on one side of the body; hemiplegia.

Hemiplegia Paralysis of one half of the body, usually due to cerebral disease or injury. The lesion is on the side of the brain opposite to the side paralysed.

Hemisacralization Abnormal development of one-half of fifth lumbar vertebra fusing with the sacrum.

Hemispasm Spasm of one side of body or face.

Hemisphere A half sphere. In anatomy, one of the two halves of the cerebrum or cerebellum.

Hemithorax One-half of the chest.

Hemivertebra Congenital absence or failure of development of half of vertebra.

Hemp *(See Cannabis)*.

Henderson Hasselbalch equation An equation for expression of pH.

Henle's loop *FGJ Henle, German anatomist, 1809–1885.* The U shaped loop of the uriniferous tubule of the kidney.

Henoch's purpura *EH Henoch, German pediatrician, 1820–1910.* Allergic purpura.

Henoch-Schonleln Purpura E.H. Henoch, German pediatrician, 1820-1910. Allergic Purpura.

Henry's law The weight of a gas dissolved by a given volume of liquid at a constant temperature is directly proportional to the pressure.

Heparin An anticoagulant formed in the liver and circulated in the blood. Injected intravenously it prevents the conversion of prothrombin into thrombin, and is used in the treatment of thrombosis.

Hepatectomy Excision of a part or the whole of the liver.

Hepatic Relating to the liver.

Hepatic coma Impaired CNS function due to liver dysfunction. Coma results from increased serum ammonia, false neurotransmitters and middle molecules, the toxic products of protein metabolism. Common precipitating factors are high protein diet, bleeding into GI tract, infections, electrolyte imbalance, diuretics and drugs.

Hepatic duct The bile channel from liver that joins with cystic duct to form common bile duct *(See figure)*.

Hepatic flexure The angle of the colon that is situated under the liver.

Hepatic veins The three veins draining right and left lobes of liver into inferior vena cava.

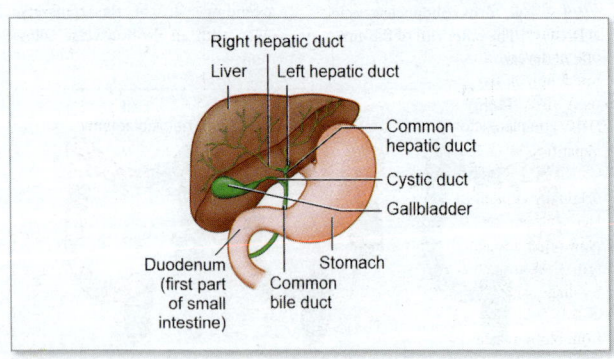

Right hepatic duct
Liver   Left hepatic duct
Common hepatic duct
Cystic duct
Gallbladder
Duodenum (first part of small intestine)   Stomach
Common bile duct

Hepatic Duct

Hepaticojejunostomy The anastomosis of the hepatic duct to the jejunum, usually created after extensive excision for carcinoma of the pancreas.

Hepaticostomy A surgical opening into the hepatic duct.

Hepatitis Inflammation of the liver.

Alcoholic hepatitis history of excessive indulgence in alcohol, with tender hepatomegaly, icterus and marked elevation of SGOT and SGPT.

Amoebic hepatitis Inflammation that may arise during amebic dysentery and lead to liver abscesses.

Anicteric hepatitis Viral hepatitis without jaundice, tending to occur chiefly in infants and young children; symptoms include mild anorexia and gastrointestinal disturbances, slight fever, and enlargement and tenderness of the liver.

Fulminant hepatitis (acute hepatitis with coma) An acute fulminating form of hepatitis resulting from extensive hepatic necrosis. It maybe due to: (a) Toxic liver injury, as in carbon tetrachloride poisoning or paracetamol overdosage; (b) A hypersensitivity reaction to a drug, such as halothane; or (c) Viral hepatitis. Death is usually caused by acute yellow atrophy of the liver.

Viral hepatitis An acute, notifiable, infectious hepatitis caused by one of several different viruses that infect human liver cells, e.g., hepatitis A virus (HAV), hepatitis B virus (HBV), hepatitis C virus (HCV) and hepatitis E virus (HEV).

Hepatitis–associated antigen It was originally applied to hepatitis B surface antigen or Australia antigen. Now other antigens like core antigen (Hbc), "e" antigen are also identified for diagnosis of hepatitis B infection.

Hepatitis B immunoglobulin Derived from blood plasma of human donors who have high titer of antibodies against hepatitis B.

Hepatitis B vaccine A recombinant vaccine with hepataitis B surface antigen given as 20 µg. Dose-3 doses, to persons at high risk.

Hepatization The alteration of lung tissue into a solid mass resembling liver, which occurs in acute lobar pneumonia.

Hepatoblastoma Malignant teratoma of liver.

Hepatogenic Having its origin in the liver.

Hepatogenous Arising in the liver. Applied to jaundice in which the disease arises in the parenchymal cells of the liver.

Hepatojugular reflex Pressure on the liver or right upper abdomen causes a rise in jugular venous pressure in patients of congestive heart failure.

Hepatolenticular Pertaining to the liver and the lentiform nucleus.

Hepatolenticular degeneration Wilson's disease; a progressive condition, usually occurring between the ages of 10 and 25 years. There are tremors of the head and limbs, pigmentation of the cornea and sometimes defective twilight vision.

Hepatology Study of liver.

Hepatoma A primary malignant tumor arising in the liver cells.

Hepatomegaly An enlargement of the liver.

Hepatorenal syndrome Kidney dysfunction with uremia secondary to acute or chronic hepatic catastrophe.

Hepatosis Non-inflammatory disease of liver.

Hepatosplenomegaly Enlargement of the liver and spleen, such as maybe found in kala-azar.

Hepatotoxic Applied to drugs and substances that cause destruction of liver cells.

Herb A plant with soft stem containing little wood, usually seasonal.

Herbal medicine A form of complementary or alternative medicine in which plants are used for their therapeutic properties. Also called phytotherapy.

Herd immunity The immunity of a population. When there is a high enough number of persons in a population immune to a particular infection, the infection fails to spread because of the absence of enough susceptibles. For example, in measles this could probably be achieved by vaccination of 90–95% of the population.

Hereditary Derived from ancestry; inherited.

Heredity The transmission of both physical and mental characteristics to the offspring from the parents. Recessive characteristics may miss one or two generations and reappear later.

Heredofamilial Any disease recurring in family members due to inherited defect or other familial factors.

Hering–Breuer reflex Reflex inhibition of inspiration resulting from stimulation of lung receptors following lung inflation.

Hering's serve Afferent nerve fibers from carotid sinus passing to brain via glossopharyngeal nerve. A rise in blood pressure stimulates these nerves to reflexly diminish heart rate.

Heritage The genetic and other characteristics transmitted from parents to offsprings.

Hermaphrodite An individual whose gonads contain both testicular and ovarian tissue. These maybe combined as an ovotestis or there maybe a testis on one side and an ovary on the other. The external genitalia maybe indeterminate or of either sex.

Pseudo-hermaphrodite One whose gonads are histologically of one sex but in whom the genitalia have the appearance of the opposite sex.

True hermaphrodite One who possesses both male and female gonads.

Hermaphroditism Existence of ovarian and testicular tissue in same individual.

Hermeneutics The study of meanings in social behavior and experience. It denotes the art, skill or theory of interpreting human behavior, speech and writings in terms of intentions and meanings.

Hermetic Airtight. A wound dressing maybe sealed to ensure that the wound is not exposed to air.

Hernia A protrusion of any part of the internal organs through the structures enclosing them.

Cerebral hernia A protrusion of brain through the skull.

Diaphragmatic hernia and *hiatus hernia* A protrusion of a part of the stomach through the esophageal opening in the diaphragm.

Femoral hernia A loop of intestine protruding into the femoral canal. More common in females.

Incisional hernia A hernia occurring at the site of an old wound.

Inguinal hernia Protrusion of the intestine through the inguinal canal. This maybe congenital or acquired, and is more common in males. A rupture.

Irreducible hernia A hernia that cannot be replaced by manipulation.

Reducible hernia A hernia that can be returned to its normal position by manipulative measures.

Strangulated hernia A hernia of the bowel in which the neck of the sac containing the bowel is so constricted that the venous circulation is impeded, and gangrene will result if not treated promptly.

Umbilical hernia Protrusion of bowel through the umbilical ring. This maybe congenital or acquired.

Vaginal hernia Rectocele or cystocele.

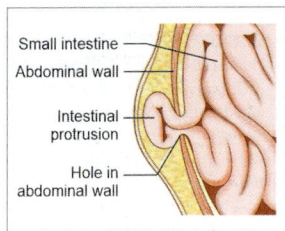

Small intestine
Abdominal wall
Intestinal protrusion
Hole in abdominal wall

Strangulated Hernia

Hernial sac The pouch of peritoneum pushed before the hernia and into which it descends.

Herniated disc Rupture of nucleus pulposus through annulus fibrosus to protrude into spinal canal.

Hernioplasty A plastic repair of the abdominal wall performed after reduction of a hernia.

Herniorrhaphy Removal of a hernia sac and repair of the abdominal wall.

Herniotomy An operation to remove a hernial sac.

Heroin A diacetate of morphine used as an analgesic and abused illicitly for its euphoriant effects. The drug readily induces physical dependence and maybe sniffed, smoked ("chasing the dragon") or injected subcutaneously or intravenously ("shooting up" or "mainlining"). Slang terms for heroin include "smack", "H" and "brown sugar".

Heroin babies Babies who have received regular heroin (morphine) via the placenta before birth and who show signs of withdrawal after birth. Withdrawal symptoms may persist for 1–4 weeks and include vomiting, diarrhea, sweating, breathing difficulties and hyperactivity.

Herpes An inflammatory skin eruption showing small vesicles caused by a herpes virus.

Herpes simplex A viral infection which gives rise to localized vesicles in the skin and mucous membranes and is characterized by latency and subsequent recurrence. It is caused by herpes simplex viruses type 1 and 2. Type 1 infection is common in children and is often symptomless. Type 2 infection is common in older age groups and is associated with sexual activity. Lesions appear on the cervix, vulva and surrounding skin in women and on the penis in men. In homosexual men rectal lesions are common. Recurrent genital herpes may follow primary infection. Type 2 virus may cause aseptic meningitis.

Herpes zoster A local manifestation of reactivation of infection of the varicella zoster virus, the causative agent of chickenpox, characterized by a vesicular rash in the area of distribution of a sensory nerve. Called also shingles.

Herpes virus One of a group of DNA containing viruses. They include the causative agents of herpes simplex, herpes zoster, chickenpox, cytomegalic inclusion disease and infective mononucleosis.

Herring bodies Neurosecretory granules in the terminal nerve endings of hypothalamus and hypophyseal tract.

Hertz A unit of frequency equivalent to one cycle per second.

Hesperidin A chemical present in orange and lemon peel that is hemostatic by strengthening the capillaries.

Hesselbach's hernia Hernia passing through cribiform fascia.

Hesselbach's triangle Triangular space bounded by Poupart's ligament below, outer border of rectus sheath and epigastric artery.

Hess's test *AF Hess, American physician, 1875–1933.* A test used to diagnose purpura. An inflated blood pressure cuff causes an increase in capillary pressure and rupture of the walls, causing purpuric spots to develop.

H

Heterochromia A difference in color in the irises of the two eyes or in different parts of one iris. It maybe congenital or secondary due to inflammation.

Heterogeneous Composed of diverse constituents.

Heterogenesis Production of offsprings that have different characteristics in alternate generations.

Heterogenous Derived from different sources.

Heterogeusia Perception of an inappropriate quality of taste when food is chewed.

Heterograft Graft from another individual.

Heterolalia The use of meaningless words.

Heterologous 1. Composed of tissue not normal to the part. 2. A tissue, cell or blood obtained from a different individual/species.

Heterometropia Two eyes with different refraction.

Heterophil An antibody reacting with other than specific antigen.

Heterophonia Change of voice occurring especially at puberty.

Heterophoria A tendency to squint when fusion is interrupted. It occurs mainly when the person is tired or in poor health.

Heterosexual 1. Pertaining to, characteristic of or directed towards the opposite sex. 2. A person with erotic interests directed towards the opposite sex.

Heterotopia Development of normal tissue at an abnormal location or displacement of an organ from its normal location.

Heterotropia A marked deviation of the eyes; strabismus or squint.

Heterotrichosis Growth of different kinds or colors of hairs on the scalp or body.

Heterotroph An organism like man who requires complex organic food for growth and development.

Heterozygous Possessing dissimilar alternative genes for an inherited characteristic, one gene coming from each parent. One gene is dominant and the other is recessive (*See Homozygous*).

Heubner's disease Syphilitic end arteritis in brain.

Hexachlorophane A detergent and germicidal compound commonly incorporated in soaps and dermatological agents. Topical preparations have been associated with severe neurotoxicity and should not be used on children under 2 years old except on medical advice. Avoid on large raw areas.

Hexachlorophene A detergent and germicidal compound commonly incorporated in soaps and dermatological agents. Topical preparations have been associated with severe neurotoxicity and should not be used on children under 2 years old except on medical advice.

Hexamine Methenamine; a urinary antiseptic which releases formaldehyde in an acid urine.

Hexokinase An enzyme catalyzing phosphorylation of glucose; present in muscle tissue and yeast.

Hexose Any monosaccharide of formula $C_6H_{12}O_6$.

Hexylresorcinol Anthelmintic agent.

Hg Symbol for mercury (L. hydrargyrum).

Hiatus A space or opening.

  Hiatus hernia A protrusion of a part of the stomach through the oesophageal opening in the diaphragm.

Hib An injectable vaccine that protects against Hemophilus influenzae type B causing severe respiratory and ear infections and meningitis. Offered to infants at ages of 2, 3 and 4 months. (*See Annexure 10*).

Hibernation Condition of remaining asleep and immobile for the winter, especially in animals.

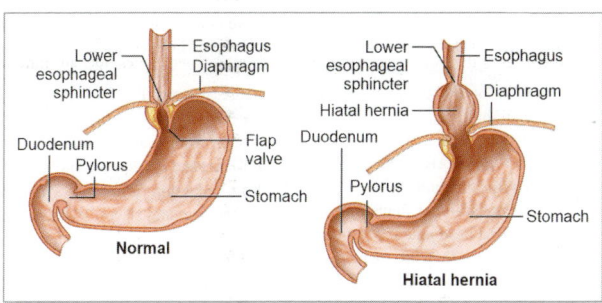

Normal

Hiatal hernia

Hiatus Hernia

Hibernoma A rare multilobular encapsulated tumor containing fetal fat tissue closely resembling fat stored in the foot pads of hibernating animals.

Hiccough Intermittent spasmodic contraction of diaphragm with closure of glottis, causing a short sharp inspiratory cough.

Hiccup Hiccough. A spasmodic contraction of the diaphragm causing an abrupt inspiratory sound.

Hick's sign Intermittent painless uterine contraction occurring after third month of pregnancy.

Hickman line Trade name for a central venous line catheter.

Hidradenoma Adenoma of sweat glands.

Hidrosis The excretion of sweat.

Hierarchy In order of importance.

High-altitude sickness The condition resulting from difficulty in adjusting to diminished oxygen pressure at high altitudes. It may take the form of mountain sickness, high-altitude pulmonary edema or cerebral edema.

High blood pressure Blood pressure above the normal range for age. Usually 140/90 mm Hg if below 50 years and above 160/90 if above 60 years.

High dependency unit Abbreviated HDU. For those patients who do not need intensive care in the clinical situation but require a greater degree of specialist monitoring and observation than in a general ward, nursing and medical care is provided in the high dependency unit.

High residue diet High fiber/cellulose diet (above 30 g/day) beneficial for colorectal diseases, diabetes and obesity.

Highly active antiretroviral therapy Abbreviated HAART. A treatment regimen that incorporates a combination of different antiviral drugs for human immunodeficiency viral infection. Sometimes also called ART, antiretroviral therapy.

Hilton's law A nerve supplying a muscle also supplies the joint that muscle moves and the skin overlying the insertion of that muscle.

Hilton's line A white line at the junction of skin of the perineum and anal mucosa.

Hilton's sac A pit along the external portion of false vocal cord.

Hilum Hilus; a recess in an organ by which blood vessels, nerves and ducts enter and leave it.

Hindbrain Part of the brain consisting of the medulla oblongata, the pons and the cerebellum.

Hind gut The caudal portion of endodermal tube giving rise to ileum, colon and rectum.

Hinge joint A joint permitting only flexion and extension in a single axis.

Hip 1. The region of the body at the articulation of the femur and the innominate bone at the base of the lower trunk. These bones meet at the hip joint. Also called coax. 2. Loosely, the hip joint.

Total hip replacement Replacement of the femoral head and acetabulum with prostheses that are cemented into the bone; also called *total hip arthroplasty*. The procedure is done to replace a severely damaged arthritic hip joint.

Hip joint The ball and socket articulation between head of femur and acetabulum.

Hippocampal commissure A thin sheet of fibers passing transversely under posterior portion of corpus callosum.

Hippocampal formation Olfactory structures including hippocampus, dentate gyrus, supracallosal gyrus, diagonal band of Broca and hippocampal commisure.

Hippocampus major Elevation of floor of inferior horn of lateral ventricle.

Hippocampus minor Small elevation on the medial wall of lateral ventricle formed by end of calcarine fissure.

Hippocrates Greek physician who first established the scientific basis of medical practice; hence known as father of medicine.

Hippocratic facies The appearance of face at the time of impending death.

Hippocratic oath The oath Hippocrates exacted from his students which reads like "I will follow that system of regimen which, according to my ability and judgment, I consider for the benefit of my patients, and abstain from whatever is deleterious and mischievous. I will give no deadly medicine to anyone if asked nor suggest any such counsel, and in like manner I will not give to a woman a pessary for abortion. With purity and holiness I will pass my life and practice my art, into whatever houses I enter, I will go into them for the benefit of the sick, and I will abstain from every voluntary act of mischief and corruption, and further from seduction of females or males, of free men and slaves. Whatever in connection with my professional practice, or not in connection with it, I see or hear in the life of men, which ought not to be spoken of abroad. I will not divulge, as reckoning that all such should be kept secret. While I continue to keep this oath unviolated, may it be granted to me to enjoy life and the practice of this art, respected by all men in all times. But should I trespass and violate this Oath, may the reverse be my lot."

Hippuric acid Endogenous acid formed in the human body from combination of benzoic acid and glycine and excreted by kidneys.

Hippus Alternate contraction and dilatation of the pupils. This occurs in various diseases of the nervous system, e.g., multiple sclerosis.

Hirschberg's reflex Adduction of foot when sole at base of great toe is stimulated.

Hirschsprung's disease *H Hirschsprung, Danish physician, 1831– 1916 (See Megacolon).*

Hirsute Hairy.

Hirsutism Excessive hairiness.

Hirudin The active principle in the secretion of the leech and certain snake venoms that prevents clotting of blood.

Herudicide Any substance that destroys leeches.

His bundle A trioventricular bundle arising in the ventricles.

Hirudo A genus of leeches.

Hirudo medicinalis The medical leech.

Histamine An enzyme that causes local vasodilatation and increased permeability of the blood vessel walls. Readily released from body tissues, it is a factor in allergy response, greatly increases gastric secretion of hydrochloric acid and increases the heart rate.

Histamine test 1. Subcutaneous injection of 0.1% solution of histamine to stimulate gastric secretion in order to measure maximal acid output. 2. After rapid intravenous injection of histamine phosphate, normal persons experience a brief fall in blood pressure, but in those with pheochromocytoma, after the fall, there is a marked rise in blood pressure.

Histamine blocking agents H_1 receptor blocking agents are antiallergic and H_2 receptor blockers reduce gastric acid production.

Histamine headache Headache after taking histamine containing foods.

Histidinemia A hereditary metabolic defect caused by an enzyme defect involving L-histidine ammonia lypase affecting the amino acid histidine. Affected persons show mild mental handicap and disordered speech development.

Histidine One of the ten essential amino acids formed by the digestion of dietary protein. Histamine is derived from it.

Histiocyte A stationary macrophage of connective tissue. Derived from the reticuloendothelial cells, it acts as a scavenger, removing bacteria from the blood and tissues.

Histiocytoma A tumor containing histiocytes, causing a vascular nodule.

Histiocytosis A group of diseases of bone in which granulomata containing histiocytes and eosinophil cells appear *(See Letterer-Siwe disease and Hand-Schüller-Christian disease).*

Histiocytosis-X A granulomatous destructive disease.

Histochemistry Light and electron microscopy and special chemical tests and stains done to study chemistry of cells and tissues.

Histocompatibility The ability of cells to be accepted and to function in a new situation. Tissue typing reveals this and ensures a higher success rate in organ transplantation.

Histocompatibility antigens A number of antigens expressed by all nucleated cells which are controlled by genes located in major histocompatibility gene complex (MCH) in chromosome 6.

Histogenesis Origin and development of tissue.

Histogram A bar-chart. Statistical values are expressed as blocks on a graph.

Histoid Resembling one of the tissues.

Histology The science dealing with the minute structure, composition and function of tissues.

Histolysis The disintegration of tissues.

Histone A class of simple proteins present in cell chromatin.

Histonomy The law governing development and structure of tissues.

Histoplasmosis Infection caused by inhalation of the spores of a yeast-like fungus.

Histoplasma capsulatum Usually symptomless, the infection may progress and produce a condition resembling tuberculosis.

Histotomy Cutting of thin sections of tissue for microscopic study.

Histozyme A renal enzyme that converts hippuric acid into benzoic acid and glycine.

Histrionic Theatrical, dramatic.

HIV disease The entire spectrum of cellular and clinical disease from initial infection and asymptomatic disease to early and late symptomatic disease (AIDS) and death, caused

H

by human immunodeficiency virus (HIV) infection. *(See Human Immunodeficiency Virus).*

HIV Human immunodeficiency virus.

Hives (hievz) Urticaria.

Hoarseness A rough quality of voice due to simple chronic laryngitis, vocal cord palsy, or infiltration of vocal cords.

Hobnail liver Liver with an irregular surface, usually cirrhosis.

Hodge pessary *HL Hodge, American gynecologist, 1796–1873.* A pessary used to maintain the position of the uterus after correction of a retroversion *(See Pessary).*

Hodgkin's disease *T Hodgkin, British physician, 1798–1866.* Lymphadenoma, a malignant condition of the reticuloendothelial cells. There is progressive enlargement of lymph nodes and lymph tissue all over the body. Treated by radiotherapy and cytotoxic drugs, this disease has a good prognosis.

Hoffman's sign Flicking the terminal phalanx of finger causes reflex flexion of other fingers of same hand in pyramidal damage.

Holism A philosophy in which the person is considered as a functioning whole rather than as a composite of several systems. Maybe spelt as wholism.

Holistic Pertaining to holism.

Holistic health Care a comprehensive approach to health care that implies body-mind-spirit consideration in all actions and interventions for the patient, while recognizing the concept of the uniqueness of the individual and the influence of external and internal environmental factors on health.

Holistic medicine Comprehensive and total care of a patient, taking into account his physical, mental, social, economic and spiritual needs.

Holodiastolic Covering entire diastole, i.e., closure of aortic valve to closure of mitral valve.

Holoendemic A disease affecting almost all population in a given area. In malaria epidemiology, spleen index rate of ≥5% in children under 10 implies the disease to be holoendemic.

Holography A method of producing three-dimensional pictures. The picture obtained is called hologram.

Holoprosencephaly Deficiency in fore brain with CSF accumulation due to trisomy of 13, 14, 15 or 18 chromosomes.

Holorachischisis Complete spina bifida.

Holosystolic Related to entire period of systole.

Holter monitor An ECG recording system capable of recording ECG for 24 hours, particularly useful for recording arrhythmias, and silent ischemia.

Homans' sign *J Homans, American surgeon, 1877–1954.* Pain elicited in the calf when the foot is dorsiflexed. Indicative of venous thrombosis.

Homatropine A short-acting mydriatic used in ophthalmology to dilate the pupil and so allow a better view of the fundus of the eye.

Home help service A branch of the social services department, which provides domestic and housekeeping assistance to those in need. It is on either a short-term or long-term basis, and payment is according to means.

Homeopathy A system of medicine promulgated by CFS Hahnemann and based upon the principle that "like cures like". Remedies are given which can produce in the patient the symptoms of the disease to be cured, but they are administered in minute doses.

Homeostasis A tendency of biological systems to maintain stability while continually adjusting to conditions that are optimal for survival.

Homicide The killing of a human being.
Culpable homicide Covers murder (malice aforethought), manslaughter (without malice aforethought), causing death by reckless driving, and infanticide.
Nonculpable homicide Covers justifiable homicide (e.g., lawful execution) and excusable homicide (misadventure or accident) *(See McNaghten's rules on insanity at law)*.

Homocystinuria A rare but serious inherited condition where the body cannot process the amino acid methionine. Babies are screened for the condition as part of the newborn blood spot screening program.

Homogeneous Uniform in character. Similar in nature and characteristics.

Homogenize To make homogeneous. To reduce to the same consistency.

Homogenous Derived from the same source.

Homogenesis Reproduction by same process in succeeding generations.

H₁ and H₂ receptor blockers Agents that block H_1 and H_2 receptors, e.g., terphenadrine and ranitidine respectively.

H5N1 Virus that causes a virulent strain of avian influenza.

Homograft A tissue or organ transplanted from one individual to another of the same species. An allograft.

Homolateral On the same side; ipsilateral.

Homologous 1. In anatomy, having the same embryological origin although performing a different function. 2. In chemistry, possessing a similar structure
Homologous chromosomes Those that pair during meiosis and contain an identical arrangement of genes in the DNA pattern.

Homologue A part or organ which has the same relative position or structure as another one.

Homonymous In ophthalmology pertains to corresponding vertical halves of visual field.

Homoplasty Surgical replacement of defective tissues with a homograft.

Homosexual 1. Of the same sex. 2. A person who is sexually attracted to a person of the same sex.

Homosexuality Sexual and emotional orientation toward persons of the same sex.

Homozygous Possessing an identical pair of genes for an inherited characteristic *(See Heterozygous)*.

Hookworm *(See Ancylostoma)*.

Hordeolum A stye; inflammation of the sebaceous glands of the eyelashes.

Hormone A chemical substance that is generated in one organ and carried by the blood to another, in which it excites activity.
Hormone replacement therapy The giving of prepared hormones as a substitute for those hormones that the body no longer produces or that have been lost as a result of surgery. A combination of estrogenic hormones is commonly given to women for the relief of menopausal symptoms and the prevention of osteoporosis. Known as HRT.

Horn Cutaneous outgrowth composed chiefly of keratin.
Horn anterior Gray substance in anterior portion of spinal cord SYN-ventral horn.
Horn dorsal Posterior projection of gray matter in spinal cord.
Horn of Ammon Hippocampus.

Horner's syndrome *JF Horner, Swiss ophthalmologist, 1831–1886.* A condition in which there is a lesion on the path of sympathetic nerve fibers in the cervical region. The symptoms include enophthalmos, ptosis, a contracted pupil and a decrease in sweating.

Horton's syndrome *BT Horton, American physician, 1895–1980.* Severe

H

headache caused by the release of histamine in the body or by its administration. Histamine cephalalgia.

Horse power A unit of power equals to 33,000 foot pounds per minute or 745.7 watts.

Horse-shoe shaped kidney A congenital renal abnormality in which both the kidneys are united at their lower poles.

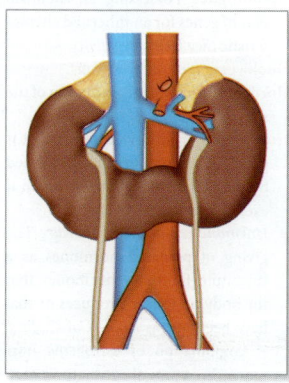

Horse-shoe Shaped Kidney

Hospice The concept of a hospice is that of a caring community of professional and non-professional people, together with the family. Emphasis is on dealing with emotional and spiritual problems as well as the medical problems of the terminally ill. Of primary concern is control of pain and other symptoms, keeping the patient at home for as long as possible or desirable, and making the remaining days as comfortable and meaningful as possible. After the patient dies, family members are given support throughout their period of bereavement.

Hospital An institution for the care, diagnosis and treatment of the sick and injured.

Hospitalization Admission of a patient into hospital.

Host The animal, plant or tissue on which a parasite lives and multiplies.
Definitive or final host One that harbours the parasite during its adult sexual stage.
Intermediate host One that shelters the parasite during a non-reproductive period.

Hostility Manifestations of anger, animosity or antagonism directed toward oneself or others. It maybe a symptom of depression.

Hotline A continuously functioning telephone connection.

Hot water bag A rubber or plastic bag for application of dry heat or keeping moist applications warm.

Hourglass contraction A contraction near the middle of a hollow organ, such as the stomach or uterus, producing an outline resembling an hourglass shape.

Housemaid's knee Prepatellar bursitis; inflammation of the prepatellar bursa, which becomes distended with serous fluid.

House physician An intern or resident responsible for patient care under direction of a senior staff.

Houston's valves Crescent shaped folds of mucous membrane in the rectum.

Howell-Jolly bodies Spherical granules in the erythrocytes seen in asplenia, thalassemia, leukemia, etc.

Howship's lacunae Grooves or pits occupied by osteoclasts during bone resorption.

HRT Hormone Replacement Therapy.

Hubbard tank Tank of suitable size and shape for active and passive underwater exercise.

Huguier's canal Canal in the base of skull through which chorda tympani nerve exists from brain.

Huhner's test Aspiration of vagina within an hour of coitus to test for sperm motility in investigation of infertility.

Hum Soft continuous sound.

Human chorionic gonadotropin *(See Gonadotropin).*

Human Fertilization and Embryology Act 2008 Act, which ensures all human embryos outside the body are subject to regulation; bans sex selection of offspring for non-medical reasons; recognizes same-sex couples as legal parents through use of donated sperm, eggs or embryos; monitors collection of data from HFEA to follow up research of infertility treatment. Termination of pregnancy must be performed before 24 weeks of pregnancy by a registered medical practitioner, agreed with a second doctor that the woman or her family would suffer physical, mental or social trauma if the pregnancy were to continue, or if the baby is at risk of gross physical or mental abnormality. Termination of pregnancy maybe performed at any time if there is serious risk to the mother's life in case of continued pregnancy *(See Abortion).*

Human Fertilization and Embryology Authority (HFEA) A UK Statutory body, its primary purpose is to independently regulate the use of gametes and embryos, infertility treatment and research. It licenses fertility clinics and centers carrying out in vitro fertilization (IVF). HFEA produces a Code of Practice and information for the public. The HFEA also regulates and monitors the storage of sperm, eggs and embryos.

Human immunodeficiency virus Abbreviated HIV. A lentivirus that belongs to a group of viruses known as retroviruses and causes AIDS in humans. There are two main types of HIV: HIV-1, the predominant AIDS-causing virus in the world, and HIV-2, also an AIDS-causing virus that is found more commonly in countries on the west coast of Africa. HIV is transmitted sexually, parenterally, from mother to child (during pregnancy, at time of birth, or in the postnatal period from breastfeeding) and more rarely, iatrogenically. Most people become infected sexually through unprotected penetrative vaginal or anal sexual intercourse. Unprotected means that the male insertive partner has not worn a good quality, intact rubber latex condom. Parenteral transmission is usually associated with injecting drug users sharing contaminated injection equipment. Blood tests to identify HIV infection detect antibodies to the virus and may not be positive for 8–12 weeks following primary infection. Because it is not possible to detect all HIV-infected patients, all health care workers in direct patient contact should practise universal infection control precautions *(See Universal precautions).*

Human insulin Insulin prepared by recombinant DNA technology using *E. coli.*

Human placental lactogen Placental secretion that helps to prepare the breast for milk secretion.

Humerus Bone of upper arm that articulates with scapula above and radius, ulna below.

Humidity The degree of moisture in the air.

    Humidity therapy The therapeutic use of water to prevent or correct a moisture deficit in the respiratory tract. The principal reasons for employing humidity therapy are: (a) To prevent drying and irritation of the respiratory mucosa; (b) To facilitate ventilation and diffusion of oxygen and other therapeutic gases being administered; and (c) To aid in the removal of thick and viscous secretions that obstruct the air passages. Another important use of water aerosol therapy is to aid in obtaining an induced sputum specimen.

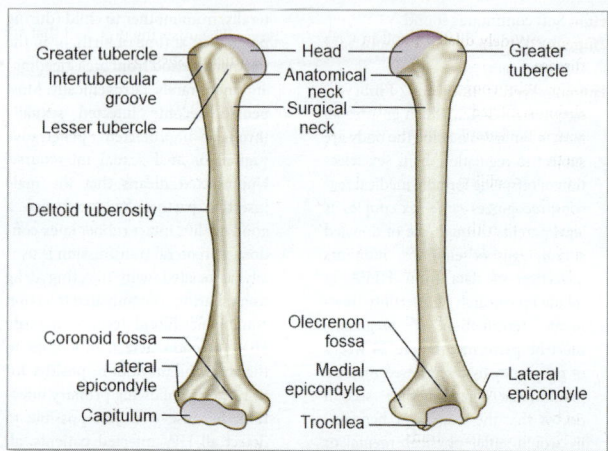

Humerus

Humour Any fluid of the body, such as lymph or blood.

Aqueous humour The fluid filling the anterior chamber of the eye.

Vitreous humour The jelly-like substance that fills the chamber of the eye between the lens and the retina.

Humoral immunity An older term for antibody mediated immunity. *(See Immunity)*.

Humour and laughter therapy An amusing intervention used by a health care professional or patient and designed to benefit the patient.

Humpback Curvature of spine or kyphosis.

Hunchback Kyphosis with prominent rounded deformity of back.

Hunger A desire to eat with dull pain in epigastrium. Appetite in contrast is pleasant sensation of seeking food to eat to enjoy it.

Hunter's canal Adductor canal.

Hunter's disease Mucopoly saccharidosis II.

Hunterian chancre Indurated syphilitic chancre.

Huntington's chorea (disease) *GS Huntington, American physician, 1851–1927.* A rare, degenerative inherited disorder of the brain in which there is progressive chorea and mental deterioration (dementia).

Huntington's disease G. S. Huntington, American physician, 1851-1927. A rare, degenerative inherited disorder of the brain in which there is progressive chorea and mental deterioration (dementia).

Hurler's syndrome *G Hurler, Austrian pediatrician.* An inherited disorder in which learning difficulties are caused by excess mucopolysaccharides being stored in the brain and reticuloendothelial system. Gargoylism.

Hurthle cells Eosinophilic staining cells of thyroid gland.

Hutchinson's teeth *Sir J Hutchinson, British surgeon, 1828–1913.* Typical notching of the borders of the permanent incisor teeth occurring in congenital syphilis.

H's pupil Widely dilated pupil in CNS disease.

H's triad In congenital syphilis this diagnostic triad consists of deafness, interstitial keratitis and Hutchinson's teeth.

Hyaline Resembling glass.

Hyaline degeneration A form of deterioration that occurs in tumors and is due to deficiency of blood supply. It precedes cystic degeneration.

Hyaline membrane disease (See Respiratory distress syndrome of newborn).

Hyaline cartilage Smooth, pearly true cartilage covering articular surface of bone.

Hyalaine casts Pale, transparent casts with homogeneous rounded ends seen in urine in nephropathy.

Hyalinization The development of an albuminioid mass in a cell or tissue.

Hyalinosis Waxy or hyaline degeneration.

Hyalitis Inflammation of vitreous humor; can be asteroid, punctuate and suppurative.

Hyalogen A protein substance in vitreous humor and cartilage.

Hyaloid artery A fetal artery supplying nutrition to the lens. It disappears after birth.

Hyaloid canal Lymph channel in vitreous extending from optic disk to posterior capsule of lens; contains hyaloids artery in fetus.

Hyaloid membrane Membrane that envelops the vitreous humor.

Hyaluronic acid An acid mucopolysaccharide forming the ground substance of connective tissue; functioning as a binding and protective agent.

Hyaluronidase An enzyme that facilitates the absorption of fluids in subcutaneous tissues. It is found in the testes of mammals, and a preparation of it is particularly used with subcutaneous infusions to promote absorption.

Hybrid The offspring of parent that are of different species.

Hybridization Production of hybrids by cross-matching.

Hybridoma It is the cell produced by fusion of an antibody producing cell and a multiple myeloma cell. The hybrid cell thus formed can be a source of continuous monoclonal antibodies.

Hydantoin A colorless base, glycolyl urea.

Hydatid A cystic swelling containing the embryo of *Echinococcus granulosus*. It maybe found in any organ of the body, e.g., in the liver. "Daughter cysts" are produced from the original. Infection is from contaminated foods, e.g., salads.

Hydatid disease The result of the presence of hydatids in the lungs, liver or brain.

Hydatidiform Resembling a hydatid cyst.

Hydatidiform mole *(See Mole).*

Hydatid of Morgagni Cyst like remnant of müllerian duct that is attached to fallopian tube.

Hydradenitis Inflammation of sweat glands.

Hydradenoma Tumor of sweat gland.

Hydraemia A modification of the blood in which there is an excess of plasma in relation to the cells. A degree of hydraemia is physiological in pregnancy.

Hydragogue Drug promoting watery evacuation of bowel like sodium sulfate or magnesium sulfate.

Hydralazine A vasodilator and antihypertensive agent used to lower blood pressure.

Hydramnios An excessive amount of amniotic fluid in the uterus in the later months of pregnancy.

Hydranencephaly Hydrocephalus due to congenital absence of cerebral hemispheres.

H

Hydrarthrosis A collection of fluid in a joint.

Hydrate A compound of an element with water.

Hydraulics The science of fluids.

Hydriatrics Application of water for treatment *SYN*-hydrotherpay.

Hydroa A childhood hypersensitivity of the skin to sunlight, resulting in the formation of a vesicular eruption on the exposed parts, with intense irritation.

Hydroa vacciniforme A rare and chronic childhood hypersensitivity of the skin to sunlight, resulting in the formation of a vesicular eruption on the exposed parts, with intense irritation.

Hydrocarbon A compound of hydrogen and carbon. Fats are of this type.

Hydrocele A swelling caused by accumulation of fluid, especially in the tunica vaginalis surrounding the testicle.

Hydrocephalus "Water on the brain". Enlargement of the skull due to an abnormal collection of cerebrospinal fluid around the brain or in the ventricles. It maybe either congenital or acquired from inflammation of the meninges during infancy. The most effective treatment is surgical correction employing a shunting technique. It frequently accompanies spina bifida.

Hydrochloric acid HCl, a colorless compound of hydrogen and chlorine. It is present, in 0.2% solution, in gastric juice and aids in digestion.

Hydrochlorothiazide A valuable oral diuretic similar to but more potent than chlorothiazide. It is used in the treatment of edema and hypertension.

Hydrocodone Opioid alkaloid, analgesic and hypnotic.

Hydrocolloid dressings Absorbent dressings with a soft spongy consistency that are applied to wounds subject to pressure, for example, those in the sacral area or on heels. They relieve pain from the site, rehydrate and encourage debridement and healing.

Hydrocolpos Retention cyst of vagina.

Hydrocortisone Cortisol, the principal glucocorticoid secreted by the adrenal gland; it is used in the treatment of inflammations, allergies, pruritus, collagen diseases, adrenocortical insufficiency, severe status asthmaticus, shock and certain neoplasms.

Hydroflumethiazide An oral thiazide diuretic used in the treatment of edema and hypertension.

Hydrogenase An enzyme that catalyzes reduction by molecular hydrogen.

Hydrogenation Addition of hydrogen to convert unsaturated fat to solid fat.

Hydrogel dressings Wound dressings that rehydrate dry necrotic tissue, reduce pain and promote healing.

Hydrogen donor In oxidation reduction reactions a substance that gives up hydrogen to another substance.

Hydrogen Symbol H. A combustible gas, present in nearly all organic compounds, which, in combination with oxygen, forms water.

Hydrogen ion concentration The amount of hydrogen in a liquid, which is responsible for its acidity. The degree of acidity is expressed in pH values: the higher the hydrogen ion concentration, the greater the acidity, and the lower the pH value. The concentration in the blood is of importance in acidosis.

Hydrogen peroxide H_2O_2, a strong disinfectant cleansing and bleaching liquid used, diluted in water, for cleansing wounds.

Hydrogen sulfide H_2S. A poisonous, gas with pungent odor of rotten egg.

Hydrolase An enzyme causing hydrolysis.

Hydrolysis The process of splitting up into smaller molecules by uniting with water.

Hydrometer An instrument for estimating the specific gravity of fluids, e.g., a urinometer.

Hydromorphone An analgesic, opium derivative.

Hydromyelia A dilatation of the central canal of the spinal cord caused by an accumulation of cerebrospinal fluid.

Hydromyelocele Protrusion of spinal CSF sac through spina bifida.

Hydromyoma Cystic uterine fibroid.

Hydronephrosis An accumulation of urine in the pelvis of the kidney, resulting in atrophy of the kidney structure, due to an obstruction to the flow of urine from the kidney. The condition maybe: (a) Congenital, due to malformation of the kidney or ureter; or (b) Acquired, due to an obstruction of the ureter by tumor or stone, or to back pressure from stricture of the urethra or an enlarged prostate gland.

Hydropathy The treatment of disease by the use of water internally and externally; hydrotherapy.

Hydropericarditis Inflammation of the pericardium resulting in serous fluid in the pericardial sac.

Hydroperitoneum *(See Ascites).*

Hydrophobia 1. Rabies. 2. Irrational fear of water.

Hydrophilic ointment Topical ointment that absorbs water and hence is emollient.

Hydropneumatois Liquid and gas in tissues producing combined edema and emphysema.

Hydropneumopericardium Fluid and gas in pericardial cavity.

Hydropneumothorax The presence of fluid and air in the pleural space.

Hydrops [L.] Abnormal accumulation of serous fluid in the tissues or in a body cavity; also called dropsy.

Fetal hydrops, hydrops fetalis Gross edema of the entire body of the newborn infant, occurring in hemolytic disease of the newborn.

Hydropyonephrosis Dilatation of renal pelvis with pus and urine.

Hydroquinone A depigmenting agent.

Hydrorrhoea Production of profuse watery discharge from any part or organ of the body, e.g., Hydrorrhoea gravidarum refers to discharge of watery fluid from the vagina during the third trimester of pregnancy.

Hydrostatic densitometry An underwater weighing technique for determination of body components, usually percentage of fat.

Hyderostatic test A test to know if the dead infant has breathed prior to death. If the infant's lungs float in water, breathing had been established prior to death.

Hydrotherapy The treatment of disease by means of water.

Hydrothorax Fluid in the pleural cavity due to serous effusion, as in cardiac, renal and other diseases.

Hydroureter An accumulation of water or urine in a ureter.

Hyderoxycobalamin A chemical with activity similar to B_{12}.

Hydroxyapatite Calcium phosphate in combination with calcium carbonate present in the bones; when it combines with fluorine, it becomes decay resistant fluoroapatite.

Hydroxybenzene Phenol

Hydroxybutyric acid A component of ketone body produced by abnormal metabolism of fat in diabetic ketosis.

Hydroxychloroquin Antimalarial agent.

Hydroxyproline An amino acid found in collagen.

Hydroxypropyl methyl cellulose A substance used to increase viscosity of solutions.

Hydroxystilbamidine isethionate Antiprotozoal antimonial.

Hydroxytryptamine Serotonin.

Hydroxyurea An orally active cytotoxic agent used mainly in the treatment of melanoma, resistant chronic myelocytic leukemia and recurrent, metastatic or inoperable ovarian carcinoma.

Hydroxyzine An antihistamine.

Hygiene 1. The science of health and its preservation. 2. A condition of practice, such as cleanliness, that is conducive to preservation of health.

Communal hygiene The maintenance of the health of the community by the provision of a pure water supply, efficient sanitation, good housekeeping, etc.

Industrial hygiene (Occupational health) care of the health of workers in an industry.

Mental hygiene The science dealing with development of healthy mental and emotional reactions and habits.

Oral hygiene The proper care of the mouth and teeth.

Personal hygiene Individual measures taken to preserve one's own cleanliness and well-being.

Hygroma A swelling caused by fluid.

Cystic hygroma A cystic lymphangioma of the neck.

Subdural hygroma A collection of clear fluid in the subdural space.

Hygrometer An instrument for measuring the water vapor in the air.

Hygroscopic Readily absorbing moisture. An example is glycerin, which is used in suppositories as a means of aiding evacuation by moistening the feces.

Hymen A fold of mucous membrane partially closing the entrance to the vagina.

Imperforate hymen A membrane which completely occludes the vaginal orifice.

Hymenectomy The surgical removal of the hymen.

Hymenolepsis A genus of tapeworm, *Hymenolepsis nana* Dwarf tapeworm, average length 1". Capable of completing life cycle within one host.

Hymenology Science of the membranes and their diseases.

Hymenoptera An order of insects that includes ants, bees, hornets and wasps.

Hymenorrhaphy Plastic surgery of hymen to restore it to preruptured state.

Hyoglossus Muscle arising from hyoid bone and inserted into dorsum of tongue. It draws sides down and retracts the tongue.

Hyoid Shaped like a U.

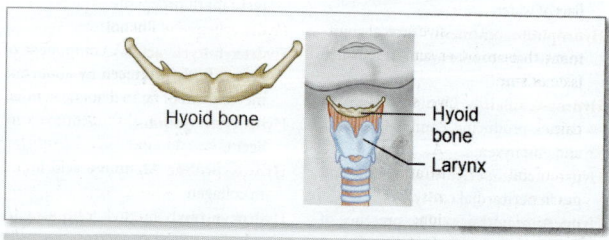

Hyoid bone

Hyoid bone — Larynx

Hyoid

Hyoid bone A U shaped bone above the thyroid cartilage, to which the tongue is attached.

Hyoscine Scopolamine; an anticholinergic drug used as an anesthetic premedicant, antispasmodic, and in the treatment of motion sickness. Should be avoided in the elderly because of its tendency to cause restlessness and confusion (central cholinergic syndrome).

Hyopharyngeus Middle pharyngeal constrictor.

Hyoscine hydrobromide Belladona alkaloid having atropine like effect.

Hypaesthesia Impairment of the sense of touch.

Hypalgesia A decrease in sensitivity to pain.

Hypamnios A deficiency of fluid in the amniotic sac.

Hyper Prefix meaning excessive, beyond.

Hyperacidity Excessive acidity.

> *Gastric hyperacidity* Hyperchlorhydria.

Hyperactive Exhibiting hyperactivity; hyperkinetic.

Hyperactivity Abnormally increased activity. Developmental hyperactivity of children (hyperkinesia) is characterized by very restless, impulsive behavior. These children are usually inattentive and have a poor concentration span. Other features that maybe associated with hyperactivity include aggression, anxiety, poor eating and sleeping patterns, and social and learning difficulties.

Hyperacusis Abnormal sensitivity to sound, e.g., in hysteria.

Hyperaemia Excess of blood in any part.

Hyperaesthesia Excessive sensitiveness to touch or to other sensations, e.g., taste or smell.

Hyperalgesia Excessive sensibility to pain.

Hyperalimentation A program of parenteral administration of all nutrients for patients with gastrointestinal dysfunction; also called total parenteral alimentation (TPA) and total parenteral nutrition (TPN). Although, the term hyperalimentation is commonly used to designate total or supplementary nutrition by intravenous feedings, it is not technically correct in as much as the procedure does not involve an abnormally increased or excessive amount of feeding *(See Nutrition (Parenteral)).*

Hyperammonemia Excess of ammonia in blood, e.g., cirrhosis can be congenital either due to deficiency of carbamyl phosphate synthetase or ornithine transcarbamylase that metabolize ammonia.

Hyperamylasemia Increased blood amylase.

Hyperasthenia Extreme weakness.

Hyperbaric At greater pressure than normal; applied to gases under greater than atmospheric pressure.

> *Hyperbaric oxygenation* Exposure to oxygen under conditions of greatly increased pressure. The patient is placed in a sealed enclosure, called a hyperbaric chamber. Compressed air is introduced; at the same time the patient is given pure oxygen through a face mask. Patients suffering from tetanus and gas gangrene, infections caused by bacteria that are resistant to antibiotics but vulnerable to oxygen, are helped by hyperbaric oxygenation. The technique is also useful in radiotherapy for cancer. When full of oxygen, cancer cells seem more vulnerable to radiation. Carbon monoxide poisoning can be treated by hyperbaric oxygenation. Carbon monoxide molecules, displacing the oxygen in the erythrocytes, usually cause asphyxiation, but hyperbaric oxygenation can often keep the patient alive until the carbon monoxide has been eliminated from the body's system.

Hyperbetalipoproteinemia Excessive amount of betalipoprotein in blood.

Hyperbilirubinemia An excess of bilirubin in the blood.

Hypercalcaemia An excess of calcium in the blood. Maybe caused by over administration of vitamin D, hyperparathyroidism, thyrotoxicosis, breakdown of bone by malignant disease, or impaired renal function.

Hypercalciuria A high level of calcium in the urine leading to renal stone formation.

Hypercapnia An increased amount of carbon dioxide in the blood, causing over stimulation of the respiratory center. Hypercarbia.

Hypercatabolism An excessive rate of catabolism leading to wasting or destruction of a part or tissue.

Hyperchloremia An excess of calcium in the blood. May rarely be caused by over administration of vitamin D, hyperparathyroidism, thyrotoxicosis, prolonged immobility, breakdown of bone by malignant disease, or impaired renal function.

Hyperchlorhydria An excess of hydrochloric acid in the gastric juice.

Hypercholesteremia, Hypercholesterolaemia Excess of cholesterol inthe blood. Predisposes to atheroma and gallstones.

Hypercusis Excessive sensitivity to sound.

Hyperchromatic Over pigmentted.

Hyperchromatopsia Defect of vision in which all objects appear colored.

Hypercorticism Excessive production of adrenocortical hormones.

Hypercyesis Presence of more than one fetus in uterus.

Hyperdontia Presence of more than normal number of teeth.

Hyperemesis Excessive vomiting. *Hyperemesis gravidarum* An uncommon, serious complication of pregnancy, characterized by severe and persistent vomiting, the aetiology of which is not fully understood.

Hyperemia Vascular congestion; can be active as in increased blood flow or passive due to venous stasis.

Hypercosinophilic syndrome Idiopathic persistent hyper–eosinophilia often with CNS and cardiac involvement.

Hyperesthesia Increased sensitivity to sensory stimuli especially pain and touch.

Hyperextension The forcible extension of a limb beyond the normal. It is used to correct orthopedic deformities.

Hyperferremia Increased iron content of blood.

Hyperflexion The forcible bending of a joint beyond the normal.

Hypergalactia, Hypergalactosis Excessive secretion of milk.

Hypergammaglobulinemia Increased gamma-globulins in the blood.

Hyperglycemia Excess of sugar in the blood (normal 4.0–5.9 mmol/L when fasting); a sign of diabetes mellitus. *(See Hypoglycemia on p. 314)*.

Hyperglycinemia Accumulation of amino acid glycine in blood manifesting with mental and growth retardation.

Hypergnosia Distorted or exaggerated perception.

Hypergonadism Excessive secretion of sex hormones.

Hyperhidrosis Excessive perspiration; hyperidrosis.

Hyperhydration Excess amount of water in the body.

Hyperinsulinism Excess of insulin in the body causing hypoglycemia that manifests with hunger, sweating, weakness, convulsion and often coma.

Hyperkalemia An excess of potassium in the blood. If untreated, this will lead to cardiac arrest.

Hyperkeratosis Hypertrophy of the horny layers of the skin.

Hyperkinesis A condition in which there is excessive motor activity *(See Hyperactivity)*.

Hyperlipaemia An excess of fat or lipids in the blood.

Hyperlipoproteinemia Increased lipoprotein content in blood due to increased synthesis or decreased breakdown.

Hypermastia 1. The presence of one or more supernumerary breasts.
2. Overdevelopment of one or both breasts.

Hypermelanosis Increased melanin content of skin either in epidermis (melanoderma) in which the coloration is brown, or in the dermis in which skin color is blue or slate gray. Conditions responsible for hypermelanosis are ACTH producing tumors, Wilson's disease, biliary cirrhosis, chronic renal failure, etc.

Hypermenorrhea Abnormal increase in duration or amount of menstrual blood loss.

Hypermetabolism Increased metabolic rate seen in hyperthyroidism, fever, following trauma and surgery.

Hypermetria Unusual range of movement as in cerebellar disease.

Hypermetropia Hyperopia; longsightedness. The light rays entering the eye converge beyond the retina. Clear vision can be obtained by the wearing of spectacles or contact lenses.

Hypermimia Making great number of gestures while speaking.

Hypermnesia Great ability to remember or memorize minute details as in mania or in conditions of temporal lobe stimulation.

Hypermobility Increased range of joint movement due to lax surrounding structures as in Ehlers-Danlos syndrome, Marafan's syndrome.

Hypermotility Excessive movement.
Gastric hypermotility Increased muscle action of the stomach wall, associated with increased secretion of hydrochloric acid.

Hypermorph Large limb length causing high standing height in comparison to sitting height.

Hypernatremia An excess of sodium in the blood, usually diagnosed when the plasma sodium is above 150 mmol/L. It is the result of loss of water and electrolytes from the body caused by diarrhea, polyuria, excessive sweating or inadequate fluid intake.

Hypernephroma A malignant tumor of the kidney; renal cell carcinoma.

Hypernormal Abnormal

Hyperosmia Abnormal sensitivity to odors.

Hyperosmolarity Increased osmolarity of blood (300 mOsm/L.)

Hyperostosis A thickening of bone; a bony outgrowth; exostosis.

Hyperoxaluria Increased oxalic acid excretion in urine.
Hyperoxaluria enteric Caused by disease or surgical removal of ileum.
Hyperoxaluria primary Defective oxalate metabolism causing oxlate calculi in urinary system.

Hyperparathyroidism Excessive activity of the parathyroid glands, causing drainage of calcium from the bones, with consequent fragility and liability to spontaneous fracture.

Hyperphagia Overeating.

Hyperpathia Hypersensitivity to sensory stimuli.

Hyperphasia Excessive talkativeness.

Hyperphenylalaninaemia An excess of phenylalanine in the blood, as in phenylketonuria.

Hyperphonia Explosive speech in stammerers.

Hyperphoria Tendency of one eye to turn upward.

Hyperphosphatasemia Raised alkaline phosphatase in blood either due to biliary obstruction or bone destruction.

Hyperphosphatemia Increased blood phosphorus content.

Hyperphosphaturia Increased amount of phosphates in urine.

Hyperphrenia Excessive mental ability as in mania.

Hyperpituitarism Overactivity of the pituitary gland.

H

Hyperplasia Excessive formation of normal cells in a tissue or organ, which increases in size.

Hyperploidy Condition having one extra chromosome, e.g., Down syndrome (trisomy 21).

Hyperpnea Overbreathing; hyperventilation; an abnormal increase in the rate and depth of breathing.

Hyperpraxia Excessive activity and restlessness.

Hyperprolactinemia Increased levels of prolactin in the blood; in women, it is associated with infertility and may lead to galactorrhea, and it has been reported to cause impotence in men.

Hyperprolinemia Excess blood proline level due to inherited metabolic defect.

Hyperproteinemia Excess of protein in plasma, as in multiple myeloma.

Hyperproteinuria Protein excretion in urine exceeding 150 mg/24 hours.

Hyperptyalism Excess salivary secretion.

Hyperpyrexia An excessively high body temperature, i.e., over 41°C.

Hyperreflexia Increased tendon reflexes.

Hyperresonance Increased resonance to percussion especially over cavity, bullae, pneumothorax and emphysematous lung tissue.

Hypersensitivity Abnormal sensitivity especially to a particular antigen. The reactions include allergies (such as asthma) and anaphylaxis.

Contact hypersensitivity Produced by contact of the skin with a chemical substance having the properties of an antigen or hapten; it includes contact dermatitis *(See Contact).*

Delayed hypersensitivity A slowly developing increase in cell-mediated immune response (involving T lymphocytes) to a specific antigen, as occurs in graft rejection, autoimmune disease, etc.

Immediate hypersensitivity Antibody-mediated hypersensitivity characterized by lesions resulting from release of histamine and other mediators of hypersensitivity from regaining sensitized mast cells, causing increased vascular permeability, edema and smooth muscle contraction; it includes anaphylaxis and atopy.

Hypersomnia Prolonged sleepiness, usually pathological, i.e., narcalepsy.

Hypersplenism Overactivity of an enlarged spleen resulting in the destruction of blood cells and platelets.

Hypersthenia Abnormal strength or excessive tension of the entire body or part of it.

Hyperthenuria Passage of abnormally concentrated urine.

Hypersusceptibility Unusual susceptibility to a disease, pathological process, parasite or chemicals.

Hypertelorism Abnormally increased distance between two organs or parts.

Ocular hypertelorism, orbital hypertelorism Increase in the interocular distance, often associated with craniofacial dysostosis and sometimes with mental handicap.

Hypertension Persistently high blood pressure. In adults, it is generally agreed that a blood pressure is abnormally high when the resting, supine arterial systolic pressure is equal to or greater than 140 mm Hg and the diastolic pressure is equal to or greater than 90 mm Hg. A diagnosis of hypertension should be based on a series of readings rather than a single measurement.

Essential hypertension High blood pressure without demonstrable change in kidneys, blood vessels or heart.

Malignant hypertension A form of hypertension which may develop at a comparatively early age, in which the prognosis is poor.

Portal hypertension Raised pressure in the portal system.

Pulmonary hypertension Increased pressure in the arteries of the lung, usually following emphysema or fibrosis.

Hyperthecosis Hyperplasia of theca interna of ovary often leading to amenorrhea and 2 nipples.

Hyperthelia Presence of more than 2 nipples.

Hyperthermia An exceedingly high body temperature.

Malignant hyperthermia A serious condition, sometimes arising during general anesthesia.

Hyperthrombinemia Increased thrombin concentration in blood.

Hyperthyroidism Excessive activity of the thyroid gland *(See Thyrotoxicosis)*.

Hypertonia Increased vascular/muscle tone.

Hypertonic 1. Showing excessive tone or tension, as in a blood vessel or muscle. 2. Describing a solution that has greater osmotic pressure than normal physiological tissue fluid *(See Hypotonic)*.

Hypertrichosis Excessive growth of hair on any part of the body.

Hypertrophy An increase in the size of a tissue or a structure caused by an increase in the size of the cells that compose it (as opposed to an increase in the number of cells) *(See Hyperplasia)*.

Hyperuricemia An excess of uric acid in the blood *(See Gout)*.

Hyperventilation 1. Increase of air in the lungs above the normal amount. 2. Abnormally prolonged and deep breathing, usually associated with acute anxiety or emotional tension. Hyperpnea.

Hyperviscosity Excess adhesiveness or stickiness property of fluid, commonly blood.

Hypervitaminosis A condition caused by the intake of an excessive quantity of vitamins, particularly vitamins A and D.

Hypervolemia Abnormal increase in the volume of circulating fluid (plasma) in the body.

Hypesthesia Lessened sensibility to touch.

Hyphaema Hemorrhage into the anterior chamber of the eye.

Hypnagogic Induced by sleep; inducing sleep; in psychiatry relates to hallucinations and dreams just before loss of consciousness.

Hypnodontics The application of controlled suggestions and hypnosis to practice of surgery.

Hypnology Scientific study of sleep.

Hypnosis An artificially induced passive state in which there is increased amenability and responsiveness to suggestions and commands. In hypnosis, a drowsy phase is followed by a sleep. It may also be used to produce painless childbirth and tooth extraction.

Hypnotherapy Treatment by hypnosis or by the induction of prolonged sleep.

Hypnotic An agent that causes sleep; a soporific.

Hypnotism The practice of hypnosis.

Hypoacusis Decreased sensitivity to sound stimuli.

Hypoalbuminemia Decreased plasma albumin manifesting with edema, usually due to malnutrition or cirrhosis.

Hypoaldosteronism Decreased plasma aldosterone with hypotension and hyperkalemia.

Hypoalimentation Insufficient nourishment.

Hypob aric Decreased atmospheric pressure.

Hypocalcemia Decreased plasma calcium manifesting with stridor and tetany.

H

Hypocalciuria Decreased calcium excretion in urine.

Hypocapnia A deficiency of carbon dioxide in the blood.

Hypocellularity Decreased cell population in any tissue.

Hypochloremia A deficiency of chloride in the blood.

Hypochlorhydria A lower than normal amount of hydrochloric acid in the gastric juice.

Hypochlorous acid (HClO), used as disinfectant/bleaching agent.

Hypochlorite Any salt of hypochlorous acid used in solution to yield chlorine, a disinfecting and germicidal agent. Milton, a proprietary preparation, is used in solution for the disinfection of equipment and infant-feeding utensils.

Hypochondria A morbid preoccupation or anxiety about one's health. The sufferer feels that first one part of the body and then another part is the seat of some serious disease.

Hypochondriac One affected by hypochondria.

Hypochondriac region The hypochondrium.

Hypochondrium The upper region of the abdomen on each side of the epigastrium.

Hypochromic Deficient in pigmentation or coloring.

Hypocomplementemia Decreased complement concentration in blood.

Hypocorticism Decreased cortical hormone.

Hypodermic Beneath the skin; applied to subcutaneous injections and to the syringes used for such injections.

Hypodontia Absence or poor tooth development.

Hypofunction Decreased function.

Hypofibrinogenemia A lack of fibrinogen in the blood. This may occur in severe trauma or hemorrhage or as an inherited condition.

Hypogammaglobulinemia A deficiency of gamma-globulin in the blood, rendering the person susceptible to infection.

Hypogastrium The lower middle area of the abdomen, immediately below the umbilical region.

Hypogeusia Blunting of taste sensation.

Hypoglossal Under the tongue.

Hypoglossal nerve The 12th cranial nerve.

Hypoglottis Under surface of tongue.

Hypoglycemia A condition in which the blood sugar level is less than normal. Usually seen in diabetic patients as a result of insulin overdosage, delay in eating or a rapid combustion of carbohydrate. *(See Hyperglycemia)*

Hypoglycemic agents Sulphonyl urea compounds causing a decrease in blood sugar.

Hypoglycemic shock Shock produced by hypoglycemia induced by insulin injection to treat schizophrenia.

Hypokalemia A low potassium level in the blood. This is likely to be present during dehydration and with the repeated use of diuretics.

Hypokinesia Decreased motor activity.

Hypolipidemic Reducing lipid concentration.

Hypomagnesemia Decreased plasma magnesium with neuromuscular excitability.

Hypomania A degree of elation, excitement and activity higher than normal but less severe than that present in mania.

Hypomelanosis Decreased melanin in epidermis, e.g., vitiligo, burn.

Hypomenorrhea Decreased menstrual flow.

Hypomorph Individual with disproportionately short legs.

Hypometropia Myopia; shortsightedness.

Hypomotility Deficient power of movement in any part.

Hyponatremia A deficiency of sodium in the blood.

Hypoparathyroidism A lack of parathyroid secretion, leading to a low blood calcium and tetany.

Hypophysis An outgrowth.

Hypophysis cerebri The pituitary gland.

Hypopharynx Lowermost portion of pharynx leading to esophagus and larynx.

Hypophonia Weak voice.

Hypophoria Tendency of one visual axis to fall below the other.

Hypophosphatasia Decreased alkaline phosphatase in serum, usually in inherited metabolic deisease manifesting with rickets, osteomalacia, poor dentition, etc.

Hypophosphatemia Decreased plasma phosphate concentration.

Hypophyseal Pertains to hypophysis or pituitary.

Hypophysectomy Excision of hypophysis.

Hypophysis The pituitary gland occupying sella turcica.

Hypophysitis Inflammation of pituitary body.

Hypopituitarism Deficiency of secretion from the anterior lobe of the pituitary gland, causing excessive deposition of fat in children *(See Frolich's syndrome)*.

Dwarfism may result. In adults asthenia, drowsiness and adiposity may occur, together with an impairment of sexual activity and premature senility.

Hypoplasia Imperfect development of a part or organ.

Hypopnea Shallow breathing.

Hypoproteinemia A deficiency of serum proteins in the blood.

Hypoprothrombinemia A deficiency of prothrombin in the blood, leading to a tendency to bleed *(See Haemophilia)*.

Hypopyon An accumulation of pus in the anterior chamber of the eye.

Hyposecretion A deficiency in secretion from any glandular structure or secreting cells.

Hyposensitivity A lack of sensitivity, especially to a particular allergen with which the patient may have been overdosed over a period.

Hypospadias A developmental anomaly in the male in which the urethra opens on the underside of the penis or on the perineum.

Hypostasis 1. A sediment or deposit. 2. Congestion of blood in a part, due to slowing of the circulation.

Hyposthenia Weakness, subnormal strength.

Hyposthenuria Secretion of low specific gravity urine.

Hypostatic Relating to hypostasis.

Hypostatic pneumonia (See Pneumonia).

Hypotension Abnormally low arterial blood pressure; hypopiesis.

Controlled or induced hypotension An artificially produced lowering of the blood pressure so that an operation field is rendered practically bloodless.

Orthostatic or postural hypotension Temporary hypotension when the patient stands up, producing giddiness and sometimes a faint.

Hypotensive Producing a reduction in tension, especially pertaining to a drug that lowers the blood pressure.

Hypothenar The fleshy prominence at the base of little finger along innerside of palm.

Hypothalamus The portion of the diencephalons lying beneath the thalamus at the base of the cerebrum, and forming the floor and part of the lateral wall of the third ventricle. It influences peripheral autonomic mechanisms, endocrine activity and many somatic functions, e.g., a general regulation of water balance,

H

body temperature, sleep, thirst and hunger, and the development of secondary sexual characteristics. It plays an important role in the regulation of protein, fat and carbohydrate metabolism, body fluid volume and electrolyte content, and internal secretion of endocrine hormones.

Hypothermia 1. A severe reduction in the body temperature. The condition usually arises gradually and may prove fatal if untreated. It is most common among babies and elderly people. 2. Artificial cooling of the body to reduce the oxygen requirements of the tissues.

Mild hypothermia A reduction of the body temperature to 34°C, which maybe induced by surface cooling with cold air. Generalized lowering of the body temperature is used in three main situations: (a) To control fever, as in malignant hyperthermia; (b) To enable certain cardiac and neurological operations to be carried out; and (c) To protect the brain from raised intracranial pressure in patients with head injuries or following drowning.

Hypothesis A supposition that appears to explain a group of phenomena and is assumed as a basis of reasoning and experimentation. A starting point for further investigations from known facts.

Hypothrombinemia A diminished amount of thrombin in the blood, with a consequent tendency to bleed.

Hypothrombinemia A diminished amount of thrombin in the blood, with a consequent tendency to bleed.

Hypothyroidism An insufficiency of thyroid secretion. In children it may produce cretinism. In adults it leads to myxoedema.

Hypotonia 1. Deficient muscle tone. 2. Deficient tension in the eyeball.

Hypotonic Describing a solution that has a lower osmotic pressure than another one *(See Hypertonic).*

Hypotrichosis Sparse hair.

Hypotrophy Degeneration and atrophy of tissues.

Hypotympanum The part of middle ear below the level of tympanic membrane.

Hypoventilation Hypopnea; shallow breathing, usually at a very slow rate. It may cause a build-up of carbon dioxide in the blood.

Hypovitaminosis Condition arising from lack of vitamins.

Hypovolemia A reduction in the circulating blood volume due to external loss of body fluids or to loss from the blood into the tissues, as in shock.

Hypoxanthine A purine derivative formed during protein decomposition to form urea and uric acid.

Hypoxemia An insufficient oxygen content in the blood.

Hypoxia A diminished amount of oxygen in the tissues.
Anaemic expand as hypoxia Low oxygen content due to deficiency of hemoglobin in the blood.

Hypsarrhythmia An abnormal EEG pattern in which there is persistent generalized slowing and very high voltage discharge; characteristic of infantile epilepsy.

Hypsiloid U or Y shaped.

Hypsiloid ligament Iliofemoral ligament.

Hypsokinesis Tendency to fall backwards when standing as seen in Parkinson's disease.

Hypsophobia Fear of being at great heights.

Hysterectomy Removal of the uterus.
Abdominal hysterectomy Removal via an abdominal incision.
Subtotal hysterectomy Removal of the body of the uterus only.
Total hysterectomy Removal of the body and cervix.
Vaginal hysterectomy Removal through the vagina.

H

Wertheim's hysterectomy Additional excision of the parametrium, upper vagina and lymph glands. Radical abdominal hysterectomy.

Hysteresis Failure of the manifestation of an effect to keep up with its cause.

Hysteria A psychoneurosis in which the individual converts anxiety created by emotional conflict into physical symptoms, e.g., tics, mutism or paralysis of an arm or leg, that have no organic basis; also called conversion reaction or conversion hysteria. The term hysteria is also used to describe a state of tension or excitement in which there is a temporary loss of control over the emotions.

Hysterical Relating to hysteria.

Hysteric chorea A form of hysteria with choreiform movements.

Hysterography Recording of frequency and intensity of uterine contractions.

Hysterogram X-ray of uterus.

Hysteroid Resembling hysteria.

Hysteromania Nymphomania.

Hysterometry Measurement of size of uterus.

Hysteromyoma A fibromyoma of the uterus.

Hysteromyomectomy Excision of a hysteromyoma.

Hystero-oophorectomy Excision of the uterus and the ovaries.

Hysteropia Hysteric visual defect.

Hysterorrhexis Rupture of pregnant uterus.

Hysterosalpingography Radiographic examination of the uterus and uterine tubes after the injection of a radio-opaque dye. Uterosalpingography.

Hysterosalpingostomy or anastomosis The operation of forming an anastomosis, or opening, between the distal portion of the uterine tube and the uterus in an effort to overcome infertility when the medical portion is occluded or excised.

Hysteroscope Instrument for examination of inside of uterus.

Hysterotomy Incision of the uterus, usually in order to remove a fetus in mid-pregnancy when it is too late to perform a therapeutic abortion *(See Caesarean section).*

Hysterotrachelectomy Amputation of uterine cervix.

Hysterotrachelorrhaphy Repair of torn cervix.

H

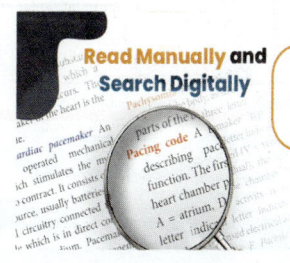

Undergraduate Packs

By **THE MASTERMINDS**

Undergraduate Pack - 1st Year

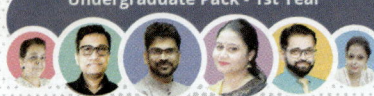

What all you will get

Main Subjects	Video Duration	No. of Questions
Anatomy	60+ Hours	600+ Qs
Physiology	60+ Hours	600+ Qs
Biochemistry & Nutrition	50+ Hours	500+ Qs
Microbiology	50+ Hours	500+ Qs
Fundamentals of Nursing	200+ Hours	400+ Qs

MRP ₹7997/-
Validity: 18 months

Bonus Subjects:- Computers & Psychology

Undergraduate Pack - 2nd Year

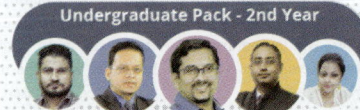

What all you will get

MRP ₹7997/-
Validity: 18 months

Main Subjects	Video Duration	No. of Questions
Pharmacology	50+ Hours	800+ Qs
MSN - Medicine	90+ Hours	900+ Qs
MSN - Surgery	50+ Hours	600+ Qs
Community Health Nursing	90+ Hours	900+ Qs
Sociology	40+ Hours	250+ Qs

Undergraduate Pack - 3rd & 4th Year

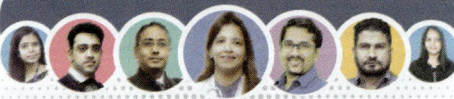

What all you will get

Main Subjects	Video Duration	No. of Questions
Pediatric Nursing	80+ Hours	900+ Qs
Midwifery & Obstetrical Nursing	100+ Hours	1000+ Qs
MSN - Medicine	90+ Hours	900+ Qs
MSN - Surgery	50+ Hours	600+ Qs
Mental Health Nursing	90+ Hours	900+ Qs
Community Health Nursing	90+ Hours	900+ Qs
Nursing Research & Statistics	35+ Hours	400+ Qs

MRP ₹12992/-
Validity: 24 months

Bonus Subjects:- Nursing Managment & Nursing Education

Special Features

- Handwritten Notes of Videos in PDF Format
- IBQs/VBQs Discussion Videos of above mentioned Subjects
- Monthly Mega Assessment Tests
- Monthly Live Doubt Session/Live Classes/Live Webinar by MM Faculty
- Best Guidance & Support
- Get your query directly resolved by MM faculty

I Symbol for iodine.

Iatrogenesis Additional patient problems, complications or disease brought about by the activities of physicians, surgeons or other health care professionals, including new infections, unwanted effects of drug therapy and psychological distress.

Ibuprofen An anti-inflammatory analgesic and antipyretic drug used in the treatment of mild rheumatic and arthritic conditions.

Ice Water in a solid state, at or below freezing point.

Dry ice Carbon dioxide snow.

Ice bag A rubber or plastic bag half-filled with pieces of ice and applied near or to a part to relieve pain or swelling.

Ichnogram A footprint taken while standing.

Ichor Fetid Discharge from an ulcer.

Ichthammol An ammoniated coal tar product, used in ointment form for certain skin diseases.

Ichthyosis A congenital abnormality of the skin in which there is dryness and roughness, the horny layer is thickened and large scales appear.

Ichthyotoxin Any toxin present in fish.

Ictal Pertains to acute attack of epilepsy or stroke.

Icteric Pertains to jaundice.

Icteroid Resembling jaundice.

ICM International Confederation of Midwives.

ICN Infection Control Nurse *(See Infection)*, International Council of Nurses.

ICP Intracranial pressure.

ICSH Interstitial cell stimulating hormone.

Icterus Jaundice.

Icterus gravis A fatal form of jaundice occurring in pregnancy. Acute yellow atrophy.

Icterus gravis neonatorum Hemolytic disease of the newborn *(See Rhesus factor).*

ICU Intensive Care Unit.

Id Part of the personality, containing the instinctive drives, which leads to gratification of primitive needs and which exists in the unconscious.

Idea A mental impression or conception.

Autochthonous idea A strange idea that comes into the mind in some unaccountable way, but is not a hallucination.

Compulsive idea An idea that persists despite reason and will and that drives one to action, usually inappropriate.

Dominant idea A morbid or other impression that controls or colors every action and thought.

Fixed idea A persistent morbid impression or belief that cannot be changed by reason.

Idea of reference The incorrect idea that the words and actions of others refer to oneself, or the projection of the causes of one's own imaginary difficulties upon someone else.

Ideal A goal regarded as a standard of perfection.

Ideation The process of thinking or formation of ideas. It is quick in mania but slow in depression, and dementias.

Identical Exactly alike.

Identical twins Twins of the same sex developing from a single fertilized ovum.

Identification A mental mechanism by which an individual adopts the attitudes and ideas of another, often admired person.

Identity Part of the 'self concept' of being distinguishable and separate from others.

Identity crisis One in which the individual loses the sense of self distinctiveness and role in society. Occurs most commonly in the transition from one phase of life to the next, e.g., during adolescence.

Ideology 1. The science of the development of ideas. 2. The body of ideas characteristic of an individual or of a social unit.

Ideomotion The association of ideas and muscle action, as in involuntary acts.

Ideomotor Muscular automatic movement regulated by a dominant idea.

Idiocy Severe mental deficiency due to defective mental development, the cause of which may be genetic, vascular or birth asphyxia.

Idioglossia Inability to articulate properly so that the language is not comprehensible.

Idiogram Graphic respresentation of chromosome karyotype.

Idiopathic Self-originated; applied to a condition the cause of which is not known.

Idiopathic pulmonary fibrosis A form of interstitial lung disease with diffuse fibrosis and rapid deterioration.

Idiophrenic Pertaining to or originating in the mind alone.

Idiosyncrasy 1. A habit or quality of body or mind peculiar to any individual. 2. An abnormal susceptibility to an agent (e.g., a drug) that is peculiar to the individual.

Idiot Person with severe mental deficiency.

Idiotropic In psychology turning inward mentally and emotionally, i.e., introvert who is satisfied with his own emotions and is content to live apart from social contacts.

Idiotype In immunology, the specific Fab region of the immunoglobulin to which the specific antigen binds.

Idioventricular A heart rhythm arising from conduction tissue or ventricular muscle without any influence from sinus node.

Idoxuridine Abbreviated IOU. An iodine containing drug used to treat infections caused by herpes virus, particularly keratitis and dendritic corneal ulcer.

Ifosfamide Anticancer drug.

Ig Immunoglobulin of any of the five classes: IgA, IgD, IgE, IgG and IgM.

Ileal Referring to the ileum.

Ileal bypass A method of treating obesity where by absorption of nutrients from intestine is decreased from anastomosis of one portion of upper small intestine to another portion down below.

Ileal conduit A surgical procedure in which the ureters are transplanted into the ileum, an isolated loop of which is then brought to the surface of the abdomen in order to allow the urine to drain into a bag.

Ileitis Inflammation of the ileum.

Regional ileitis Crohn's disease. A chronic condition of the terminal portion of the ileum in which granulation and oedema may give rise to obstruction.

Ileocecal valve A muscular ring at the terminal ileum that regulates passage of food from small intestine to large intestine and prevents re-entry of food back into small intestine.

Ileocolitis Inflammation of the ileum and colon.

Ileocecostomy Surgical formation of an opening between ileum and cecum.

Ileocolostomy The making of a permanent opening between the ileum and some part of the colon.

Ileoileostomy Surgical formation of an opening between two parts of ileum.

Ileocystoplasty Repair of the wall of the urinary bladder with an isolated segment of the ileum.

Ileoproctostomy Surgical anastomosis between the ileum and the rectum; ileorectal anastomosis.

Ileorrhaphy Surgical repair of ileum.

Ileosigmoidostomy An operation carried out when most of the colon has to be removed and an anastomosis is made between the ileum and the sigmoid colon.

Ileorectal Referring to the ileum and rectum.

Ileorectal anastomosis Ileoproctostomy.

Ileostomy An artificial opening (stoma) created from the ileum and brought to the surface of the abdomen for the purpose of evacuation. Ileostomy is an inevitable part of proctocolectomy. An ileostomy maybe temporary or permanent.

Ileostomy bags Disposable bags to collect the liquid fecal matter discharged from an ileostomy. The bags can be adhesive or worn on a belt.

Ileum The last part of the small intestine, terminating at the cecum.

Ileus Intestinal obstruction, especially failure of peristalsis. The condition frequently accompanies peritonitis and usually results from disturbances in neural stimulation of the bowel. The principal symptoms of ileus are abdominal pain and distension, vomiting (the vomitus may contain fecal material) and constipation. If the intestinal obstruction is not relieved, the patient becomes extremely ill with shock and dehydration.

Iliac Pertaining to the ilium.

Iliac artery The right and left arteries form the terminal branches of the abdominal aorta and supply blood to the pelvic region and the lower limbs.

Iliac crest The crest of the hip bone.

Iliac fossa The depression on the concave surface of the iliac bone.

Iliac vein The right and left veins join to form the inferior vena cava and drain the blood from the lower limbs and pelvis.

Illiotibial band A thick wide fascial layer from the iliac crest to knee point.

Illizarov method A method of bone lengthening by distraction using external fixators.

Ilium The haunch bone; the upper part of the hip bone.

Illness A condition marked by pronounced deviation from the normal healthy state; sickness.

Illness behaviour The way in which ill individuals regard the structure and function of their own body, interpret symptoms and seek treatment for their condition.

Illusion A mistaken perception due to a misinterpretation of a sensory stimulus; believing something to be what it is not.

Image 1. The mental recall of a form former precept. 2. The optical picture transferred to the brain cells by the optic nerve.

Image intensifier Device that increases brightness of an image and permits discrimination of much smaller objects in the image.

Imagery The calling up of events or mental pictures pertaining to sound, smell, taste, etc.

Imagination Formation of mental images of things, persons or situations.

Imaging Production of image of an object by X-ray, ultrasound, magnetic resonance, etc.

Imago [L.] 1. In psychoanalysis, a childhood memory or fantasy of a loved person that persists in adult life. 2. The adult or definitive form of an insect.

Imbalance Lack of balance, e.g., of endocrine secretions, between water and electrolytes, or of muscles.

Autonomic imbalance Sympathetic – parasympathetic imbalance.

Vasomotor imbalance Excessive vasoconstriction or dilatation.

Imatinib Anticancer agent for CML.

Imbecile Severe mental deficiency.

Imbed In histology, to surround with a firm substance such as paraffin or colloidium.

Imbibition The absorption of fluid by a solid.

Imbricated Overlapping as tiles.

Imidazole An organic comound with heterocyclic ring as in histamine and histidine.

Imipenem An antibiotic, betalactamase resistant.

Imipramine A drug, chemically related to chlorpromazine, that may be effective in relieving depression *(See Antidepressant)*. Also used to treat nocturnal enuresis in children.

Immature Unripe; not fully developed, as in a cataract when only a part of the lens is opaque.

Immedicable Incurable.

Immersion Placing body or object under water or fluid; in microscopy the act of immersing the objective (lens) in oil.

Immersion foot A form of cold injury due to dampness and cold.

Immiscible Incapable of being mixed, e.g., oil and water.

Immobilize To render incapable of being moved, as by a plaster of Paris cast.

Immune Protected against a particular infection or allergy.

Immune response The (10 general) helpful events that follow activation of the immune system, including T-lymphocyte activity (cell-mediated responses) and B-lymphocyte activity (humoral responses). Immune responses are involved in protecting persons from disease following infection and are also involved in the rejection of transplanted organs and tissues that the body recognizes as foreign, or non-self.

Immunifacient Making immune.

Immunity The resistance possessed by the body to infectious diseases, foreign tissues, foreign nontoxic substances and other antigens. The opposite of susceptibility. Immunological responses in humans can be divided into two broad categories: humoral immunity, which takes place in the body fluids and is concerned with antibody and complement activities; and cell mediated or cellular immunity, which involves a variety of activities designed to destroy or at least contain cells that are recognized by the body as alien and harmful. Both types of response are instigated by lymphocytes that originate in the bone marrow as stem cells and later are converted into mature cells having specific properties and functions. The two kinds of lymphocyte that are important to the establishment of immunity are T-lymphocytes *(T-cells)* and B-lymphocytes (B-cells).

B-lymphocytes mature into plasma cells that are primarily responsible for forming antibodies, thereby providing humoral immunity. Cellular immunity is dependent upon T-lymphocytes and is primarily concerned with a delayed type of immune response as occurs in the rejection of transplanted organs, defence against some slowly developing bacterial diseases, allergic reactions and certain autoimmune diseases.

Immunization The act of creating immunity by artificial means.

Immunization schedule A standard schedule for immunization against infectious diseases *(See Appendices)*.

Immunoassay A quantitative estimate of the proteins contained in the blood serum.

Immunobiology Study of immune phenomena in biological systems.

Immunochemistry The chemistry of antigen, antibodies and their relation to each other.

Immunocompetence Being capable of developing antibody response stimulated by an antigen.

Immunocompromised Unable to have adequate immunological response because of genetic defect of T and B cells, immunosuppressive drugs or AIDS virus infection.

Immunodiagnosis Use of specific immune response in diagnosing medical conditions.

Immunodeficiency A deficiency of the immune response, either that mediated by humoral antibody or by immune lymphoid cells.

Immunodeficiency disorders Acquired or congenital conditions in which the body's immune system fails to protect against infection, foreign material and some forms of cancer.

Immunodiffusion A test method in which antigen and antibody are place in a gel where they diffuse towards each other and when they meet a precipitate is formed.

Immunoelectrophoresis A method of investigating the amount and character of antibodies and immunoproteins present in body fluids.

Immunofluorescence The use of fluorescein stained or fluorescein labeled in tissues. The sample is examined in fluorescent microscope.

Immunogen A substance that stimulates formation of antibody.

Immunogenetics The study of genetics by use of immune responses.

Immunogenic Capable of inducing immunity.

Immunogenicity The capability to stimulate antibody formation.

Immunoglobulin Antibody. A variety of chemical compound found mainly in gamma-globulin *(See Gamma)*. Immunoglobulins are major components of the humoral immune response system. They are synthesized by lymphocytes and plasma cells and found in the serum and in other body fluids and tissues. The five classes of immunoglobulin (Ig) are: IgA, IgO, IgE, IgG and IgM. There are two types of IgA and both are known to have antiviral properties. Secretory IgA is present in nonvascular fluids such as colostrum and breast milk. IgD is found in trace quantities in serum. It serves as a B-lymphocyte surface receptor. IgE is called the reaginic antibody and may be increased in persons with allergy. IgG is the most abundant of the five classes of immunoglobulin and is the major antibody in the secondary humoral response of immunity. It is the only immunoglobulin to cross the placenta. IgM is principally concerned with the primary antibody response.

Immunology The study of immunity and the body's defence mechanisms.

Immunopathology Study of tissue alterations resulting from immune or allergic reactions.

Immunoselection Selective survival of cell populations due to their having least amount of cell surface antigenicity.

Immunostimulant Agent capable of stimulating antibody production.

Immunosuppression Inhibition of the formation of antibodies to antigens that may be present; used in transplantation procedures to prevent rejection of the transplanted organ or tissue.

Immunosuppressant Agent suppressing body immune response, usually employed in treatment of autoimmune diseases.

Immunosuppressive 1. Pertaining to or inducing immunosuppression. 2. An agent that induces immunosuppression.

Immunotherapy 1. Treatment by immunization. Sometimes used in the treatment of leukemia. 2. The establishing of passive immunity.

Immunotransfusion Transfusion of blood from a donor previously rendered immune to the disease affecting the patient.

Imodium Trade name for preparations of loperamide hydrochloride, an antidiarrheal.

Impaction A state of being wedged.

Dental impaction The condition in which a tooth, usually a molar, is unable to erupt through the gum because it is lodged in position by bone or the other teeth.

Faecal impaction A collection of putty-like or hardened faeces in the rectum or sigmoid colon.

Impairment Any loss or abnormality of psychological, physiological or anatomical structure or function.

Impalpable Incapable of being felt by manual examination. May apply to an organ or a tumor.

Impedance Resistance met by alternating current while passing through a conductor.

Impedance acoustic Resistance to the passage of sound waves.

Imperative Obligatory, involuntary.

Imperception Lack of perception, inability to form a mental picture.

Imperforate Without an opening.

Imperforate antis A congenital defect in which this opening is closed.

Imperforate hymen Complete closure of the vaginal opening by the hymen.

Impermeable Not permitting the passage of fluid or molecules.

Impervious Difficult to be penetrated.

Impetigo An acute contagious inflammation of the skin marked by pustules and scabs; of streptococcal or staphylococcal origin. It occurs mainly on the face and limbs, particularly those of children.

Implant Any substance grafted into the tissues.

Hormone implant A hormonal pellet which may be implanted subcutaneously.

Intraocular lens implant A plastic lens which may be implanted in the eye after lens extraction.

Plastic implant A silicone implant which may be used in plastic surgery, e.g., to reshape the breast.

Implantable cardioverter defibrillator (ICD) An implanted device that automatically terminates life-threatening arrhythmias by delivering low energy shocks to the heart, restoring normal rhythm. Some devices have inbuilt pacing capabilities.

Implantation The act of planting or setting in. 1. The embedding of the fertilized ovum in the wall of the uterus. 2. The placing of a drug within the tissues. 3. The surgical introduction of healthy tissue to replace tissue that has been damaged.

Implementation The third phase of the nursing process signifying the giving of care in relation to defined nursing interventions and goals. During implementation the nursing care plan is tested for effectiveness and accuracy. Data gathering continues and plans may change on the basis of new information obtained. The implementation phase concludes with the recording of the activities performed and the response of the patient (*See Assessment and Evaluation*).

Implosion In behavior therapy, a form of desensitization used in the treatment of phobias and related disorders (*See Flooding*).

Impotence Inability in a man to carry-out sexual intercourse from either psychological or physical causes.

Impotent Inability to copulate and procreate.

Impregnation Insemination; rendering pregnant.

Impression A hollow or depression of surface; effect produced upon mind by external stimuli, the imprint of dental arch.

Impression material Materials appropriate for dental impression work, like plaster of paris, zinc oxide paste, reversible colloids.

Impression tray A tray to carry impression material to mouth and hold it in opposition to jaw/teeth.

Impulse 1. A sudden pushing force. 2. A sudden uncontrollable act. 3. Nerve impulse.

Cardiac impulse Movement of the chest wall caused by the heartbeat.

Nerve impulse The electrochemical process propagated along nerve fibers.

Impulsion Idea to do something or commit some act suddenly imposed upon the subject that tortures him until the accomplishment of that act.

IMV Intermittent Mandatory Ventilation.

In situ [L] In the original position.

In vitro [L] In a glass. Refers to observations made outside the body *(See In vitro)*.

In vivo [L.] Within the living body *(See In vitro)*.

Inactivate To make inactivate or to cause loss of activity.

Inaccessibility A state of unresponsive characteristic of certain psychiatric patients, e.g., schizophrenics.

Inadequacy Insufficiency, incompetence.

Inanimate Dull, lifeless.

Inapparent Not noticeable.

Inarticulate 1. Without joints. 2. Unable to speak intelligibly.

Inassimilable Not capable of being utilized by body.

INC Indian Nursing Council.

Incarcerated Held fast. Applied to (a) a hernia that is immovable, and therefore only curable by operation, and (b) a pregnant uterus held under the sacral brim.

Incarnation To grow in (e.g., toe nails); the process of being converted to flesh.

Inception The beginning, ingestion.

Incest Sexual intercourse between close blood relatives, e.g., brothers and sisters; marriage between them is legally or culturally prohibited. Some form of incest taboo is found in all known societies, although the relationships prohibited vary.

Incidence The number of particular new events which occur in a population in a given period of time. For example, the number of new cases of a disease, such as measles, expressed per 1,000 of population per year.

Incident A happening, event or occurrence, falling or striking ray of light.

Incident report A report or form that is required to be filled in any health care facility, such as hospital following any accident or unfortunate incident or near miss involving a patient, visitor or member of staff. These incidents may be clinical, e.g., cardiac arrest or the incorrect administration of a medication, but can also include such issues as the loss of a patient's belongings.

Incipient Beginning to exist.

Incise To cut, as with a sharp instrument.

Incision 1. In surgery, a cut into soft tissue. 2. The act of cutting.

Incisor One of the four front teeth in the center of each jaw.

Incisura Indentation at edge of any structure, e.g., stomach incisura at distal end of lesser curvature.

Incitant The stimulus that sets off a reaction, disease.

Inclination Leaning from normal or from a vertical as in case of tooth, vertebra or pelvis.

Inclinometer Device for measuring ocular diameter from vertical and horizontal lines.

Inclusion Something that is enclosed or the act of enclosing.

Inclusion bodies Particles that are temporarily enclosed in the cytoplasm of a cell. For example, in trachoma virus particles can be seen in the conjunctival epithelial cells.

Inclusion conjunctivitis Chlamydia trachomatis infection of the conjunctiva.

Incoercible Uncontrollable, not able to be held in check.

Incoherent 1. Unconnected; inconsistent. 2. Uttering speech that is disconnected and rambling.

Incombustible Unfit for burning.

Incompatibility The state of two or more substances being antagonistic, or destroying the efficiency of each other. Applied to mixtures of drugs, and to blood (*See Blood group*).

Incompetence Inefficiency.

Aortic incompetence Failure of the aortic valves to regulate the flow of blood.

Mitral incompetence Failure of the mitral valve to close properly.

Incompetent One legally unable to execute; incapable.

Incompetent palatal syndrome Distortion of speech (whinolalia) due to ineffective function of soft palate.

Incontinence Inability to control natural functions or discharges.

Faecal incontinence Mobility to control the movements of the bowels.

Overflow incontinence That from an overfull bladder, most common in elderly men with urinary obstruction

Paralytic incontinence Loss of control of anal and urethral sphincters due to injury to nerve centers.

Stress incontinence That which is due to a defect in the urethral sphincters and is liable to occur when intra-abdominal pressure is increased, as in coughing or lifting heavy weights; most common in women with weak pelvic muscles.

Urinary incontinence Inability to control the outflow of urine.

Incoordination Inability to adjust various muscle movements harmoniously.

Incorporation Combining two substances to produce a homogeneous mass.

Increment Something added or gained; an addition in number, size or extent.

Incremental To build up as in the contractions of labor or to add in stages.

Incrustation The formation of a crust or scab on a wound.

Incubation The development and growth of microorganisms and animal embryos.

Incubation period The period between the date of infection and the appearance of symptoms of an infectious disease.

Incubator 1. A warmed servo-controlled Perspex box for nursing ill and preterm babies. 2. An apparatus used to develop bacteria at a uniform temperature suitable to their growth.

Incus The small anvil-shaped bone of the middle ear. The second auditory ossicle.

Indicator 1. The index finger, or the extensor muscle of the index finger. 2. Any substance that indicates the appearance or disappearance of a chemical by a color change or attainment of a certain pH.

Indecision Inability to make up one's mind.

Indentation A depression or hollow.

Index case In hereditary disease, the initial patient whose condition led to investigation of the disease.

Index The forefinger, the ratio of the measurement of a given substance with that of a fixed standard.

Cardiac index Cardiac output expressed as L/min divided by body surface area in m^2.

Cephalic index Skull breadth to length multiplied by 100.

Cerebral index Ratio at greatest transverse to anteroposterior diameter of skull.

Pelvic index Ratio of pelvic conjugate and transverse diameters.

Therapeutic index The maximum tolerable dose of a drug divided by minimum curable dose.

Indicator In chemical analysis a substance that can be used to determine pH.

Indifferent Not responsive to normal stimuli, apathetic, neutral.

Indigenous Occurring naturally in a certain locality.

Indigestion (See *Dyspepsia*).

Indium A rare metallic element, its isotope ^{113}I used in scanning.

Indocyanine green A dye used in testing hepatic and renal excretory function.

Indocin Trade name for indomethacin.

Indole A solid crystalline substance found in feces, a bacterial decomposition product of tryptophan.

Indolent Slow growing. Reluctant to heal. Largely painless.

Indolent ulcer A chronic ulcer of the skin or mucous membrane.

Indomethacin An anti-inflammatory analgesic used in the treatment of arthritis and of acute attacks of gout.

Induction The act of initiating something.

Electromagnetic induction The production of an electric current in a body because of its nearness to an electrified (or magnetized) body.

Induction of abortion The intentional bringing about of an abortion

Induction of anesthesia The start of the administration of a general anesthetic.

Induction of labor The artificial starting of the process of childbirth.

Inductor Any substance that will cause cells exposed to it to differentiate into an organized tissue.

Induratio penis plastica (IPP) *(See PEYRONIE'S DISEASE).*

Induration The abnormal hardening of a tissue or organ.

Industrial Referring to industry.

Industrial diseases Those that are caused by the nature of the work.

Prescribed industrial diseases Those for which sickness benefit is payable, including those that are notifiable under the Factories Act (1961).

Inebriant Any intoxicant; making drunk.

Inebriation The condition of being intoxicated by alcohol; drunkenness.

Inelastic Not elastic.

Inert Having no action.

Inert gas A gas which does not react with other elements, e.g., neon.

Inertia Sluggishness; inability to move except when stimulated by an external force.

Uterine inertia. Lack of muscle contraction during the first and second stages of labor.

Infant A child under 1 year of age. Educationally, a child under 7 years of age.

Floppy infant, floppy infant syndrome A congenital myopathy of infants, marked clinically by myotonia and muscle weakness.

Infant feeding The supplying of nutrition to an infant. Breast milk is the ideal food for the baby and if breast-feeding is established satisfactorily for the first few months it can aid physical and emotional development. Where it is not possible an infant food formula can be given.

Infant mortality rate The number of deaths of children under 1 year of age per 1,000 live births in any one year.

Premature infant One born before the state of maturity *(See Preterm infant).*

Infanticide The killing of a child during the first year of its life.

Infantile Concerning an infant; childish.

Infantile paralysis Poliomyelitis.

Infantilism Persistence of the characteristic; of childhood into adult life, marked by underdevelopment of the reproductive organs, and often short stature.

Infarct The wedge-shaped area of necrosis in an organ produced by the blocking of a blood vessel, usually due to an embolus.

Red infarct A hemorrhage infarct. Red blood cells infiltrate the area.

White infarct An anemic infarct. The area is suddenly deprived of blood and is pale.

Infarction The formation of an infarct.

Myocardial infarction An infarct of the heart muscle following a coronary thrombosis.

Pulmonary infarction An infarct resulting from obstruction of a branch of the pulmonary artery by embolism or thrombosis.

Infection 1. Invasion and multiplication of microorganisms in body tissues, especially that causing local cellular injury due to competitive metabolism, toxins, intracellular replication or antigen-antibody response. 2. An infectious disease.

Aerobic infection Infection caused by an aerobe.

Air-borne infection Infection by inhalation of organisms suspended in air on water droplets, droplet nuclei or dust particles.

Anaerobic infection Infection caused by an anaerobe.

Cross infection Infection transmitted between patients infected with different pathogenic microorganisms.

Droplet infection Infection due to inhalation of respiratory pathogens suspended on liquid particles exhaled by someone already infected.

Hospital-acquired infections Those acquired during hospitalization; also called nosocomial infections. A recent prevalence survey showed that 10% of patients in hospitals in England and Wales acquired an infection while in hospital. The most common causative agents are *Escherichia coli, Proteus, Pseudomonas* and *Klebsiella,* among the Gram-negative organisms, and *Staphylococcus* and *Enterococcus* among the Gram-positive organisms *(See also Infection (Control))*

Infection control The utilization of procedures and techniques in the surveillance, investigation and compilation of statistical data in order to reduce the spread of infection, particularly hospital-acquired infections. Practitioners in infection control have titles such as Infection Control Officer and Infection Control Nurse, and they function as liaison between staff, nurses, doctors, department heads of the infection control committee and the health authority. Such practitioners also assume some responsibility for teaching patients and their families, as well as employees.

Mixed infection Infection with more than one kind of organisms at the same time.

Opportunistic infection An infection with a microorganism that does not usually cause disease but may do so when the patient's resistance to infection is lowered, e.g., after surgery.

Secondary infection Infection by a pathogen superimposed upon an infection by a pathogen of another kind.

Sexually transmitted infection An infection transmitted by sexual intercourse or by intimate contact with the genitals, mouth and rectum *(See Sexually transmitted infection).*

Subclinical infection Infection associated with no detectable symptoms but caused by microorganisms capable of producing easily recognizable diseases, such as poliomyelitis or mumps; it is detected by the production of antibody, or by delayed hypersensitivity exhibited in a skin test reaction to such antigens as tuberculoprotein.

Infection prevention and control The utilization of procedures and techniques in the surveillance, investigation and compilation of statistical data in order to reduce the spread of infection, particularly hospital-acquired infections. Practitioners in infection prevention and control are frequently nurses with specialist qualifications who are employed by NHS Trusts and other health care facilities. They have titles such as Director of Infection Prevention and Control (DIPC), Consultants in Infection Prevention and Control, and Infection Prevention and Control Practitioners/Nurses, and they function as liaison between staff, nurses, doctors, department heads and infection prevention and control committees. Such practitioners also assume some responsibility for teaching patients and their families, as well as employees.

Infectious Caused by or capable of being communicated by infection.

Infectious disease Disease resulting from multiplication of microorganisms in the body. Most are communicable, but not all *(See also Communicable disease).*

Infectious mononucleosis Glandular fever. An acute virus infection characterized by sore throat and glandular enlargement, caused by the Epstein-Barr (EB) virus. A common infection worldwide, particularly prevalent in older children and young adults in Western countries. The source of infection is human and is spread by oropharyngeal secretions: for example, during kissing. The incubation period is 4–6 weeks and infectivity after the disease may be prolonged.

Infective Infectious, capable of producing infection; pertaining to or characterized by the presence of pathogens.

Inferior Lower

Inferior vena cava The lower large vein.

Inferiority Lesser rank, stature, position or ability.

Inferiority complex (See Complex).

Infertility Inability of a woman to conceive or of a man to bring about conception.

Infestation The presence of animal parasites, e.g., mites, ticks or worms, in or on the body, in clothing or in a house.

Infibulation An extensive form of female circumcision performed in some cultures in which the clitoris and labia are removed and the vaginal entrance narrowed. Also known as Type III female genital mutilation according to the WHO classification system. *(See Circumcision).*

Infiltration The entrance and diffusion of some substance not usually found there, either fluid or solid, into tissues or cells.

Infiltration analgesia The injection into tissues of a local analgesic solution.

Infinity Space, time and quantity without limits.

Infirmary A small hospital, a place for care of sick.

Inflammation A localized protective response elicited by injury or destruction of tissues, which serves to destroy, dilute or wall off both the injurious agent and the injured tissue. The cardinal signs are heat, swelling, pain and redness.

Acute inflammation Sudden onset of inflammation, with marked and progressive symptoms.

Catarrhal inflammation Inflammation in which mucous surfaces are attacked, with stimulation of exudation.

Chronic inflammation Inflammation that develops slowly. Granulation tissue forms and tends to localize the infection.

Diffuse inflammation Extensive inflammation, as in nephritis and cellulitis.

Suppurative inflammation One marked by pus formation.

Traumatic inflammation That which follows an injury.

Inflammatory bowel disease Abbreviated IBD. Collective term for a group of chronic disorders affecting the small and/or large intestines that result in pain, bleeding and diarrhea. *(See Crohn's Disease).*

Inflation Distention of a part by air, gas or fluid.

Inflator Device used to force air into an organ.

Inflection An inward bending; change of tone or pitch of the voice.

Influenza An acute viral infection of the respiratory tract, occurring in isolated cases, epidemics and pandemics. Also called flu. Transmission is by droplet inhalation and the period of infectivity lasts from 1 day before the onset of symptoms up to 7 days later. There is fever, headache, pain in the back and limbs, anorexia and sometimes nausea and vomiting. The fever subsides in 2–3 days, leaving a feeling of lassitude. There is no specific drug cure for influenza, but an influenza vaccine is available, the formulation of which is changed annually to include recently circulating strains of viruses on recommendation of the WHO. Annual vaccination is advised for persons with chronic heart, lung or renal disease, those with diabetes, and patients on immunosuppressive therapy. It should also be advised for the elderly and residents of residential and nursing homes.

Influenza virus vaccine Vaccine containing inactivated influenza virus A and B; given every year with different strains of A and B.

Infolding Process of enclosing within a fold.

Informal patient A patient who has entered hospital voluntarily, i.e., without any statutory requirements for detention.

Informatics Discipline that integrates science, computer science and information science in systematizing, identifying, collecting, processing and managing data.

Nursing i. The way in which nurses, managers, researchers and practitioners use information systems in their work, enabling technology to develop a body of readily available knowledge to support the practice of nursing and the delivery of health care.

Informed choice In order to make decisions about their own health care and treatment, mentally competent patients need to be given information regarding their own condition that is accurate, non-judgmental and valid, in language that is jargon free and understandable. This enables the patient to make an informed choice from the treatment options. In some situations, an interpreter may be required.

Informed consent Competent and voluntary permission for a medical test, procedure or medication.

Infra Prefix meaning below, under, beneath.

Infrared Rays of a lower wave length than those in the visible spectrum. They can produce radiant heat which is used in the treatment of rheumatic conditions *(See Ultraviolet rays)*.

Infracotyloid Beneath the cotyloid cavity of the acetabulum of hip.

Infraction An incomplete fracture of bone.

Infradentale The bony point between the mandibular central incisors.

Infundibulum 1. Funnel-shaped passage or structure. 2. Tube connecting the frontal sinus with middle nasal meatus. 3. Stalk of pituitary gland. 4. Peritoneal end of fallopian tube. 5. Upper end of cochlear canal.

Infusion 1. The process of extracting the soluble principles of substances (especially drugs) by soaking in water. 2. The solution thus produced. 3. The slow therapeutic introduction by gravity of fluid other than blood into a vein.

Ingestion The taking in of food and drugs by mouth.

Ingravaescent Becoming more severe.

Ingredient Any unit or part of a complex compound or mixture.

Ingrowing Growing inward.

Ingrown nail Growth of nail edge deep into soft tissues causing pain and inflammation.

Inguinal Relating to the groin.

Inguinal canal The channel through the abdominal wall, above Poupart's ligament, through which the spermatic cord and vessels pass to the testis in the male, which contains the round ligament of the uterus in the female.

Inguinal glands Lymph nodes of groin draining from lower limb and perineum.

Inguinal ligament Poupart's ligament; that connecting the anterior superior spine of the ilium to the tubercle of the pubis.

Inguinal region The iliac region on either side of pubes.

Inguinal ring Interior and exterior openings of inguinal canal, termed as internal and external inguinal rings.

INH *(See Isoniazid)*.

Inhalation 1. The drawing of air or other substances into the lungs. 2. Any drug or solution of drugs, administered (as by means of nebulizers or aerosols) by the nasal or oral respiratory route.

Inhaler An apparatus used for administering an inhalation.

Inherent A characteristic that is innate or natural and essentially a part of the person.

Inheritance The acquisition of qualities and characteristics from parents and ancestors.

Inhibin A testicular hormone that inhibits LH secretion by pituitary.

Inhibition Arrest or restraint of a process. In psychiatry, the unconscious restraining of an instinctual drive.

Inhibitor That which inhibits.

Inhomogeneity Lack of uniform quality or consistency.

Inion External occipital protruberance.

Iniopagus Twins fused at the occipital.

Initials Beginning or commencement.

Initis Inflammation of fibrous tissue.

Inject To introduce.

Injection 1. The forcing of a liquid into a part, as into the subcutaneous tissues, the vascular tree or an organ. 2. A substance so forced or administered; in pharmacy, a solution of a medicament suitable for injection. 3. Prominence of small blood vessels on the surface of an organ or tissue, frequently indicating the vascular phase of an inflammatory response.

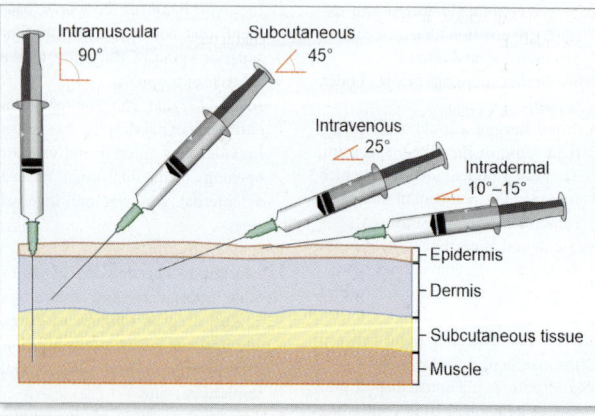

Sites and Angles of Injection

Depot injection The giving of a medication by injection, usually intramuscularly that can be absorbed slowly over a period of time. Many drugs and hormones are given in this way.

Hypodermic injection That made just below the skin; a subcutaneous injection.

Intramuscular injection That made into a muscle.

Intrathecal injection That made into the subarachnoid space of the spinal cord.

Intravenous injection That made into a vein.

Subcutaneous injection That made into the subcutaneous tissues, a hypodermic injection.

Injectors Instruments used for injection of fluids.

Injury Damage or trauma to some body part.

Injury steering wheel Automobile accidents where victims lung and heart are contused by pressure of steering wheel.

Inlay Material inserted to replace a defect in a tissue: For example, a bone graft or a filling cast in metal to fit a hole in a tooth.

Innate Inborn; present in the individual at birth.

Innervation Nerve supply to a part.

Innocent As applied to a tumor, benign or nonmalignant.

Innocuous Harmless.

Innominate Unnamed.

Innominate artery A branch of the aorta, now termed the brachiocephalic trunk.

Innominate bone The hip bone, formed by the union of the ilium, ischium and pubis.

Innominate vein Formed by union of internal jugular and subclavian veins.

Inoculate To inject microorganism, serum or toxic materials into body.

Inoculation 1. Introduction of pathogenic microorganisms, injected material, serum or other substances into tissues of living organisms or into culture media. 2. Introduction of a disease agent (usually a live infectious agent) into a healthy individual to produce a mild form of the disease, followed by immunity.

Inoculum Substance introduced by inoculation.

Inocyte Fibroblast.

Inogenesis Formation of fibrous tissue.

Inoperable Unsuitable for surgery.

Inopexia Tendency of blood to coagulate spontaneously.

Inorganic Of neither animal nor vegetable origin.

Inorganic compound A chemical compound without carbon.

Insemia An excessive amount of fibrin in the blood.

Inositis Inflammation of fibrous tissue.

Inositol A form of muscle or plant carbohydrate that has the same formula as simple sugar but not its other properties.

Inosital nicotinate A vasodilator used in peripheral vascular disease.

Inotropes An agent capable of altering the force or energy of muscular contractio ins inside the body of the living organism after administration.

Inotropic Affecting the force or energy of muscular contractions, particularly the heart muscle, e.g., beta-blocking drugs are said to be inotropic.

Inpatient Hospitalized patient.

Inquest A legal inquiry held by a coroner, with or without a jury, into the cause of sudden or unexpected death.

Insalubrious Not healthy.

Insanitary Not conducive to health.

Insanity A legal term for mental illness, roughly equivalent to psychosis and implying inability to be responsible for one's acts.

Insatiable Unable to be appeared or satisfied.

Inscription A prescription slip with name of the drug and its doses.

Insect bites and stings The venom of stinging insect, may be more toxic than that of poisonous snake but fortunately the quantity injected is small.

Insecta A class of phylum Arthropoda characterized by three distinct body divisions like head, thorax and abdomen, two pairs of wings and three pairs of jointed legs.

Insecticide One of a large group of chemical compounds that kill insect pests.

Insectifuge Insect repellant.

Insecurity Feeling of helplessness, apprehension.

Insemination 1. Fertilization of an ovum by a spermatozoon. 2. Introduction of semen into the vagina.

Artificial insemination Insemination by means other than sexual intercourse. The semen can be either the husband's (AIH) or some other donor's (AID).

Insenescence Process of growing old.

Insensible 1. Unable to perceive with the senses. 2. Unconscious. 3. Imperceptible to the senses.

Insertion 1. The act of implanting. 2. Something that is implanted. 3. The attachment of a muscle to the bone that it moves.

Insidious Approaching by stealth. A term applied to any disease that develops imperceptibly.

Insight Mental awareness. The capacity of individuals to estimate a situation or their own behavior or the connection between their present attitudes and past experiences. In psychiatry, a recognition by patients that they are ill. Insight in this connection may be complete, partial or absent, and may alter during the course of the illness.

Insipid Lacking in spirit, without taste.

Insolation Heat stroke.

Insoluble Not capable of being dissolved in a liquid.

Insomnia Inability to sleep.

Inspect To examine visually.

Inspection Visual examination.

Inspersion Sprinkling with power or a fluid.

Inspiration The act of drawing in the breath.

Inspissated Thickened through evaporation or absorption of fluid.

Insterscapular reflex Scapular muscular contraction following percussion between the scapula.

Instillation The act of pouring a liquid into a cavity drop by drop, e.g., into the eye.

Instinct A complex of unlearned responses characteristic of a species.

Death instinct In psychoanalysis, the latent instinctive impulse toward death; the drive to reduce tensions by reaching the ultimate tensionless state of death.

Herd instinct The instinct or urge to be one of a group and to conform to its standards of conduct and opinion.

Institutionalization A condition of apathy and withdrawal occurring in residents of long-stay institutions, prisons, etc. as a result of rigid routines and lack of independence. The person may resist leaving because the routine has become predictable and familiar, making minimal demands.

Instruction Directions or command.

Instrumentation The use of instruments.

Insufficiency Inadequacy. Used to describe the failure of function of an organ, such as the heart, stomach, liver or muscles.

Insufflate The act of blowing into or pumping air into a cavity/lung as in infants.

Insufflation The act of blowing air, gas or powder into a cavity of the body.

Insula Triangular area of the cerebral cortex lying in the floor of the lateral fissure.

Insulator That which insulates.

Insulin A protein hormone formed in the beta cells of the pancreatic islets of Langerhans. The major fuel regulating hormone, it is secreted into the blood in response to a rise in concentration of blood glucose or amino acids. A deficiency results in diabetes mellitus. Various types of commercially prepared insulin are available. There are three main groups: rapid-acting, intermediate acting and long-acting. Diabetic patients react differently in the rate at which they absorb and utilize insulin; therefore, the duration of action varies from patient to patient. Insulin is measured in units. The concentration used is 100 units/mL. This strength allows for accurate measurement of dosage and reduces the possibility of error in calculating an individual dose.

Insulin pump A device consisting of a syringe filled with a predetermined amount of short-acting insulin, a plastic canula and a needle, and a pump that periodically delivers the desired amount of insulin.

Human insulin Synthesized by recombinant DNA technology using *E. coli.*

Monocomponent insulin Highly purified insulin containing impurity 10 parts per million.

Isophane insulin (NPH) intermediate acting insulin with 18–28 hours of action.

Insulin dependent diabetes mellitus Type 1 diabetes mellitus although insulin is prescribed to people with Type 2 diabetes if oral medication is ineffective.

Insulin lipodystrophy Atrophy or hypertrophy of skin fat at the insulin injection site.

Insulin sensitivity test A test used to determine the body's response to hypoglycemia induced by a small intravenous dose of insulin. It is used to test anterior pituitary function, particularly the ability to secrete growth hormone.

Insulin shock Hypoglycemic shock due to overdose of insulin.

Insulinase An enzyme that destroys the action of insulin.

Insulinemia Excess of blood insulin.

Insulinogenesis Production of insulin by the pancreas.

Insulinogenic Pertains to production of insulin.

Insulinoid Resembling or having properties of insulin.

Insulinoma A benign adenoma of the islet cells of the pancreas, causing hypoglycemia.

Insult Any trauma, irritation, poisoning or injury to the body.

Intake Things taken up like food and liquids.

Integrated care Care that is person centered and coordinated within healthcare settings, across mental and physical health and across health and social care.

Integrated therapy A combination of complementary therapies with orthodox medicine to facilitate healing and promote the wellbeing of the patient. A biopsychosocial approach to care.

Integration The bringing together of various parts or functions for harmonious working.

Integrator Device for measuring body surfaces.

Integument 1. The skin. 2. A layer of tissue covering a part or organ of the body.

Integumentary system The skin and its appendages.

Intellect The mind, thinking faculty or understanding.

Intelligence 1. The capacity to understand. 2. General mental ability.

Intelligence quotient Abbreviated IQ. The ratio of the mental age to the chronological age expressed as a percentage.

Intelligence test A test designed to measure the level of intelligence, usually expressed as an IQ.

Intemperance Lack of moderation, excess in use of anything.

Intensity The degree or extent of activity, strength, force.

Intensive Related to or marked by intensity.

Intensive care unit Abbreviated ICU. A hospital unit in which are concentrated special equipment and specially trained personnel for the care of seriously ill patients requiring immediate and continuous monitoring and treatment. Also called critical care unit (CCU), intensive therapy unit (ITU).

Neonatal ICU (NICU) An intensive care unit that is designated solely for small, preterm neonates and those neonates requiring surgery or other specialized care.

Intention A process of healing.

Intention tremor Occurrence of tremor on attempted coordinated movements.

Intercadence A supernumerary pulse wave between two regular beats.

Intercalated ducts Short narrow ducts that lie between secretory ducts and the terminal alveoli in the parotid and submandibular glands and in the pancreas.

Intercalated Inserted between.

Intercellular Between the cells of a structure. May be applied to the connective tissue or to fluid bathing the cells.

Intercilium The space between the eyebrows.

Intercostal Between the ribs.

Intercostal muscles Muscles situated between the ribs and controlling their movements during inspiration and expiration.

Intercourse 1. Social exchange. 2. Coitus.

Intercurrent Occurring at the same time. Describes a disease occurring during the course of another disease in the same person.

Interdent A specially designed knife used for removing interdental tissue.

Interdentium The space between contiguous teeth.

Interdisciplinary Joint working between professional disciplines: nursing, social work, clergy, medical staff, physiotherapy and other professions allied to medicine (PAMs) or health care professions (HCPs).

Interface Clashing.

Interferon A protein, produced by cells infected by a virus, which has an inhibitory effect on the multiplication of the invading viruses.

Intergemmal Between taste buds.

Interglobular spaces Gaps in dentin due to failure of calcification.

Intergluteal Between the two buttocks.

Interictal Between the two seizure attacks.

Interleukin 15 variety of interleukins have been discovered, IL-3 stimulates hematopoitic and lymphoid stem cells, IL-4 regulates IgE and eosinophil-mediated reactions, IL-5 stimulates growth and differentiation of eosinophils; IL-6 and IL-7 are differential factors for B-cells, IL-8 is a chemotactic and activator for neutrophils, IL-9 is a growth factor for T-cells, IL-10 inhibits cytokine production by T-cells, IL-11 stimulates megakaryocytes, IL-12 stimulates production of IFN-gamma, IL-13 inhibits inflammatory cytokine production, and IL-15 promotes NK-cell proliferation.

Interleukin I Substance from monocytes and macrophages responsible for acute phase response.

Interleukin II A lymphokine that stimulates growth of T-lymphocytes, often used in treatment of metastatic renal cancer.

Interlobular Between lobules.

Interlobular veins Branches of the portal vein in the liver.

Intermarriage Marriage between persons of two distinct populations.

Intermediary Situated between two bodies; occurring between two periods of time.

Intermediary metabolism The series of intermediate products formed during process of digestion and excretion.

Intermediate care The purpose of services designed to assist the transition for a patient or client from medical and social dependence to day-to-day independence. A range of services have the potential to fulfill this function as people move from hospital to home, where the objective of care are not primarily medical, the patient's discharge destination is anticipated, and a clinical outcome of recovery (or restoration of health) is desired. Intermediate care is also used to prevent hospital admission through provision of care at home.

Intermedin A substance secreted by pituitary controlling pigmentation of skin in lower animals.

Intermenstrual Occurring between two menstrual periods.

Intermission A temporary interruption, particularly of a feverish condition.

Intermittent Occurring at intervals.

Intermittent claudication (See Claudication).

Intermittent fever One in which the temperature drops to normal or lower, at times.

Intermittent mandatory ventilation Abbreviated IMV. A type of mechanical ventilation in which the ventilator is set to deliver a prescribed tidal volume at specified intervals, and a high-flow gas system permits the patient to breathe spontaneously between cycles.

Intermittent positive airway ventilation Abbreviated IPAV; also known as intermittent positive pressure ventilation, abbreviated IPPV. A method of assisted ventilation in which oxygen or air is used under pressure to inflate the lungs when the patient is unable to breathe spontaneously.

Intermural Between the walls or sides of an organ.

Internal Situated on the inside.

Internal haemorrhage One occurring in a cavity or into the tissues.

Internal ear The cochlea, semi-circular canals, vestibule.

Internal injury Any injury not visible from outside.

Internal secretion One in which the hormones pass directly into the bloodstream from the secreting gland.

International classification of diseases A classification code devised by WHO, helpful for international comparison.

International Council of Nurses Abbreviated ICN. Founded in 1899 to represent worldwide international nurses' associations as a corporate organization.

International unit Internationally accepted amount of substances like vitamins, hormones, vaccines, etc.

Internalization The unconscious mental mechanism in which the values and standards of society and one's parents are taken as one's own.

Internet A global computer network with millions of connected computers. By connecting to this network, it is possible to access a wide range of information and provide for the transmission of electronic mail. NHS Net links all NHS Trusts and can securely exchange information with other health care organizations and agencies.

I. Addiction syndrome (See Problematic Internet Use).

Interneuron A neuron situated in between neurons.

Internist Physician specializing in internal medicine.

Intermittent self-catheterization (ISC) A procedure carried out by the patient or their carer to drain urine from the bladder. This procedure is recommended for patients who cannot empty their bladder completely but can retain urine for 2 to 4 hours at a time and who have mental cognition, some manual dexterity and the ability to insert a catheter into the urethra. It can be used successfully by women, men and children. This is a clean rather than a sterile procedure.

Intermuncial Acting as a connecting medium.

Interocclusal Between the occlusal surfaces or cusps of opposite teeth.

Interoceptive Sensations arising within body itself, not those arising from outside the body.

Interceptor A receptor activated by stimuli within the body.

Interoinferior Inward and downward position.

Interparietal Between the parietal bones; between the parietal lobes of cerebrum, between walls.

Interpersonal Concerning the relations and interactions between persons.

Interphase The period between two cell divisions during which the chromosomes are not easily visible.

Interpolation 1. In surgery transfer of tissue from one site to another. 2. In statistics the calculation of an intermediate value from the observed values.

Interposition The state of being interposed or inserted between.

Interpretation Analysis, significance.

Interradicular Between the roots of teeth.

Intersection Site where one structure crosses another or joins similar structure.

Intersex 1. A congenital abnormality in which anatomical features of both sexes are evident. 2. A person displaying intersexuality.

Intersexuality An intermingling of the characters of each sex, including physical form, reproductive tissue and sexual behavior, in one individual, as a result of some flaw in embryonic development.

Interspinal Between the two spinous processes of the spine.

Interstitial Situated within the tissue spaces or between the tissues.

Intertitial cell stimulating hormone Abbreviated ICSH. Luteinizing hormone.

Interstitial cystitis Idiopathic inflammation of bladder.

Interstitial fluid The fluid in which body cells are bathed. It acts as an intermediary between the cells and the blood. Extracellular fluid.

Interstitial keratitis (See Keratitis).

Interstitial lung disease A large group of diseases, chronic non-infectious oxygen transfer from alveoli to the capillaries.

Interstitial nephritis Chronic nephritis associated with fibrosis and hypertension.

Interstitial tissue Intercellular connective tissue.

Interstitium Space or gap in a structure or an organ.

Intertransverse Joining the transverse processes of vertebrae.

Intertriginous Having similarity with intertrigo.

Intertrigo An irritating, eczematous skin eruption caused by the chafing of two moist skin surfaces.

Intertrochanteric Between greater and lesser trochanter of femur.

Intertrochanteric line Ridge between greater and lesser trochanter of femur.

Intervaginal Between the sheaths.

Interval Space, time or period between two objects or happenings.

Interval AV Interval between beginning of atrial systole and ventricular systole.

Interval cardio-arterial Time between apex beat and radial pulse.

Interval isometric Time between onset of ventricular systole and opening of semilunar (aortic pulmonary) valves.

Interval lucid Brief remission of symptoms in head injury and psychosis.

Interval PR Period between onset of P wave and beginning of QRS complex. Normal less than 0.2 sec.

Interval QR Period between onset of Q wave and peak of R wave.

Interval QRS – QRS duration from beginning of Q wave to end of S wave. Normal 0.12 sec.

Interval QT Interval between beginning of Q wave and end of T wave.

Intervention In health-care any act carried out to prevent harm to patients or to improve, promote or enhance their physical, mental or spiritual well-being.

Intervertebral Between the vertebrae.

Intervertebral disc The pad of fibro cartilage between the bodies of the vertebrae. Protrusion of the contents of the disc may give rise to sciatica by exerting pressure on the nerve roots.

Interviewing Process involving a structured, semi-structured or conversational style meeting that allows the interviewer to probe for information and is widely used in research as well as in everyday situations. This technique is also used at the initial stage of patient assessment. Interviews are used as a method of data collection involving face-to-face or telephone questioning by the researcher; most often used in qualitative research.

Intervillous Between the villi.

Intestinal Referring to the intestine.

Intestinal bypass Surgical short circuiting of small intestine to produce controlled malabsorption to treat massive obesity.

Intestinal flora Bacteria present in intestine that synthesize vitamins.

Intestinal gas H_2, methane, CO_2, H_2S and methyl mercaptan produced in GI tract during digestive process.

Intestinal juice Secretion of small intestine containing a number of enzymes like maltase, lipase, peptidase, sucrose, etc.

Intestinal obstruction Blockage of intestinal lumen due to stricture, worms, fibrous band, foreign body, stone, fecolith, etc. producing absolute constipation, abdominal distension, dehydration and pain.

Intestinal perforation Soiling of peritoneal cavity with intestinal content; commonly a complication of enteric fever, tuberculosis or prolonged intestinal obstruction.

Intestinal putrefaction The putrefying effect of intestinal bacteria producing indole, skatole, para-cresol, phenol, phenylpropionic acid, phenyl acetic acid and gases.

Intestinal reflex Intestinal contraction and relaxation above the portion of bowel that is stimulated.

Intestinal tubes Plastic or rubber tubes placed in intestinal tract through nose or mouth to suck gas, fluids or solids.

Intestine Part of the alimentary canal that extends from the stomach to the anus.

Small intestine The first 6 m from the pylorus to the cecum, consisting of the duodenum, the jejunum and the ileum.

Large intestine The final 2 m, consisting of the cecum, the ascending, transverse and descending colon, and the rectum.

Intima The innermost coat of an artery or vein.

Intolerance Lack of power to endure. Applied to the effect of some drugs on individuals, e.g., iodine and quinine *(See Idiosyncrasy)*.

Intorsion Rotation of eye inward.

Intoxication 1. Poisoning by drugs or harmful substances. 2. The condition produced by excessive use of alcohol.

Intra-abdominal Within the abdomen.

Intra-aortic balloon counterpulsation Placement of an inflatable balloon in aortic root to lower/decrease systolic work of LV and to promote coronary blood flow; useful in treating shock. The balloon is inflated with helium during diastole and deflated during systole.

Intra-articular Within a joint capsule.

Intra-articular injection Injection into a joint capsule, applicable to hydrocortisone.

Intra-atrial Within the atrium.

Intra-atrial thrombosis A blood clot formed in the atrium of the heart.

Intracardiac Within the heart.

Intracapsular Within a capsule, usually of a joint.

Intracapsular extraction The removal of the whole lens with its capsule in the treatment of cataract.

Intracellular Within a cell.

Intracellular fluid The water and its dissolved salts found within the cells.

Intracerebral Within the brain substance.

Intracerebral haemorrhage An escape of blood in the cerebrum, most often a rising from the middle cerebral artery or from an aneurysm.

Intracisternal Within cistern of brain.

Intracranial Within the skull.

Intracranial abscess One arising within the brain or meninges.

Intacranial aneurysm Dilatation of one of the cerebral vessels. It may be congenital or acquired.

Intracranial pressure Abbreviated ICP. The pressure exerted by the cerebrospinal fluid within the subarachnoid space and ventricles of the brain.

Intractable Not able to be relieved, controlled or cured.

Intradermal Between the layers of the skin.

Intradural Within the dura mater.

Intradural haemorrhage (See Haemorrhage).

Intragastric Within the stomach.

Intragastic balloon Placement of inflatable balloon in stomach to treat obesity.

Intrahepatic Within the liver. Referring to a condition of the liver cells or connective tissue.

Intralipid Trade name for an intravenous fat emulsion used to prevent or correct deficiency of essential fatty acids and to provide calories in high-density form during total parenteral nutrition.

Intralobular Within a lobule.

Intralobular veins Veins which collect blood from within the lobules of the liver.

Intralocular Within the cavity of any structure.

Intramedullary 1. Within the medulla oblongata. 2. Within the bone marrow.

Intramedulllary nail A metal pin used for the internal fixation of fractures.

Intramural With the walls of a hollow organ or cavity.

Intramuscular Within muscle tissue.

Intranasal Within the nose.

Intracapsular Within a capsule, usually of a joint.

I. extraction The removal of the whole lens with its capsule in the treatment of cataract.

Intracerebral Within the brain substance.

I. hemorrhage An escape of blood in the cerebrum, most often arising from the middle cerebral artery or from an aneurysm.

Intracranial Within the skull.

I abscess One arising within the brain or meninges.

I. Aneurysm dilatation of one of the cerebral vessels. It may be congenital or acquired.

I. pressure Abbreviated ICP. The pressure exerted by the cerebrospinal fluid within the subarachnoid space and ventricles of the brain.

Intranet A computer network designed to meet the internal needs of a single organization, e.g., an NHS Trust. It is not necessarily open to the internet and is not accessible by individuals from outside the organization.

Intraocular Within the eyeball.

Intraorbital Within the orbit of the eye.

Intraosseous Within a bone.

Intraosseous infusion The process of supplying fluid into the narrow cavity of a bone in a life-threatening situation.

Intrapartum Occurring during childbirth.

Intraperitoneal Within the peritoneal cavity.

Intrathecal Within the meninges of the spinal cord, usually in the subarachnoid space.

Intratracheal Endotracheal; within the trachea.

Intratracheal anaesthesia Inhalation anaesthesia *(See Anaesthesia).*

Intrauterine Within the uterus. *Intrauterine contraceptive device* Abbreviated IUCD. A contraceptive device introduced into the uterine cavity.

Intrauterine douche Irrigation of the uterine cavity. A special grooved nozzle is used, so that the fluid can return and is not forced into the uterine tubes.

Intrauterine growth retardation Associated with a poor blood supply to the placenta, or maternal disease. Other factors include infection during pregnancy, maternal smoking or drug addiction. The infant at birth is "small for dates" and falls below the tenth percentile of appropriate gestational age for infants.

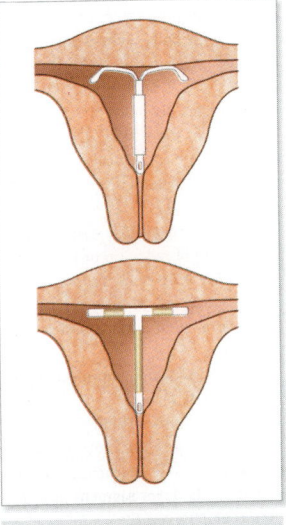

IUCD

Intrauterine life Fetal development in the uterus.

Intravasation Entry into blood vessels.

Intravenous Within a vein. *Intravenous flow rate* The rate at which fluids, medications and blood products flow into the bloodstream during intravenous infusion. The flow rate is usually ordered by the doctor as total volume (mL) per total hours or, in the case of drugs, total dose per total hours.

Intravenous infusion The therapeutic introduction of a fluid, such as saline, into a vein. The infusion works by gravity, in that the container of fluid is higher than the blood vessel into which the fluid is being introduced.

Intravenous urography Radiographic examination of the urinary tract after the injection of a radiopaque contrast medium into a vein.

Intraventricular Within a ventricle; may apply to a cerebral or a cardiac ventricle.

Intravesical Within urinary bladder.

Intravitreous With the vitreous of eye.

Intrinsic Particular to or contained within an organ.

Intrinsic factor A glycoprotein, contained in the gastric juices, which is necessary for the absorption of extrinsic factor (Vitamin B_{12}).

Intrinsic muscles Muscles having their origin and insertion entirely within a structure, e.g., intrinsic muscles of eye, tongue and larynx.

Introducer Device for controlling, directing and placing intubation tube within trachea, blood vessels or heart.

Introitus [L.] An opening or entrance into a hollow organ or cavity.

Introitus vaginae The vulva.

Introjection A mental process by which individuals take into themselves the personal characteristics of another person, usually those of someone much loved or admired.

Intromission An insertion or placing of one part into another.

Introns The noncoding region between the coding regions (exons) of the DNA in gene.

Introspection A subjective study of the mind and its processes, in which individuals study their own reactions.

Introversion 1. A turning inward within itself of a hollow organ. 2. Preoccupation with oneself, with reduction of interest in the outside world.

Introvert A person whose interests are turned inward upon the self *(See Extrovert)*.

Intubation The introduction of a tube into a part of the body, particularly into the air passages to allow air to enter the lungs.

Intuition Knowing something spontaneously in advance.

Intumescence A swelling or increase in bulk, as of nasal mucous membrane in catarrh.

Intussusception Prolapse of one part of the intestine into the lumen of an immediately adjacent part, causing obstruction (intestinal).

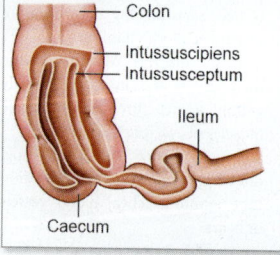

Colon
Intussuscipiens
Intussusceptum
Ileum
Caecum

Intussusception

Intussusceptum The inner segment of intestine in intussusceptions.

Intussuscipiens That portion of intestine that receives the intussusceptum.

Inunction 1. Rubbing an oily or fatty preparation containing a medicinal ingredient into the skin, with absorption of the drug. 2. Any preparation so applied.

Inulase Enzyme that converts inulin to levulose.

Inulin A polysaccharide found in plants yielding levulose on hydrolysis. Used in study of renal function (GFR).

Invagination 1. The folding inwards of a part, thus forming a pouch. 2. Intussusception.

Invalid A sick person confined to bed or wheelchair.

Invasion 1. The entry of bacteria into the body. 2. The entrance of parasites into the body of a host.

Invasive 1. Having the quality of invasiveness. 2. Involving puncture or incision of the skin or insertion of an instrument or foreign material into the body; said of diagnostic techniques.

Invasive procedure Procedure in which the body cavity is entered that could interfere with bodily function.

Invasiveness 1. The ability of micro organisms to enter the body and spread in the tissues. 2. The ability to infiltrate and actively destroy surrounding tissue, a property of malignant tumors.

Inverse square law Law stating that the intensity of radiation or light at any distance is inversely proportional to the square of the distance between the irradiated surface and a point source.

Inversion A turning upside down or inside out.

Sexual inversion Homosexuality.

Uterine inversion The condition of the uterus after parturition when a part of its upper segment protrudes through the cervix.

Invert sugar A mixture of levulose and dextrose, formed by inversion of sucrose by the enzyme invertase.

Invertase A sugar – splitting enzyme found in GI tract.

Invertebrate 1. Without a spinal column. 2. An animal without a spinal column.

Investigations Procedures performed to establish a diagnosis, to monitor a person's health, disease or the effectiveness of treatment. They are classified as non-invasive where there is no direct entry into the body, e.g., recording body weight, or as invasive, e.g., endoscopy or blood sampling.

Investment A covering or sheath.

Inveterate Chronic, firmly seated habit.

In vitro Outside the living body, e.g., tests done in laboratory involving isolated tissue or cell preparation.

In vivo Within the living body or organism.

Involucrum New bone which forms a sheath around necrosed bone, as in chronic osteomyelitis.

Involuntary Independent of the will *(See Voluntary)*.

Involuntary muscle One that acts without conscious control; for instance, the heart and stomach muscles.

Involution 1. Turning inward; describes the contraction of the uterus after labor. The process where by the uterus returns to its normal size. 2. The progressive degeneration occurring naturally with advancing age, resulting in shrivelling of organs or tissues.

Involutional melancholia Depression visiting in men and women between 50–65 years and 40–55 years of age.

Iodameba A genus of ameba seen in GI tract.

Iodide A compound of iodine, e.g., pot iodide.

Iodine Symbol I. A nonmetallic element with a distinctive odor, obtained from seaweed. Iodine is essential in nutrition, being specially prevalent in the colloid of the thyroid (gland). It is used in the treatment of hypothyroidism and as a topical antiseptic. It is a frequent cause of poisoning. Iodine is opaque to X-rays and can be combined with other compounds for use as contrast media in diagnostic radiology.

Iodine tincture Preparation of iodine in alcohol and water.

Iodipamide meglumine Agent used for gallbladder X-ray.

Iodism Condition resulting from excess and prolonged use of iodine.

Iodized salt Salt containing 100 mg of sodium or potassium iodide per gram.

Iododerma Dermatitis due to iodine.

Iodoform A compound formed by action of iodine on acetone in the presence of an alkali. Used topically for mild antibacterial action.

Iodohippurate sodium A radio-active dye used in renal studies.

Iodophilia Unusual pronounced affinity of polymorphs for iodine in some infections and anemia.

Iodophor Iodine in a solubilizing agent, e.g., povidone iodine.

Iodopsin A violet pigment found in the retinal cones of the eyes.

Iodoquinol Antiamebic agent, can cause subacute myelooptic neuropathy.

Iodosorb Trade name for a preparation of cadexomer iodide used to cleanse venous leg ulcers and pressure sores.

Iodotherapy Use of iodine medication.

Iodoxyl A radiopaque contrast medium *(See Intravenous (Urography))*.

Ion An atom or group of atoms having a positive (cation) or negative (anion) electric charge by virtue of having gained or lost one or more electrons. Substances forming ions are electrolytes *(See Electrolyte, Hydrogen)*.

Ion exchange resins Resins that bind to some ions, e.g., cholestyramine.

Ionization The breaking up of molecules into electrically charged particles or ions when an electric current is passed through an electrolytic solution.

Ionizing radiation iontophoresis (See Radiation)

Ionometer A device to measure amount of radiation and intensity of rays.

Iontophoresis The introduction through the skin of therapeutic ions by ionization.

Iopanoic acid Radioopaque dye used for gallbladder studies.

Iophendylate Radioopaque dye used in myelography.

Iothalamate meglumine Radiopaque material for angiography.

IPAV Intermittent Positive Airway Ventilation.

Ipatropium bromide An anti-cholingergic given by inhalation in bronchial asthma.

Ipecacuanha The dried root of a Brazilian shrub, given in small doses as an expectorant and in larger doses, as an emetic.

Ipodate calcium Radioopaque material for X-ray studies of gallbladder.

IPPV Intermittent Positive Pressure Ventilation.

Iproniazid Antitubercular drugs.

Ipsilateral Occurring on the same side. Applied particularly to paralysis or other symptoms occurring on the same side as the cerebral lesion causing them.

IQ Intelligence Quotient *(See Intelligence).*

IRDS Infant Respiratory Distress Syndrome *(See Respiratory).*

Iridalgia Pain in the iris.

Iridauxesis Increase in thickness of iris as in glaucoma.

Iridectome Instrument for cutting iris in iridectomy.

Iridectomy Excision of a part of the iris, usually for the treatment of glaucoma.

Irideremia Partial or total congenital absence of iris.

Iridencleisis An operation to make a drain out of a part of the iris, used in the treatment of glaucoma.

Irides Pleural of iris.

Iridium Symbol Ir, radioactive metal, often used in the form of wires or hairpins to treat superficial malignancies, e.g., those of the tongue, cheek or breast.

Iridoavulsion Tearing away of iris.

Irido capsulitis Inflammation of iris and capsule of lens.

Iridocele Herniation of a part of the iris through a corneal wound.

Iridocoloboma Congenital defect or fissure in iris.

Iridocyclectomy Surgical removal of iris and ciliary body.

Iridocyclitis Inflammation of the iris and ciliary body.

Iridodialysis Separation of outer margin of iris from its ciliary attachment.

Iridodonesis Trembling of the iris due to lack of support from the lens in dislocation of the lens or after a cataract extraction.

Iridokinesis Contraction and expansion movement of iris.

Iridorrhexis Rupture of or tearing of the iris from its attachment.

Iridoptosis Prolapse of the iris.

Iridotomy The making of a hole in the iris to form an artificial pupil.

Iris The colored part of the eye, made of two layers of muscle, the contraction of which alters the size of the pupil and so controls the amount of light entering the eye.

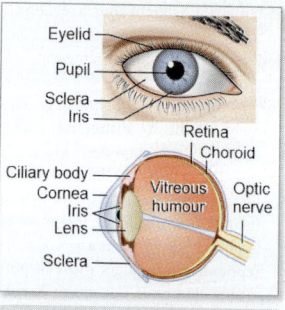

Iris

Iris bombe A bulging forward of the iris due to pressure of the aqueous humour when its passage into the anterior chamber is obstructed.

Iritis Inflammation of the iris, causing pain, photophobia, contraction of the pupil and discoloration of the iris *(See Uveitis).*

Iron Symbol Fe. A metallic element, present in the body in small quantities and essential to life. A deficiency may produce anemia.

Iron-dextran Injectable form of iron.

Iron storage disease Hemochromatosis.

Irradiation The treatment of disease by electromagnetic radiation.

Irrational Contrary to what is reasonable or logical.

Irreducible Incapable of being replaced in a normal position. Applied to a fracture or a hernia.

Irrelevance Unrelated to, inappropriate.

Irreversible Impossible to reverse.

Irrigation The washing out of a cavity or wound with a stream of lotion or water.

Irrigator Devise used to flush or irrigate.

Irritable Reacting excessively to a stimulus.

Irritable bowel syndrome Mucous colitis; spastic colon. The patient complains of disordered bowel function with abdominal pain, but no organic disease can be found.

Irritant An agent causing stimulation or excitation.

Irritation 1. A condition of undue nervous excitement resulting from abnormal sensitiveness. 2. itching of the skin.

Cerebral irritation A stage of excitement present in many brain conditions and typical of the recovery stage of concussion.

Ischaemia A deficiency in the blood supply to a part of the body. *Myocardial ischaemia* Ischaemia of the heart muscles, which causes angina pectoris.

Ischiocavernosus An erectile muscle extending from ischium to penis or clitoris.

Ischiococcygeus Coccygeus muscle forming posterior portion of levator ani.

Ischiorectal Concerning the ischium and the rectum

Ischiorectal abscess A collection of pus in the ischiorectal connective tissue. An anal fistula may result.

Ischium The lower posterior bone of the pelvic girdle.

Ischium ischiorectal fossa Pararectal fat filled fossa bounded laterally by obturator internus and ischial tuberosity, posteriorly by gluteus maximus and medially by levator ani.

Ischloanal Concerning the ischium and the anus.

I. abscess A collection of pus in the ischiorectal connective tissue. An anal fistula may result.

Ishihara colour charts S. Ishihara, Japanese ophthalmologist, 1879–1963. Patterns of dots of the primary colors on similar backgrounds which make numbers or patterns. The numbers or patterns can be seen by a normal-sighted person, but one who is color blind will only be able to identify some of them, depending on the type of color blindness.

Island A structure detached from surrounding structures or a tiny, isolated mass of one kind of cells within another type.

Islet of Langerhans P. Langerhans, German pathologist, 1847–1888. One of a group of cells in the pancreas that produce insulin and glucagon; islet of the pancreas.

Ismelin Guarnethideine sulphate.

Isoagglutination Agglutination of red blood cells by agglutinin from blood of another person.

Isoagglutinin Antibody in the serum that agglutinates RBC of same species.

Isoantigen A substance present in certain individuals that stimulates production of antibody in other members SYN-alloantigen.

Isobucaine hydrochloride A local anesthetic agent.

Isocarboxazid A monoamine oxidase inhibitor used in the treatment of depressive illness.

Ishochromatic Having the same color.

Isochromosomes A chromosome with arms that are morphologically identical and contain the same genetic loci.

Isochronal Taking place at regular intervals or in uniform time.

Isochronia The correspondence of events with respect to time, rate or frequency.

Isocoria Equality in size of both pupils.

Isocytosis Cells of equal size.

Isodontic Having teeth of equal size.

Isoelectric Having equal electric potentials.

Isoelectric period The time or point when no electric energy is produced.

Isoenzyme A form of an enzyme.

Isoetharine hydrochloride A sympathomimetic agent, used as bronchodilator.

Isoflurophate An anticholinesterage drug used to treat glaucoma and atony of intestinal and vesical smooth muscles.

Isogamete A cell which on fusion with a similar cell reproduces.

Isogamy Reproduction resulting from conjugation of isogametes or identical cells.

Isogel Proprietary, bulk forming laxative prepared from the husks of mucilaginous seeds. Used in chronic constipation.

Isograft A tissue graft from one identical twin to another.

Isohemaglutin Blood group antibody normally present in blood that causes clumping of incompatible blood.

Isoimmunization The development of antibodies against an antigen derived from an individual of the same species, e.g., a rhesus-negative woman may immunize herself against her fetus, if it is rhesus-positive, by forming specific antibody.

Isolation The separation of a person with an infectious disease from those non-infected.

Isolation period Quarantine; the length of time during which a patient with an infectious fever is considered capable of infecting others by contact.

Isoleucine One of the ten essential amino acids that are vital for health in the adult.

Isomer Substances having same molecular formula but different chemical and physical properties, e.g., dextrose is an isomer of levulose.

Isomerase Any enzyme that catalyzes isomerization of its substrate.

Isomerism Compounds with equal number of atoms but with different atomic arrangements.

Isomerization Conversion of a substance to its isomer.

Isometric Having equal dimensions. 1. Exercises the contraction and relaxation of muscles without producing movement; used to maintain muscle tone after a fracture.

Isoniazid INH. A drug, given orally in combination with streptomycin or para-aminosalicylic acid (PAS), which is effective in treating tuberculosis.
Combined therapy reduces the risk of bacterial resistance.

Iso-osmotic Having the same total concentration of osmotically active molecules.

Isophoria Equal tension of vertical muscles of each eye with visual lines in the same horizontal plane.

Isoprenaline A sympathomimetic drug which has an action like adrenaline and can be used to treat asthma.

Isopropamide iodide A synthetic antimuscarinic drug with actions similar to belladonna. Isopropyl alcohol

Isopropyl alcohol C_3H_8O, an alcohol used in medical preparations for external use, antifreeze, cosmetics, and as a solvent.

Isoproterenol A sympathomimetic, used in bronchial asthma.

Isosexual Concerning or characteristic of same sex.

Isospora A genus of sporozoa, e.g., *I hominis*, a nonpathogenic protozoa inhabiting small intestine.

Isosorbide dinitrate A short-acting vasodilator similar in action to glyceryl trinitrate and used in the treatment of angina pectoris.

Isosthenuria Passage of urine having constant specific gravity; a sign of advanced renal disease.

Isotherapy Treatment of a disease by the same causative agent.

Isotonic Having uniform tension.

Isotonic exercise Contraction of a muscle during which the force of resistance to the movement remains constant throughout the range of motion.

Isotonic solution A solution of the same osmotic pressure as the fluid with which it is compared. Normal saline (0.9% solution of salt in water) is isotonic with blood plasma.

Isotope One of the several forms of an element with the same atomic number but different atomic weights.

Radioactive isotope An unstable isotope which decays and emits alpha, beta or gamma rays. May be used in the diagnosis and treatment of malignant disease.

Isotretionin A retinoid used in acne.

Isotropic Possessing similar qualities in every direction; having equal refraction.

Isovaleric acidemia A rare hereditary condition where the body cannot process the amino acid leucine. Screening for the condition takes place as part of Newborn Blood Spot Screening.

Isoxsuprine hydrochloride A vasodilator and smooth muscle relaxant.

Isradipine A calcium channel blocking agent, anti hypertensive.

Issue Offspring.

Isthmoplegia Paralysis of fauces.

Isthmus A narrow connection between two larger bodies or parts, e.g., the band of tissue between the two lobes of the thyroid gland.

Isuprel hydrochloride Isoproterenol hydrochloride.

Itch A skin eruption with irritation.

Baker's itch Eczema of the hands due to the proteins of flour.

Barber's itch Sycosis; tinea barbae.

Dhobi itch Tinea (cruris). The name is derived from the belief in India that the spread of infection was due to washermen (*dhobis*) wearing their clients' clothes.

Itch mite The cause of scabies, *Sarcoptes scabiei*.

Washerwomen's itch Dermatitis of the hands due to the constant use of detergents.

Itraconazole Antifungal agent.

ITP Idiopathic Thrombocytopenic Purpura.

ITU Intensive Therapy Unit.

IUCD Intrauterine Contraceptive Device.

IVF In vitro fertilization *(See Fertilization).*

Ivy method A method for estimation of bleeding time.

IVP Intravenous pyelography *(See Urography).*

Ivy poisoning Poison ivy dermatitis.

IVU Intravenous Urography *(See Urography).*

Ixodes A genus of ticks.

Nursing Next Live
The Next Level of NURSING EDUCATION

PREPARE ANYTIME, ANYWHERE FOR
Nursing Officer/Staff Nurse/CHO/ Nursing Undergraduate & Postgraduate Exams

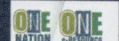

THE COMPLETE PACKAGE

50,000+
MCQs with their Rationale

2000+
Hours of Recorded video lectures (Covering All Subjects/All Topics/ Imp Topics Chanting Videos/Exam Discussions/LMR/IBQ & VBQs Discussions)

150+
Previous years' question papers covering all National and State Level Exams (2021-2010)

Monthly/Weekly/Daily
Live Doubt Sessions & Faculty-Students' Meet (Forthcoming)

200+
Newly Created Subject-wise cum Topic-wise Test, Mini Test & Grand Tests based on all important National Exams like AIIMS, PGIMER, JIPMER, DSSSB, RRB & ESIC, also State level exams like Kerala PSC

1500+
E-Notes/Flash cards of all the subjects for Last-minute Revision

1000+
Image-based Questions with their Rationale

200+
Video-based Questions with their Rationale

Monthly
Special Mega Assessment Tests, National Scholarship Test with up to 100% Scholarship & Reward points

200+
CBS Nursing Books available for purchase

Special Features

Live Classes

Live Doubt Sessions

Mega Assessment Tests

Live Webinars

Faculty-Student Meet on Zoom Sessions

Study Plans

Success Stories

Daily Dose of Knowledge

Blogs

National Scholarship Test with upto 100% scholarship

Any Doubt Ask Us

Exam Notifications

Buy CBS Nursing Books

Bookmark Your Imp Topics

Download Videos/ Notes

Follow us:

CALL US +91- 999-911-7411
www.nursingnextlive.com

Scan the QR Code to download the app

J Symbol for joule.

Jacket A bandage usually applied to the trunk to immobilize the spine or correct deformities.

Jacket Minerva A plaster of Paris jacket used for fracture cervical spine.

Jacket porcelain Crown restoration with porcelain.

Jacket Sayre's Plaster of Paris jacket to support spinal deformity.

Jackscrew A threaded screw used for expanding the dental arch.

Jacksonian epilepsy *JH Jackson, British neurologist, 1835–1911.* Focal motor epilepsy.

Jackson's syndrome Unilateral muscular and structural paralysis which are innervated by tenth, eleventh, and twelth cranial nerves.

Jacobson Danish anatomist,

J's cartilage Cartilage lying along anterior inferior border of nasal septum.

J's Nerve Tympanic nerve.

Jacksonian epilepsy *J.H. Jackson, British neurologist, 1835-1911.* Focal motor Epilepsy.

Jacquemier's sign *JM Jacquemier, French obstetrician, 1806–1879.* Blueness of the lining of the vagina seen from the early weeks of pregnancy.

Jactitation The extreme restlessness of an acutely ill patient.

Jaegers test types A reading test type for near vision.

Jamais vu Feeling of being placed in a strange environment or unfamiliarity; a feature of temporal lobe epilepsy.

James fiber Preexcitation of ventricles by fibers connecting atria to ventricle or distal. His bundle, bypassing AV node.

Janeway lesion Small painless red blue macular lesions in palms and soles in bacterial endocarditis.

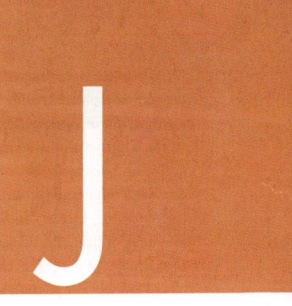

Japanese encephalitis A severe inflammation of the brain caused by the Japanese encephalitis virus that is transmitted by the bite of infected mosquitoes. Around 75% of those affected are under the age of 15 years. There is currently no cure and around 1 in 250 people who contract the disease become severely ill. Of those who develop serious complications around one third will die and others will have permanent brain damage. There is a vaccine that gives protection against the disease.

Jargon 1. The terminology used and generally understood only by those who have knowledge of that speciality, e.g., medical jargon/legal jargon. 2. Gibberish talked by the insane.

Jarvi's snare Snare for removing growth in nasal cavity.

Jaundice icterus A yellow discoloration of the skin and conjunctivae, due to the presence of bile pigment in the blood. It may be one of the following types:

(a) Haemolyticjaundice Due to excessive destruction of red blood cells, causing increase of bilirubin in the blood. The liver is not involved. Acholuric jaundice is of this type. It is characterized by increased fragility of the red blood cells,

(b) Hepatocellular jaundice The liver cells are damaged by either infection or drugs,

(c) Obstructive jaundice The bile is prevented from reaching the duodenum owing to obstruction by a gallstone, a growth or a stricture of the common bile duct.

(d) Physiological jaundice (icterus neonatorum) Occurs within the first few days of life, and is caused by the breakdown of the excessive number of red blood cells present in the newborn.

Jaw A bone of the face in which the teeth are embedded.

Lower jaw The mandible.

Upper jaw The two maxillae.

Jealousy Intense concern for the loss of affection or attention of another person; may also be exhibited as being envious of someone else's achievements or advantages.

Morbid J. Also known as Othello syndrome, it is concerned with the potential sexual infidelity of one's partner. Morbid jealousy is usually caused by a personality disorder but may also occur in those suffering from organic brain disease or alcohol dependency.

Jejunal biopsy Removal of a small piece of the jejunum for histological and enzyme examination. Used to confirm Crohn's disease, celiac disease and other malabsorption syndromes. The biopsy is taken using a flexible endoscope passed down through the mouth into the jejunum. *(See Crosby Capsule)*.

Jejunectomy Excision of a part or the whole of the jejunum.

Jejunocolostomy Anastomosis of colon with jejunum.

Jejunoileitis Inflammation of jejunum and ileum as in Crohn's disease.

Jejunoileostomy The making of an anastomosis between the jejunum and the ileum.

Jejunorrhaphy Surgical repair of jejunum.

Jejunostomy The making of an opening into the jejunum through the abdominal wall.

Jejunotomy An incision into the jejunum.

Jejunum The portion of the small intestine from the duodenum to the ileum; about 2.4 m in length.

Jelly A soft, coherent, resilient substance; generally, a colloidal semisolid mass.

Contraceptive jelly A non-greasy jelly used in the vagina for prevention of conception *(See also Contraception)*.

Petroleum jelly A purified mixture of semisolid hydrocarbons obtained from petroleum (also called petrolatum).

Wharton's jelly The soft, jelly-like intracellular substance of the umbilical cord, which insulates the vein and arteries, preventing occlusion and fetal hypoxia.

Jendrassik's maneuver Facilitation of deep tendon reflexes of lower extremity by hooking the fingers of both hands by the patient and trying to pull them apart.

Jenner, Edward British physician who invented cowpox vaccine for immunization against smallpox.

Jenner's stain Eosin methylene blue stain.

Jerk A sudden muscular contraction.

Knee jerk A kicking movement produced by tapping the tendon below the patella. Used with other jerks, such as the ankle jerk, to test the nervous reflexes.

Jervell and Lange-Nielsen syndrome *(See Long QT Syndrome)*.

Jessner's solution Combination of resorcinol, lactic acid, and salicylic acid that acts as a peeling agent.

Jet lag The lack of balance that occurs between local time and the person's biological rhythms that results from air travel over a long distance, especially in an easterly direction and to a lesser extent westwards. Sleep, memory and concentration are disturbed and there is a persistent feeling of tiredness usually lasting 2–3 days as the body adjusts to the time change.

Jigger A sand flea, found in the tropics, which burrows into the soles of the feet and causes severe irritation.

Jogger's heel Irritation of fibrofatty tissue of heel in joggers.

Jogger's nipple Soreness of the nipple(s) caused by friction of clothing against them; occurs in runners and athletes. Prevention is by applying petroleum jelly before running.

Jogging Running at a slow even pace. A popular form of street exercise.

Joint An articulation; the point of junction of two or more bones, particularly one which permits movement of the individual bones relative to each other.

Ball and socket joint Rounded end of one bone fits into cavity of another.

Charcot's joint Denervated joint with increased range of movement as in syringomyelia and tabes dorsalis.

Condyloid joint Joint permitting all forms of angular movements except axial rotation.

Hinge joint Joint having only forward and backward motion.

Pivot joint Joint permitting rotation.

Saddle joint Joint in which the opposing surfaces are reciprocally concavoconvex.

Joint capsule The sac like covering enclosing the articulating ends of bones in a diarthrodial joint. It consists of an outer fibrous layer and inner synovial layer.

Joint strategic needs assessment Abbreviated JSNA, involves scrutiny of a wide range of indicators to identify the needs of local populations in order to support the planning of ser-

vices based on need.

Jones criteria USA physician who devised the major and minor criteria for diagnosis of acute rheumatic fever. The major criteria include 1. Fleeting polyarthritis 2. Chorea, 3. Erythema marginatum and 4. Subcutaneous nodules.

Joule Symbol J. The SI unit of energy.

Judgement The ability of an individual to estimate a situation, to arrive at reasonable conclusions and to decide on a course of action.

Judicial review A legal process by which individuals or organizations can challenge government or public body decisions. Any person or organization with sufficient interest and concern regarding a decision that has been made, e.g., by a health sector organization, can apply for a review to the Administrative Court. This relates to the legal process in England and Wales only.

Jugular Relating to the neck.

Jugular foramen Opening formed by jugular notches of the occipital and temporal bones.

Jugular ganglion Nodes of vagusroot and glossopharyngeal nerve in jugular foramen.

Jugular process Projection of occipital bone toward the temporal bone.

Jugular veins Several veins in the neck which drain the blood from the head.

Junction The place of union of two parts.

Jung Carl Gustav *Swiss psychologist and psychiatrist, 1875–1961.*

Jungian theory C.G. Jung Swiss psychologist and psychiatrist, 1875-1961. The concept that certain ideas from past experiences are present in the unconscious and are controlled by the way in which the person views the world. Jung called these shared ideas the 'collective unconscious' containing personal life experiences.

Jung separated individuals into personality types: the externally sensitive type who directs energy outwards, and the introvert whose energies are directed inwardly. The goal of Jungian Psychotherapy is to permit the individual to become what they essentially are, i.e., to encourage individual development.

Junk food Non-nutritious or fast food high in monosodium glutamate.

Jurisprudence The science of law. Medical jurisprudence is another name for forensic medicine.

Jury-mast Apparatus for support of head in diseases of spine.

Juster's reflex Finger extension instead of flexion when palm of the hand is irritated.

Juvenile chronic arthritis A rare form of inflammatory arthritis affecting children, most often girls, between the ages of 2 and 4 years or at puberty; usually affects four or more joints. Management is based around the relief of pain, suppression of the inflammatory process and the prevention of deformity. Formerly known as Still's disease.

Juvenile Relating to young people.

Juxta Close proximity.

Juxta-articular Near a joint.

Juxtaglomerular Near to a glomerulus of the kidney.

Juxtaglomerular apparatus The myoepithelioid cell structure cuffing afferent renal arteriole concerned with production of rennin.

Juxtaglomerular cells Specialized cells found in the kidney which appear to play an important part in the control of aldosterone release.

Juxtangina Inflamed condition of pharyngeal muscles.

Juxtaposition An adjacent, or side by side position.

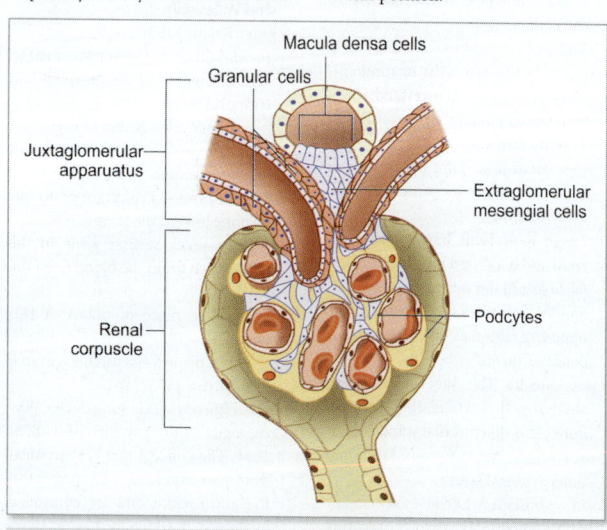

Juxtaglomerular Apparatus

K Symbol for potassium.

Kader's operation Surgical formation of gastric fistula with the feeding tube inserted through a valve like flap.

Kahn test *BL Kahn, American bacteriologist, 1887–1979.* An agglutination test for syphilis.

Kakidrosis Unpleasant odor of the sweat.

Kakosmia Perception of bad odor that does not exist.

Kakotrophy Malnutrition.

Kala-azar; Visceral leishmaniasis. A tropical disease caused by the protozoan parasite *Leishmania donovani* which is carried by the sand fly. Symptoms include enlargement of the liver and spleen, anemia and wasting. The disease is often fatal.

Kalimeter Device for determining alkalinity of a substance.

Kalium A mineral (potassium).

Kaaliuresis Excretion of potassium in urine.

Kallikrein An enzyme, when activated is a potent vasodilator.

Kanamycin A broad spectrum antibiotic for use against severe infections with Gram-negative organisms where penicillin is ineffective.

Kangaroo care The use of skin-to-skin contact between the premature but stable infant and parent or caregiver. The infant in nappy and cap rests on the mother's or father's exposed chest either in a sling or a blanket; vital signs can be kept monitored. The skin contact has a soothing effect, calming and warming the infant while promoting bonding between the parent and baby.

Kanner syndrome Infantile autism.

Kaolin Powdered clay containing aluminium silicate. It is taken orally in the treatment of diarrhea and is also used as a dusting powder and for poultices.

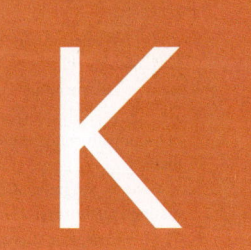

Kaolinosis Pneumoconiosis caused by inhalation of kaolin particles.

Kaposi Hungarian physician.

Kaposi's disease Xeroderma pigmentosum.

Kaposi's sarcoma *MK Kaposi, Austrian dermatologist, 1837–1902.* A multifocal, metastasizing, malignant reticulosis with angiosarcoma-like features, involving chiefly the skin. Rarely seen in the developed world until the outbreak of AIDS. Kaposi's sarcoma is a major feature of this disease.

Kaposi's spots A serious complication of infantile eczema occurring on exposure to herpes simplex virus infection. More commonly known as Kaposi's varicelliform eruption.

Kaposi's varicelliform Herpes or vaccinia infection in presence of pre-existing eczema.

Karaya A gum made from certain species of *Sterculia*, a genus of tropical trees and shrubs. Used as an aid to applying ostomy bags to the skin.

Karman catheter Catheter used in performing suction curettage of uterus.

Karnofsky's index A tool used in studying chronic illnesses and cancers to clinically estimate the physical state, performance, and prognosis of a patient after a therapeutic procedure.

Kartagener's syndrome Hereditary syndrome consisting of bronchiectasis, sinusitis and transposition of viscera.

Karyocyte Nucleated red blood cell, normoblast.

Karyolysis Destruction of cell nucleus.

Karyopyknosis Shrinkage of nucleus of a cell with condensation of chromatin.

Karyorrhexis Fragmentation of chromatin in nuclear lysis.

Karyosome Irregular clumps of nondividing chromatin in cell nucleus.

Karyotype 1. The chromosomal constitution and arrangement of a cell of an individual. 2. The pattern that is seen when human chromosomes are photographed during metaphase. The pictures are then enlarged and paired according to the length of their short arm.

Kasabach-Merritt syndrome Capillary hemangioma associated with thrombocytopenic purpura.

Kata (Cata) Prefix meaning down, wrongly, back, against.

Kawasaki disease Mucocutaneous lymphnode syndrome; children are the prime victims and run a risk of coronary arteritis with infarction.

Kayser-Fleischer ring The green ring around the cornea due to deposition of copper in Descemet's membrane in Wilson's disease.

Kcal Kilocalorie.

Kegel exercises Specific exercises named after Dr Arnold H Kegel, a gynecologist who first developed them to strengthen the pelvic-vaginal muscles as a means of controlling stress incontinence in women.

Keith-Wagener-Barker classification A classification of hypertensive changes of retina. Grade I moderate narrowing of retinal arterioles Grade II retinal hemorrhages Grade III cotton wool exudates and grade IV papilledema.

Kell blood group One of the human blood groups, composed of three forms of antigens.

Keller's operation *WL Keller. American surgeon, 1874–1959.* An operation for correcting hallux valgus.

Keloid Hard, raised scar tissue in the skin, common in people with dark skins. A type occurs in a healed wound due to overgrowth of fibrous tissue, causing the scar to be raised above the skin level.

Kelvin scale Temperature scale in which absolute zero is equal to minus 273 degree on Celsius scale.

Kemadrin Procyclidine hydrochloride, used in Parkinsonism for anticholinergic effect.

Kenalog Triamcinolone hydrochloride.

Kennedy's syndrome *F Kennedy, American neurologist, 1884–1952.* Ipsilateral optic atrophy caused by a frontal lobe tumor which involves one of the optic nerves.

Kenny treatment Physical therapy for treating poliomyelitis consisting of application of hot moist packs, early muscle education.

Kenophobia Fear of empty spaces.

Kent's bundle Accessory conduction pathway joining atria with ventricles.

Kerasin A cerebroside.

Keratectasia Protrusion of the cornea following inflammation.

Keratectomy Excision of a portion of the cornea.

Keratic l. Horny. 2. Relating to the cornea.

Keratic precipitates Inflammatory exudates adhering to the back of the cornea; a sign of iritis and cycitis.

Keratin An albuminoidal substance which forms the principal constituent of all horny tissues.

Keratinize To make or become horny.

Keratinization The process of keratin formation within keratinocytes and its progress upward through the layers of epidermis to the surface stratum corneum.

Keratinocyte Cell synthesizing keratin.

Keratitic precipitates Inflammatory cells in anterior chamber that stick to inner endothelial surface of cornea.

Keratitis Inflammation of the cornea. The causes may be physical (trauma, exposure to dust, vapors or ultraviolet light) or due to infectious conditions such as corneal and dendritic ulcers.

Interstitial keratitis Deep chronic keratitis, usually arising in congenital syphilis.

Striate keratitis Inflammation that appears in lines due to the folding over of the cornea after injury or operation, particularly one for cataract.

Keratoacanthoma A papular keratin filled lesion resembling squamous cell carcinoma but subsiding spontaneously.

Keratocele; Descemetocele Protrusion of Descemet's membrane through the base of a corneal ulcer. A horny growth of the skin.

Keratoconjunctivitis Inflammation of both the cornea and the conjunctiva of the eye.

Keratoconus Conical protrusion of center of cornea without inflammation.

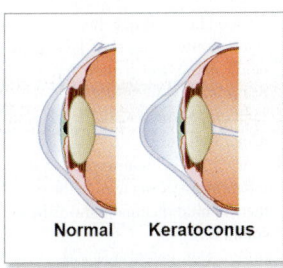

Normal   Keratoconus

Keratoconus

Keratoderma blenorrhagica Prominent hyperkeratotic scaling lesions of palms, soles associated with Reiter's syndrome.

Keratodermia Hypertrophy of stratum corneum of palms and soles of feet.

Keratinize To make or become horny.

Kerato iritis Inflammation of both the cornea and iris.

Keratoiritis Inflammation of both the cornea and iris.

Keratoma A callosity, a horny growth, Keratosis.

Keratomalacia Ulceration and softening of the cornea due to a deficiency of vitamin A.

Keratometer; Ophthalmometer An instrument by which the amount of corneal astigmatism can be measured accurately.

Keratometry Measurements of cornea.

Keratomileusis Plastic surgery of cornea in which a portion of cornea is removed, frozen, its curvature is reshaped and then reattached in its place.

Keratonosis Any non-inflammatory disease or deformity of horny layer of skin.

Keratonyxis Surgical puncture of cornea.

Keratopathy band Calcium deposit in superficial layer of cornea and Bowman's capsule, occurring in hypercalcemia or chronic intraocular inflammation.

Keratophakia Keratoplasty in which a slice of donor's cornea is shaped to a desired curvature and inserted between layers of the recipient's cornea to change its curvature.

Keratoplasty A plastic operation on the cornea, including corneal grafting.

Keratoprotein The protein of hair, nail and epidermis.

Keratorrhexis Rupture of cornea.

Keratoscope An instrument for examining the eye to detect keratoconus placido's disc.

Keratosis A skin disease marked by excessive growth of the epidermis or horny tissue.

K

Keratosis actinic A horny keratotic premalignant lesion due to prolonged exposure to sunlight.

Keratosis follicularis SYN – Darier's disease, characterized by verrucous papular growths that coalese into plaques affecting face, neck, axillae and scalp.

Keratosis pilaris Chronic inflammation of unknown etiology involving hair follicle.

Keratotome A knife for corneal incision.

Keratotomy Incision of the cornea.

Keratotomy radial Very shallow, bloodless, hairline incisions are made in outer portion of cornea thereby allowing it to flatten; a treatment modality for axial myopia upto 5 diopters.

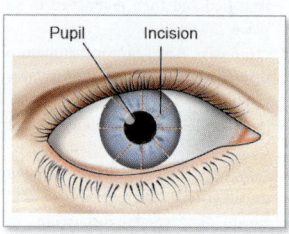

Pupil   Incision

Radial Keratotomy

Keraunophobia Morbid fear of thundering and lightening.

Kerion A complication of ring worm of the scalp, with formation of pustules.

Kerley lines Thickening of inter alveolar septa due to pulmonary edema.

Kernicterus A condition in the newborn marked by severe neural symptoms, associated with high levels of bilirubin in the blood; it is commonly a sequela of icterus gravis neonatorum.

Kernig's sign *VM Kernig, Russian physician, 1840–1917.* A sign of meningitis. When the thigh is supported at right angles to the trunk, the patient is unable to straighten the leg at the knee joint.

Kerosene An inflammable liquid fuel distilled from petroleum. Fumes of it can cause pneumonitis.

Ketamine A rapidly acting, nonbarbiturate general anesthetic which is given by intramuscular or intravenous injection.

Ketanserine 5 HT antagonist.

Keto acid Any organic acid containing ketone (CO) radical.

Ketoacidosis Acidosis due to excess of ketone bodies.

Keto aciduria Presence of ketoacids in urine.

Ketoconazole Systemic antifungal agent.

Ketogenic Forming or capable of being converted into ketone bodies.

Ketogenic diet Diet insufficient in calories to produce mild ketosis helpful in some cases of childhood epilepsy.

Ketohexose A nonsaccharide consisting of a six carbon chain and containing a ketone group in addition to alcohol group (e.g., fructose).

Ketone An organic compound containing the carbonyl group (CO) attached to two hydrocarbon groups. Ketones are produced by the metabolization of fats.

Ketonemia Presence of ketone bodies in blood in excess quantity.

Ketone threshold Level of ketones in blood above which they appear in urine.

Ketonuria The presence of ketones in urine; acetonuria.

Ketoprofen A nonsteroidal anti-inflammatory drug used in the treatment of mild rheumatic and arthritic conditions.

Ketorolac Non-opioid analgesic.

Ketose A carbohydrate containing the ketones.

Ketosis The condition in which ketones are formed in excess in the body and accumulate in the blood. Severe acidosis may occur.

K

Ketosteroid A steroid hormone which contains a ketone group attached to a carbon atom.

17 ketosteroid Are excreted in the urine and formed from the adrenal corticosteroids, testosterone and, to a lesser extent, oestrogens.

Ketotifen Mast cell stabilizer used in asthma.

Key worker A person (commonly a social worker) designated as coordinator for action where several people are involved in the care of a person or family. The key worker is also responsible for calling a case conference to consider relevant issues for the client.

Kick chart A method of fetal assessment carried out by the mother. The number of kicks or movements felt during the day is counted and noted. If fewer than 10 kicks are felt in a 12 hrs daytime period on two consecutive occasions, the mother is advised to contact her midwife or doctor immediately. If no movements are felt in any day, the mother is advised to contact the hospital at once. The value of this test is that it can highlight a potential case of fetal distress and alert medical attention before it is too late.

Kidney One of two organs situated in the lumbar region, which purify the blood and secrete urine. The kidney secretes renin and renal erythropoietic factor.

Artificial kidney The apparatus used to remove retained waste products from the blood when kidney function is impaired.

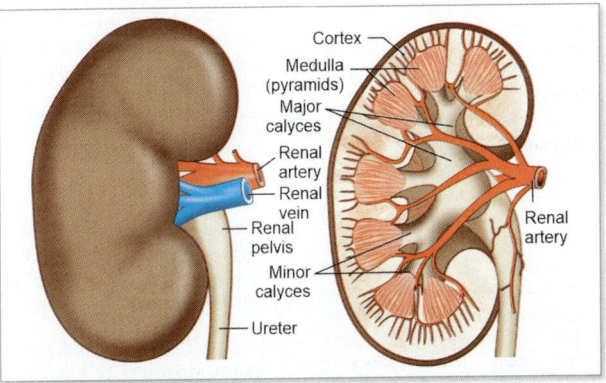

Structure of Kidney

Granular kidney The small fibrosed kidney of chronic nephritis.

Horseshoe kidney A congenital defect producing a fusion of the two kidneys into a horseshoe shape.

Kidney failure The condition in which renal function is severely impaired and the organs are unable to maintain the fluid and electrolyte balance of the body.

Kidney transplant The surgical implantation of a kidney taken from a live donor or from one who has recently died. Used in the treatment of renal failure.

Polycystic kidney A congenital bilateral condition of multiple cysts replacing kidney tissue.

Kidney stone Calculus present in renal parenchyma, calyx or renal pelvis, composed principally of calcium, urate, oxalate, phosphates and carbonates, ranging from small granular masses to 5 cm or more in diameter. Most common in patients of hyperparathyroidism, oxaluria, gout and chronic pyelonephritis.

Kiesselbach's plexus A rich network of capaillaries on the anteroinferior part of nasal septum; the most common site of bleeding in epistaxis.

Kilocalorie Symbol kcal. One thousand calories, a unit of food energy.

Kilocycle One thousand cycles as in electricity.

Kilogram One thousand gram.

Kilohertz One thousand cycles as in electricity.

Kilojoule Symbol kJ. One thousand joules, a unit of food energy (1 kcal = 4.184 kJ).

Kilometer 1,000 meters, 3,281 feet or 0.61 mile.

Kilowatt A unit of electrical energy equivalent to 1000 watts.

Kimmelstiel-Wilson syndrome P. Kimmelstiel, German pathologist, 1900-1970; C. Wilson, British physician, 1906-1997. A degenerative complication of Diabetes (Mellitus) with albuminuria, edema, hypertension, renal insufficiency and retinopathy. May lead to kidney failure. Called also intercapillary glomerulosclerosis.

Kinaesthesia The combined sensations by which position, weight and muscular position are perceived.

Kinanaesthesia An inability to perceive the sensation of movements of parts of the body.

Kinase An enzyme activator' *(See Enterokinase and Thrombokinase).*

Kinematograph Device for viewing photographs of objects in motion.

Kineplasty Plastic amputation; amputation in which the stump is so formed as to be utilized for producing motion of the prosthesis.

Kinoscope Device for conducting refraction of eye.

Kinesiatrics Treatment involving active and passive movements.

Kinesics Systematic study of the body and use of its static and dynamic position as a means of communication.

Kinesiology The study of muscles and body movement.

Kinesthesia Ability to perceive extent, direction and weight of movement.

Kinetic Producing or pertaining to motion.

Kinetosis Any disorder caused by motion, such as sea sickness.

King's evil A historic term for tuberculosis of the tonsillar lymph glands in the neck (scrofula) thought to be cured by the touch of the king.

King's Fund King Edward's Hospital Fund for London was founded in 1897 for the support, by the giving of grants, of voluntary hospitals in London. Since the inception of the National Health Service in 1948, it has been concerned with the funding of experimental schemes, particularly relating to the management of services.

Kings's bed A Bed fitted with jointed springs which may be adjusted to various positions, developed as the result of research undertaken on behalf of and funded by the King's Fund.

Kinin A polypeptide which occurs naturally and is a powerful vasodilator.

Kininogen Precursor of kinin.

Kinky hair disease Congenital autosomal recessive syndrome consisting of short, sparse kinky hair, poor physical and mental development, associated with degenerative changes of cerebral gray matter.

Kinomometer Device for measuring degree of motion in a joint.

Kinship Relationship.

Kinship studies In anthropology the study of kin (relatives) and their patterns of marriage, descent, inheritance, habitation, social values and economics.

Kirschner wire *M Kirschner, German surgeon, 1879–1942.* A thin wire that may be passed through a bone to apply skeletal traction.

Kisch's reflex Closure of an eye from stimulation of auditory meatus.

Kiss of life The expired air method of artificial respiration, by either mouth-to-nose or mouth-to-mouth breathing *(See Appendices).*

Kite apparatus Apparatus for reeducation of weak muscles and prevention of contractures around forearm, wrist and fingers.

KJ Kilojoule.

Klebs-Loffler bacillus *TAE Klebs, German bacteriologist, 1834–1913; FAJ Loffler, German bacteriologist, 1852–1915.*

Corynebacterium diphtheriae, the causative agent of diphtheria.

Klebsiella A genus of Gram-negative bacteria (family Enterobacteriaceae).

Kleihauer test A microscopic test to detect fetal cells in the maternal circulation, usually done immediately after delivery so that, if the mother is rhesus-negative and the fetus rhesus-positive, anti-D immunoglobulin may be given to prevent isoimmunization.

Klepto To steal.

Kleptolagnia Sexual gratification obtained from stealing.

Kleptomania An irresistible urge to steal when there is often no need and no particular desire for the objects. Often associated with depression.

Kleptomaniac A psychopathic personality suffering from impulsive stealing.

Kleptophobia Morbid fear of stealing.

Klieg eye Conjunctivitis, lacrimation and photophobia from exposure to intense lights as used in making television, film shooting.

Klinefelter's syndrome *HF Klinefelter, American physician, b. 1912.* A congenital chromosome abnormality in which each cell has three sex chromosomes, XXY, rather than the usual XX or XY, making a total of 47 (normal is 46). Affected men have female breast development and small testes and are infertile.

Klippel's disease Pseudoparalysis due to generalized arthritis.

Klippel-Feil syndrome *M Klippel, French neurologist, 1858–1942; A. Feil, French physician; b. 1884.* A congenital abnormality in which the neck is very short as a result of the absence or fusion of several vertebrae in the cervical region.

Kllocalorle Symbol kcal. One thousand calories, a unit of food energy.

Klumpke's paralysis Atrophic paralysis of forearm usually due to birth trauma with stretching, avulsion of brachial plexus.

Kluver-Bucy syndrome Behavioral syndrome usually following bilateral temporal lobectomy, manifesting with hypersexuality, rage, memory deficit, hyperreligiosity, hyperphagia, failure of visual recognition, etc.

Knapp's forceps Forceps with roller like blades for expressing trachomatous granulations on the palpebral conjunctiva.

Kneading A form of massage consisting of grasping, wringing, lifting, rolling, pressing.

Knee The joint between the femur and the tibia.

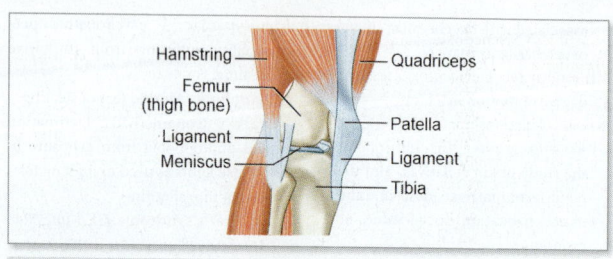

Knee

Housemaid's knee Prepatellar bursitis.

Knee jerk An upward jerk of the leg obtained by striking the patellar tendon when the knee is passively flexed.

Knock-knee A condition in which the knees turn inward towards each other; genu valgum.

Knee cap The patella.

Knee chest position Position in which patient is on knees with thighs straight, head and upper part of chest resting on table and arms crossed in front of head. Employed for sigmoidoscopic examination of colon and rectum, repositioning of retroverted uterus or displaced ovary.

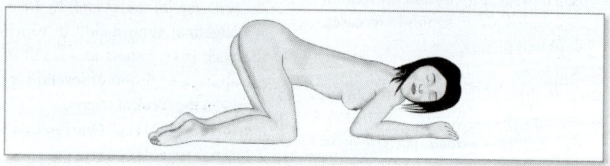

Knee Chest Position

Kneecap The patella.

Knemometry A precise method of determining the length of a limb.

Knob A mass or nodule.

Knot 1. In surgery, the intertwining of the ends of a suture, ligature, bandage so that the ends will not slip or get loose. 2. An intertwining of a cord or cord-like structure to form a knob or lump.

Knuckle Prominence of the dorsal aspect of any of the phallangeal joints.

Knocher's reflex Contraction of abdominal muscles following moderate compression of testicle.

Koch's bacillus *R Koch, German bacteriologist, 1843–1910.*

Mycobacterium tuberculosis, the causative organism of tuberculosis.

Koebner phenomenon Appearance of skin lesion as a result of on specific trauma.

Kohler's disease *A Kohler, German physician and radiologist. 1874–1947.* Osteochondritis of the navicular bone of the foot, occurring in children.

Koilocyte An abnormal cell of squamous epithelium of the cervix, a forerunner of cervical intraepithelial neoplasia.

Koilonychia The development of brittle, spoon-shaped nails which may occur in iron-deficiency anemia.

Koniology Science of dust and its effect.

Koniometer Device for estimating amount of dust in air.

Koplik's spots *H Koplik, American pediatrician, 1858–1927.* Small white spots that sometimes appear on the mucous membranes inside the mouth in measles on the second day of onset, before the general rash.

Korotkoff's method *NS Korotkoff, Russian physician, 1874–1920.* A method of finding the systolic and diastolic blood pressure by listening to the sounds produced in an artery while the pressure in a previously inflated cuff is gradually reduced.

Korsakoff's syndrome or psychosis *SS Korsakoff, Russian neurologist, 1854–1900.* A chronic condition in which there is impaired memory, particularly for recent events, and the patient is disorientated for time and place. It may be present in psychosis of infective, toxic or metabolic origin, or in chronic alcoholism.

Kosher Food that is prepared and cooked in accordance with Jewish dietary laws; it is eaten by practising Jews.

Krabber's disease Globoid cell leukodystrophy due to collection of galactocerebrocides in the tissues. Clinically manifesting with seizure, deafness, blindness and mental retardation.

Kraurosis Dryness and shrinking of a part of the body.

Kraurosis vulvae A degenerative condition of the vulva. May be treated by giving oestrogen preparations.

Krause's glands Accessory lacrimal glands opening into fornix of eye.

Krause's valves Fold of mucous membrane of the lacrimal sac at the junction of lacrimal duct.

Krause's end bulbs Encapsulated nerve endings present in skin.

Krebs cycle *Sir HA Krebs. German-British biochemist, 1900–1981.* A series of reactions during which the aerobic oxidation of pyruvic acid takes place. This is part of carbohydrate metabolism.

Krebs urea cycle The way in which urea is formed in the liver.

Krukenberg's tumor A malignant tumor of ovary, usually bilateral and frequently secondary to malignancy of GI tract (through peritoneal seedling).

Krypton A gaseous element in the atmosphere.

Kufs' disease Adult form of cerebral sphingolipidosis with dementia, retinitis pigmentatosa, blindness and myoclonic jerks.

Kugelberg-Welander disease Juvenile spinal muscular atrophy.

Kummell's disease Spondylitis following compression fracture of vertebra.

Kuntscher nail *G Kuntscher, German orthopedic surgeon. 1902–1972.* An intramedullary nail used in treating fractures of long bones, especially the shaft of the femur.

Kupffer's cells *KW von Kupffer, German anatomist, 1829–1902.* Phagocytic reticuloendothelial cells of the liver which form bile from haemoglobin released by disintegrated erythrocytes.

Kuru A progressively fatal encephalopathy probably of slow virus infection spreading by practice of cannibalism.

Kussmaul's breathing Very deep and gasping respiration in acidosis.

Kveim test *MA Kveim, Norwegian physician, b. 1892.* A test for sarcoidosis in which antigen from the lymph nodes or spleen of a sarcoidosis patient is injected intradermally.

Kwashiorkor A condition of protein malnutrition occurring in children in under-privileged populations. Fatty infiltration of the liver arises and may cause cirrhosis.

K

Kyasanur forest disease (KFD) Tick born encephalitis of South India.

Kymograph An instrument for recording variations or undulations, arterial or other.

Kymoscope Device for measuring variations in blood flow and pressure.

Kyphoscoliosis An abnormal curvature of the spine in which there is forward and sideways displacement.

Kyphosis Posterior curvature of the spine. May be congenital or secondary to compression fracture or malignancy; hump back, hunch back.

⊙⊙⊙

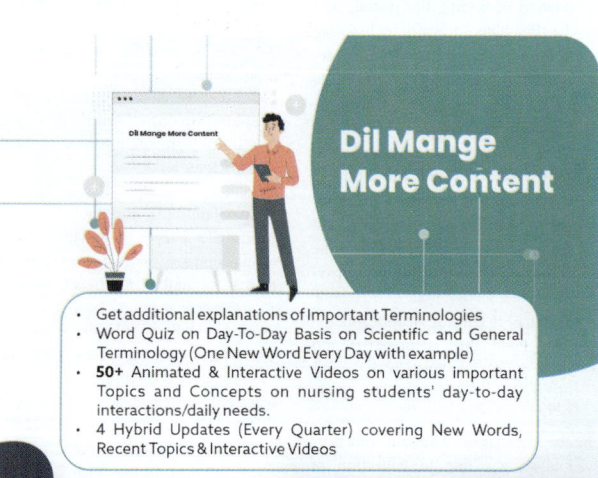
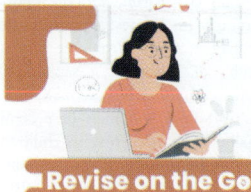

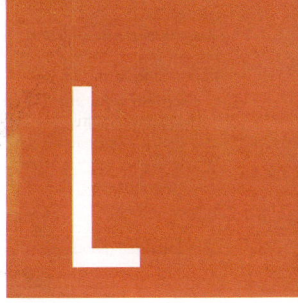

L Symbol for litre.

LA 50 The total body surface size of a burn that will kill 50% of victims, used for statistical analysis of mortality figures in burn patients.

Labelling The process or procedure followed using chemical or radioactive labels as an aid in reaching diagnosis or for experimental study.

Labetalol An alpha- and beta-adrenergic receptor blocker used in the treatment of hypertension.

Labial Pertaining to the lips or labia.

Labile Unstable. Applied to those chemicals that are subject to change or readily altered by heat.

Lability Instability.

Lability of mood The tendency to sudden changes of mood of short duration.

Labioplasty Plastic surgery of labium majus or minus.

Labium A lip.

Labium majus pudendi The large fold of flesh surrounding the vulva.

Labium minus pudendi The lesser fold within the labium majus.

Labour Parturition or childbirth, which takes place in three stages: (a) Dilatation of the cervix uteri; (b) Passage of the child through the birth canal; and (c) Expulsion of the placenta.

Arrested labour Failure of progression of labour.

Dry labour Premature rupture of membranes with escape of liquor.

False labour Uterine contractions that do not progress.

Induced labour Labour brought on by artificial means before term, as in cases of contracted pelvis, or if overdue.

Obstructed labour Labour in which there is a mechanical hindrance.

Precipitate labour Labour in which the baby is delivered extremely rapidly.

Premature labour Labour which occurs before term.

Prolonged labour Extended duration of labor as first phase exceeding 20 hours in nullipara, 14 hours in multipara or cervical dilatation less than 1.2 cm/hr in nullipara and 1.5 cm in multipara.

Spurious labour Ineffective labor pains which sometimes precede true labor pains.

Labrum Lip like structure.

Labrum acetabulare Traingular rim of fibrocartilage, base of which is fixed to acetabular margin, deepening its cavity.

Labrum glenoidale A triangular rim of fibrocartilage, the base of which is fixed to circumference of glenoid cavity of scapula.

Labyrinth The structures forming the internal ear, i.e., the cochlea and semicircular canals.

Bony labyrinth The bony canals of the internal ear.

Membranous labyrinth The soft structure inside the bony canals.

Labyrinth vestibularis The portion of membranous labyrinth comprising sacculus, utriculus and their connections and the three semicircular canals.

Labyrinthectomy Excision of the labyrinth.

Labyrinthitis Inflammation of the labyrinth, causing vertigo.

Laceration A wound with torn and ragged edges.

Lacrimal Relating to tears.

Lacrimal apparatus The structures secreting the tears and draining the fluid from the conjunctival sac.

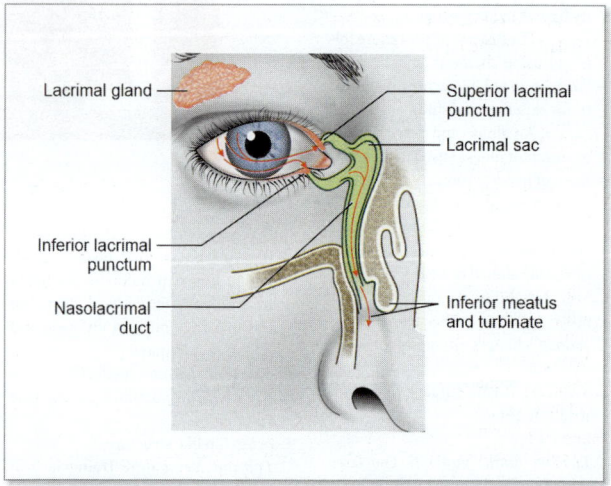

Lacrimal gland

Superior lacrimal punctum

Lacrimal sac

Inferior lacrimal punctum

Nasolacrimal duct

Inferior meatus and turbinate

Lacrimal Apparatus

Lacrimal gland A gland that secretes tears, which drain through two small openings in the eyelids *(L. puncta)* into a pair of ducts *(L. canaliculi)* into the sac and finally into the nasal cavity through the nasolacrimal duct. Situated in the outer and upper corner of the orbit.

Lacrimation An excessive secretion of tears.

Lacrimator A substance that causes excessive secretion of tears, e.g., tear gas.

Lactagogue Any agent that promotes the secretion or flow of milk; galactagogue.

Lactalbumin An albumin of milk.

Lactase An enzyme, produced in the small intestine, which converts lactose into glucose and galactose.

Lactate 1. Any substance given to promote lactation. 2. Any salt of lactic acid. 3. To secrete milk.

Lactate dehydrogenase Abbreviated LD, LDH. An enzyme that catalyses the interconversion of lactate and pyruvate. Widespread in tissues and particularly abundant in kidney, skeletal muscle, liver and myocardium. It has five isoenzymes denoted LD1 to LD2. The "flipped" pattern, in which the serum LD1 level is greater than the LD2 level, is indicative of an acute myocardial infarction. This pattern occurs within 12–24 hours after the attack.

Lactation 1. The period during which the infant is nourished from the breast. 2. The process of milk secretion by the mammary glands.

Lacteal 1. Consisting of milk. 2. A lymphatic duct in the small intestine which absorbs chyle.

Lactic Pertaining to milk.

Lactic acid An acid formed by the fermentation of lactose or milk sugar. It is produced naturally in the body as a result of glucose metabolism. An excess of the acid accumulating in the muscles may cause cramp.

Lactiferous Conveying or secreting milk.

Lactobacillus A genus of Gram-positive, rod-shaped bacteria, many of which produce fermentation.

Lactoferrin An iron-binding protein found in neutrophils and bodily secretions (milk, tears, saliva, bile, etc.), having bactericidal activity and acting as an inhibitor of colony formation by granulocytes and macrophages.

Lactogenic Stimulating the production of milk *(See Luteotrophin).*

Lactometer An instrument for measuring the specific gravity of milk.

Lactoglobulin A milk protein with a concentration of 3 g per liter in cow's milk, second only to case in among milk proteins.

Lactose Milk sugar consisting of glucose and galactose.

Lactose intolerance The ingestion of milk containing lactose results in the patient experiencing severe abdominal colic and diarrhea due to deficiency of the lactose-splitting enzyme (betagalactosidase) in the lining of the small intestine. Asian and African people who have a change in diet to one with a higher milk content are often affected in this way.

Lactose synthetase Enzyme helping in synthesis of lactose, found in mammary glands.

Lactosuria Lactose in the urine.

Lactovegetarian 1. A person who subsists on a diet of milk or milk products and vegetables. 2. Pertaining to such a diet.

Lactulose A synthetic disaccharide which is used as a laxative.

Lacuna A small cavity or depression in any part of the body.

Lacuna cerebral Hypertensive lipohyalunosis causing minor infarction with lacune formation within cerebral hemisphere (lacunar syndrome).

Lacuna Howship's Bony pits occupied by osteoclasts.

Laennec's disease *RTH Laennec, French physician, 1781–1826.* The most common type of cirrhosis of the liver, frequently attributable to high alcohol consumption.

Laetrile American trade name for a substance derived from apricots, almonds and other fruit; alleged to have antineoplastic activity.

Laevulose Fruit sugar; fructose.

Lag Slowness to act or react, the interval between an expected action or reaction and its occurrence.

Lag anaphase A retarded movement of chromosome during mitosis.

Lag eyelid Failure of upper eyelid to descend promptly while looking down as in Grave's disease.

Lag globe While looking upward, upper eyelid pulls faster than the eyeball is raised, thus exposing the sclera above the iris.

Lag jet Altered biological rhythms like sleep, satiety, hunger, after rapid jet transport.

Lagophthalmos Inability to close the eyelids completely as in facial palsy.

Laking Hemolysis of the red blood cells. The cells swell and burst and the hemoglobin is released.

Lallation A babbling, infantile form of speech.

Lamaze method *F Lamaze. French obstetrician, 1890–1957.* A method of preparing for natural childbirth developed by Fernand Lamaze, and based on the technique of training the mind and body for the purpose of modifying perception of pain during labor and delivery.

Lambdoid Shaped like the Greek letter Λ or λ.

Lambdoid suture The junction of the occipital bone with the parietals.

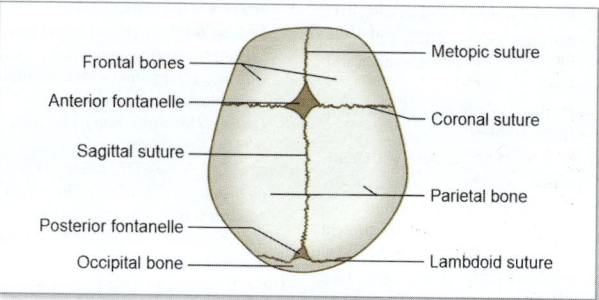

Frontal bones

Anterior fontanelle

Sagittal suture

Posterior fontanelle

Occipital bone

Metopic suture

Coronal suture

Parietal bone

Lambdoid suture

Lambdoid Suture

Lambert-Eaton myasthenic syndrome (LEMS) A rare condition affecting signals sent from nerves to muscles resulting in muscles not being able to contract properly. Some cases are associated with lung cancer.

Lambliasis Giardiasis.

Lamella 1. A thin layer, membrane or plate, as of bone. 2. A thin medicated disc of gelatin used in applying drugs to the eye. The gelatin dissolves and the drugs are absorbed.

Lamina A bony plate or layer.

Lamina dental A flat band of epithelial cells that develops in the embryos along which develop the tooth germs giving rise to primary and secondary dentition.

Lamina of rexed Lamination of cells in spinal gray matter marked 1 to 9, arranged in dorsoventral direction and lamina 10 situated centrally.

Lamina terminalis A membrane formed in the developing embryo remaining to adulthood as a thin layer of gray matter extending from superior surface of optic chiasma to rostrum of corpus callosum.

Laminated Arranged in layers.

Laminectomy Excision of the posterior arch of a vertebra, sometimes performed to relieve pressure on the spinal cord or nerves.

Lamotrigine Antiepileptic.

Lamp A device producing light artificially.

Eldridge green lamp Color vision testing device using spectral filters.

Finsen lamp Carbon arc lamp utilized for treating lupus vulgaris.

Kromayer lamp Mercury quartz ultraviolet lamp for treatment of skin ulcers.

Wood's lamp Lamp producing ultraviolet rays at 365 nm giving characteristic fluorescence of some fungi. Infected hairs have bright green fluorescence.

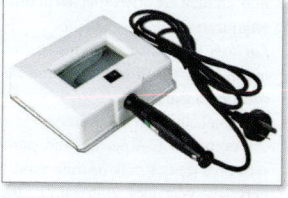

Wood's Lamp

Lancefield's groups *RC Lancejield, American bacteriologist, 1895– 1981.* Divisions of B-haemolytic streptococci, which are classified on the basis of serological action into groups A–R. Most human infections are due to group A.

Lancet A small surgical blade, used for making small drainage incisions.

Lancinating Sudden sharp transient pain as if tearing into pieces.

Landry's paralysis *JBG Landry, French physician, 1826–1865.* Guillain-Barre syndrome; acute ascending polyneuritis.

Landsteiner's classification *K Landsteiner, Austrian biologist, 1868– 1943.* A system of blood groups; the ABO system, consisting of groups A, B, AB and O.

Lange colloidal gold test *CFA Lange, German physician, 1883–1953.* A test made on cerebrospinal fluid to detect syphilis, disseminated sclerosis, meningitis and other neurological conditions.

Langerhans cell histiocytosis A rare disease of childhood where Langerhans cells proliferate and migrate from the skin to lymph nodes.

Langerhans *P Langerhans, German pathologist, 1847–1888. Islet of Langerhans* One of the group of cells in the pancreas that produce insulin.

Langers lines The structural orientation of fibrous tissues of skin. Incision made parallel to them produce less scar.

Language The means of human communication consisting of the use of spoken or written word in a structured way. Gestures of hands, head and even the body may be involved, although this is reflected differently from one setting to another, e.g., from a formal presentation to the greeting of a friend. Cultural background too plays a part in the use or absence of gestures.

L. disorders Problems affecting the ability to communicate and/or comprehend the spoken and/or written word. *(See Speech).*

Lanolin A fat obtained from sheep's wool, and used as a basis for ointments, salves, creams and cosmetics.

Lansoprazole Proton pump inhibitor, used in peptic ulcer.

Lanugo The fine hair that covers the body of the fetus and newly born infants, especially those who are premature.

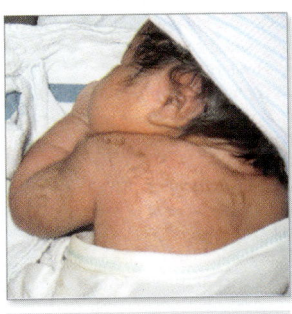

Lanugo

Laparoscopy Viewing of the abdominal cavity by passing an endoscope through the abdominal wall.

Laparotomy Incision of the abdominal wall for exploratory purposes.

Laplace's Law Pressure within a tube is inversely proportional to its radius.

Larva Motile developing stage of worms, maggots, caterpillars.
1. Fillariform: Infective larva of nematodes.

Larva migrans Migratory phase of the cycle of helminth in an abnormal host/site with random wandering.

Larva migrans cutaneous Linear eruption caused by hookworm larva.

Larva migrans visceral Disorder of visceral larval migration from normal, i.e., intestine to liver, heart, lungs, trachea, mouth and back to intestine so that the larva migrate in random with ultimate encapsulation in aberrant site.

Larvicide Medication effective against larval form.

Larviparous Deposition of hatched larvae than eggs.

Laryngeal Pertaining to the larynx.

Laryngectomy Excision of the larynx.

Laryngismus A spasmodic contraction of the larynx.

Laryngismus stridulus A crowing sound on inspiration, following a period of apnea, due to spasmodic closure of the glottis. It occurs in children, particularly those suffering from rickets. Croup.

Laryngitis Inflammation of the larynx causing hoarseness or loss of voice due to acute infection or irritation by gases.

Laryngocele An air containing pouch, usually bilateral in wind instrument players and glass blowers.

Laryngomalacia A flaccid supraglottic larynx in babies causing inspiratory stridor but with spontaneous cure.

Laryngopharynx The lower portion of the pharynx connecting with the larynx.

Laryngoplasty Reconstruction of larynx to improve airway as in bilateral abductor palsy.

Laryngoscope An endoscopic instrument for examining the larynx or for aiding the insertion of endotracheal tubes or the bronchoscope.

Laryngospasm A reflex, prolonged contraction of the laryngeal muscles that is liable to occur on insertion or withdrawal of an endotracheal tube.

Laryngostenosis Contraction or stricture of the larynx.

Laryngostomy The making of an opening into the larynx to provide an artificial air passage.

Laryngotomy An incision into the larynx to make a temporary opening in an emergency when the larynx is obstructed. Tracheostomy.

Laryngotracheal Referring to both the larynx and trachea.

Laryngotracheitis Inflammation of both the larynx and trachea.

Laryngotracheobronchitis An acute viral infection of the respiratory tract which occurs particularly in young children.

Larynx [Gr.] The muscular and cartilaginous structure, lined with mucous membrane, situated at the top of the trachea and below the root of the tongue and the hyoid bone. The larynx contains the vocal cords and is the source of the sound heard in speech; it is also called the voice box.

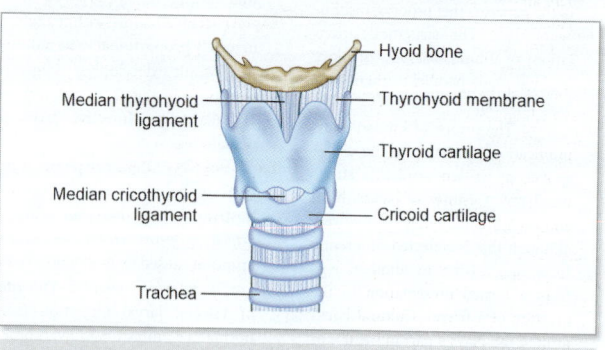

Hyoid bone
Median thyrohyoid ligament
Thyrohyoid membrane
Thyroid cartilage
Median cricothyroid ligament
Cricoid cartilage
Trachea

Larynx

Laser Light amplification by stimulated emission of radiation. An apparatus producing an extremely concentrated beam of light that can be used to cut metals. Used in the treatment of neoplasms, detached retina, diabetic retinopathy and macular degeneration, and some skin conditions.

Lassa fever A West African viral hemorrhagic fever with insidious onset and an incubation period of 6–21 days. It is a zoonosis, the reservoir of infection of which is the multimammate rat. Devastating outbreaks of person-to-person transmission have occurred in hospitals in West Africa by accidental inoculation of blood and tissue fluid from infected patients. Prevention is dependent on the early detection of cases and their isolation, and strict precautions to protect health-care staff caring for febrile patients from Mica from inoculation or other accidents.

Lassar's paste *G Lassar, German dermatologist, 1849–1907.* A soothing paste used in skin diseases, containing salicylic acid, zinc oxide, starch and soft paraffin.

Lassitude A feeling of extreme weakness and apathy.

Lasting powers of attorney (LPA) There are two types of LPA-one for financial decisions and one for health and care decisions. These decisions are registered with the Office of the Public Guardian and give the attorney the authority to make treatment decisions in the event that the patient is unable to make such decisions due to incapacity.

Latency The period between stimulation application and onset of response.

Latent Temporarily concealed; not manifest.
  Latent heat The heat absorbed by a substance during a change in state, e.g., from water into steam. When condensation occurs this heat is released.
  Latent period 1. The incubation period of an infectious disease. 2. The time between the application of a nerve stimulus and the reaction.

Lateral Situated at the side; therefore, away from the center.

Lateralization The tendency to perform an act predominantly on left or right side of the body.

Lateroversion A turning to one side, such as may occur of the uterus.

Latex A milky fluid derived from tapping the rubber tree Hevea brasiliensis found mainly in Thailand, Indonesia and Malaysia. It comprises an aqueous suspension of globules of rubber hydrocarbon coated with proteins.
  L. Allergy A reaction to latex proteins, varying in severity. It is a significant occupational health problem for health care workers. Latex is a component of many medical supplies, e.g., various tubes, materials and gloves. Latex gloves have been frequently implicated due either to the latex or to the proteins used in the powders that lubricate the gloves for ease of use.

Lathyrism Spastic paraplegia with sensory impairment due to consumption of khesari dal containing fungus *Lathyrus sativatus.*

Laudanum Tincture of opium; a preparation formerly used as a narcotic.

Laughing gas Nitrous oxide.

Laurence-Moon-Biedl syndrome An autosomal recessive disorder affecting especially males and characterized by obesity, polydactyly, mental retardation, subnormal development of genitals, and retinitis pigmentosa.

Lauric acid A fatty acid found in neutral fat like butter.

Lavage The washing out of a cavity.

Colonic lavage The washing out of the colon.

Gastric lavage The washing out of the stomach.

Law An accepted and tested phenomena.

Laxative A medicine that loosens the bowel contents and encourages evacuation. A laxative with a mild or gentle effect on the bowels is also known as an aperient; one with a strong effect is referred to as a cathartic or a purgative.

Lean body mass Body weight without fat content.

LE Lupus Erythematosus.

LE cell A mature neutrophilic polymorphonuclear leukocyte that has phagocytized a large, spherical inclusion derived from another neutrophil; a characteristic of lupus erythematosus, but also found in analogous connective tissue disorders.

Lead Symbol Pb. A metallic element, many of the compounds of which are highly poisonous.

Lead lotion Lead subacetate solution used externally on bruises.

Lead poisoning A condition that usually occurs in children as the result of excessive lead in the atmosphere, or from chewing objects covered with paint containing lead. The symptoms and signs include malaise, diarrhea and vomiting, and sometimes encephalitis. There is often pallor and a blue line around the gums.

Learning Knowledge or skills gained, or behavior modified through being taught or from study. Learning occurs as a result of using intelligence, memory, insight and understanding.

L. curve A person's rate of progress in gaining experience or new skills, which can be represented as a graph.

L. difficulties Problems with learning arising from a result of a range of mental and physical problems.

L. disability The preferred term to the one formerly used, 'mental handicap'. Essentially disorders are characterized by substantial deficits in scholastic or academic skills.

Leber's disease TB Leber, German ophthalmologist, 1840–1917. Hereditary optic atrophy.

Lecithin One of a group of phospholipids that are found in the cell tissues and are concerned in the metabolism of fat.

Lecithin-Sphyngomyelin ration This ratio in amniotic fluid indicates fetal maturity. Level more than 1 occurs in full term. Low level is associated with hyaline membrane disease in newborn.

Leech Hirudo medicinalis An aquatic worm which sucks blood and secretes hirudin (an anticoagulant) in its saliva. On rare occasions used to withdraw blood from patients.

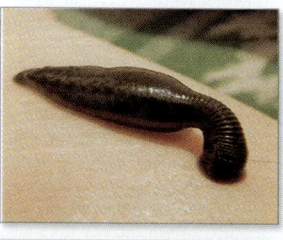

Leech

Leflunomide Used in rheumatoid arthritis.

Leg The lower limb, from knee to ankle.

Barbados leg Elephantiasis.

Bow leg Genu varum.

Scissor leg Condition in which the patient is cross-legged, such as occurs in cerebral diplegia.

White leg Phlegmasia alba dolens.

L

Legionella pneumophila A species of Gram-negative, non-acid-fast, rod shaped bacteria which require both cysteine and iron for growth; it is the causative agent of Legionnaires and pontiac fever.

Legionellosis A disease caused by infection with *Legionella* species, such as *L pneumophila*. A notifiable disease in Scotland.

Legionnaires' disease A pulmonary form of legionellosis, resulting from infection with *Legionella pneumophila*. It is contagious and symptoms include fever, pain in the muscles and across the chest, a dry cough and a partial loss of kidney function. The prevalence of Legionnaires' disease is not certain.

Leiomyoma A benign smooth muscle tumor (fibroid) most commonly found in the uterus.

Leiomyosarcoma A malignant muscle tumor.

Leishmania A genus of parasitic flagellated protozoa which infect the blood of humans and are the cause of leishmaniasis.

Leishmaniasis A group of diseases caused by one of the protozoans, *Leishmania* parasites *(See Kalaazar)*.

Leishmanoid Facial cutaneous lesion containing leishmania.

Lembert's suture *A Lembert, French surgeon, 1802–1851.* A series of stitches used for wounds of the intestine. So arranged that the edges are turned inwards and the peritoneal surfaces are in contact.

Lemniscus A ribbon, band, bundle of axons.
Lemniscus lateral Longitudinal tract of auditory system terminating in inferior colliculus and medial geniculate body.
Lemniscus medial Myelinated tract emerging from nucleus gracilis and cuneatus and crossing over to oppo-

site side in medulla and terminating in ventrobasal thalamic nucleus.
Lemniscus trigeminal A large band of myelinated axons originating from principal trigeminal nucleus and crossing over to opposite side in pons to join medial lemniscus.

Length *Cranial length* Skull length between glabella and inion.
Crown heel length Fetal or infant length from crown to heel
Foot length Toe to heel length for estimation of age of fetus.
Sitting length Distance between vertex and coccyx.

Lens 1. A piece of glass or other material shaped to transmit light rays in a particular direction. 2. The transparent crystalline body situated behind the pupil of the eye. It serves as a refractive medium for rays of light.
Contact lens A thin sheet of glass or plastic molded to fit directly over the cornea. Worn instead of spectacles.

Lentiasis Bilateral symmetrical hypertrophy of bones of face and cranium of unknown cause.

Lentiform Shaped like a lentil or lens of eye.

Lentigo A brownish or yellowish spot on the skin. A freckle.
Lentigo maligna Hutchinson's melanotic freckle *(See Freckle)*.

Lentivirus From Latin *lentus* (slow) + virus. A group of retroviruses that cause disease in animals and humans, including HIV-1 and HIV-2 *(See Human Immunodeficiency Virus)*. These viruses are associated with slowly progressive diseases.

Leontiasis An osseous deformity of the face which produces a lion-like appearance. It occurs sometimes in leprosy and rarely in osteitis deformans.

Leopold's maneuver A method to determine position, presentation, and engagement of fetus.

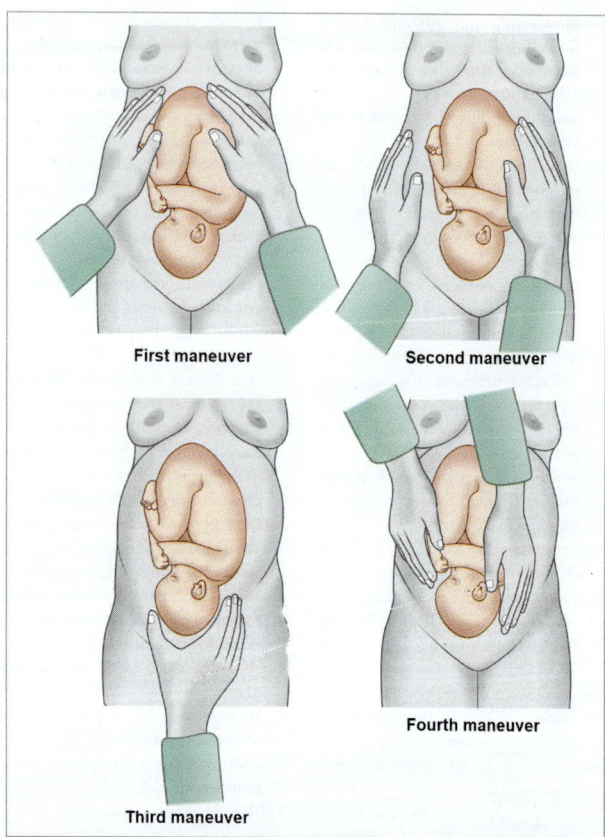

First maneuver

Second maneuver

Third maneuver

Fourth maneuver

Leopold's Maneuver

Lepidosis Any scaly eruption of the skin.

Lepothrix A superficial corynebacterium infection of axillary or pubic hair in which nodules form on hair.

Leprosy Hansen's disease. A chronic infection of the skin, mucous membrane and nerves with *Mycobacterium leprae*. It is predominantly a tropical disease which is transmitted by direct contact. There is an insidious onset of symptoms, mainly involving the skin and nerves, after an incubation period of between 1 and 30 years. The disease can be classified into three types: (a) Lepromatous, which is a steadily progressive form, often resulting in paralysis, disfigurement and deformity. This form is often complicated by tuberculosis. (b) Shaped to transmit light rays in a tuberculoid, which is often self-limiting and generally runs a more benign course, (c) Indeterminate, in which there are skin symptoms representative of both lepromatous and tuberculoid forms. Leprosy is now treated with a range of drugs including dapsone, rifampicin, and clofazimine.

Leptocyte A thinner erythrocyte, appearing hypochromic, seen in iron deficiency, anemia, thalassemia, etc.

Leptodactyly Unusual slenderness of fingers.

Leptomeningitis Inflammation of the pia mater and arachnoid membranes of the brain and spinal cord.

Leptophonia A weak thin quality of voice.

Leptospira A genus spirochaetes.

Leptospira icterohaemorrhagiae The cause of spirochaetal jaundice (Weil's disease).

Leptospirosis Any of a group of notifiable infectious diseases due to serotypes of *Leptospira*. The best known is Weil's disease, or leptospiral jaundice; others are mud fever, autumn fever and swineherd's disease. The etiological agent is a spiral organism that is common in water. Initially the symptoms include fever, rigors, vomiting, headache and often jaundice. Diagnosis may be difficult because the symptoms resemble those of several other diseases. Jaundice is a key symptom. Sanitation measures can reduce the spread of the disease in both humans and animals.

Lergotrile Ergot alkaloid.

Leriche's syndrome *R Leriche, French surgeon, 1879–1955.* A condition in which atherosclerosis of peripheral arteries is accompanied by obstruction of the lower end of the aorta.

Lesbianism Sexual and emotional orientation of one woman to another; female homosexuality.

Lesch-Nyhan syndrome *M Lesch, American physician, b, 1939; WI Nyhan Jr, American physician, b. 1926.* A hereditary disorder of purine metabolism transmitted as an X-linked recessive trait with physical and mental handicap, compulsive self-mutilation of fingers and lips by biting, spasticity, cerebral palsy and impaired renal function.

Lesion Any pathological or traumatic discontinuity of tissue or loss of function of a part. Lesion is a broad term, including wounds, sores, ulcers, tumors, cataracts and any other tissue damage. Lesions range from the skin sores associated with eczema to the changes in lung tissue that occur in tuberculosis.

Lethal Deadly, capable of causing death.

Lethargy A condition of drowsiness or stupor that cannot be overcome by the will.

Lithotomy position Common position for surgical procedures and medical examinations involving the pelvis and the lower abdomen and a common position for child birth in western nations. The patient lies on back, thighs flexed on abdomen and abducted.

Letrozole Aromatose inhibitor.

Letterer-Siwe disease *E Letterer, German physician, 1895–1982; SA Siwe, German physician, 1897–1966.* Reticuloendotheliosis of early childhood, marked by a haemorrhagic tendency, eczematoid skin eruption, hepatosplenomegaly with lymph node involvement, and progressive anemia.

Leucine A naturally occurring essential amino acid, vital for growth in infants and for nitrogen equilibrium in adults.

Leuco For words beginning thus, *(See Leuko)*.

Leukorrhea A viscid, whitish discharge from the vagina.

Leucovorin A calcium salt of folinic acid that counteracts toxic effects of folic acid antagonists.

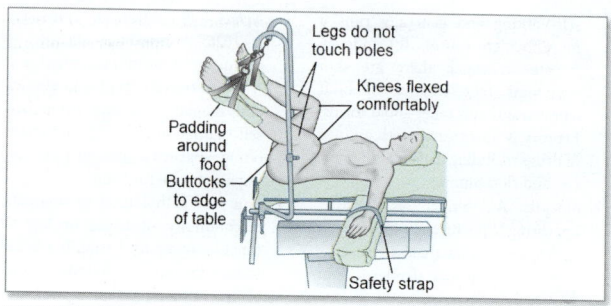

Labels: Legs do not touch poles; Knees flexed comfortably; Padding around foot; Buttocks to edge of table; Safety strap

Lithotomy Position

Leukapheresis Selective removal of leukocytes by hemopheresis, useful in treatment of blast crisis or to obtain leukocyte donation.

Leukaemia A progressive, malignant disease of the blood-forming organs, marked by abnormal proliferation and development of leukocytes and their precursors in the blood and bone narrow. It is accompanied by a reduced number of erythrocytes and blood platelets, resulting in anemia and increased susceptibility to infection and hemorrhage. Other typical symptoms include fever, pain in the joints and bones and swelling of the lymph nodes, spleen and liver. Leukaemia is classified clinically on the basis of (a) the duration and character of the disease (acute or chronic), and (b) the cell line involved, i.e., myeloid (myelocytic, myeloblastic, granulocytic) or lymphoid (lymphatic, lymphoblastic, lymphocytic). A widely used classification of acute leukaemia based on cell type is the French American British (FAB) classification. The incidence of the disease is growing and the increase is only partially explained by increased efficiency of detection. Treatment is primarily with chemotherapy but this may also be combined with radiotherapy, removal of the spleen and bone narrow transfusions. Antibiotics are commonly required.

Leukapheresis Withdrawal of blood for the selective removal of leukocytes. The remaining blood is retransfused.

Leukemid A nonspecific cutaneous lesion containing infiltration of leukemic cells.

Leukemoid Resembling leukemia with appearance of immature leukocytes in peripheral blood and leukocytosis. Seen in some infectious diseases.

Leukoblastosis Any malignant disorder of while cells including leukemia and lymphoma.

Leukocyte A white blood corpuscle. There are three types: (a) Granular (polymorphonuclear cells) formed in bone narrow, consisting of neutrophils, eosinophils and basophils; (b) Lymphocytes (formed in the lymph glands); and (c) Monocytes.

Leukocytoblast The earliest recognizable leukocyte precursor.

Leukocytoma Tumorous accumulation of leukocytes including chloroma, granulocytic leukemia and lymphoma.

Leukocytolysis Destruction of white blood cells.

Leukocytopoiesis Leukopoiesis.

Leukocytosis An increase in the number of leukocytes in the blood. Often a response to infection.

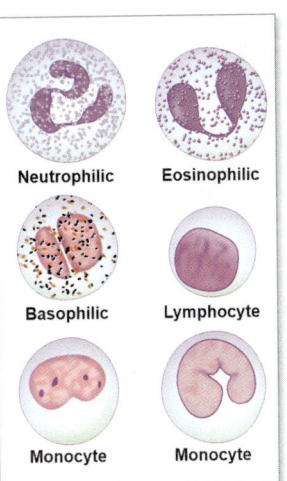

Neutrophilic   **Eosinophilic**

Basophilic   **Lymphocyte**

Monocyte   **Monocyte**

Leukocyte

Leukocytotoxin Any substance that selectively damages leukocytes.

Leukoderma An absence of pigment in patches or bands, producing abnormal whiteness of the skin. Vitiligo.

Leukodystrophy A degenerative disorder of the brain which starts during the first few months of life and leads to mental, visual and motor deterioration.

Leukoencephalitis Encephalitis predominantly involving cerebral white matter.

Leukoencephalopathy Any disease of cerebral white matter; may be hemorrhagic, necrotizing.

Leukoerythroblastosis Presence in the blood of numerous normoblasts together with precursors of granulocyte series.

Leukokoria White reflex of pupil as in retinopathy or any pathological condition posterior to crystalline lens.

Leukoma A white spot on the cornea, usually the result of an injury to the eye.

Leukopedesis Migration of lymphocytes through walls of blood vessels.

Leukonychia White patches on the nails due to air underneath.

Leukopenia A decreased number of white cells, usually granulocytes, in the blood.

Leukopoiesis Formation, growth and maturation of leukocytes.

Leukophoresis Withdrawal of blood for the selective removal of leukocytes. The remaining blood is retransfused.

Leukoplakia A chronic inflammation, characterized by white thickened patches on the mucous membranes, particularly on the tongue, gums and inside of the cheeks.

Leukoplakia vulvae Thickening of the mucous membrane of the labia with the appearance of scattered white patches.

Leukopsin The colorless product of bleaching of rhodopsin.

Leukopoiesis The formation of white blood cells. Leukocytopoiesis.

Leukorrhea Abnormal white non-bloody discharge from vagina.

Leukotactic Capable of attracting leukocytes.

Leukotaxis Active ameboid, unidirectional movement of leukocytes towards an attractant.

Leukotomy Trans orbital frontal lobotomy.

Leukotrienes Mediators of inflammation derived from arachidonic acid.

Leukotriene $C_4D_4E_4$ Play roles in anaphylaxis (slow reacting substance) and B_4 is a chemoattractant and aggregator of neutrophils.

Leuprolide Gonadotropin releasing hormone analog for prostatic carcinoma.

Levallorphan tartrate A narcotic antagonist for treatment of respiratory depression caused by narcotics.

Levamisole The I-form tetramisole, used for treatment of roundworm, hookworm, strongyloides. Also used as an immunopotentiator.

Levarterenol Norepinephrine.

Levator A muscle that raises a structure or organ of the body.

Levels of care The six divisions of the Health Care System: preventive care, primary care, secondary or acute care, tertiary care, restorative care and continuing care.

Levobunolol Antiglaucone drug.

Levocardia Visceral situs inversus with a normally positioned left sided heart. Such a heart often has aortic arch and valvular malformations.

Levodopa L-dopa; a synthetic drug used in the treatment of Parkinsonism.

Levonorgestrel A potent.

Levorotatory Capable of rotating the plane of polarized light counter clockwise.

Levorphanol An analgesic somewhat resembling morphine in its action and addiction potentialities. It is used to relieve severe pain.

Levothyroxine L-thyroxine; yellow crystalline powder for oral supplement in hypothyroid cases.

Levoxadrol L-isomer of dioxadiol, used as local relaxant.

Levulinic acid 4-oxopentanoic acid, source of aminolevulinic acid which is an intermediate in biosynthesis of porphyrins.

Levulose Levorotatory glucose.

Lewy body dementia A type of dementia where there is a build-up of Lewy bodies, which are clumps of alpha-synuclein protein in neurons.

LH Luteinizing hormone.

Lhermitte's sign Also sometimes known as the Barber Chair phenomenon. There is a production of electrical sensation which runs down the back, arms and legs when the person flexes his head. It is usually present in lesions of dorsal columns of the cervical cord, e.g., multiple sclerosis,

Behcet's disease, vitamin B_{12} deficiency, etc. It may persist for a few days or weeks and then disappear on its own without treatment.

Li Symbol for lithium.

Liaison Communication and contact between groups, units and/or agencies and organizations.

Liaison officer Appointed to facilitate communications between the hospital and the community services for the benefit of the patient's care at home after discharge from the inpatient unit.

Libido 1. The vital force or impulse which brings about purposeful action. 2. Sexual drive in Freudian psychoanalysis, the motive force of all human beings.

Lichen A group of inflammatory infections of the skin in which the lesions consist of papular eruptions.

Lichen planus Raised flat patches of dull, reddish-purple color, with a smooth or scaly surface.

Lichenification The stage of an eruption when it resembles lichen.

Lid Eyelid.

Granular lid Trachoma.

Lid lag Jerky movement of the upper lid when it is being lowered. A sign of exophthalmic goitre (thyrotoxicosis).

Lidocaine A local anesthetic applied as sprays, creams to skin and mucous membrane.

Lidoflazine A coronary vasodilator.

Lie A position or direction.

Lie of fetus The position of the fetus in the uterus. The normal lie is longitudinal.

Lieberkuhn's glands JN *Lieberkühn, German anatomist, 1711–1756.* Tubular glands of the small intestine.

Lien The spleen.

Lienculus An accessory spleen.

Lienorenal Relating to the spleen and kidneys; splenorenal; splenonephric.

Life assessment The choice of the most appropriate method to use when moving a patient, as from bed to chair. Factors that need to be taken into account include whether the patient is conscious or unconscious; if there is a visual, hearing or cognitive impairment present; the presence of equipment, e.g., urinary drainage, IV lines or monitors and the body weight of the person. No particular method is suggested as correct or appropriate in all situations; rather, that safe moving and handling practices should be used at all times. Lifting devices are the first option when implementing moving and handling activities

Life crisis An unpleasant experience, which may often be unforeseen and sudden such as being robbed or mugged, redundancy, early retirement, divorce, bereavement and sudden and severe ill health.

Life event A sociological term used to describe major events in a person's life, e.g., leaving home for the first time, getting married, moving house, changing a job.

Life expectancy The average length of life based upon prevailing mortality trends.

Life long learning A process of personal, social and professional development throughout the lifespan of an individual.

Life support system The equipment and technology used to maintain the life of a patient who is not otherwise able to survive.

Lifestyle The pattern of daily living that an individual develops. On the initial assessment of a person entering the health care services, this is considered in relation to the delivery of care by health care workers in order that the aims and objectives for care can be individualized.

Ligament 1. A band of fibrous tissue connecting bones forming a joint. 2. A layer or layers of peritoneum connecting one abdominal organ to another or to the abdominal wall.
Annular ligament The ring-like band that fixes the head of the radius to the ulna.
Cruciate ligament Crossed ligaments within the knee joint.
Inguinal ligament That between the pubic bone and anterior iliac crest.
Round ligament For example, one of the two anterior ligaments of the uterus, passing through the inguinal canal and ending in the labia majora. There are also round ligaments of the femur and of the liver.

Ligand Any of the molecules or ions, identical or different that bind to same central entity by multiple coordination bonds. E.g., O_2 and N_2 attaching to same iron molecule contained in Hb.

Ligate To tightly tie a thread to compress a vessel, pedicle of a tumor.

Ligation The application of a ligature.
Tubal ligation Both fallopian tubes are tied and cut or crushed for the purpose of sterilization.
Ligator Surgical instrument facilitating ligation, superficial or deep.

Ligature A thread of silk, catgut or other material used for tying round a blood vessel to stop it bleeding.

Light Electromagnetic waves which stimulate the retina of the eye.
Light adaptation The changes that take place in the eye when the intensity of the light increases or decreases.
Light coagulation A method of treating retinal detachment by directing a beam of strong light from a carbon arc through the pupil to the affected area.

Lightening The relief experienced in pregnancy, 2–3 weeks before labor, when the uterus sinks into the pelvis and ceases to press on the diaphragm.

Lignocaine A local anesthetic administered by injection and by surface application. Also used intravenously in cases of cardiac arrhythmia, especially myocardial infarction.

Limbic system The parts of brain including hippocampus amygdala, dentate gyrus, cingulated gyrus responsible for emotion, arousal, behavior and motor autonomic functions.

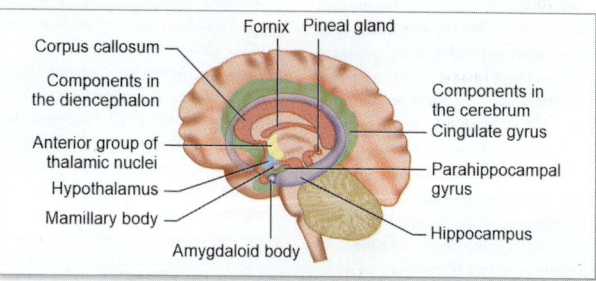

Corpus callosum

Components in the diencephalon

Anterior group of thalamic nuclei

Hypothalamus

Mamillary body

Fornix Pineal gland

Amygdaloid body

Components in the cerebrum

Cingulate gyrus

Parahippocampal gyrus

Hippocampus

Limbic System

Limbus An edge or border.

  Corneal limbus The border where the cornea joins the sclera.

Liminal Pertaining to the threshold of perception.

Lincomycin An antibiotic derived from the *Streptomyces* genus. Used in the treatment of streptococcal bone and joint infections, including osteomyelitis.

Linctus A thick syrup given to soothe and allay coughing.

Lindane Gamma benezene hexachloride, used in pediculosis.

Linea [L.] A line.

  Linea alba The tendinous area in the center of the abdominal wall into which the transversalis and part of the oblique muscles are inserted.

  Linea albicanes White streaks that appear on the abdomen when it is distended by pregnancy or a tumor.

  Linea aspera The rough ridge on the back of the femur into which muscles are inserted.

  Linea nigra The pigmented line that often appears in pregnancy on the abdomen between the umbilicus and the pubis.

Lineage The direct descendants of an individual.

Linear Pertaining to a line.

  Linear accelerator A megavoltage machine for accelerating electrons so that powerful X-rays are given off for use in the treatment of deep-seated tumors.

Lingual Pertaining to the tongue.

Lingula A tongue-like structure, such as the projection of lung tissue from the left lower lobe.

Lingulectomy Surgical resection of lingual of left upper lobe.

Liniment A liquid to be applied externally by rubbing on to the skin.

Linin Fine thread like achromatic substance of the cell nucleus that interconnects the chromatin granules.

Lining In dentistry, the coating applied to the walls of a tooth cavity to protect the pulp from irritation by restorative filling, e.g., zinc oxide, eugenol, zinc phosphate and calcium hydroxide.

Linitis Inflammation of cellular tissue of stomach.

  Linitis plastica Extensive thickening of stomach wall due to infiltration by scirrhous carcinoma.

Linkage 1. The force that holds together the atoms in a chemical compound. 2. The relationship existing between two or more genes in the same chromosome.

Linoleic acid An essential fatty acid, precursor of prostaglandin.

Linseed The oil acts as a demulcent and laxative.

Lip 1. The upper or lower fleshy margin of the mouth. 2. Any lip-like part; labium.

Cleft lip Congenital fissure of the upper lip.

Lip reading Understanding of speech through observation of the speaker's lip movements; called also speech reading.

Lipaemia The presence of excess fat in the blood. Sometimes a feature of diabetes.

Lipaemia retinalis Condition in which the retinal blood vessels appear to be filled with milk owing to the presence of an excess of fat in the blood.

Lipase Fat-splitting enzyme; any enzyme that catalyses the splitting of fats into glycerol and fatty acids. Measurement of the serum lipase level is an important diagnostic test for acute and chronic pancreatitis.

Lipemia Increased turbidity of plasma due to increased lipids.

Lipid One of a group of fatty substances that are insoluble in water but soluble in alcohol or chloroform. They form an important part of the diet and are normally present in the body tissues.

Lipidosis Disease state with abnormal lipid storage by RE cells, e.g., metachromatic leukodystrophy (sulfatide); Niemann-Pick disease (sphingomyelin), gangliosidosis, cerebral lipidosis.

Lipoadenoma A tumor with mixture of glandular and fat tissue, e.g., parathyroid adenoma.

Lipoatrophy Atrophy of subcutaneous tissue of sites of insulin injection.

Lipoblast A polyhedral cell with small lipid droplets which becomes a fat cell.

Lipoblastomatosis A benign lobulated tumor of fetal fat cell, may be localized or diffuse.

Lipochondrodystrophy A congenital condition affecting the metabolism of fat and producing bone deformities, short stature, facial abnormalities and learning difficulties. Hurler's syndrome.

Lipodermatosclerosis A browny pigmented fibrosis of the skin and subcutaneous tissue of lower leg resulting from venous stasis.

Lipodystrophy A disorder of fat metabolism.

Progressive lipodystrophy A rare condition, occurring mainly in females, in which there is progressive loss of fat over the upper half of the body.

Lipoedema An abnormal build-up of fat cells in the legs and buttocks and occasionally in the arms.

Lipofuscin A brown pigment, partially soluble in fat, occurring in nerve and muscle cells.

Lipogranulomatosis A rare metabolic disorder in which ceramides and gangliosides accumulate as a result of ceramidase deficiency.

Lipohyalin Lipoid material sometimes seen in hyalinized beta cells of pancreatic islets of Langerhans in diabetes.

Lipoidosis Any one of a group of diseases in which there is an error in lipoid metabolism producing reticuloendothelial hyperplasia. Xanthomas are common.

Lipolysis The breakdown of fast by the action of bile salts and enzymes to a fine emulsion and fatty acids.

Lipoma A benign tumor composed of fatty tissue, arising in any part of the body, and developing in connective tissue.

Diffuse lipoma A tumor of fat in an irregular mass, without a capsule, occurring above the pelvis.

Lipomatosis Presence of multiple or diffuse lipoma.

Lipomatosis dolorosa Presence of multiple painful lipomas.

Lipophilic Fat soluble.

Lipophore A pigmented cell whose color is caused by lipochrome pigment.

Lipopolysaccharide Any substance made up partly from lipid and partly from polysaccharide e.g., bacterial cell wall which is highly antigenic.

Lipoprotein One of a group of fatty proteins present in blood plasma.

Liposarcoma A malignant tumor of the fat cells.

Liposis Diffuse fatty infiltration of body tissues. *SYN-* adiposis.

Liposome A small vesicular structure which forms spontaneously when phospholipids are placed in water.

Liposuction The removal of excess fat in the body by suction through a small skin incision. Most commonly used method cosmetically as a means of contour reduction or reshaping. Also called lipectomy.

Lipoteichoic acid The teichoic acid found in bacterial membranes.

Lipotropin Any hormone that causes release of fatty acids from fat.

Lipoxygenase An oxidizing enzyme for linoleate group.

Lippe's loop A type of intrauterine contraceptive device.

Liquefaction Reduction to liquid form.

Liquid 1. A substance that flows readily in its natural state. 2. Flowing readily, neither solid nor gaseous.

Liquid diet A diet limited to the intake of liquids or foods that can be changed to a liquid state. A liquid diet may be restricted to clear liquids or it may be a full liquid diet.

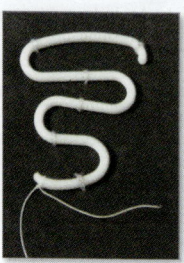

Lippe's Loop

Liquor A watery fluid; a solution.

Liquor amnii The fluid in which the fetus floats; amniotic fluid.

Lisch nodule A hamortoma of iris, seen in neurofibromatosis.

Listeria *Lister, British surgeon, 1827–1912.* A genus of Gram-negative bacteria which produce upper respiratory disease, septicemia and encephalitic disease in humans. They can be transmitted by the consumption of infected, unpasteurized dairy produce, or by direct contact with infected animals or contaminated soil. Newborn infants, pregnant women, the elderly and the immune-suppressed are more susceptible to infection.

Listeriosis Infection with organisms of the genus *Listeria*.

Lithagogue A drug that helps to expel calculi.

Lithiasis The formation of calculi.

Conjunctival lithiasis The formation of small white chalky areas on the inner surface of the eyelids.

Lithium Symbol Li. An alkaline metallic element.

Lithium carbonate A drug used in the treatment of manic depressive illness.

Lithocholic acid Bile acid, found conjugated with taurine and glycine.

Lithogenesis Formation of calculi.

Litholysis Fragmentation or dissolution of stones.

Litholyte An instrument designed to administer stone dissolving agents directly inside bladder.

Lithopedion A retained calcified fetus.

Lithosis Pneumoconiosis resulting from inhalation of particles of silica, etc. into the lungs.

Lithotomy An incision into a duct or organ for removing stone.

Lithotony Formation of bladder fistula for stone removal.

Lithotripsy The crushing of calculi in the bladder; lithotrity.

Lithotrite Surgical instrument designed to crush or fragment stones and help their removal.

Lithuresis Passage of small calculi or gravel in the urine.

Litmus A blue pigment obtained from lichen and used for testing the reaction of fluids.

Blue litmus Turned red by an acid.

Red litmus Turned blue by an alkali.

Litmus paper A blotting paper impregnated with blue pigment obtained from lichen and used for testing the reaction of fluids.

Blue L. Turned red by an acid.

Red L. Turned blue by an alkali.

Litre Symbol L. The SI unit of capacity. One cubic decimetre.

Litter A stretcher for transporting the invalid.

Little's disease *WJ Little, British surgeon, 1810–1894.* Spastic diplegia. A congenital muscle rigidity of the lower limbs causing "scissor leg" deformity.

Livedo A discoloration, skin erythema that follows a reticular pattern of the cutaneous vascular network.

Livedo reticularis Circulatory disorder of unknown origin causing constant bluish discoloration on large areas of extremity.

Liver The large gland situated in the right upper area of the abdominal cavity. Its chief functions are: (a) The secretion of bile; (b) The maintenance of the composition of the blood; and (c) The regulation of metabolic processes.

Cirrhotic liver Fibrotic changes which occur in the liver as the result of degeneration of the liver cells, often as a result of alcoholism.

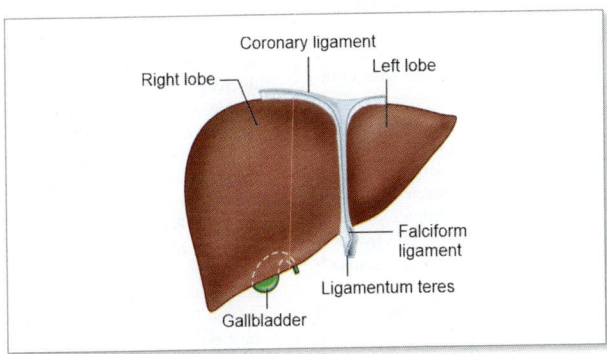

Liver

Fatty liver Yellow soft greasy liver with increased cytoplasmic fat within hepatocytes.

Liver biopsy The taking of a small core of liver tissue through a liver biopsy needle under a local anesthetic. Allows for microscopic examination to aid diagnosis of a wide range of disorders of the liver.

Liver transplant The transplantation of a liver from a suitable donor who has recently died.

Nutmeg liver Liver affected by chronic vascular congestion as in CHF.

Polycystic liver Liver with multiple congenital cysts, often associated with polycystic kidney, usually asymptomatic.

Liverpool Care Pathway for the Dying Patient (LCP) Was a UK pathway providing palliative care options for patients in final days or hours of life but no longer in use. (See *End of Life Care Pathways*).

Livid Descriptive of the bluish-gray discoloration of the skin produced, by congestion of blood.

Living will A statement signed by a person requesting and indicating what should be done in the event of becoming totally incapacitated or terminally ill. It enables the writer, while still alive, to refuse resuscitation or other measures to maintain life.

LOA Left occipitoanterior. Refers to a possible position of the fetus in the uterus.

Loading dose In pharmacotherapeutics, loading dose is the administration of a drug in larger doses than the body can eliminate in order to bring the concentration of the drug within the body to an effective level. After this, the daily dose is gradually reduced.

Loa–loa The thread like eye worm of Africa causing blindness and calabar swelling. The microfilarae with nuclei extending right up to tail are found only during day.

Lobar Relating to a lobe.

Lobe A section of an organ, separated from neighboring parts by fissures.

The liver, lungs and brain are divided into lobes.

Lobectomy Removal of a lobe, e.g., of the lung.

Lobeline Ganglionic stimulant.

Lobotomy Incision of a lobe.

Prefrontal lobotomy A psychosurgical procedure with division of fibers connecting prefrontal and frontal lobes with thalamus. Also called prefrontal leukotomy.

Lobular Relating to a lobule.

Lobulated Consisting of or divided into lobules.

Lobule A small lobe, particularly one making up a larger lobe.

Local anesthetic Numbing of a part of the body, with no loss of consciousness using medication administered by injection or tropically, which blocks pain signals from nerves to the brain.

Local authority The local government.

Localize 1. To limit the spread, e.g., of disease or infection, to a certain area. 2. To determine the site of a lesion.

Lochia The discharge of blood and tissue debris from the uterus after childbirth, lasting for 2–3 weeks. Initially lochia is bright red and gradually becomes paler.

Lochia alba Light colored uterine discharge consisting of leukocytes.

Lochia rubra Bloody uterine discharge immediately after delivery.

Lochiometra The retention of lochia in the uterus, causing its distension.

Lockjaw Tetanus.

Locomotor Pertaining to movement from one place to another. *Locomotor ataxia*

Tabes dorsalis *(See Ataxia).*

Loculated Divided into small loculi or cavities.

Loculus A small cystic cavity, one of a number.

Locum tenens A person, usually a doctor, who substitutes for another over a period of time; usually referred to as a locum.

Locus A place or spot, as the specific site occupied by a gene in the chromosome.

Locus ceruleus A bluish gray area in the floor of fourth ventricle.

Locus histocompatibility One of the genes located within major histocompatibility complex that specifies transplantation antigens or immune response functions.

Locus operator A regulator locus that governs the transcription of adjacent structural genes of the operon and is the binding site of a repressor protein molecule.

Locus of control The ideas and beliefs that people have about the way in which they can control external events in their lives. Those with an internal locus of control tend to expect that any change or reinforcement is the result of their own efforts or behavior and will want to be actively involved in any health care measures. Those with an external locus of control see themselves as being dependent upon luck, fate or the actions of 'powerful others' and are therefore fatalistic about any health care provision or treatment.

Loeffler's syndrome Disorder lasting less than a month, characterized by transient infiltrates in lungs, low fever and eosinophilia.

Loeffler's disease Also called eosinophilic endomyocardial disease with eosinophilic coronary arteritis, congestive cardiac failure, eosinophilia and multiple systemic emboli.

Log roll A nursing technique used to turn a reclining patient from one side to the other. The patient lies on the back with arms folded across the chest, and legs extended. The nurses manipulate the underlying drawsheet so that the patient is rolled on to one side or the other.

Logorrhoea Excessive and often unintelligible volubility.

Loiasis Infestation of the conjunctiva and eyelids with a parasite worm.

Loin The area of the back between the thorax and the pelvis.

Lomotil Trade name for preparations of diphenoxylate, an antidiarrheal.

Lomustine Antineoplastic agent.

Long QT syndrome Irregularity of the electrical activity of the heart as a result of a faculty gene, which can cause blackouts, seizures, arrhythmia and cardiac arrest. It is a leading cause of sudden death in young and otherwise healthy people and is thought to be an underlying cause in cases of Sudden Infant Death Syndrome.

Long sight Hyperopia.

Longitudinal study An investigation that involves making observations of the same group at sequential time intervals. Longitudinal studies are valuable as a means of studying human development or change and may also be used to observe change over time within an institution or organization.

Loop A bend in a cord or cord like structure, the arched dermal ridges in dermatoglyphics.

Lippe's loop S-shaped intrauterine contraceptive device.

Meyer's loop The portion of geniculo-calcarine radiation that loops around inferior horn of lateral ventricle.

Loop of recurrent laryngeal nerve The arching of recurrent laryngeal nerves after their origin from vagus in the chest. The left one hooks below the arch of aorta behind attachment of ligamentum arterisoum and then up the left side of trachea while the right one hooks around first part of subclavian artery.

Loperamide A meperidine congener, intestinal smooth muscle relaxant.

Lophophorine An extreme toxic alkaloid found in cactus.

Lophotrichous Bacteria possessing multiple flagella at one pole only.

LOP Left occipitoposterior. Refers to a possible position of the fetus in the uterus.

Lorazepam A minor tranquillizer used to treat anxiety and insomnia.

Loraadine H_1 receptors, blockers, anti-allergic.

Lorbamate A cyclopropane carbamate ester used as muscle relaxant.

Lorcainide Antiarrhythmic agent, for ventricular tachycardia.

Lordosis A form of spinal curvature in which there is an abnormal forward curve of the lumbar spine.

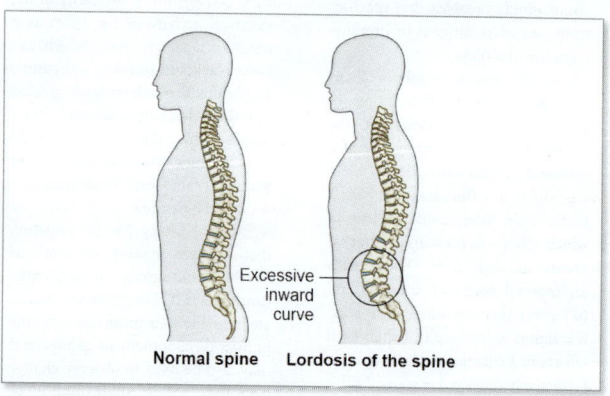

Excessive inward curve

Normal spine   Lordosis of the spine

Lordosis

Larnoxican Analgesic, anti-inflammatory.

Losartan Angiotension receptor blocker used in hypertension.

Loosening In psychiatry, a disorder of thinking in which associations of ideas become so shortened, fragmented and disturbed as to lack logical relationship.

Loss *Dissociated sensory loss* Pain and temperature severely lost with preservation of touch as in syringomyelia or central cord tumors.

Hearing loss 1. Sensory neural due to ageing or autoimmune. 2. Conductive due to disease of middle ear or external ear.

Lotion A medicinal solution for external application to the body. Lotions usually have a soothing or antiseptic effect.

Calamine lotion A soothing mixture containing calamine and zinc oxide.

Evaporating lotion A dilute alcoholic solution applied to bruises.

Lead lotion A weak solution of lead acetate used for sprains and bruises where the skin is unbroken.

Loudness The intensity of noise or sound.

Loupe A magnifying lens, which may be used in eye examination.

Louse A general term covering a number of small insects that are parasitic to humans and to other mammals and birds. Three varieties are parasitic to humans:

(a) Pediculus capitis, the head louse;

(b) Pediculus corparis, the body louse; and

(c) Phthirus, pubis, which infects the coarse hair on the body and also the eyebrows. Diseases known to be transmitted by lice are typhus fever, relapsing fever and trench fever.

Lovastatin Ester of methyl butanoic acid, given orally for increased LDL and cholesterol.

Lowe's syndrome Oculocerebrorenal syndrome.

Loxapine A tricyclic anti-psychotic agent with tranquilizing properties.

Loxotomy Surgical amputation by means of an oblique incision.

Lozenge A medicated tablet with a sugar basis, used to treat mouth and throat conditions.

LSD *(See Lysergide).*

Lubb-dupp Representation of the sounds heard through the stethoscope when listening to the normal heart: *lubb* when the atrioventricular valves shut, and *dupp* when the semilunar valves meet each other.

Lubricant Agent used to reduce friction.

Lucid Clear, particularly of the mind.

Lucid interval Period of clear thinking that may occur in cerebral injury between two periods of unconsciousness or as a sane interval in a mental disorder.

Luciferase An enzyme which catalyzes the transfer of an electron from luciferin to oxygen with emission of light. (Bioluminescence of fire flies, glow worms and bacterial fungi).

Lues Syphilis

Luetic Syphilitic.

Lumbago Pain in the lower part of the back. It may be caused by muscular strain or by a prolapsed intervertebral disc (slipped disc).

Lumbar Pertaining to the loins.

Lumbar puncture Insertion of a trocar and cannula into the spinal canal in the lower back and withdrawal of cerebrospinal fluid for diagnostic purposes.

Lumbarization Fusion between the transverse processes of the lowest lumbar and adjacent sacral vertebra.

Lumbosacral Relating to both the lumbar vertebrae and the sacrum.

Lumbosacral support A corset aimed at both supporting and restricting movement in that region.

Lumbosacral vertebra One of the five vertebrae in the lower back lying between the thoracic vertebrae and the sacrum.

Lumbrical Resembling an earth worm, lumbrical muscles of hand.

Lumbricoid Earthworm like appearance.

Lumefantrine An antimalarial.

Lumen The space inside a tube.

Luminescence Emission of infrared, visible light or ultraviolet by matter from any cause except incandescence.

Luminiferous Capable of transmitting light.

Lumiracoxib Anti-inflammatory, analgesic.

Lumpectomy The surgical excision of only the local lesion (benign or malignant) of the breast.

Lunate Moon or crescent shaped, semilunar.

Lunacy An obsolete term formerly applied to insanity.

Lund and Browder chart A chart that has been adopted by many burn centers in the UK for calculation of the surface area of a burn. At birth the size and area of the head is large compared with the adult, and the legs and thighs constitute a much smaller proportion of the total body surface. On admission to a burn unit or ward the area of the body burned is mapped on to the Lund and Browder chart and the area of the burn affecting each portion of the body surface is calculated.

Lung One of a pair of conical organs of the respiratory system, consisting of an arrangement of air tubes terminating in air vesicles (alveoli) and filling almost the whole of the thorax. The right lung has three lobes and the left lung two. They are connected with the air by means of the bronchi and trachea.

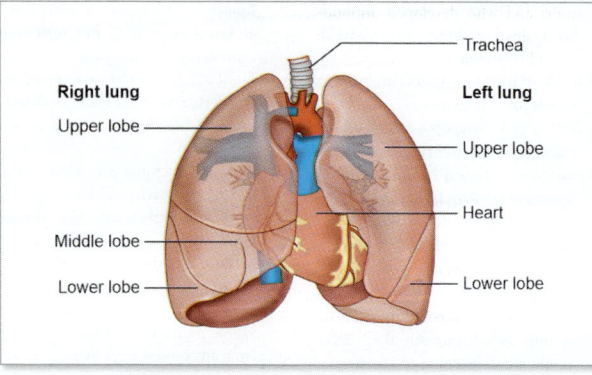

Lung

Lupoma A small granulomatous nodule characteristic of lupus vulgaris.

Lunula The white semicircle near the root of each nail.

Lupus A chronic skin disease having many manifestations.

Lupus erythematosus Abbreviated LE. An inflammatory disease, affecting both the internal organs and the skin, which finally produces a round plaque-like area of hyperkeratosis. It is thought to be due to an autoimmune reaction to sunlight, infection or other unknown cause.

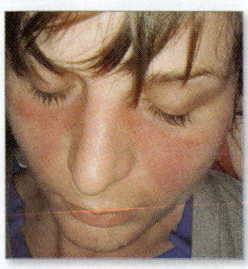

Lupus Erythematosus

Lupus vulgaris A tuberculous disease of the skin producing brownish nodules, frequently on the nose or cheek, and severe scarring.

Luteal Relating to corpus luteum of ovary.

Luteinizing hormone Abbreviated LH. One of three hormones produced by the anterior pituitary gland which control the activity of the gonads.

Lutembacher's syndrome Congenital cardiac abnormality with ASD and mitral stenosis.

Luteoid Acting like progesterone.

Luteolysis Involution or destruction of corpus luteum.

Luteoma Growth of lutein cells of ovary during third trimester with regression after parturition, often may secrete androgens.

Luteotrophin An anterior pituitary hormone which stimulates the formation of the corpus luteum and the production of milk. Prolactin.

Lutetium Element No. 71, isotopes used in nuclear medicine.

Lutheran blood group Antigens of red blood cells, specified by lugene that react with antibodies designated with anti – Lu a and anti-Lu b, first detected in serum of an individual who had received many transfusions and who developed antibodies against erythrocyte of a donor named Lutheran.

Lux A unit of illumination, equal to one lumen per square meter.

Luxation The dislocation of a joint.

Luxation of the lens Displacement of the lens of the eye into the anterior chamber or posteriorly into the vitreous humor.

Lye Sodium potassium hydroxide.

Lying –in Confinement of a woman during childbirth.

Lyme disease A zoonosis transmitted by ticks and characterized by a rash (erythema chronicum migrans), arthritis and aseptic meningitis, caused by the spirochaete *Borrelia burgdoiferi.*

Lymph The fluid from the blood which has transuded through capillary walls to supply nutriment to tissue cells. It is collected by lymph vessels which ultimately return it to the blood.

Lymph nodes or glands Structures placed along the course of lymph vessels, through which the lymph passes and is filtered of foreign substances, e.g., bacteria. These nodes also make lymphocytes.

Plastic lymph An inflammatory exudate which tends to cause adhesion between structures and so limit the spread of infection.

Vaccine lymph A lymph preparation obtained from calves or other animals and used for vaccination.

Lymphaden Lymph node.

Lymphadenectasia Enlargement of lymp nodes with excessive lymph.

Lymphadenectomy Excision of a lymph gland or nodes.

Lymphadenitis Inflammation of a lymph gland.

Lymphadenography X-ray examination of lymph nodes.

Lymphadenoma Lymphoma.

Multiple Lymphadenoma Hodgkin's disease.

Lymphadenomatosis Presence of numerous enlarged lymph nodes.

Lymphadenopathy Any disease condition of the lymph nodes.

Lymphadenosis Generalized enlargement of lymph glands and lymphatic tissue, may be benign (e.g., infectious mononucleosis) or malignant.

Lymphagogue An agent that increases formation and flow of lymph.

Lymphangiectasia Abnormal dilatation of lymphatic vessels.

Lymphangiectasia intestinal Dilatation of intestinal lymphatic with subsequent protein losing enteropathy, steatorrhea and diarrhea. It may be congenital due to hypoplasia of thoracic duct or acquired due to inflammation or malignancy of lymphatics. Small intestinal biopsy is diagnostic with dilated lacteals in intestinal villi.

Lymphangiectasis Dilatation of the lymph vessels due to some obstruction of the lymph flow. It may be congenital.

Lymphangioendothelioma A tumor composed of small masses of endothelial cells and aggregation of tubular structures thought to be lymphatic vessels.

Lymphangiography Radiographic examination of lymph vessels after the insertion of a radiopaque contrast medium.

Lymphangioleiomyomatosis A proliferation of lymphatic and smooth muscle cells typically affecting lung and lymph node, a lesion of women in reproductive age, with honey combing and respiratory insufficiency.

Lymphangioma A swelling composed of dilated lymph vessels.

Lymphangiosarcoma Malignant tumor of lymphatic tissue, mainly associated with chronic lymph stasis usually secondary to radical mastectomy.

Lymphangitis Inflammation of lymph vessels, manifested by red lines on the skin over them. It occurs in cases of severe infection through the skin.

Lymphatic Referring to lymph.

Lymphatic system The system of vessels and glands through which the lymph is returned to the circulation. The vessels end in the thoracic duct and the right lymphatic duct.

Lymphedema Chronic unilateral or bilateral swelling of extremities caused by obstruction of lymph vessels or disease of lymph nodes, usually congenital.

Type 1: Autosomal dominant, associated intestinal protein loss and pleural effusion (Millroy's disease).

Type II: Slowly progressive form with onset around puberty.

Lymphedema praecox Lymphedema occurring in girls approaching puberty.

Lymph node A rounded body consisting of accumulations of lymphatic tissue found in the course of lymphatic vessels.

Lymphoblast An early developmental cell that will mature into a lymphocyte.

Lymphoblastoma A form of malignant lymphoma, composed mainly of lymphoblasts.

Lymphocyte A white blood cell formed in the lymphoid tissue. Lymphocytes produce immune bodies to overcome and protect against infection.

Lymphocythemia An excessive number of lymphocytes in the blood. Lymphocytosis.

Lymphocytoma A tumor of low grade malignancy arising in a lymph node, composed mainly of mature lymphocyte.

Lymphocytopenia Absence or scarcity of lymphocytes in the blood. Lymphopenia.

Lymphocytosis Greater than normal number of lymphocytes to peripheral blood.

Lymphocytosis acute infections An acute benign infectious disease of obscure etiology in children with headache, upper respiratory symptoms, and lymphocytosis.

Lymphocytotoxin A complement fixing antilymphocyte antibody.

Lymphoedema A condition in which the intercellular spaces contain an abnormal amount of lymph due to obstruction of the lymph drainage.

Lymphoepithelioma A malignant tumor derived from epithelium around tonsils and nasopharynx containing abundant lymphoid tissue.

Lymphogranuloma Hodgkin's disease.

Lymphogranuloma venereum A sexually transmitted disease, caused by a virus; primarily a tropical condition.

Lymphokine A hormone like factor produced by sensitized lymphocytes when they come in contact with antigen to which they were sensitized, acts as an intercellular messenger to regulate immunologic and inflammatory responses.

Lymphokinesis 1. Circulation of lymph through lymphatic vessels and nodes. 2. Movements of endolymph in the membranous labyrinth of the internal ear.

Lymphoma Lymphadenoma. Used to denote any malignant condition of the lymphoid tissue. Generally these diseases are classified as either Hodgkin's or non-Hodgkin's lymphomas.

Burkitt's lymphoma A type of lymphoma found predominantly in East Africa and affecting the jaws of children.

Lymphopoietin A soluble factor required for maturation of lymphocytes.

Lymphopoiesis The production of lymphocytes. Occurs chiefly in the bone marrow, lymph nodes, thymus, spleen and gut wall.

L

Lymphorrhea Flow of lymph from ruptured lymph channel.

Lymphosarcoma A term formerly used to denote a malignant lymphoma (with the exception of Hodgkin's disease).

Lymphotaxis The induction of lymphocyte movement.

Lymphotoxin Substance destructive to lymphocytes.

Lymphotrophic Attracted to lymphatic system.

Lynestrenol A semisynthetic progestin.

Lyon hypothesis Inactivation of one X chromosome in female during embryogenesis forming the barr body.

Lyophilic Dispersing or dissolving easily because of affinity for solvent.

Lyophobic Difficult to disperse because of poor affinity for solvent.

Lyophilization A method of preserving biological substances in a stable state by freeze drying. It may be used for plasma, sera, bacteria, viruses and tissues.

Lypressin Vasopressin with lysine in place of arginine in position 8. An antidiuretic and vasopressor.

Lysergic acid diethylamide Also known as acid and LSD. A powerful hallucinogenic drug, manufactured from lysergic acid, which is found in the ergot fungus. LSD is mainly used for recreational purposes and is a Class A drug making it illegal to possess.

Lysergide Lysergic acid diethylamide (LSD). A hallucinogenic drug that can cause visual hallucinations and increased auditory acuity but may prove very disrupting to the personality and affect mental ability.

Lysin A specific antibody present in the blood that can destroy cells *(See Bacteriolysin)*.

Lysine An essential amino acid formed by the digestion of dietary protein. It is vital for normal health.

Lysis 1. The gradual decline of a disease, especially of a fever. The temperature falls gradually, as in typhoid *(See Crisis)*. 2. The destruction of cells.

Lysochrome A lipid soluble pigment that is suitable for staining fat.

Lysogen An antigen that stimulates the formation of specific lysine.

Lysogeny A form of viral parasitism in which viral DNA becomes incorporated in a (bacterial) cell genome, without destroying the cell, thereby permitting transmission of virus to subsequent bacterial generations.

Lysokinase An activator agent of fibrinolytic system.

Lysolecithin A lecithin without unsaturated fatty acid residue. It is strongly hemolytic, a good detergent.

Lysosome A particle, found in the cytoplasm of cells, which causes the breakdown of metabolic substances and foreign particles, (e.g., bacteria) within the cell.

Lysozyme An enzyme present in tears, nasal mucus and saliva that can kill most bacteria coming into contact with it.

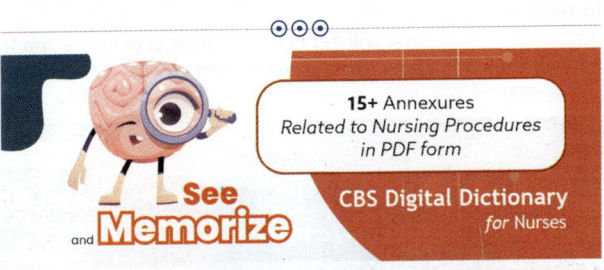

Why To Choose
Nursing Next Live
The Next Level of NURSING EDUCATION

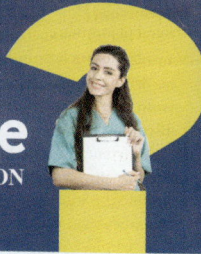

- India's 1st Digital Learning Platform for all nursing competitive, nursing undergraduate and nursing postgraduate exams (One-in-All, All-in-One)
- User friendly interface with unique & advanced features
- Most Up-to-date & Quality Content based on New INC Syllabus
- Conceptual learning with an integrated and futuristic approach
- Smart Study under the guidance of India's Top Educators who are the masterminds of their subjects
- Enhance your learning from Basic To Advance level with a 360-degree approach
- Regular Live Doubt Sessions and Live Tests based on real-time exam pattern
- TOP Selections in AIIMS NORCET, AIIMS MSc, BFUHS, CHO, SGPGI, JIPMER, RRB, DSSSB etc (From Rank 1 to 1000)
- Study Planner that helps you to organize your study
- Faculty-Student Meet (Forthcoming) that provides you an opportunity to meet with faculty and get clarify your doubts
- Printed Booklet: You will get the printed notes of the video lectures that will save your time in notes making and organize your time in a better way
- Customize Study which helps you to create your own pack depending on your needs and wants
- Daily dose of information keeps you updated everyday with new information
- One-in-all all-in-one: You will get exam oriented plan in the app for whatever exams you are targeting. Simulation Videos

Follow us:

 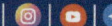

CALL US +91- 999-911-7411
www.nursingnextlive.com

Scan the QR Code to download the app

M Symbol for metre.

M Symbol for molar.

McBurney's point *C McBurney, American surgeon, 1845–1913.* The spot midway between the anterior iliac spine and the umbilicus where pain is felt on pressure if the appendix is inflamed.

Maceration Softening of a solid by soaking it in liquid.

Neonatal maceration The natural softening of a dead fetus in the uterus.

Machine A device for accomplishing a specific objective.

Heart - Lung machine A combination of pump and oxygenator to affect extracorporeal circulation and oxygenation of blood during open heart surgery.

Holtz machine A machine for developing high voltage static electricity by multiplication of an induced charge.

Panoramic rotating machine An X-ray machine capable of radiographing all the teeth and surrounding structures by using a reciprocating motion of the tube and extraoral film.

Mackenrodt's ligaments *AK Mackenrodt, German gynecologist, 1859–1925.* The transverse or cardinal ligaments that support the uterus in the pelvic cavity.

Macmillan nurses Qualified nurses who have also received special training in the management of pain relief, palliative care and the provision of emotional support to cancer patients and their families. This nursing service is provided either in the patient's home through the Macmillan home visiting service, in hospital or in a hospice.

Mckee Farrar prosthesis The first widely used total hip replacement to employ metal-on- metal articulation.

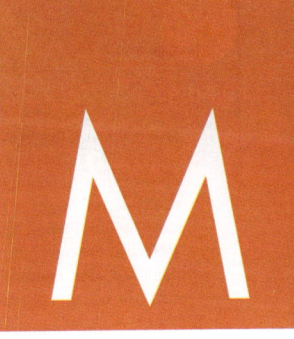

McNaghten's Rules on Insanity at Law The rules that define the factors on which a defence to a charge of murder on grounds of insanity maybe established. These were evolved after Sir Robert Peel's Secretary was killed by McNaghten in 1843. He was suffering from delusions and the judge ordered that he be found not guilty. The Homicide Act 1957 provided for a defence based on diminished responsibility, i.e., the accused was suffering from such abnormality of mind as to impair mental responsibility and was not responsible for any actions undertaken in that state.

Macroamylase A form of amylase that occurs as a complex joined to a serum globulin.

Macrocheilia A congenital condition in which there is excessive development of the lips.

Macrocyte An abnormally large red corpuscle found in the blood in some forms of anaemia.

Macrocythaemia The presence of abnormally large red cells in the blood. Macrocytosis.

Macroencephaly Malformation and increase in size and weight of brain due to proliferation of glia with small ventricles and mental retardation.

Macrogamete The female gamete, larger egg fusing with microgamete, leading to zygote formation.

Macrogametocyte The mother cell producing macrogamete.

Macroglia The astrocyte and oligodendrocyte, the two neuroglial elements of ectodermal origin.

Macroglobulin Plasma globulin with molecular weight of 10,00,000, increased in multiple myeloma, cirrhosis, collagen disorders.

Macroglobulinemia Plasma cell myeloma, a disorder with excessive production of IgM with anemia and bleeding, also called Waldenstrom's macroglobulinemia.

Macroglossia Enlarged tongue.

Macrogyria Congenital malformation in which the cerebral gyri are large due to few sulci.

Macrolides A group of antibiotics having molecules made-up of large ring lactones e.g., erythromycin.

Macromastia An abnormal increase in the size of the breast.

Macromelia Enlarged limbs.

Macromolecule Any molecule composed of several monomers.

Macronutrient An essential nutrient that has a large minimal daily requirement (greater than 100 mg); calcium, phosphorus, magnesium, potassium, sodium and chloride are macronutrients.

Macrophage A large reticulo-endothelial cell which has the power to ingest cell debris and bacteria. It is present in connective tissue, especially when there is inflammation.

Macrophthalmia A congenital condition of abnormally large eyes.

Macropsia Condition of seeing objects larger than their actual size.

Macroscopic Discernible with the naked eye. The opposite of microscopic.

Macrostomia An abnormal development of the mouth in which the mandibular and maxillary processes do not fuse and the mouth is excessively wide.

Macrotia Abnormally large ears.

Macula A spot or discolored area of the skin, not raised above the surface; a macule.

Macula corneae A small area of opacity in the cornea, seen through an ophthalmoscope as a deeper red.

Macula lutea The yellow central area of the retina, where vision is clearest.

Macule A nonelevated discolored lesion on the skin.

Maculoerythematous Both red and spotted.

Maculopapular Displaying both maculae and papules.

Maculopapular eruption A rash comprising both maculae and papules as in measles.

Maculopathy Any disease of macula of retina.

Mad Suffering from mental disorder, rabid, angry.

Maddox rod Multiple parallel cylindrical rods of glass fused side to side and shaped into a trial lens used for testing of squint and fusion.

Madelung deformity Subluxation of distal radioulnar joint secondary to abnormal growth and curvature of distal radius.

Madarosis Loss of eye lashes.

Madura foot Mycetoma of the foot.

Madurella A genus of fungi causing madura mycosis.

Maduromycosis A chronic disease caused by various fungi or actinomycetes which usually effect the feet.

Madurella mycetoma. The most common form is Madura foot.

Maffucci's syndrome A combination of multiple cutaneous hemangiomas and dyschonderoplasia.

Magaldrate Hydroxy magnesium aluminate, an antacid.

Magendie's foramen *F Magendie, French physiologist, 1783–1855.* Aperture in the roof of the fourth ventricle of the brain through which

M

cerebrospinal fluid passes into the subarachnoid space.

Maggots Worm-like larvae of flies that feed on organic matter and are occasionally found in wounds *(See Myiasis)*.

Magma 1. A paste like preparation of any organic matter. 2. Finely divided material suspended in a small quantity of water.

Magnesia Magnesium oxide, it neutralizes acids to give soluble magnesium salts.

Magnesium Symbol Mg. A bluish-white metallic element. It occurs widely in mineral sources and is present in some of the body tissues.
Magnesium carbonate and *Magnesium hydroxide* Neutralizing antacids used in hyperacidity.
Magnesium sulphate A saline purgative. Epsom salts.
Magnesium trisilicate An antacid powder taken after food for dyspepsia and peptic ulceration.

Magnet In ophthalmology, an instrument used for removing metallic foreign bodies that have penetrated the eye.

Magnetic resonance imaging Abbreviated MRI. An imaging technique based on the nuclear magnetic resonance properties of the hydrogen nucleus. Cross-sectional images in any plane of the body for examination may be obtained. MRI is without hazard to the patient.

Magnetism 1. The properties of mutual attraction, or repulsion produced by magnet or electric current. 2. Study of magnet and their properties. 3. The force exhibited by a magnetic field.

Magneton A unit of measure of the magnetic movement of an atomic or subatomic particle.

Magnification An enlargement of an object by an optical element or instrument.

Maim To disable, mutilate, cripple by injury.

Main lining Term used by drug addicts denoting IV injection of heroin or other drugs.

Malnutrition The condition in which nutrition is defective in quantity or quality.

Majocchis' disease Annular telangiectatic purpura.

Majority The age at which a person becomes legally entitled to full civil rights of an adult. It is 18 in UK, 21 in India, USA, Canada and 20 in Japan.

Makaton One of the sign languages. **mal** [Fr.] Disease.
Grand makaton, petit makaton Forms of epilepsy.
Makaton demer Sea sickness.

Makeshift Denoting a shunt from a large variceal collateral vessel to a systemic vein when a standard shunt cannot be employed. Employed for portal hypertension.

Mal A disease

Mala The cheek bone, cheek.

Malabsorption Inability of the small intestine to absorb certain substances. It may be the cause of a deficiency disease due to the lack of an essential factor.

Malachite green Green crystalline substance used as a pH indicator.

Malacia Softening of tissues *(See also Keratomalacia and Osteomalacia)*.

Malady Illness.

Maladaptation The inability to make normal adjustments in personal relationships and in society, which may result in stress, ill health and abnormal behavior.

Maladjustment In psychiatry, a failure to adjust to the environment.

Malaise A feeling of general discomfort and illness.

Malakoplakia The formation of soft, fungus like growths on the mucous membrane of a hollow organ, especially urinary bladder.

Malalignment Displacement, especially of the teeth from their normal relation to the line of the dental arch.

M

M

Malar Relating to cheek or cheek bone.

Malaria A serious, notifiable infectious illness characterized by periodic chills, fever, sweating and splenomegaly. Serious and often fatal complications may arise in falciparum malaria. It is endemic in parts of Africa, Asia and Central and South America and is estimated to occur at the rate of 100 million cases each year throughout the world. Treatment is with antimalarial drugs. Epidemics usually occur in areas where mosquitoes persist in large numbers. The disease is caused by a parasite of the genus *Plasmodium* introduced into the blood by mosquitoes of the genus *Anopheles*. The attacks are periodic, every 48–72 hours according to the type of plasmodium. For *P. vivax* it lasts 48 hours, *P. malarie* 71 hours, and *P. falciparum* 36–48 hours.

Airport malaria A term sometimes used to describe malaria occurring at or near an airport, in a country normally free of the disease, and spread by infected mosquitoes brought in on an aeroplane from an endemic area. Control measures include disinsectization of aircraft where appropriate.

Malassizia furfur Fungus that causes tinea versicolor.

Malate Salt of malic acid.

Malathion Insecticide.

Male pattern baldness *(See Alopecia)*.

Male Sex of an individual containing organs that produce spermatozoa, with one X- and one Y-chromosome.

Malformation Deformity; a structural defect.

Klippel–Feil malformation Short webbed neck due to malformation of cervical vertebrae.

Mondini malformation Congenital deafness due to hypoplasia of latter part of cochlea.

Malfunction Abnormal or inadequate function.

Malic acid An intermediate in carbohydrate metabolism, present in unripe apples, cherries, tomatoes, etc.

Malignant Tending to become progressively worse and to result in death; having the properties of anaplasia, invasiveness and metastasis; said of tumors.

Malingering Wilful, deliberate and fraudulent feigning or exaggeration of the symptoms of illness or injury to attain a consciously desired end.

Malleable Liable, capable of being made into small sheets.

Malleation A spasmodic movement.

Malleolar Relating to one or both prominences on either side of ankle.

Malleolus One of the two protuberances on either side of the ankle joint.

Lateral malleolus That on the outer surface at the lower end of the fibula.

Medial malleolus That on the inner surface at the lower end of the tibia.

Malleus The hammer-shaped bone in the middle ear.

Mallory–Weiss syndrome *G Kenneth Mallory, US Pathologist, b. 1900; Soma Weiss, US internist, 1898-1942.* Hemorrhage from the upper GI tract due to a tear in the mucosa of the esophagus or gastroesophageal junction. The syndrome is associated with chronic alcoholism and is usually preceded by severe vomiting.

Malnutrition The condition in which nutrition is defective in quantity or quality.

Malocclusion An abnormality of dental development which causes overlapping of the bite.

Malonic acid It competitively inhibits the oxidation of succinate to fumarate.

Malonyl - Coenzyme A Formed from acetyle COA, helpful in fatty acid biosynthesis.

Malpighian body M *Malpighi, Italian anatomist, physician and physiologist, 1628–1694.* The glomerulus and Bowman's capsule of the kidney.

Malposition An abnormal position of any part of the body.

Malpractice Failure to maintain accepted ethical standards. Professional misconduct.

Malpresentation Any abnormal position of the fetus at birth that renders delivery difficult or impossible.

Malrotation Developmental failure of rotation in the normal direction and to normal degree, most common to digestive tract.

Malt Grain, especially barley, containing dextrin, maltose.

Malta fever Brucellosis; undulant fever.

Maltase A sugar-splitting enzyme which converts maltose to glucose. Present in pancreatic and intestinal juice.

Maltose The sugar formed by the action of digestive enzymes on starch.

Malunion Faulty repair of a fracture.

Mamma Breast, rudimentary in male and containing milk producing glands in female.

Mammal Vertebrates that nourish their offspring with milk.

Mammary Relating to the breasts.

Mammilities Inflammation of the nipples.

Mammila Nipple, nipple like protruberance.

Mammilate Having nipple like structures.

Mammilliplasty Plastic surgery of the nipples and the areola.

Mammitis Also known as mastitis. This is the infection or inflammation of the breast tissue which occurs commonly among breast feeding women.

Mammogram X-ray of mammary gland.

Mammography Radiographic or infrared examination of the breast to detect abnormalities.

Mammoplasty A plastic operation to reduce the size of abnormally large, pendulous breasts or augment the size of very small breasts.

Mammothermography An examination of the breast that depends on the more active cells producing heat that can be shown on a thermograph; it may indicate abnormalities of the breast tissue.

Memmotrophic Promoting development and growth of mammary glands.

Manchester operation Also known as Fothergill operation. A technique used for uterine prolapse.

Mandelate Salt of mandelic acid.

Mandelic acid Urinary antibacterial agent.

Mandible The lower jawbone.

Mandibullectomy Removal of lower jaw.

Maneuver A skillful movement.

Manganese Element Atomic no. 25, an essential micronutrient.

Manganous Bivalent salts of manganese.

Mange Scabies.

Mania A disordered mental state of extreme excitement, especially the manic type of manic depressive psychosis. Also used as a word termination to denote obsessive preoccupation with something, as in kleptomania.

Maniac Colloquial term for one suffering from a violent or extreme form of insanity.

Manic Pertaining to mania.

Manic depressive psychosis A mental illness characterized by mania or endogenous depression. The attacks may alternate between mania and depression or the patient may just have recurrent attacks of mania or depression.

Manifestation Display of characteristic signs and symptoms of a disease.

M

Neurotic manifestation The use of various defense mechanisms like conversion, dissociatioin, depression in an attempt to resolve emotional conflicts.

Psychotic manifestation Loss of contact with reality, personality disintegration.

Manikin An anatomic model of human body for practice of certain manipulations as those of obstetrics and dentistry.

Manipulation Use of the hands to produce a desired movement, such as in reducing a fracture or a hernia or changing the position of a fetus. A skillfully applied forced movement upon a joint in order to relocate the joint or increase its range of movements by tearing adhesions round it.

Manna The dried sugary exudates of ash tree, rarely used as a laxative.

Mannerism Distinctive characteristic or behavioral trait.

Mannitol A sugar alcohol occurring widely in nature; an osmotic diuretic used for forced diuresis in drug overdose and in cerebral edema.

Manometer An instrument for measuring the pressure of liquids or gases.

Mansonia A genus of mosquitoes transmitting filaria.

Manual Involving the use of the hands.

Manual evacuation of the bowel A nursing technique used to evacuate the bowel following use of fecal softening agents *(See Laxatives)* in a severely constipated patient. This procedure is rarely used now due to the possibility of causing rectal trauma and distress to the patient.

Manual expression of urine Pressure is placed upon the abdomen by using the hands at regular intervals to encourage the patient to void when the bladder is paralyzed.

Manubrium A structure that resembles a handle but when used alone refers to manubrium sterni.

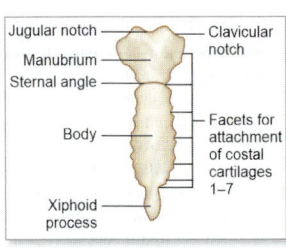

Manubrium Sterni

Manus The hand.

Mantle A covering.

Mantoux test *C Mantoux, French physician, 1877–1947.* A tuberculin skin test in which a solution of purified protein derivative (PPD) - tuberculin is injected intradermally into either the anterior or posterior surface of the forearm. The test is read 48–72 hours after injection. It is considered positive when the induration at the site of injection is more than 10 mm in diameter, 5–10 mm is doubtful and less than 5 mm is negative.

Manubrium The upper part of the sternum to which the clavicle is attached.

MAOI *(See Monoamine oxidase).*

Maple syrup urine disease An inborn error of metabolism in which there is an excess of certain amino acids; in the urine the urine smells like maple syrup. There are learning difficulties, spasticity and convulsions.

Mapping In genetics, locating the position and order of gene loci on a chromosome by analyzing the frequency of recombination between the loci.

Maprotiline Tricyclic antidepressant.

Marasmus Severe and chronic malnutrition producing a gradual wasting of the tissues, owing to insufficient or unassimilated food, occurring especially in infants. It is not always possible to discover the cause.

Marburg virus disease A Central African viral hemorrhagic fever with acute onset and characteristic morbilliform rash. The incubation period is 3–7 days. It was first reported in Europe in 1967, associated with the importation of green monkeys from Uganda. Since then several isolated incidents have occurred in Africa. The reservoir of infection is not known. Person to person transmission by inoculation of blood and tissue fluid and by sexual intercourse has been reported.

Marble bone disease Abnormally calcified bone with spotted appearance in X-ray.

Marcus Gunn's phenomenon Closing of the eyes when mouth is closed and exaggerated opening of the eyes when mouth is opened. *SYN*-Jaw winking syndrome.

Marfan's syndrome *BJA Marfan, French pediatrician, 1858–1942.* A hereditary disorder in which there is excessive height with very long digits, a high arched palate, hypertonus and dislocation of the lens of the eyes; heart disease commonly occurs.

Margin The edge or border of a structure or organ.

Margin of safety A measure of drug safety based on the dose required to produce an effective, therapeutic response in most individuals versus the dose required to produce toxic effects in few individuals. It is similar to but not same as therapeutic index.

Margination Adhesion of leukocytes to the interior of capillary wall during early stages of inflammation.

Marihuana *Cannabis indica*; Indian-hemp or hashish *(See Cannabis)*.

Marfan's syndrome B.J.A. Marfan, French pediatrician, 1858-1942. A hereditary disorder in which there is excessive height with very long digits, a high arched palate, hypertonus and dislocation of the lens of the eyes; heart disease commonly occurs.

Marie strumpel disease Ankylosing spondylitis.

Marijuana Cannabis indica; Indian hemp. *(See Cannabis)*.

Mark A blemish, a spot.

Mark port wine Congenital discoloration of skin, usually on the face varying from pink to purple.

Marker 1. A characteristic factor by which a cell or molecule can be identified or a disease can be recognized. 2. A general term for any trait that helps to throw light on the genetic nature of a disorder.

Maroteaux Lamy syndrome.

Marmot Ticks that transmit rocky mountain spotted fever.

Maroteaux-Lamy syndrome A form of mucopolysaccharidosis characterized by dwarfism, chest deformity, knock knee, stiff joints, cloudy cornea, short hands and fingers, inherited as autosomal recessive and there is excessive dermatan sulphate excretion in urine.

Marrow The substance contained in the middle of long bones and in the cancellous tissue of all bones.

Puncture marrow Investigatory procedure in which marrow cells are aspirated from the sternum or iliac crest.

Red marrow That found in all cancellous tissue at birth. Blood cells are made in it.

Yellow marrow The fatty substance contained in the center of long bones in later life.

Masculinization The development of male secondary sexual characteristics in a woman.

Masculine Relating to characteristics of male sex.

Mask 1. A covering for the face and nose to prevent spread of infection. 2. An expressionless appearance of face, e.g., Parkinson facies. 3. A metal frame covered with gauze placed over face for giving inhalation anesthesia. 4. To cover metal parts of denture with an opaque material.

BLB mask An oxygen mask used at high altitudes, having a combination of inspiratory and expiratory valves in a rebreathing bag.

Venturi mask Mask that develops a constant concentration of oxygen, using the Venturi Principle of entrainment of air to dilute the flow of pure oxygen.

Masking 1. The introduction of noise in one ear for the purpose of excluding that ear from a hearing test given to the other ear. 2. The opaque material placed over the metal or any other part of a dental prosthesis.

Maslow's hierarchy of needs *AM Maslow, American psychologist, 1908–1970.* A hierarchical ranking, in ascending order of importance, concerning human needs and the aim of realizing one's full potential. Physiological needs for oxygen, nutrition, shelter, sleep, etc. are the most basic and need to be met first before one is able to deal in successive order with the need for safety, security, love and belonging, self-esteem and ultimately the need for self-actualization.

Masochism A sexual perversion in which pleasure is derived from suffering mental or physical pain.

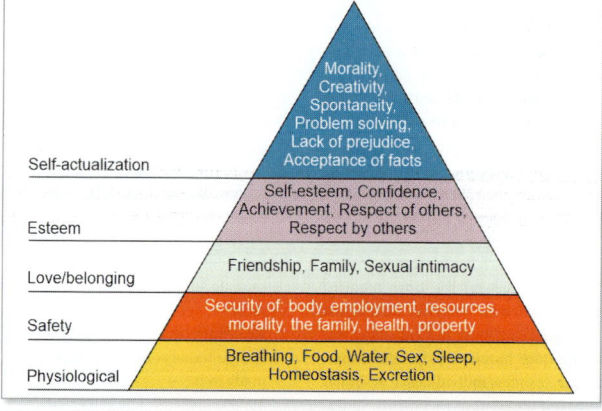

Maslow's Hierarchy

Masochist 1. The passive partner in practice of macochism. 2. One who for psychological purposes exposes himself unnecessarily to sufferings.

Mass A collection of tissue; in pharmacology, a soft pasty mixture of drugs suitable for rolling into pills.

Massage A method of stroking, rubbing, kneading and manipulating the body to stimulate circulation and to promote a sense of well-being.

External cardiac massage The application of rhythmic pressure to the lower sternum to cause expulsion of blood from the ventricles and restart circulation in cases of cardiac arrest.

Carotid sinus massage Massage of carotid sinus at the angle of jaw for treatment of SVT or identification of tachycardia.

Prostatic massage Massage of prostate through rectum to express its

M

secretions into prostatic urethra (examination for gonococci).

Masseur A person trained in or who practices the art of massage.

Masseter A muscle which runs through the rear part of the cheek from the temporal bone to the lower jaw on each side and closes the jaw in chewing.

Mast cell A large connective tissue cell found in many body tissues, including the heart, liver and lungs. Mast cells contain granules which release heparin, serotonin and histamine in response to inflammation or allergy.

Mastalgia Pain in the breast.

Mastectomy Amputation of the breast.
Radical mastectomy Removal of the breast, axillary lymph glands and the pectoral muscle.
Halstead radical mastectomy Removal of breast, chest muscles and lymph nodes of axilla.
Modified radical mastectomy Removal of breast and axillary lymph nodes without removal of pectoralis muscle.
Total mastectomy Removal of breast only.

Masticate To chew.

Mastication The act of chewing food.

Mastigophora The process of chewing.

Mastitis Inflammation of the breast, usually due to bacterial infection.

Mastochondroma A benign breast tumor composed chiefly of cartilaginous tissue.

Mastocytogenesis The formation of mast cells.

Mastocytoma A nodule resembling a tumor, composed chiefly of mast cells.

Mastocytosis Disorder characterized by yellow, brown macules and papules on skin due to skin infiltration by mast cells.

Mastodynia Pain in the breast.

Mastoid Breast or nipple shaped.

Mastoid antrum The cavity in the mastoid process which communicates with the middle ear, and contains air.

Mastoid cells Hollow spaces in the mastoid bone.

Mastoid operation Drainage of mastoid cells when infection spreads from the middle ear.

Mastoid process The breast-shaped prominence on the temporal bone which projects downward behind the ear and into which the sternocleidomastoid muscle is inserted.

Mastoidectomy Removal of diseased bone and drainage of the mastoid antrum in severe purulent mastoiditis.

Mastoiditis Inflammation of the mastoid antrum and cells.

Mastomenia Vicarious menstruation from breast.

Mastoptosis Drooping or pendulous breasts.

Mastoplastia Hypertrophy or enlargement of the breast.

Masturbation The production of sexual excitement by friction of the genitals.

Materia (Latin) For substance or matter.

Materia alba White cheese like deposit along gum line.

Material The substance from which something is made or composed.
Material impression Substances taken for making impressions like plaster of Paris, hydrocolloid compounds.

Materia medica The science of the source and preparation of drugs used in medicine.

Maternal Pertaining to the mother.
Maternal mortality rate The number of deaths in childbirth per 1,000 births.

Maternity Pertaining to pregnancy, the state of being pregnant.

M

Mating The union of male and female for reproduction.

Matrilineal Relating to inheritance of traits through the maternal line rather than the paternal.

Matrix Tissue in which cells are embedded.

Matter Substance.

Gray matter A collection of nerve cells or nonmedullated nerve fibers.

White matter Medullated nerve fibers massed together, as in the brain.

Maturation Ripening or developing.

Mature Complete in natural development, the reproductive cell which has undergone meiosis.

Matron The chief nursing officer in a hospital

Mattress ripple Mattress containing transverse inflatable tubes linked in a series to pump so that alternate tube is inflated. Thus, the area of compression between skin and mattress changes which prevents formation of decubitus ulcer/bedsore.

Maxilla One of the pair of bones forming the upper jaw and carrying the upper teeth.

Maxillary Pertaining to the upper jaw bones.

Maxillofacial Pertaining to the maxilla and the face.

MACE Abbreviation for Mothers and babies: Reducing Risk through Audit and Confidential Enquires in the UK. It is a collaboration led by the University of Oxford to undertake surveillance of maternal and deaths in utero or in young infants.

MCADD Medium-chain acyl-CoA dehydrogenase deficiency. A rare disease screened in the Newborn Blood Spot test resulting in an inability to properly break down fat.

Maximum 1. The greatest quantity, value or degree. 2. The height of a fever or any acute state.

Maximum glucose transport The maximum rate at which kidneys can reabsorb glucose (300 mg/min).

Maximum tubular (Tm) The maximum ability of renal tubules either to excrete or secrete a substance.

Maze An intricate labyrinth of walled pathways frequently used to study the learning process in laboratory animals.

Mazindol A CNS stimulating agent with properties similar to amphetamine, hence used as anorexogenic agent.

Mcburney's sign A sign of acute appendicitis, characterized by tenderness over the Mcburney's point, located in right lower quadrant, during palpation.

MCHC Mean Corpuscular Hemoglobin Concentration.

MCV Mean Corpuscular Volume.

ME Myalgic encephalomyelitis. *(See Chronic Fatigue Syndrome)*.

Meal Food.

Boyden meal Meal used to test the evacuation time of gallbladder; it consists of flour, egg yolks, and milk mixed with sugar.

Meal test Bland food given before analysis of gastric secretion.

Mean An average of a set of values.

Arithmetic mean The ratio of the sum of the terms in a statistical series to their number.

Geometric mean A value indicating the central tendency of a statistical series of 'n' terms, equal to the positive 'n'th root of their products.

Harmonic mean For a given set of values, the reciprocal of the mean of the reciprocals of the individual values.

Measles Morbilli; rubeola. An acute, infectious, statutorily notifiable disease of childhood caused by a virus spread by droplets. Endemic and worldwide in distribution. Onset is catarrhal before the rash appears on the fourth day. Koplik's spots are diagnostic earlier. Secondary infection may give rise to the serious complication of otitis media or bronchopneumonia. Vaccination provides a high degree of immunity.

German measles (See Rubella).

Measles, mumps and rubella vaccine Abbreviated MMR. An injectable vaccine offered to children aged 12 months and 40 months. *(See Annexure 10).*

Measure 1. The dimensions, quantity, capacity like length, area, volume, etc. 2. The act of determining such dimensions, quantity or capacity. 3. A device used for measuring like graduated glass, tape.

Measurement The act of measuring.

Skinfold measurement Skinfold measurement by caliper for assessing body fat percentage.

Meatometer Apparatus for measuring urinary meatus.

Meatoplasty Reconstructive surgery usually of external auditory meatus.

Meatorrhaphy Enlarging the urethral meatus by suturing the urethral membrane to glans penis.

Meatotomy An incision of a meatus to increase its diameter.

Meatus An opening or passage.

Auditory meatus The opening leading into the auditory canal.

Urethral meatus The opening of the urethra to the exterior.

Mebendazole A benzimidazole given for hookworm, roundworm, trichuriasis and enteriobiasis.

Mebeverine A smooth muscle relaxant used for gastrointestinal motility disorder like irritable bowel syndrome (IBS).

Mebutamate Orally acting hypotensive agent.

Mecamylamine An orally acting ganglion blocking agent rarely used to treat severe hypertension.

Mechanics The branch of physics concerned with the interaction of force and matter.

Mechanism of labour The sequence of movements whereby the fetus adapts itself to pass through the maternal passages during the process of birth.

Mechlorethamine Alkylating agent used in treatment of lymphomas.

Meckel's diverticulum *JF Meckel, German anatomist and surgeon, 1781–1833.* The remains of a passage which, in the embryo, connected the yolk sac and intestine, evident as an enclosed sac or tube in the region of the ileum.

Meclizine Drug used in treatment and prevention of motion sickness.

Meclocycline A topically applied antibiotic closely related to chlortetracycline.

Mecloqualone A compound with hypnotic and sedative properties.

Mecobalamine Neuroprotective agent, congener of methyl cobalamine.

Mecometer Instrument used to measure newborn infant.

Meconism Opium addiction or opium poisoning.

Meconium The first intestinal discharges of a newly born child. Dark green and consisting of epithelial cells, mucus and bile.

Meconium ileus Intestinal obstruction due to blockage of the bowel by a plug of meconium in a neonate with cystic fibrosis.

Medallion A circumscribed red, scaly patch, characteristic of pityriasis rosea.

Medazepam A weak tranquilizer, anxiolytic agent.

Medial 1. Toward the midline. 2. Relating to tunica media or middle layer.

Median 1. Placed in the center. 2. In a series of values, the value middle in position.

Mediastinitis Inflammation of mediastinum.

M

Mediastinography X-ray visualization of mediastinum by injection of NO_2.

Mediastinoscope An endoscope to visualize superior mediastinum, introduced through a small suprasternal incision.

Mediastinum The space in the middle of the thorax, between the two pleurae.

Medical Pertaining to medicine.

Medical audit An evaluative process applied to the quality of clinical practice, often by peer review of routine or specially collected records of individual cases. Judgments are frequently made on the appropriateness of the processes carried out during the management of the case, in light of the outcome. Deaths are frequently the subject of medical audit, two established examples being the confidential enquiry into maternal deaths (carried out at national level), and local reviews of perinatal deaths *(See Audit)*.

Medical certificate (See Medical statement below).

Medical jurisprudence Medical-science as applied to aid the law, e.g., in the case of death by poisoning, violence, etc.

Medical laboratory scientific officer Abbreviated MLSO. An allied health professional skilled in the theory and practice of clinical laboratory procedures.

Medical model The traditional approach to the diagnosis and treatment of disease in the Western world. The medical practitioner, using a problem-solving approach, focuses on the disease process and the deficits identified in the body organs and tissues.

Medical social worker A professionally qualified worker who looks after the patients' socioeconomic and welfare needs.

Medical statement Replaced the medical certificate in 1976. Advises how long a patient should refrain from work. When the patient is claiming sickness benefit, the statement must be sent to the local social security office.

Medical statistics Branch of statistics concerned with data relating to health and health services. Traditionally these include the use of routine data relating to death, illness and use of hospitals, clinics, etc. The term is also often used to encompass statistics derived from aspects of medical research, such as the conduct of trials of newdrugs or procedures.

Medicalization 1. The extension of medical authority into areas previously regarded as being non-medical, where the lay or a popular approach prevailed, e.g., pregnancy and childbirth. 2. The tendency to view undesirable conduct as illness and therefore requiring medical intervention.

Medically unexplained symptoms Also known as functional symptoms. Various symptoms such as pain or dizziness for which no cause can be found.

Medicament Any medicinal substance used in treatment.

Medicate To treat disease with medicine, to impregnate with a medicinal substance.

Medicated Impregnated with a medicinal substance.

Medication 1. A substance administered to a patient for therapeutic purposes. 2. The treatment of a patient by means of drugs.

Medicinal 1. Having therapeutic qualities. 2. Pertaining to a medicine.

Medicine 1. Any drug or remedy. 2. The art and science of the diagnosis and treatment of disease and the maintenance of health 3. The non-surgical treatment of disease.

M

Community medicine Specialty which deals with all aspects of medical care in the community, including notification and control of infectious diseases, preschool and school health care, and factors affecting the health of the population as a whole.

Emergency medicine Specialty which deals with the acutely ill or injured who require immediate medical treatment.

Family medicine Family practice; the medical specialty concerned with the provision of comprehensive primary health care.

Forensic medicine The application of medical knowledge to questions of law; medical jurisprudence. Also called legal medicine.

Geriatric medicine Medicine dealing with diagnosis, treatment and prevention of disease in elderly.

Group medicine The practice of medicine by a group of doctors, usually representing various specialties, who are associated together for the cooperative diagnosis, treatment and prevention of disease.

Holistic medicine An approach to health care based on theory that health is the result of harmony between body, mind and spirits and that stress of any kind including physical, psychological and social are causes for illness.

Legal medicine Forensic medicine.

Nuclear medicine Branch of medicine concerned with the use of radionuclides in the diagnosis and treatment of disease.

Physical medicine Branch of medicine using physical agents in the diagnosis and treatment of disease. It includes the use of heat, cold, light, water, electricity, manipulation, massage, exercise and mechanical devices.

Preventive medicine The science aimed at preventing disease.

Proprietary medicine Any chemical, drug or similar preparation used in the treatment of diseases, if such article is protected against free competition as to name, product, composition or process of manufacture by secrecy, patent, trademark or copyright, or by other means.

Psychosomatic medicine The study of the interrelations between bodily processes and emotional life.

Space medicine Branch of aviation medicine concerned with conditions to be encountered in space.

Sports medicine The field of medicine concerned with injuries sustained in athletic endeavors, including their prevention, diagnosis and treatment.

Medicines and Healthcare Products Regulatory Agency In the UK abbreviated MHRA. Responsible for the regulation of medicines and health care products. Its primary objective is to promote and protect public health by taking all possible steps to ensure that medicines, health care products and medical equipment meet agreed standards for quality, performance, effectiveness, and are safe for those who use them. MHRA is also responsible for reporting, investigating and monitoring of adverse drug reactions to medicines and incidents with medical devices.

Medicolegal Pertaining to a matter that involves both medicine and law.

Medicosocial Applying to both medicine and the social factors involved.

Medionecrosis Necrosis of middle layer (tunica media) of an artery.

Meditation (transcendental) (TM) An exercise of contemplation that induces a temporary hypometabolic state; a sense of well being, and a feeling of complete relaxation; this hypometabolic state is associated with change in physiologic function

M

including a reduction in oxygen consumption, a decrease in cardiac output and altered EEG activity.

Medium In bacteriology, a preparation for the culture of microorganisms.

Contrast medium A substance used in radiography to make structures visible that could not be seen otherwise.

Medlars (Medical Literature Analysis and Retrieval System). A computerized system of online database containing citations of world's biomedical schools, hospitals, Government organizations, which are connected by telephone to central library's computers. Any data required can be retrieved; only available in advanced countries.

Medline An electronic database providing abstracts of thousands of bio-medical studies.

Medroxyprogesterone A synthetic female sex hormone used to treat menstrual disorders, endometrial carcinoma and endometriosis, an as a short-term contraceptive.

Medulla 1. Bone marrow. 2. The innermost part of an organ, particularly the kidneys, lymph glands and suprarenal glands.

Medulla oblongata Portion of the spinal cord that is contained inside the cranium. In it are the nerve centers which govern respiration, the action of the heart, etc.

Medullary Pertaining to the marrow or a medulla.

Medullary cavity The hollow in the center of long bones.

Medullated Having a myelin covering.

Medullated nerve fibre One enclosed in a myelin sheath.

Medulloblast An undifferentiated cell of embryonic neural tube. It is rounded, poor in cytoplasm without processes found in middle layer of neural tube and is derived from germinal cells of inner ependymal layer.

Medulloblastoma A rapidly growing tumor of neuroepithelial origin occurring in childhood and appearing near the fourth ventricle of the brain. The tumor is highly radiosensitive.

Medulloepithelioma A tumor of eye, primarily of children, characterized by formation of multilayered sheets of undifferentiated cells resembling primitive medullary epithelium of optic vesicle. The malignant form resembles retinoblastoma.

Mefenamic acid An analgesic and antipyretic drug used in the treatment of mild to moderate pain.

Mefexamide A CNS stimulant, used to treat fatigue and depression.

Mefloquine Antimalarial agent, schizonticide.

Mefruside A diuretic with use similar to chlorthiazide.

Megabecquerel A unit of activity in radionuclide equal to 10^6 becquerel. Symbol MBq.

Megacolon Extreme dilatation and hypertrophy of the large intestine. When the condition is congenital it is known as Hirschsprung's disease.

Megadyne Unit of force equal to 1 million dynes.

Megaelectronvolt (MeV) One million electron volts.

Megaesophagus Abnormal enlargement of lower esophagus.

Megakaryoblast A primitive cell of megakaryocyte series with a large oval or kidney shaped nucleus and scanty cytoplasm. It develops into a promegakaryocyte and then finally to megakaryocyte.

Megakaryocyte A large cell of the bone marrow, responsible for blood platelet formation.

Megaloblast An abnormally large nucleated cell from which mature red blood cells are derived.

Megaloblastoid Having some features resembling megaloblastic maturation.

An erythrocyte precursor is said to be megaloblastoid when nuclear chromatin condensation is in clumps but with a prominent parachromatin, i.e., open, transparent, unstained cleft are prominent in the nucleus and the contours of nucleus are irregular.

Megalocephaly 1. Abnormal largeness of the head. 2. Leontiasis ossea.

Megalomania Delusions of grandeur or self-importance characteristic of general paralysis of the insane.

Megaloureter Dilatation of the ureter.

Megavitamin A vitamin dose for in excess of daily recommended dose.

Megavolt A unit of electromotive force equal to 1 million volts.

Megavoltage Electromotive force in the range of 2–10 MeV, used in radiotherapy.

Megastrol acetate A synthetic progestin used as anti neoplastic agent in palliation of metastatic endometrial cancer.

Meglitinide Antidiabetic agent.

Meglumine A substance used in the preparation of radiopaque compounds.

Meibomian cyst A small swelling of the gland caused by obstruction of its duct. If untreated, it may become infected. A chalazion.

Meibomian glands *H Meibom, German anatomist, 1638–1700.* Small sebaceous glands situated beneath the conjunctiva of the eyelid; tarsal glands.

Meibomianitis A bilateral chronic inflammation of the meibomian glands.

Meig's syndrome Polyserositis associated with ovarian fibroma.

Meiosis 1. A stage of reduction cell division when the chromosomes of a gamete are halved in number ready for union at fertilization. 2. Contraction of the pupil of the eye; miosis.

Meissner's corpuscle End-organ for touch present in epidermis.

Meissner's plexus Autonomic plexus in submucosa of alimentary tract regulating intestinal secretions.

Melagia Pain in the lower extremity.

Melancholia A state of extreme depression.

Involutional melancholia A major depression occurring in the involutional period, i.e., 40–55 years in female and 50–65 years in males. Its characteristic triad of symptoms are delusions of guilt or poverty, obsession with death, and delusional fixation on gastrointestinal functioning all within a setting of depression and agitation.

Melanic Having a dark color.

Melanin A dark pigment found in the hair, the choroid of the eye, the skin and in melanotic tumors.

Melanism A condition marked by an abnormal deposit of dark pigment in the skin or other tissue. Melanosis.

Melanoameloblastoma Benign tumor of anterior maxilla, usually occurring in infants.

Melanoblast A derivative of neural crest which differentiates in an embryo into a melanocyte.

Melanocyte A cell of the skin pigment melanin.

Melanocyte stimulating hormone Abbreviated MSH. Hormone produced in the pituitary gland which stimulates the formation of melanin.

Melanoderma A patchy pigmentation of the skin.

Melanoma A malignant tumor arising in any pigment-containing tissues, especially the skin and the eye.

Amelanotic melanoma An unpigmented malignant melanoma.

Juvenile melanoma A benign lesion which usually occurs on the face before puberty. May be mistaken for a malignant melanoma.

M

Melanophore A pigment cell carrying melanin.

Melanosis Abnormal deposits of dark pigment in various organs.

Melanosome A single melanin containing organelle that has finished synthesizing melanin.

Melanuria The presence of black pigment in the urine. Occurs in melanotic sarcoma and porphyria.

Melarsoprol A trivalent arsenic containing antiprotozoal drug for trypanosomiasis.

Melasma Dark discoloration of the skin; chloasma.

Melatonin A hormone believed to be secreted by pineal gland. It has action opposite to that of MSH. It stimulates aggregation of melanosomes in melanophores, thus lightening the skin.

Melena Black tarry stool due to GI bleed.

Melena spuria Melena in breast-fed babies where blood originates from fissures in mother's nipple.

Meleney's ulcer Incision of an operative site which typically appears after one to two weeks after surgery.

Melioidosis An infectious disease primarily affecting rodents. Caused by *Pseudomonas pseudomallei*, often transmitted to man via open wounds, manifesting with fever, pneumonia and metastatic abscess formation.

Melisma Formation of light to dark brown or greyish pigmentation of the skin, mainly on the face. The cause is not known.

Melitis Inflammation of cheek.

Mellitum Any pharmaceutical preparation having honey as excipient.

Mellitus (Latin) for honeyed.

Melomelia A condition of unequal conjoined twins in which both normal limbs and rudimentary accessory limbs are present.

Melphalan A cytotoxic drug that is particularly useful in the treatment of multiple myeloma.

Membrane A thin elastic tissue covering the surface of certain organs and lining the cavities of the body.

Basement membrane The interface between epithelial cells and the underlying connective tissue.

Mucous membrane A membrane that secretes mucus and lines all cavities connected directly or indirectly with the skin.

Serousmembrane Membrane lining the abdominal cavity and thorax and covering most of the organs within.

Memory The mental faculty that enables one to retain and recall previously experienced sensations, impressions, information and ideas. The ability of the brain to retain and to use knowledge gained from past experience is essential to the process of learning. The exact way in which the brain remembers is not completely understood; it is believed that a portion of the temporal lobe of the brain acts as a memory center, drawing on memories stored in other parts of the brain.

Menadiol sodium diphosphate A synthetic derivative of menadione.

Menadione (Vit. K$_3$) Methyl naphthoquinone, parent substance of various forms of vitamin K.

Menadione sodium bisulfate The water soluble form of menadione, used in the treatment of hemorrhage consequent to hypoprothrombinemic states.

Menaquinone Any of the several substituted menadiones with vitamin K activity.

Menarche The first appearance of menstruation.

Mendel's theory *GJ Mendel, Abbot of Brunn, 1822–1884.* The theory that the characters of sexually reproducing organisms are handed on to the offspring in fixed ratios and without blending.

Menetrier's disease/syndrome A disease of unknown etiology characterized by large gastric rugae, and pseudopolyps which may be associated with ulcer like symptoms, bleeding or idiopathic hypoproteinemia, *SYN* – Hypertrophic gastritis.

Meniere's disease or syndrome *P Meniere, French physician, 1799–1862.* A disease of the inner ear causing attacks of vertigo and tinnitus with progressive deafness.

Meninges The membranes covering the brain and spinal cord. There are three: the dura mater (outer), arachnoidmater (middle) and pia mater (inner).

Meningioma A slow-growing, usually benign tumor developing from the arachnoid and pia mater.

Meningiomatosis Presence of multiple meningiomas.

Meningism A condition in which there are signs of cerebral irritation similar to meningitis but where no causative organism can be isolated.

Meningitis Inflammation of the meninges due to organisms such as bacteria, viruses and fungi; chemical toxins such as lead and arsenic; contrast media used in myelography; and metastatic malignant cells. Meningitis is a notifiable disease, and its causal organism, if known, should also be stated.
Meningococcal meningitis Cerebrospinal fever. An epidemic form with a rapid onset caused by *Neisseria meningitides* infection.
Tuberculous meningitis Inflammation of tuberculous origin.

Meningocele A protrusion of the meninges through the skull or spinal column, appearing as a cyst filled with cerebrospinal fluid *(See Spina (Bifida)*.

Meningococcus *Neisseria meningitidis.* A diplococcus, the microorganism of cerebrospinal meningitis.

Meningococcemia Presence of meningococci in blood, often associated with petechial rash, cardiovascular collapse and meningitis/(Waterhouse-Fredrichson syndrome), chronic persistent meningococcemia may be associated with low grade fever, rash and arthritis.

Meningocyte A mesenchymal epithelial cell of subarachnoid space.

Meningoencephalitis Inflammation of the brain and meninges.

Meningoencephalomyelitis Combination of meningitis, encephalitis and myelitis.

Meningomyelocele A protrusion of the spinal cord and meninges through a defect in the vertebral column. Myelomeningocele *(See Spina (Bifida).*

Meningoencephalomyelopathy Any disease involving brain, meninges and spinal cord.

Meningoencephalomyelitis radiculoneuritis Inflammation of brain, spinal cord, meninges, nerve roots and peripheral nerves.

Meningoencephalopathy A diffuse disorder of function of brain and meninges; commonly relates to toxic and metabolic encephalopathies.

Meningomyelitis Inflammation of spinal cord and its covering membranes.

Meningomyelocele A protrusion of spinal cord and associated meninges through a developmental defect in spinal canal.

Meningovascular Concerning meninges and adjacent blood vessels.

Meniscectomy Surgical removal of a semilunar cartilage from the knee joint.

Meniscus 1. The convex or concave surface of a liquid as observed in its container. 2. A lens having one convex and one concave surface. 3. A semi-lunar cartilage of the knee joint.

Menolipsis The temporary cessation of menstruation.

Menometrorrhagia Abnormal bleeding during or between menstrual periods.

Menopause The span of time during which the menstrual cycle wanes and gradually stops; also called change of life and climacteric. It is the period when ovaries stop functioning and therefore menstruation and child-bearing cease. Usually occurs between the 45th and 50th years of life. There may be an associated hormonal imbalance which causes symptoms such as night sweats, hot flushes, diminished libido and extreme lethargy.

Artificial menopause An induced cessation of menstruation by surgery or by irradiation.

Premature menopause Early menopause, idiopathic or secondary to pituitary disease, systemic illness.

Menorrhagia An excessive flow of the menses; menorrhea.

Menoschesis Suppression of menses.

Menostasis Amenorrhea

Menses The discharge from the uterus during menstruation.

Menstrual Relating to the menses.
Menstrual cycle The monthly cycle commencing with the first day of menstruation, when the endometrium is shed, proceeding through a process of repair and hypertrophy till the next period. It is governed by the anterior pituitary gland and the ovarian hormones, oestrogen and progesterone.

Menstruation The monthly discharge of blood and endometrium from the uterus, starting at the age of puberty and lasting until the menopause.

Anovular menstruation, anovulatory menstruation Periodic uterine bleeding without preceding ovulation.

Vicarious menstruation Discharge of blood at the time of menstruation from some organ other than the uterus, e.g., epistaxis, which is not uncommon.

Mensal Monthly.

Mensuration Measurement by immediate comparison.

Mental 1. Pertaining to the mind. 2. Pertaining to the chin.

Mental age The measurement of the intelligence level of an individual in terms of the average chronological age of children showing the same mental standard, as measured by a scale of mental tests.

Mental disorder A term defined by the Mental Health Acts, 1983. The Acts of Parliament govern the care and treatment of the mentally disordered and cover all forms of mental illness and disability including mental impairment and psychopathic disorder.

Mental handicap Arrested or incomplete development of mind in which the patient does not require compulsory detention.

Mental Health Review Tribunal A board to whom persons detained under compulsory admission orders or taken into guardianship have the right of appeal at stated intervals for discharge from hospital. Also responsible to the Secretary of State for providing a Code of Practice for all mental health-care practitioners.

Mental health welfare officer A social worker who carries out the requirements of the Mental Health Acts.

Mental hygiene The science that deals with the development of healthy mental and emotional reactions.

Mental illness A term used to describe a number of disorders of the mind that affect the emotions, perceptions, reasoning or memory of the individual, e.g., psychoses and neuroses.

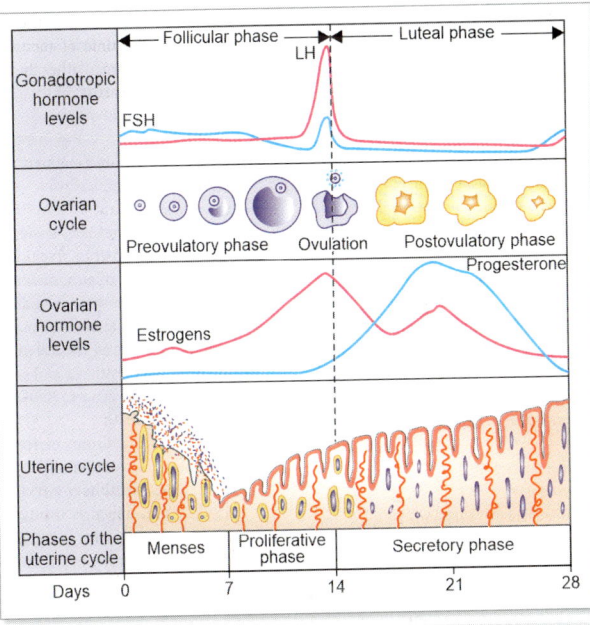

Menstrual Cycle

Mental impairment Arrested or incomplete development of mind associated with abnormally aggressive or socially irresponsible conduct. If the patient is considered treatable, hospital admission may be arranged, if necessary compulsorily.

Mental mechanism An unconscious and indirect manner of gratifying a repressed desire.

Mental subnormality This term has been superseded by mental handicap, mental impairment or learning difficulties.

Mentation Mental activity.

Menthol A crystalline substance derived from oil of peppermint and used in neuralgia and rhinitis and as a local anodyne and antiseptic.

Menoanterior In a face presentation, having the fetal chin pointing anteriorly in relation to maternal pelvis.

Mentoplasty Plastic operation on chin.

Mentoposterior In face presentation, having fetal chin pointing posteriorly in relation to maternal pelvis.

Mentor 1. A wise or trusted adviser or guide. 2. In nursing, a professional colleague who assists with the career development of a colleague, and facilitates and encourages that person's professional growth and awareness.

Mentotransverse In face presentation, having the fetal chin pointing laterally in relation to maternal pelvis.

Mentum The anterior prominence of mandible produced by mental protruberance; the chin.

Mepacrine A synthetic drug used as an antimalarial agent and in the treatment of giardiasis.

Maperidine A synthetic narcotic analgesic, with spasmolytic properties and high addiction potential.

Mephenesin An agent used for skeletal muscle relaxation.

Mephenoxalone A skeletal muscle relaxant, also has mild anxiolytic properties.

Mephentermine An adrenergic agent used as a nasal decongestant or in certain hypotensive states to augment vascular tone.

Mephenytoin Anticonvulsant agent for focal, Jacksonian, grandmal and psychomotor seizure.

Mephobarbitol Long acting barbiturate with anxiolytic and anticonvulsant properties.

Mepivacaine An analogue of lidocaine for local anesthesia, peripheral nerve block or epidural block.

Meprednisone A synthetic glucocorticoid used to treat corticosteroid responsive diseases, allergic conditions.

Meprobamate A tranquillizer used in the treatment of nervous anxiety.

Meprylcaine A local anesthetic for infiltration and nerve block anesthesia.

Mepyramine malleate An antiallergic.

Meralein sodium A water soluble topically applied antibacterial agent.

Meralgia Pain in the thigh.

Meralgia Paresthetica is troublesome tingling, pricking or numbness in lateral aspect of thigh due to compression of lateral femoral cutaneous nerve while it passes beneath or through the inguinal ligament just medial to anterior superior iliac spine.

Meralluride A mercurial salt of succinamic acid used as a parenterally administered diuretic.

Merbromin Topically used antibacterial and antiseptic. Syn mercurochrome.

Mercaptan Used in dentistry as an elastic impression compound.

Mercaptoethylamine A component of coenzyme A, used in treatment of radiation sickness and chronic leukemia.

2–Mercaptoimidazole A thiourea group of antithyroid drug, five times more potent than methylthiouracil.

Mercaptomerin sodium A mercurial diuretic given subcutaneous or IM.

Mercaptopurine A drug which prevents nucleic acid synthesis and may be used in the treatment of some types of leukaemia.

Mercurial poisoning From mercury (mercurialism). Can occur in people in close contact with the metal over a period of time through the skin, by inhalation or ingestion. This may present with a variety of symptoms ranging from gastrointestinal and dental problems, ataxia, visual and auditory disturbances.

Mercurialism Poisoning by mercury or its compounds.

Mercuric Bivalent mercury.

Mercurous Monovalent mercury.

Mercury Symbol Hg, quicksilver; a heavy liquid metallic element, the salts of which are used occasionally as antiseptics and disinfectants. Also used in the manufacture of various types of thermometer and manometer.

Mercury 197 (^{197}Hg) A radioactive mercury isotope used in brain tumor localization and in the study of renal function.

Meridian A conceptual channel along which qi energy flows in the body. *(See Acupuncture)*.

Merocrine Denoting secretory cells that remain intact during discharge of secretory products as those in the salivary glands.

Merocyte An incompletely isolated cell found in the vicinity of the yolk of a fertilized ovum during segmentation. Its nucleus is generally derived from accessory spermatozoa.

Meropenem Highly potent antibiotic.

Merotomy Cutting into parts.

Merozoite The product of a sexual schizogony of a protozoan in the body of host; in malaria merozoites are liberated from rupture of RBC to invade fresh RBC or form gametocyte, the sexual form in man, infective to mosquito.

Merogony The development of only a portion of an egg. If the egg contains only male pronucleus, the development is called andromerogony and if only female pronucleus gynomerogony.

Merology Study of rudimentary tissue.

Meromycin One of the two proteins - heavy meromycin and light meromycin formed by enzymatic digestion of muscle protein mycin.

Merphalon A racemic mixture of melphalan and medphalan; antineoplastic drug.

Mersalyl sodium A mercurial diuretic given parenterally.

Mesangium The framework of glomerulus which arises from vascular pole and extends into intercapillary spaces. It contains matrix and mesangial cells which are phagocytic in nature.

Mescaline An alkaloid drug which produces intoxication and hallucinations. It is a drug of addiction.

Mesencephalaon The embryonic mid brain; the second cephalic dilatation of neural tube that develops into corpora quadrigemina, the cerebral peduncles and aqueduct of sylvius.

Mesenchyme Embryonic connective tissue consisting of an aggregation of cells in close contact by means of long processes thus forming a loose network. (stellate cells).

Messenchymoma A rare benign or malignant tumor consisting of two or more clearly identifiable mesenchymal elements in addition to fibrous tissue.

Mesentery A fold of the peritoneum which connects the intestine to the posterior abdominal wall.

Mesial Situated in, near, or toward the midline or apex of dental arch.

Mesmerism *FA Mesmer, Austrian-physician, 1734–1815.* Hypnotism, mesoderm, the middle of the three primary layers of cells in the embryo from which the connective tissues develop.

Mesna Uroepithelial protector.

Mesoappendix A triangular fold of peritoneum around the vermiform appendix, attaching the latter of posterior surface of the mesentery of the ileum. The artery to appendix runs along the free margin of this fold.

Mesocardium The double layer mesoderm attaching the embryonic heart to the wall of pericardial cavity.

Mesocephalic Denoting a skull having cephalic index between 75 and 80; intermediate between dolichocephalic and brachy cephalic.

Mesocolon The double layer of peritoneum attaching colon to posterior abdominal wall. Only the transverse colon and sigmoid colon have actual mesentery.

Mesocolopexy Surgical procedure in which the mesocolon is fixed or resuspended to prevent ptosis or torsion of transverse colon.

Mesocoloplication A surgical procedure of folding back the mesocolon on itself and stitching in place in order to restrict mobility of transverse colon.

Mesocord An umbilical cord, a segment of which is bound to placenta by an accessory fold.

Mesocortex The cerebral cortex of the cingulate and retrosplenial gyri that

M

does not pass through a six layered developmental stage.

Mesoderm The middle of primary germ layers, in between outer ectoderm and inner endoderm. From this layer are derived the majority of skeletal system, the circulatory system, the musculature, the excretory system and most of the reproductive system in vertebrates.

Mesoduodenum A part of the primitive midline dorsal mesentery in relation to embryonic duodenum.

Mesoepididymis A fold of tunica vaginalis that connects the testis to the epididymis.

Mesogastrium That part of primitive dorsal mesentery which is related to developing stomach and becomes greater omentum.

Mesometrium The broad ligament connecting the uterus with the abdominal wall.

Mesomorph A stocky individual of medium height with well-developed muscles.

Mesonephroma Rare ovarian tumor believed to be formed from displaced mesonephric tissue.

Mesonephros An intermediate excretory organ of the embryo, it is replaced by permanent metanephros (kidney). While its ductal system is retained in male as epididymis and deferent duct and in female as tubules of epoophoron. Also known as wolffian body.

Mesorchium A thick fold of peritoneum which connects the developing testis to the mesonephric fold in embryo. It contains testicular vessels and nerves.

Meso-ovarium It is that part of the broad ligament which encloses the ovary. It lies between the mesosalpinx and the mesometrium.

Mesosalpinx Part of the broad ligament investing the fallopian tube. It represents the upper free part of the broad

ligament which is above its attachment to the uterus.

Mesorectum A short peritoneal fold investing the upper part of rectum and connecting it to sacrum.

Mesoridazine Antipsychotic agent.

Mesosigmoidopexy Attaching the sigmoid mesocolon to anterior abdominal wall to prevent sigmoid volvulus or rectal prolapse.

Mesotendon The connective tissue fold of synovial membrane extending from a tendon to the wall of its synovial tendon sheath.

Mesothelioma A rapidly growing tumor of the pleura, peritoneum or pericardium which may be seen in patients with asbestosis. However, this tumor may also occur in people who have no history of exposure to asbestos.

Messenger RNA Abbreviated mRNA. The ribonucleic acid which acts as a template for the linking of aminoacids during the formation of protein in the cells.

Mesterolone Anabolic androgen.

Mestranol A synthetic oestrogen commonly used in combination with a progesterone in contraceptive pills.

Mesurpine HCl A vasodilator and smooth muscle relaxant.

Meta Prefix means 1. Changed in form, or position transformed, 2. After, behind, following, 3. Next to.

Meta-analysis An attempt to improve the findings of research by combining and analysing the results of all discoverable trials on the same subject.

Metabiosis The dependence of an organism upon the preexistence of another for its development.

Metabolic Referring to metabolism.

Metabolism The sum of the physical and chemical processes by which living organized substance is built up and maintained (anabolism), and by which large molecules are broken down into smaller molecules to make energy available to the organism (catabolism). Essentially, these processes are concerned with the disposition of the nutrients absorbed into the blood after digestion.

Basal metabolism The minimal energy expended for the maintenance of respiration, circulation, peristalsis, muscle tonus, body temperature, glandular activity and the other vegetative functions of the body.

Inborn error of metabolism A genetically determined biochemical disorder in which a specific enzyme defect produces a metabolic block that may have pathological consequences at birth, as in phenylketonuria, or in later life.

Metabolite Any product or substance taking part in metabolism.

Essential metabolite A substance that is necessary for normal metabolism, e.g., a vitamin.

Metabutethamine Used in dentistry as a local anesthetic for nerve block/ infiltration anesthesia.

Metacarpal One of the five bones of the hand which join the fingers to the wrist.

Metacarpophalangeal Relating to the metacarpal bones and the phalanges.

Metacarpus The five bones of the hand uniting the carpus with the phalanges of the fingers.

Metacentric Pertaining to chromosome with centromere in the middle.

Metachromasia 1. The property by which some cells stain in a color different from the dye with which they are stained. 2. The property through which a single dye stains different tissues in different colors.

Metachromatic Term applied to cells and dyes exhibiting metachromasia.

Metacercaria The encysted stage of a digenetic trematode which occurs in the tissues or on the surface of inter-

mediate host such as snail. This stage is usually infective or is the transfer stage to definitive host.

Metacresol A local antiseptic.

Metacryptozoite A member of a second or subsequent generation of the extra erythrocytic, tissue dwelling malarial parasite; it develops from sporozoites.

Metacyesis Extrauterine pregnancy.

Metafemale A female with 3 X chromosomes (trisomy X) usually short statured, mentally retarded and obese.

Metagonimus A genus of small flukes which may infect man upon eating fish containing the larvae.

Metakinesis The separation of two chromatids of a chromosome during the anaphase of mitosis.

Metal Any of the several chemical elements that share a group of characteristic properties, arc good conducts of electricity, malleable and liberate cations.

Heavy metal Any metal 5 times or more heavier than water.

Noble metal Metal that cannot be oxidized by heat nor can be easily dissolved.

Rare earth metal Any metal with atomic no. 57 through 71.

Metaldehyde A polymer of acetaldehyde formerly used as an antiseptic.

Metalloenzyme An enzyme having a metal ion as an integral part of its active form, e.g., cytochrome (Fe^{2-}, Fe^{3+}). Cytochrome oxidase (Cu^{2-}, Cu^2) or alcohol dehydrogenase (Zn^{2+}).

Metalloprotein A protein with metal ion bound to it. Many enzymes are metalloproteins.

Metamale A male with one X-chromosome but 2 Y-chromosomes; usually tall, lean, often having tendency towards aggressive behavior.

Metamorphopsia Distortion of visual image as in parietal lobe disease, retinal lesion or intoxication.

Metamorphosis A structural change or transformation.

Metamucil Trade name for preparations of ispaghula, a bulk laxative.

Metamyelocyte An immature granulocyte, an early stage of granulocyte derived from myelocyte with kidney shaped nucleus and finely granulated cytoplasm containing azurophilic granules.

Metanephrine One of the catabolic products of epinephrine excreted in urine.

Matanephros The permanent kidney in the human fetus, formed caudal to mesonephros close to termination of cloaca. It is composed of metanephric duct (primitive ureter) and the metanephrogenic tissue.

Metaphase The second stage of mitosis or cell division.

Metaphysis The junction of the epiphysis with the diaphysis in along bone.

Metaplasia Abnormal change in the structure of a tissue. May be indicative of malignant change.

Metaproterenol A potent beta-adrenergic stimulant used a bronchodilator.

Metarhodopsin An intermediate formed in retina from degradation of lumirhodopsin. It is unstable and degrades to scotopsin and transretinine.

Metaraminol A compound with vasopress or activity used to treat acute hypotension.

Metastasis The transfer of a disease from one part of the body to another, through the blood vessels, via the lymph channels or across the body cavities. Secondary deposits may occur from a primary malignant growth. Septic infection may arise in other organs from some original focus.

Metatarsal One of the five bones of the foot which join the tarsus to the toes.

Metatarsalgia Pain in the metatarsal bones.

Metatarsus The five bones of the foot uniting the tarsus with the phalanges of the toes.

Metathalamus That portion of thalamus composed of medial and lateral geniculate bodies.

Metathrombin A thrombin-antithrombin complex formed during clotting and is inactive.

Metaxalone Orally administered smooth muscle relaxant.

Metazoa The division of the animal kingdom that includes the multicellular animals, i.e., all animals except the Protozoa.

Metazoonosis A type of zoonosis requiring both a vertebrate and in invertebrate host stage in the life cycle of causative organism.

Metencephalon The more rostral part of brain in embryo that develops into cerebellum and pons.

Meteorism Distention of intestine with gas.

Meter Symbol m. The fundamental SI unit of length. Measure of length equal to 39.37 inches or 100 cm.

Metformin A biguanide hypoglycemic used in the treatment of diabetes mellitus.

Methacholine A derivative of acetyl choline with only muscarinic effect.

Methacycline A semi synthetic antibiotic of tetracycline group given orally.

Methadone A powerful analgesic with no sedative action. Similar in action to morphine, it is used to relieve pain in terminal illness and also in withdrawal programs for heroin addicts. Methadone is addictive, but less socially disabling than heroin. Amidone.

Methallenestril A synthetic nonsteroidal estrogenic agent.

Methamphetamine A sympathomimetic amine similar to amphetamine; used as a CNS stimulant.

Methandriol Anabolic steroid.

Methandrostenolone A compound of methyl testosterone with anabolic and androgenic properties.

Methane CH_4, Marshy gas, the simplest hydrocarbon.

Methanol Methyl alcohol, prepared synthetically or from distillation of wood. Toxic and causes blindness when drunk.

Methantheline bromide An anticholinergic agent used to suppress gastric motility and secretion.

Methapyrilene Antihistaminic of medium potency and short duration; used as fumarate or hydrochloride.

Methaqualone A sedative and hypnotic, chronic use can lead to psychologic and physical dependence.

Metharbital A barbiturate used as anticonvulsant for grandmal, petitmal and myoclonic seizures.

Methazolamide An agent inhibiting carbonic anhydrase, hence used in glaucoma; given orally.

Methaemalbumin A compound of haem with plasma albumin found in the blood in some types of anaemia.

Methaemoglobin An altered form of hemoglobin found in the blood and usually produced by the action of a drug on the red blood corpuscles, causing a reduction in their oxygen carrying ability. May be associated with the use of phenacetin and other aniline derivatives.

Methaemoglobinaemia Cyanosis and inability of the red blood cells to transport oxygen owing to the presence of methemoglobin.

Methenamine $C_6H_{12}N_4$ Used in treatment of infections of urinary tract.

Methetoin An analog of phenytoin used as oral anticonvulsant.

Methicillin A form of penicillin that is resistant to staphylococcal penicillinase.

Methicillin resistant Staphylococcus aureus Abbreviated MRSA. A strain of *S. aureus* that is distinguished from others by its resistance to the special beta-lactose drugs ('methicillin-like' drugs) that are usually used to treat these organisms. MRSA can affect people in different ways. People can carry the organism in the nose or on the skin without showing any symptoms of illness. This is called MRSA colonization. MRSA can also cause infections such as boils, wound infections or infected decubitus ulcers. There is no evidence that properly treated infections caused by MRSA are more or less serious than other *S. aureus* infections. MRSA is spread from person to person by direct contact. This means that if persons have MRSA on their skin (especially on the hands) and touch another individual, they may spread MRSA. A person may have MRSA on the hands as a result of being a carrier or from touching another person who is a carrier or infected with MRSA. General infection control measures are appropriate for preventing spread. Persons who are colonized with MRSA do not usually need to be treated but in severe MRSA infections vancomycin is given intravenously. It can have severe side effects.

Methicillin sodium A semisynthetic derivative of penicillin given IM, in infections resistant to penicillin G.

Methimazole Potent, widely used antithyroid drug. It acts by interfering with incorporation of iodine.

Methiodal sodium Iodine containing contrast for urinary tract.

Methionine 1. A sulfur-containing essential amino acid occurring in proteins that is a vital component of the diet. 2. A drug used orally in the treatment of paracetamol poisoning.

Methixene hydrochloride Anticholinergic agent used orally in gastrointestinal hypermotility and spasm.

Methocarbamol A muscle relaxant, given orally IM and SC.

Method A set form or mode of procedure, a systemic way of performing an examination, test or operation.

Methohexital sodium Short acting barbiturate used IV like pentothal sodium.

Methohexitone A barbiturate anesthetic agent; given intravenously it has a quick recovery time.

Methotrexate A cytotoxic drug that antagonizes folic acid and prevents cell formation. It is used to treat various types of malignant disease.

Methotrimeprazine A phenothiazine with sedative and analgesic properties. Useful in schizophrenia and terminal illness.

Methoxamine A sympathomimetic amine used for its vasopressor effects in restoring blood pressure during anesthesia.

Methoxsalen A psoralen compound used in association with ultraviolet exposure to vitiligo. It is also used to precipitate a phototoxic response in the treatment of psoriasis.

Methoxychlor An insecticide used to control mosquito larva and flies.

Methoxyflurane A colorless non-explosive liquid used as a slow anesthetic.

Methoxyphenamine An adrenergic agent used as bronchodilator.

Methoscopolamine A quaternary derivative of scopolamine with anticholinergic actions; used as gastrointestinal sedative.

Methsuximide An anticonvulsant for petitmal and psychomotor epilepsy.

Methyl clothiazide A thiazide antihypertensive diuretic.

Methylal Dimethoxymethane.

Methyl chloride A refrigerant, used in spray form for local anesthesia, also same property by methyl iodide.

Methyl chloride methacrylate An acrylic resin for dental use.

Methyl chloride salicylate An antipyretic, analgesic, used in pain killing ointments.

Methylate To combine with methyl alcohol or the methyl radical.

Methyl benzenethonium chloride A topical anti-infective agent.

Methyl cellulose A bulk-forming drug used as a laxative and to control diarrhea.

Methylcholanthrene One of the carcinogenic polycyclic hydrocarbons of coaltar.

Methyldopa A hypotensive drug whose action is increased if used with thiazide diuretics.

Methylated spirit A mixture of 95% ethyl alcohol and 5% methyl alcohol. An industrial spirit which, taken as a drink, is poisonous.

Methylene blue A synthetic organic compound, in dark-green crystals or lustrous crystalline powder, used in treatment of methemoglobinaemia, as an antidote in cyanide poisoning, as a stain in pathology and bacteriology, and as an antiseptic.

Methylene dioxyamphetamine (MDA) A hallucinogen commonly referred as the love drug.

Methylene green A synthetic metachromatic dye used to distinguish mast cell granules.

Methylergonovine maleate An oxytocic agent used to induce uterine contraction to reduce postpartum hemorrhage.

Methyl glucamine ditrizoate An organic compound used as a contrast medium in the making of X-ray transperencies.

Methyl malonic aciduria Elevation of methyl malonic acid in blood with excessive excretion in urine. Caused due to congenital enzymatic deficiency or B_{12} deficiency.

Methyl malony CoA Formed from propionyl CoA, helpful for utilization of fatty acids.

Methyl metharcylate Acrylic resin used to make denture bases, artificial teeth, crowns and restorations.

Methylphenobarbitone A white crystalline powder used as an anticonvulsant with a slight hypnoticaction. Especially useful for senile tremor.

Methyl phenidate Mild psycho motor stimulant, used to treat hyperkinetic children, and narcolepsy.

Methylprednisolone A corticosteroid of the glucogenic type, having an anti-inflammatory action similar to that of prednisolone.

Methyl salicylate A compound used externally for rheumatic pains, lumbago, etc. Oil of wintergreen.

Methyl testosterone Orally given androgenic steroidal agent as a replacement therapy for androgen deficiency states.

Methyl tetraphydrofolic acid An intermediate sub serving as a donor of methyl group to homocystine to form methionine.

Methyl violet Dye for staining amyloid.

Methyprylon A compound with sedative and hypnotic properties.

Methysergide A potent serotonin antagonist used in the prophylaxis of migraine.

Metitepine 5 HT antagonist.

Metmyoglobin Oxidized (Fe^{3+}) myoglobin.

Metoclopramide A drug which speeds up gastric action and is used to treat nausea, heartburn and vomiting.

Metocurine A derivative of tubocurarine which is more potent and longer acting.

Metolazone A diuretic acting on proximal and distal tubules.

Metoprolol A cardioselective betablocker having a greater effect on β1-adrenergic receptors of the heart than on the β2-adrenergic receptors of the bronchi and blood vessels; used for treatment of hypertension *(See Beta (Blockers)).*

Metorchis A genus of flukes in animals, occasionally transmitted to man.

Metra The uterus.

Metrectomy Hysterectomy.

Metrifonate A drug effective against bladder flukes *(Schistostoma hematobium)*.

Metritis Inflammation of the uterus.

Metrizamide A non-ionic radiographic contrast agent.

Metrizoate sodium A contrast medium for coronary angiography.

Metrizoic acid A compound used as contrast medium in diagnostic procedures.

Metrocolpocele The protrusion of the uterus into the vagina, the wall of the latter also being pushed forward.

Metrodynamometer Instrument used to measure the strength of uterine contractions.

Metronidazole A drug that is effective in overcoming *Trichomonas* infection of the genital tract of both sexes. Also used in the treatment of giardiasis, of acute amoebic dysentery and of infection by anaerobic bacteria.

Metropathia hemorrhagica Excessive prolonged bleeding from uterus associated with cyst formation in the endometrium.

Metrorrhagia Irregular uterine bleeding not associated with menstruation.

Metyrapone An inhibitor of adrenocortical steroid C-11 beta hydroxylation, administered orally or IV as a diagnostic test to determine the capability of pituitary to increase production of corticotrophin.

Mevalonic acid A product of methyl valeric acid produced in the pathway of biosynthesis of sterols.

Mevinolin HMG CoA reductase inhibitor used as lipid lowering agent.

Mexiletine An antiarrhythmic agent used to treat ventricular arrhythmias.

mg Milligram(s).

Mg Symbol for magnesium.

MHRA Medicines and Healthcare Products Regulatory Agency.

Micelle 1. A submicroscopic unit of a protoplasm. 2. A molecular aggregate as that of a colloid often formed by action of detergents on a hydrocarbon in water.

Michel's suture clips *G Michel, French surgeon, 1875–1937.* Small metal clips used for suturing wounds.

Miconazole An antifungal agent used topically for dermatophytic infections such as athlete's foot or vulvovaginal candidiasis, orally for candidiasis of the mouth and gastrointestinal tract, and systemically by intravenous infusion for systemic fungal infections.

Micrencephaly A condition in which the brain is abnormally small and underdeveloped.

Micro One millionth (10^{-6}); very small, minute.

Microabscess A small abscess usually less than an mm, often multiple.

Microabscess of Munro One of the characteristic lesions of psoriasis consisting of focal accumulation of polymorphonuclear leukocytes in the upper layer of epidermis.

Microabscess Pautrier's Focal collection of atypical T lymphocytes in the epidermis in mycosis fungoides.

Microadenoma A small (≤ 10 mm diameter) non-malignant glandular tumor, as associated with Cushing's disease.

Microaerophil An anaerobe that can tolerate low O_2 tension.

Microaerosol A suspension in the air of minute particles of $1-10$ μ.

Microalbuminuria Excretion in urine of less than 100 μgm per minute of albumin.

Microanalysis Analysis using small amounts of material than classical methods of chemical analysis that involves weighing precipitated material.

Microaneurysm An aneurismal dilatation affecting small arteries, arterioles and capillaries, a feature of diabetes mellitus, thrombotic thrombocytopenic purpura.

Microangiopathy A disease process affecting small blood vessels.

Diabetic microangiopathy Thickening of capillary basement membrane, heart with microaneurysm formation.

Microbe A minute living organism, especially one causing disease. A microorganism.

Microbiology The study of micro organisms and their effect on living cells.

Microcephalic Having an abnormally small head.

Micrococcus A genus of bacteria, each of which has a spherical shape. The bacteria occur in pairs or in groups and are Gram-positive. Found in soil and water.

Microcurie A unit of activity of radio nuclides equal to 10^{-6} curie, ICi = 3.7 × 10^{10} Bq = 37 GBq.

Microcyte A small red blood cell at least 2μ smaller than normal, as seen in iron deficiency.

Microcythaemia The presence of abnormally small red cells in the blood; microcytosis.

Microcytosis Condition in which RBCs are abnormally small.

Microfilaria A prelarval or embryonic form of filarial worms.

Microgamete The smaller male element in the conjugation of cells of unequal size.

Microgametocyte The mother cell that produces microgametes.

Microgamy Conjugation between two young cells in certain protozoans.

Microgila The smallest neuroglial cell, the macrophage of brain and spinal cord that remove cellular debris in CNS.

Micrognathia Failure of development of the lower jaw, causing a receding chin.

Microgram Symbol μg. One millionth of a gram.

Micrometre Symbol mm. One millionth of a metre. Formerly called micron.

Micron *(See Micrometre).*

Micronutrient A dietary element essential only in small quantities.

Microorganism A minute animal or vegetable, particularly a virus, a bacterium, a fungus, a rickettsia or a protozoon.

Microphage A minute phagocyte.

Microphonics Electrical potentials generated in the cochlea by passage of sound waves.

Microphthalmos A condition in which one or both eyes are smaller than normal. Their function may or may not be impaired.

Micropipette A pipette calibrated for accurate delivery of very small quantities less than 0.5 mL.

Micropore A submicroscopic break in the membrane of a protozoan cell or microbe through which exchange of materials, pinocytosis occur.

Microprobe An ultra fine probe used for exploration and fixation of tissues in microsurgical procedures.

Micropsia Perception of objects as smaller in comparison to their actual size. It occurs in retinal detachment, temporal lobe epilepsy, delirium and drug intoxication.

Microradiograph A recorded image obtained by microradiography, used in high resolution imaging of thin objects like tissue sections.

Microscope An instrument which produces a greatly enlarged image of objects that are normally invisible to the human eye.

Electron microscope A microscope in which a beam of electrons is used instead of a light beam, allowing magnification of as much as 5,00,000 diameters.

Microscopic Visible only by means of the microscope. The opposite of macroscopic.

Microscopy The study of objects using a microscope.

Microsecond One millionth of a second.

Microsection A thin slice of tissue prepared for examination under a microscope.

Microspectrography Study of composition of an object, especially of cellular constituents using a spectroscope. That makes a photographic record of the spectrum.

Microspectrophotometer An instrument used to measure the absorption, reflection or emission of light by objects under a microscope, especially used for spectral analysis of individual cells.

Microsporum A genus of fungi. The cause of some skin diseases, especially ringworm.

Microstomia Disproportionately small oral orifice.

Microsurgery The carrying out of surgical procedures using a microscope and miniature instruments.

Microtia Abnormally small auricle or pinna.

Microtome A mechanical device used for preparing histologic sections for microscopic examinations can be microtome freezing or microtome rotary.

Microtomography A technique for rotating a small sample in an electron microscope through 90°, processing the data by computer and displaying three dimensional images.

Microtonometer An instrument for measuring the partial pressure of gases in minute quantities of material.

M

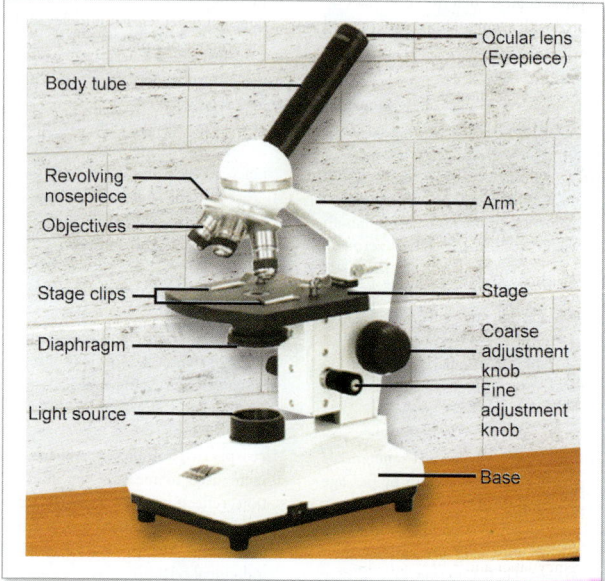

Parts of Microscope

M

Microtubule A small, hollow, cylindrical structure found in the cell cytoplasm. During cell division they increase greatly in number to form the mitotic spindle, play an important role in intracellular movements and in maintaining shape of the cell.

Microvilli Submicroscopic finger like projections on the surface of cell membrane which greatly increase the surface area.

Microvolt One millionth of a Volt, 10^{-6} volt.

Microwave Any electromagnetic radiation having a very short wavelength between 1 mm and 30 cm. Wavelength 1 mm are in infrared region and that beyond 30 cm. are radio waves. Sources of emission include radar, cathode ray tubes, induction furnaces, and electrotherapy devices.

Microwave exposure can cause cataract.

Micturition The act of passing urine.

Midazolamv A benzodiazepine.

Midbrain Portion of the brain that connects the cerebrum with the pons and cerebellum.

Middle lobe syndrome A form of chronic atelectasis marked by collapse of middle lobe of the lung resulting from compression of bronchus by enlarged lymph nodes/tumor. Symptoms include chronic cough and recurrent respiratory infections. *SYN* - Brock's syndrome.

Midlife crisis Experienced by many people during the fifth decade of life, resulting in doubt, anxiety and sometimes depression. During this time men and women may reflect on their lives, review the past and be aware of physiological deterioration associated with ageing. This is experienced when children are growing up, moving away from home and establishing their own adult relationships. Empty nest syndrome.

Midfoot The middle portion of foot consisting of navicular, cuboid and cuneiform bones.

Midgut 1. The small intestine comprising jejunum and ileum. 2. The middle segment of embryonic intestine, precursor of stomach to transverse colon.

Midpelvis The area of pelvis extending from the posterior inferior aspect of symphysis in a line through ischial spines to sacrum intersecting it at S_2 or S_3 vertebra.

Midwife The title and legal description of a person who is so certified under the Midwives Acts.

Midwifery The art and science of caring for women undergoing normal pregnancy, labor and the period following childbirth (usually 6–8 weeks).

Midwifery process The application of the nursing process to midwifery. It is the systematic, cyclical method of organizing midwifery care, and is carried out by the assessment of actual and potential problems, and the planning, implementation and evaluation of care.

Midwife's Code of Practice (1994) A code issued by the UK Central Council for Nurses, Midwives and Health Visitors (UKCC) as guidance to all midwives practising in the UK. It is not a legal document but failure to comply with its guidance may, in the event of a disciplinary hearing before the UKCC, be used in evidence against the midwife. It covers matters directly relating to the Midwives Practice Rules, and advice on home births, complementary and alternative therapies, arranging for a substitute, and maternal, intrauter-

ine and neonatal death, as well as notes on other legislation relevant to the practice of a midwife.

Midwives Acts A number of Acts of Parliament to regulate the practice of midwives, passed in the years 1902, 1918, 1926 and 1936. All this legislation was consolidated by the Midwives Act, 1951. The Nurses, Midwives and Health Visitors Acts of 1979 and 1992 replaced the former Midwives Acts, and established a new statutory structure for nursing, midwifery and health visiting in the UK.

Migpristone Progestine antagonist.

Miglitol Alphaglucosidase inhibitor for diabetes.

Migraine Paroxysmal attacks of severe headache, often with nausea, vomiting and visual disturbance.

Migravess Trade name for combination preparations containing aspirin and metoclopramide, used in migraine.

Migril Trade name for a combination preparation containing ergotamine, cyclizine and caffeine, used in migraine attacks.

Mikulicz's disease Benign bilateral swelling of the lacrimal and salivary glands associated with dryness of mouth and reduced, lacrimation, identical to Sjogren's syndrome.

Mikulicz's drain A procedure used in emergency medicine as a last resort to control bleeding while all the other methods fail.

Mikulicz's syndrome Painless bilateral enlargement of salivary and lacrimal glands with dryness of mouth and decreased lacrimation as in sarcoidosis.

Milestone One of the 'norms' against which the motor, social and psychological development of a child is measured.

Milia Small white spots usually occurring in clusters around the nose and cheeks resulting from obstruction of a sebaceous gland. May occur in young adults.

M. neonatorum Milia occurring in newborns' faces soon after birth.

Miliaria Prickly heat, an acute itching eruption common among white people in tropical and subtropical areas.

Miliary Resembling millet seed. *Miliary tuberculosis (See Tuberculosis).*

Milieu Environment, surroundings.

Milium [L.] A whitish nodule in the skin, especially of the face, usually 1–4 mm in diameter. Milia are spheroidal, epithelial cysts of lamellated keratin lying just under the epidermis, often associated with vellus hair follicles. Popularly called whitehead.

Milk 1. A nutrient fluid produced by the mammary gland of many animals for nourishment of young mammals. 2. A liquid (emulsion or suspension) resembling the secretion of the mammary gland.

Milk sugar Lactose, a disaccharide present in the milk of all mammals.

Milk teeth The first set of teeth.

Witch's milk Milk secreted from the breast of a newborn child.

Milking A manual or mechanical technique for removing fluid from body part.

Milk alkali syndrome Hyper calcemia without hypercalciuria or hypophosphaturia induced by prolonged ingestion of large quantity of milk and soluble alkali as in therapy of peptic ulcer.

Milk teeth Deciduous teeth.

Milkman's syndrome Osteoporosis with multiple fractures as seen in postmenopausal women.

Millard-Gubler syndrome Paralysis of facial muscles on one side and extremities on opposite side by brainstem lesions.

Miller-Abbott tube *TG Miller. American physician, 1886–1981; WO Abbott, American physician, 1902–1943.* A double-channel intestinal tube for treating obstruction, especially that due to paralytic ileus of the small intestine. It has an inflatable balloon at its distal end.

Millicurie A measure of radioactivity, one thousandth of a curie.

Milliequivalent A quantity equal to 10^{-3} of the equivalent weight of an element or compound.

Milligram Symbol mg. One thousandth of a gram.

Milligray A unit of absorbed dose in the field of ionizing radiation equal to 10^{-3} gray.

Milliliter Symbol mL. One thousandth of a litre (one cubic centimetre).

Millimeter Symbol mm. One thousandth of a metre.

Millimicrogram One billionth of a gram, biller called a nano gram.

Millimole Symbol mmol. The amount of a substance that balances or is equivalent in combining power to 1 mg of hydrogen. A method of assessing the body's acid-base balance or needs during electrolyte upset.

Millipore filter Trade name for a device used to filter nutrient solutions as they are administered intravenously.

Millirad A unit of absorbed dose of ionizing radiation equivalent to 10^{-3} rad, 10^{-3} gray.

Millirem A unit of radiation dose equivalent to 10^{-3} rem, 10^{-3} Joule/kg, 10^{-3} silvert.

Milliroentgen A unit of ionization exposure equal to 10^{-3} roentgen, $2.58 \leq 10^{-7}$ coulomb/kg.

Milrinone Sympathomimetic, cardiac stimulant.

Milroy's disease Familial and congenital swelling of subcutaneous tissues usually confined to extremities with large accumulation of lymph.

Milton Trade name for an antiseptic consisting of a standardized 1% solution of electrolytic sodium hypochlorite. It is used especially for the sterilization of babies' feeding bottles and teats in the home.

Milwaukee brace A brace consisting of a leather girdle and neck ring connected by metal struts; used to brace the spine in the treatment of scoliosis.

Mimesis State in which one disease presents the symptoms of another.

Mimetic Of or relating to mimesis.

Mimicry The imitation of one species by another in an adaption tending to improve its chances of survival.

Minaserine 5HT antagonist, antidepressant.

Mind The organized total of psychological processes and contents that allow the individual to respond to external and internal stimuli in an integrated and dynamic way, relating response of present to both past and future of the individual. The principal processes of mind are perceiving, learning, thinking, remembering, feeling and behaving with intelligence.

Mineral Any naturally occurring homogenous inorganic substance, having a characteristic crystalline structure and chemical composition.

Mineralocorticoid A hormone produced by the adrenal cortex. Its function is to maintain the salt and water balance in the body.

Mineralization The conversion of organic material to inorganic material.

Minims Trade name for eye drops packaged in single-use containers.

Minimal brain dysfunction syndrome A complex of symptoms that involve impairment of some or all of the following functions: language, perception, memory, concentration, and motor functions.

Minimal change disease A form of nephritic syndrome in which minimal or no glomerular abnormalities are noted by light microscopy but fusion of foot processes of podocytes in electron microscopy.

Minocycline A semisynthetic broad spectrum antibiotic of the tetracycline group.

Minoxidil Vasodilator; used for alopecia locally as 2% solution.

Miopus Unequal conjoined twins united at head in such fashion that face of one member is rudimentary.

Miosis Contraction of the pupil of the eye, as in reaction to a bright light; meiosis.

Miotic A drug which causes contraction of the pupil.

Miracidium A free swimming ciliated larva of a trematode that penetrates a small intermediate host where it develops into a sporocyst.

Mirror A polished surface that forms optical images by reflection.

Head mirror A concave mirror worn on a headband or spectacle frame used for focusing beam of light.

Laryngeal mirror A circular plane mirror used to examine the interior of larynx and hypopharynx.

Mirtazapine Antidepressant.

Miscarriage Abortion; the expulsion of the fetus before the 24th week of pregnancy, i.e., before it is legally viable.

Miscarry To give birth to a nonviable fetus.

Misce Mix, a direction given in pharmacy.

Miscible Capable of being mixed.

Misdiagnosis Wrong diagnosis.

Misogyny Hatred of women.

Misophobia Abnormal fear of contamination.

Mistura Mixture, used in pharmacy.

Misuse of Drugs Act 1971 and subsequent regulations Controls the manufacture, possession, prescription and sale of certain habit-forming drugs, including narcotic drugs that are liable to misuse with the development of dependence. These are called controlled drugs and are available for treatment only on medical prescription. Heavy penalties invariably follow the illegal sale or supply of these drugs.

Mite A minute animal, frequently parasitic on humans and animals, and causing various forms of dermatitis.

Mithramycin An antitumor antibiotic which is particularly helpful in the treatment of hypercalcaemia.

Miticide An agent for killing mite.

Mitigate To make or become milder.

Mitochondrion A body which is found in the cytoplasm of cells and is concerned with energy production and the oxidation of food.

Mitogen Agent promoting cell mitosis and lymphocyte transformation.

Mitogenesis The induction of mitosis in a cell.

Mitomycin C A highly toxic antineoplastic; indicated for palliative treatment of certain neoplasms that do not respond to surgery radiation and other drugs.

Mitosis A method of multiplication of cells by a specific process of division.

Mitoxantrone Antineoplastic agent.

Mitotane Antineoplastic agent.

Mitral Shaped like a mitre.

Mitral incompetence The result of a defective mitral valve, when there is a back flow, or regurgitation, after closure of the valve.

Mitral stenosis The formation of fibrous tissue, causing an arrowing of the valve; usually due to rheumatic heart disease and endocarditis.

Mitral valve The bicuspid valve between the left atrium and left ventricle of the heart.

Mitral valvotomy An operation for overcoming stenosis by dividing the fibrous tissue to free the cusps.

Mitralization Straightening of left cardiac border due to enlarged left atrial appendage and pulmonary artery in mitral stenosis.

Mittelschmerz Pain occurring between the menses, accompanying ovulation.

Ml Milliliter(s).

MLNS Mucocutaneous lymph node syndrome.

MLSO Medical Laboratory Scientific Officer.

mm Millimeter(s).

mmol Millimole(s).

MMR Measles mumps rubella vaccine.

Mn Symbol for manganese.

Mixture 1. An aggregation of two or more substances that are not chemically combined. 2. A pharmaceutical preparation consisting of an insoluble substance suspended in a liquid viscid material such as sugar, glycerol, etc.

Mizolastine Antiallergic agent.

M. mode A motion B mode tracing of ultrasound to visualize moving structures.

Minemonic The use or devising of techniques to facilitate memory.

MNS blood groups A system of erythrocyte antigen determined by the allelic genes, M, N and S; the grouping is primarily used to solve identification problems such as disputed paternity and genetic linkage, population studies.

Mobility The capacity for movement.

Electrophoretic mobility The velocity at which ions of a substance migrate in an electric field.

Mobilization The bringing back into mobility of a limb, joint or person following illness or injury.

Mobius sign Convergence weakness of eyes occurring in exophthalmic goiter.

Mobius syndrome A congenital disorder characterized by bilateral paralysis of both external recti and hypotrophy of facial musculature due to a genesis of ganglion cells in the brain stem of occulomotor and facial nerve nuclei.

M

Moclobemide Antidepressant.

Modality 1. Any of the several forms of therapy. 2. Any of the main forms of sensation.

Modafinil Wakefullness promoting agent.

Mode In statistics, the value occurring most often.

Model A conceptual paradigm, framework or theory, which can be used as an example to illustrate a problem, process or situation.

Modelling Providing an example that can be imitated and used as a means of teaching others to learn new behavior.

Modem A device that modulates carrier wave signals to encode digital information for transmission and demodulates signals to decode transmitted information.

Modiolus The central pillar or column of bone around which the spiral canals of cochlea turn.

MODS Multiple organ dysfunction syndrome.

Modulation The changes that take place in response to changes in the environment.

Moiety One of two, more or less equal parts. One of two or more main components, such as the groups of atoms in a complex molecule.

Molality The amount of substance of a solute divided by mass of the solvent, expressed in mole per kg.

Molar A back tooth used for grinding. There are three on either side of each jaw, making 12 in all (only eight in children).

Molar solution The concentration of a solution expressed in terms of the weight of the dissolved substance in gram per litre divided by its molecular weight.

Molarity The concentration of a substance expressed in moles/L.

Mole 1. The molecular weight of a substance expressed in gram. 2. A pigmented naevus or dark-colored growth on the skin. Moles are of various sizes, and are sometimes covered with hair. 3. A uterine tumor.

Carneous mole An organized blood clot surrounding a shriveled fetus in the uterus.

Hydatidiform mole (*vesicular mole*) A condition in pregnancy in which the chorionic villi of the placenta degenerate into clusters of cysts like hydatids. Malignant growth may follow if any remnants are left in the uterus *(See Choriocarcinoma)*.

Molecular Pertaining to or composed of molecules.

Molecular weight The weight of a molecule of a substance compared with that of an atom of carbon.

Molecule The chemical combination of two or more atoms which form a specific chemical substance, e.g., H_2O (water). The smallest amount of a substance that can exist independently.

Molindone Antipsychotic agent.

Molluscum A skin disease characterized by the development of soft, round tumors.

Molluscum contagiosum A benign tumor arising in the epidermis caused by a virus, transmitted by direct contact or fomites.

Molt To cast off.

Molybdenum Element No. 42, a silvery white hard metal required for many animal enzyme function.

Moment of death The point in time when an individual is declared dead. This determination is based on criteria which are defined by law and which differ according to situation. For autopsy and burial purposes, criteria include the clinical judgment that respiration and circulation have ceased and rigor mortis has started.

For organ transplantation brain death is employed even though functional circulatory and respiratory activities may persist.

Momentum The product of mass and velocity of a body, an index of quantity of motion.

Mometasone A steroid for topical use.

Momism The state of being excessively dependent on or subordinate to one's mother.

Monoamine oxidase inhibitors A group of drugs for treatment of depression.

Monarticular Referring to one joint only.

Monday disease The return of symptoms after a weekend away from work, as in the case of an allergic reaction to a substance encountered while at work.

Mondor's disease Inflammation of the subcutaneous veins of the chest and breast, usually extending from epigastric region to the axilla and occurring in both sexes.

Mongolian spots Blue-grey birth marks present from birth usually appearing on the lower back and buttocks. They will usually disappear by the time child is 5 years old. They resemble bruises.

Mongolism Outdated term for Down's syndrome.

Mongoloid Having characteristics or resembling mongolism.

Monilethrix Beaded hair, an anomalous condition in which the hair shaft exhibits nodosities or points of thickening alternating with normal or constricted areas.

Monilia Former name for the genus of fungi now known as Candida.

Moniliasis Infection with any fungus of genus *Monilia*.

Moniliform Having the shape of a necklace.

Monitor 1. To check constantly on a given condition, state or phenom-enon, e.g., blood pressure, heart, respiration rate or standards of care. 2. An apparatus by which such conditions or phenomena can be constantly observed and recorded.

Patient monitor The use of electrodes or transducers attached to the patient so that information such as temperature, pulse, respiration and blood pressure can be seen on a screen or automatically recorded.

Monkey rhesus Macaca mulatta widely distributed in India and China; easily raised in captivity, hence amply used in medical and biological research.

Monoamine oxidase An enzyme that breaks down noradrenaline and serotonin in the body.

Monooxidase inhibitor Abbreviated MAOI. A drug that prevents the breakdown of serotonin and leads to an increase in mental and physical activity.

Monoblast An immature cell of monocytic series, 18-22 in diameter, having many nucleoli, formed primarily in spleen and lymphoid tissue.

Monochromatism Color blindness. The patient sees all colors as black, gray or white.

Monoclonal Derived from a single cell.

Monoclonal antibodies Antibodies derived from a single clone of cells. All the antibody molecules are identical and will react with the same antigenic site.

Monocrotic Forming a smooth single crest on the downward line of a curve, e.g., pulse.

Monocular Pertaining to, or affecting, one eye only.

Monocyte A white blood cell having one nucleus, derived from the reticular cells, and having a phagocytic action.

Monocytosis Abnormal increase in number of monocytes in blood.

Monograph A detailed written account of one particular subject or a small area of a special field of learning.

M

Monohybrid A cross between parents that differ in one character.

Monoiodotyrosine (MIT) An amino acid formed by iodination of tyrosine at C_3, the first step in production of thyroxin.

Monokine A hormone like factor produced by activation of mono cytes; acts as an intercellular messenger to regulate immunologic and inflammatory responses.

Monomania Pathologic preoccupation with only one idea.

Monomer A single unit or molecule which can polymerize with similar units to form a chair or polymer.

Monomorphic Having but one shape, unchangeable in size and form.

Mononeuritis Inflammation or degeneration of a single nerve trunk or some of its branches.

Mononeuritis multiplex Neuritis involving single nerves at several distant sites, usually vascular origin (PAN).

Mononuclear Unicellular.

Mononucleosis An excessive number of monocytes in the blood; monocytosis.

Infectious mononucleosis An infectious disease due to the Epstein-Barr virus; glandular fever.

Monophasia Disorder in which the individual's vocabulary is limited to a single word or sentence.

Monoplegia Paralysis of one limb or of a single muscle or a group of muscles.

Monorchid An individual with only one testis.

Monosaccharide A simple sugar. The end result of carbohydrate digestion. Examples are glucose, fructose and galactose.

Monosodium glutamate (MSG) A chemical food flavor enhancer commonly added to Chinese dishes. May result in nausea, faintness, facial flushing and headache (sometimes called the Chinese restaurant syndrome).

Monosome A chromosome without its homologous chromosome.

Monosomy A congenital defect in the number of human chromosomes. There is one less than the normal 46.

Monoxide An oxide containing only one oxygen atom.

Monozygotic Denoting identical twins, or twins formed by division into two of the embryo derived from a single fertilized egg.

Mons A prominence or mound.

Mons pubis or mons veneris The eminence, consisting of a pad of fat, that lies over the pubic symphysis in the female.

Monster A congenitally severely deformed individual.

Montelukast Leukotriene antagonist for asthma.

Montgomery's glands or tubercles *WF Montgomery, Irish obstetrician, 1797–1859.* Sebaceous glands around the nipple, which grow larger during pregnancy.

Montgomery strap A band of adhesive tape featuring a lace-up design, used to secure dressings that must be changed frequently.

Mood Emotional reaction. Variations in mood are natural, but in certain psychiatric conditions there is severe depression in some cases and wild excitement in others, or alternations between both.

Moon face One of the features occurring in Cushing's syndrome and as a result of prolonged treatment with steroid drugs.

Moraxella Short, aerobic, Gram-negative bacteria.

Morbid Diseased or relating to an abnormal or disordered condition.

Morbidity The state of being diseased.

M

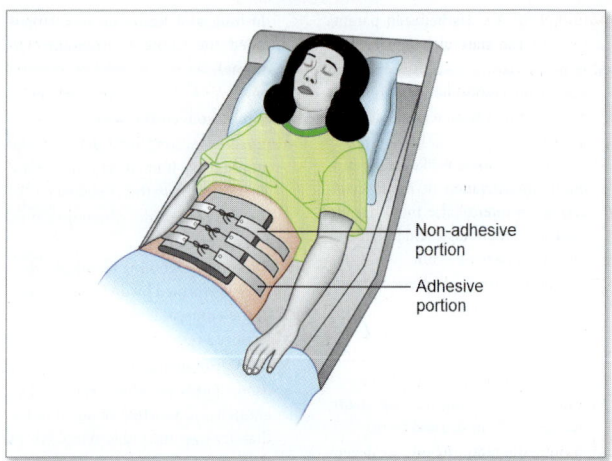

Non-adhesive portion

Adhesive portion

Montgomery Strap

M

Morbidity rate A figure that shows the susceptibility of a population to a certain disease. Usually shown statistically as the number of cases which occur annually per 1000 or other unit of population.

Morbilli Measles.

Morbilliform Resembling measles.

Morbus Latin for disease.

Morgan (m) the unit of map distance on a chromosome.

Morgue A place where dead bodies are kept pending for identification, autopsy or burial/cremation.

Moribund In a dying condition.

Morning sickness Nausea and vomiting which sometimes occurs in early pregnancy.

Moro reflex *E Moro, German pediatrician, 1874–1951.* The reaction to loud noise or sudden movement which should be present in the newborn. Startle reflex.

Morphea A circumscribed form of scleroderma presenting as acentral atrophic lesion with a pigmented border occurring chiefly on the chest, face or neck.

Morphine The principal alkaloid obtained from opium and given mainly to relieve severe pain. It is a drug of addiction. Morphia.

Morphogenesis The embryonic differentiation of cells leading to formation of characteristic structure or form of the organism or its parts.

Morphologic Relating to structure or form of organism.

Morphology 1. The study of configuration or structure of living organism. 2. The form or structure of an organism.

Morquio's syndrome A form of mucopolysaccharidosis characterized by dwarfism, knock knee, pectus carinatum, flat vertebra, corneal clouding, deformed wrist and hands. There is excess excretion of keratin sulfate in urine and the disease is autosomal recessive, also called mucopolysaccharidosis IV.

Morrhuate sodium The oily salt used as sclerosing agent and is injected into veins.

Mortal Subject to death, deadly.

Mortality The state of being liable to die.

Neonatal mortality Death during first month or four weeks of life.

Perinatalmortality The combined mortality from stillbirths and deaths in first week of life.

Mortality rate The number of deaths, per 1000 or other unit of population, occurring annually from a certain disease or condition.

Mortar A small receptacle in which substances are crushed or pulverized with a pestle.

Mortification Gangrene or death of tissue; necrosis.

Morton's neuroma A painful foot condition affecting one of the nerves between the toes. Also known as Morton's metatarsalgia.

Mortuary A funeral home where bodies of deceased are prepared for cremation *SYN* – morgue.

Morula An early stage of development of the ovum when it is a solid mass of cells.

Morula A cluster of cleaving bastomeres resulting from early division of zygote; a stage in the development of the embryo prior to the blastula.

Morulus The lesion characteristic of yaws, resembling a mulberry or raspberry.

Mosaic An individual who has cells of varying genetic composition.

Mosapride GI prokinetic agent.

Mosquito Blood sucking winged insects of family culicidae, responsible for transmission of malaria, dengue, etc.

Mother surrogate One who replaces an individual's mother in emotional feelings. A mother who bears offspring of another.

Motile Capable of movement.

Motion 1. The process of moving. 2. Evacuation of the bowels; defecation.

Motion sickness Sickness occurring as the result of travel by land, sea or air. Appears to be caused by excessive stimulation of the vestibular apparatus within the inner ear.

Motilin A gastrointestinal peptide of 22 amino acids located in enterochromaffin cells, chiefly of duodenum and upper jejunum that stimulates gastric and colonic motility.

Motility The capacity for spontaneous movement.

Segmental motility Regularly spaced ring like contractions of small intestine.

Motivation The reason or reasons, conscious or unconscious, behind a particular attitude or behavior.

Motive The incentive that determines a course of action or its direction.

Motor Something that causes movement.

Motor end-plate The nuclei and cytoplasm of muscle fibers at the termination of motor nerves.

Motor nerve One of the nerves which convey an impulse from a nerve center to a muscle or gland to promote activity.

Motor neurone disease A disease in which there is progressive degeneration of the anterior cells in the spinal cord, the motor nuclei of cranial nerves and the corticospinaltracts. The cause is unknown.

Mottling 1. A condition marked by spotty coloration. 2. Macular lesions of varying shades and hues.

Moulage The making of a mold of a bodily structure, especially for identification, prosthetics and teaching models.

Mould 1. A species of fungus. 2. The plastic shell used to immobilize apart of the body, usually the head, during radiotherapy.

Moulding The alteration in shape of the infant's head as it is forced through the maternal passages during labor.

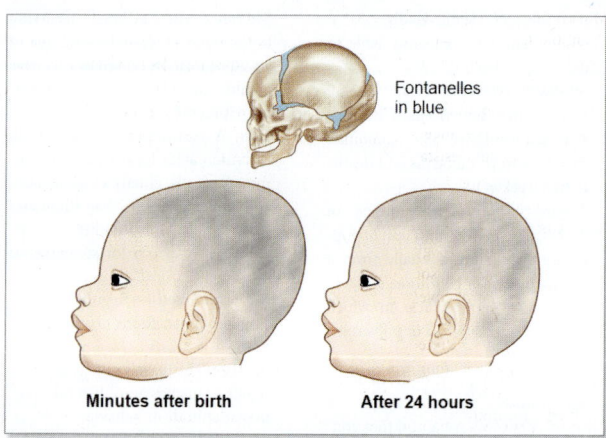

Fontanelles in blue

Minutes after birth   After 24 hours

Moulding

Mount To prepare slides of tissues for microscopic examination.

Mounting A dental laboratory procedure in which a maxillary or mandibular cast is attached to an articulator.

Mourning *(See Bereavement).*

Mountain sickness Dyspnea, headache, rapid pulse and vomiting, which occur on sudden change to the rarefied air of high altitudes.

Mouse pleural A round soft tissue density seen in chest X-ray representing a fibrin body in the pleural space.

Mouth An opening, particularly the external opening (in the face) of the alimentary canal.

Tapir mouth The characteristic pouting appearance of lips seen in facioscapulo humoral muscular dystrophy.

Trench mouth Necrotizing ulcerative gingivitis.

Mouth ulcers Painful, grayish white sores occurring inside the mouth. Most are of unknown cause and usually disappear after afew days. Aphthous ulcers.

Mouth wash A solution for rinsing the mouth.

Movement 1. An act of moving; motion. 2. An act of defecation.

Active movement Movement produced by the person's own muscles.

Associated movement Movement of parts that act together, as the eyes.

Passive movement A movement of the body or of the extremities of a patient performed by another person without voluntary motion on the part of the patient.

Vermicular movements The worm-like movements of the intestines in peristalsis.

Moving and handling Technically the moving, lifting or supporting of a load. In the work environment, this is now subject to state (Health & Safety at Work Act 1974) to enforce the regulations and guidelines to reduce the risk of back injuries for nurses.

Moxa A small mass of combustible material placed near the skin and ignited to produce counter irritation.

Moxalactam A cephalosporin group antibiotic.

Moxibustion Counter irritation by means of a moxa.

Moxifloxacin A quinolone antibiotic.

MRI Magnetic Resonance Imaging.

MRSA Methicillin-resistant *Staphylococcu saureus*.

Muciferous Secreting or producing mucus.

Mucilage In pharmacology, a thick viscous liquid, a water solution of the mucilaginous principles of certain vegetable substances.

Mucin A substance secreted by mucous membranes containing mucopolysaccharide which raises the viscosity of medium around it.

Mucinase An enzyme which acts upon mucin. Contained in some aerosols and useful in the treatment of cystic fibrosis.

Mucinosis An abnormal accumulation of mucopoly saccharides in the skin.

Mucocele A mucous tumor.

Lacrimal mucocele A distension of the lacrimal sac caused by a blockage of the nasolacrimal duct.

Mucocele of the gallbladder Occurs if a stone obstructs the cystic duct.

Mucoclasis The surgical removal or destruction of the inner lining of any hollow organ.

Mucocyte An amorphous extracellular basophilic metachromatic mass averaging 100 µ found in white matter of normal and abnormal brains; probably artifactual, derived from precipitation of myelin during tissue fixation.

Mucocutaneous Pertaining to mucous membrane and skin.

Mucocutaneous lymph node syndrome (Kawasaki disease) Condition affecting mainly infants and young children; marked by fever, conjunctivitis, reddening of oral cavity and lips, cervical lymphadenopathy, peeling of hands and feet.

Coronary arteritis with infarction is a complication and aneurysms in coronary circulation may occur.

Mucoenteritis Inflammation of intestinal mucous membrane.

Mucoid Resembling mucus.

Mucolipidosis Any inborn error of metabolism that has characteristics of both mucopolysaccharidosis and sphyngolipidosis. 4 distinct types of disease known and are autosomal recessive.

Mucolytic A drug that has a mucous-softening effect and so reduces the viscosity of the bronchial secretion in chest disorders.

Mucopolysaccharidase Enzyme that catalyzes hydrolysis of polysaccharides.

Mucopolysaccharide Polysaccharide that forms chemical bonds with water. It is thick, gelatinous and forms intercellular ground substance. It is found in mucous secretions and synovial fluid. *SYN* – Glycosaminoglycan.

Mucopolysaccharidosis (MPS) A group of inherited disorders with accumulation of mucopolysaccharides in reticuloendothelial system, intimal smooth muscle cells and fibroblasts within body; manifesting with coarse facies, mental retardation, corneal clouding, skeletal dysplasia, joint stiffness, etc.

Mucopurulent Containing mucus and pus.

Mucoprotein A complex of protein and mucopolysaccharide.

Mucoprotein Tamm-Horsfall It is secreted in renal tubules (not from plasma) and is contained in most urinary casts.

Mucor A genus of fungi seen on dead or decaying matter; often causes infection of external ear, skin and respiratory passage.

Mucosa Mucous membrane.

Mucous Pertaining to or secreting mucus.

Mucous membrane A membrane that secretes mucus and lines many of the body cavities, particularly those of the respiratory and alimentary tracts.

Mucositis Inflammation of mucous membrane.

Mucoviscidosis Fibrocytic disease of the pancreas *(See Fibrocystic)*.

Mucus The viscous secretion of mucous membrane.

Multi Prefix indicating many or much.

Multicellular Consisting of manycells.

Multidisciplinary Involving two or more professional disciplines.

Multigravida A pregnant woman who has had two or more pregnancies.

Multilocular Having manly locules.

Multilocular cyst A cyst, usually in the ovary, containing many compartments.

Multinuclear Possessing many nuclei.

Multipara A woman who has had two or more children.

Multiple Manifold, occurring in many parts of the body at once.

Multiple myeloma Malignant disease of the plasma cells which invade the bone marrow and suppress its functioning.

Multiple sclerosis (See Sclerosis).

Multiple organ dysfunction syndrome Abbreviated MODS and also known as multiple organ failure (MOF). A situation usually precipitated by shock or trauma in which the functioning of interdependent body systems is severely affected, e.g., respiration, gastrointestinal tract, kidneys, blood circulation and coagulation. This multiple organ failure causes physiological disturbances requiring vital system support to maintain life. Other systems too may be compromised.

Multiple personality Condition in which the subject may develop more than one personality.

Multivariate analysis The analysis of data collected on several different variables but all having a relevance to the study; e.g., in a survey of the provision of community nursing services for a specific population, data may be collected on age, family size and previous use of the services. In analysing the data the softening effect of each of these variables and their interaction can be examined and considered.

Multivitamin A brown, sugar-coated tablet containing vitamin A (2500 units), thiamine hydrochloride (500 mg), ascorbic acid (12.5 mg)and vitamin D (250 units).

Mummification Drying and shriveling of body; mortification producing a dry hard mass.

Mumps A communicable paramyxovirus disease, which is statutorily notifiable. It attacks one or both of the three pairs of salivary glands; also called epidemic parotitis or epidemic parotiditis. Most common amongst children; characterized by inflammation and swelling of the parotid glands. The symptoms are fever, and a painful swelling in front of the ears, making mastication difficult.

Munchausen's syndrome *Baron von Muchausen, 16th century German traveler noted for his lying tales.* Habitual seeking of hospital treatment for apparent acute illness, the patient giving a plausible and dramatic history, all of which is false.

Munchausen's syndrome by proxy An uncommon situation in which a parent's fabricate symptoms or signs in a child, who is then presented for hospital treatment; overlaps with other forms of child abuse, and fatal outcomes have been reported.

Münchhausen's syndrome Münchhausen's syndrome Baron von Munchhausen, 16th century German traveller noted for his lying tales. Habitual seeking of medical treatment for apparent acute illness, the patient giving a plausible and dramatic history, all of which is false. M.s. by proxy A situation in which a parent (usually the mother) or both parents fabricate symptoms or signs in a child, who is then presented for hospital treatment; overlaps with other forms of child abuse, and fatal outcomes have been reported.

Mupirocin Broad spectrum topical antibacterial.

Muramidase *SYN* – lysozyme. An enzyme richly present in leukocytes. Level increased in leukemias.

Murmur A sound, heard on auscultation, usually originating in the cardiovascular system.

Aortic murmur One indicating disease of the aortic valve.

Diastolic murmur One heard after the second heart sound.

Friction murmur One present when two inflamed surfaces of serous membrane rub on each other.

Mitral murmur A sign of incompetence of the mitral valve.

Systolic murmur One heard during systole.

Murphy's sign *JB Murphy. American surgeon, 1857–1916.* A sign denoting inflammation of the gallbladder. Continuous pressure over the organ will cause the patient to 'catch breath' at the zenith of inspiration.

Musca domestica The common house fly transmitting cholera, typhoid, amebic/bacillary dysentery, and other diseases.

Muscae volitantes Black spots floating before the eyes. They do not obscure the sight.

Muscarine A poisonous alkaloid found in certain fungi, and causing muscle paralysis.

Muscle Strong tissue composed of fibers which have the power of contraction, and thus produce movements of the body.

Cardiac muscle Muscle composed of partially striped interlocking cells. Not under the control of the will.

Muscle relaxant One of a group of drugs used to reduce muscular spasm and also to relax the muscles during surgery.

Smooth or *non-striated muscle* Involuntary muscle of spindle-shaped cells, e.g., that of the intestinal wall. Contracts independently of the will.

Striped or *striated muscle* Voluntary muscle. Transverse bands across the fibers give the characteristic appearance. It is under the control of the will.

Muscle cramp Painful contraction of muscle, idiopathic or due to electrolyte imbalance.

Muscular 1. Pertaining to muscle. 2. Well provided with strong muscles.

Muscular dystrophy One of a number of inherited diseases in which there is progressive musclewasting *(See Duchenne dystrophy).*

Musculocutaneous Referring to the muscles and the skin.

Musculocutaneous nerve One of the nerves which supply the muscles and the skin of the arms and legs.

Musculoskeletal Referring to both the osseus and muscular systems.

Mushbite Making a dental impression by asking the patient to bite into a soft wax.

Mushroom Umbrella – shaped fungus growing on decaying material.

Mussel's sign Nodding movement of head synchronous with ventricular contraction as in gross aortic incompetence.

Mussilation The muttering of delirium or moving of the lips without production of sound.

M

Mustard Powder of mustard seeds used as counter-irritant, rubefacient, emetic, stimulant, and condiment.

Mustine hydrochloride Nitrogenmustard. A cytotoxic drug which may be given intravenously for malignant disease of lymph glands and reticuloendothelial cells, such as Hodgkin's disease.

Mutagent Any agent that causes gene mutation, e.g., ionizing radiation

Mutant 1. In genetics, a variation owing to genetic changes. 2. Produced by mutation.

Mutase Enzyme that accelerates oxidation – reduction reactions.

Mutation A chemical change in the genes of a cell causing it to show a new characteristic. Some produce evolutional changes, others disease.

Mute Without the power of speech.
Deaf mute One who cannot hear and therefore cannot speak.

Mutilation Deliberate infliction of bodily injury.

Mutism Inability or refusal to speak. In almost all cases mutes are unable to speak because deafness has prevented them from hearing the spoken word. Speech is learned by imitating the speech of others. May also result from disease, the most common being a stroke.
Elective mutism Psychological disorder of childhood.

Myalgia Pain in the muscles.

Myalgic Encephalomyelitis Abbreviated ME. *(See Chronic Fatigue Syndrome).*

Myiasis Infestation with larva of flies or maggots.

Myasthenia Muscle weakness.
Myasthenia gravis An extreme form of muscle weakness which is progressive. There is a rapid onset of fatigue, thought to be due to the too rapid destruction of acetylcholine at the neuromuscular junction. Commonly affected muscles are those of vision, speaking, chewing and swallowing.

Mycetes The fungi

Mycetoma A chronic fungus infection of the tissues, both external and internal but most commonly affecting the hands and feet. There is swelling and the formation of sinuses. Madura foot.

Mycobacterium A genus of slender, rod-shaped, acid-fast Gram-positive bacteria.
Mycobacterium leprae Causative organism of leprosy.
Mycobacterium tuberculosis Causative organism of tuberculosis.

Mycology The study of fungi.

Mycoplasma Organisms in between bacteria and viruses, responsible for a typical pneumonia, urethritis; common forms are – *Mycoplasma hominis, Mycoplasma orale, Microplasma salivarium.*

Mycosis Any disease that is caused by a fungus.
Mycosis fungoides A rare malignant lymphoreticular neoplasm of the skin which later progresses to the lymph nodes and viscera.

Mydriasis Abnormal dilatation of the pupil of the eye. Usually caused by injury to the pupil sphincter or by the use of mydriatic drugs.

Mydriatic Any drug that causes mydriasis. Used in examination of the eye and in the treatment of inflammatory conditions.

Myelencephalon The embryonic hindbrain giving rise to medulla oblongata.

Myelin The fatty covering of medullated nerve fibers.

Myelinosis Fatty degeneration during which myelin is produced.

Myelitis 1. Inflammation of the spinal-cord, causing pain in the back and sometimes numbness and paralysis of the legs and the lower part of the trunk. 2. Inflammation of the bone marrow; osteomyelitis.

M

Myeloblast A primitive cell in the bone marrow, from which develop the granular leukocytes.

Myelocele Protrusion of spinal cord through a defect in spinal arch – usually spina bifida.

Myelocyte A cell of the bone marrow, derived from a myeloblast.

Myelofibrosis A condition cursor in bone marrow.

Myelography Radiographic examination of the spinal cord after the introduction of a radiopaque substance into the subarachnoid space by means of lumbar puncture.

Myelolysis Dissolution of myelin.

Myeloid 1. Pertaining to, derived from or resembling bone marrow. 2. Pertaining to the spinal cord. 3. Having the appearance of myelocytes, but not necessarily derived from bone marrow.

Myeloid leukaemia A malignant disease in which there is excessive production of leukocytes in the bone marrow.

Myeloid tissue Red bone marrow.

Myeloma A tumor composed of plasma cells.

Multiple myeloma A primary malignant tumor of plasma cells, usially arising in bone marrow, and usually associated with anemia and with a paraprotein in the blood or Bence Jones protein in the urine.

Myelomalacia Abnormal softening of spinal cord.

Myelomatosis A malignant disease of the bone marrow in which multiple myelomas are present.

Myelomeningocele Meningomyelocele.

Myelopathy Any pathological condition of spinal cord.

Myelopoiesis Development of bone marrow.

Myeloproliferative Concerning proliferation of bone marrow elements.

Myenteric reflex Intestinal contraction above and relaxation below the pin dot stimulation.

Myoblast Embryonic cell developing into muscle fiber.

Myiasis Infestation of wounds or body openings by fly larvae (maggots); more commonly seen in the tropics.

Myocardial Pertaining to the myocardium.

Myocardial infarction Necrosis of a part of the myocardium usually following a coronary thrombosis. Ventricular fibrillation may occur, followed by death.

Myocarditis Inflammation of the myocardium.

Myocardium The muscle tissue of the heart.

Myoclonus Spasmodic contraction of the muscles.

Myocyte A muscle cell.

Myodynamometer Device for determining muscle strength.

Myoepithelial cells Spindle shaped contractile cells found between glandular elements and basement membrane of sweat, mammary and salivary glands.

Myoepthelium Tissue containing contractile epithelial cells.

Myofibrosis A degenerative condition in which there is some replacement of muscle tissue by fibrous tissue.

Myofilament Electron microscopic picture of muscle showing thick *myosin* and thin *actin* filaments, essential for muscle contraction.

Myograph Instrument for graphic recording of muscle contraction.

Myohaemoglobin A substance, resembling hemoglobin, which is present in muscle cells. It is a pigment and is responsible for the color of muscle. It acts as an oxygen store. Myoglobin.

Myokymia A benign condition in which there is persistent quivering of the muscles.

M

Myoma A benign tumor of muscletis-sue *(See Fibromyoma)*.

Myomectomy Removal of a myoma; usually referring to a uterine fibroma.

Myometrium The muscular tissue of the uterus.

Myoneural Relating to both muscle and nerve.

Myoneural junction The point at which nerve endings terminate in a muscle; neuromuscular junction.

Myopathy Any disease of the muscles. Muscular dystrophy is one of a group of inherited myopathies in which there is wasting and weakness of the muscles.

Myope One suffering from myopia or short sightedness.

Myopia Short sightedness. The light rays focus in front of the retina and a biconcave lens is needed to focus them correctly.

Myoplasm The contractile part of the muscle cell.

Myoplasty Any operation in which muscle is detached and utilized, as may be done to correct deformities.

Myorrhaphy Suture of a muscle wound.

Myosarcoma A sarcomatous tumor of muscle.

Myosin Muscle protein.

Myositis Inflammation of a muscle.

Myositis ossificans A condition in which bone cells deposited in muscle continue to grow and cause hard lumps. It may occur after fractures.

Myotomy The division or dissection of a muscle.

Myotonia Lack of muscle tone.

Myotonia congenita A hereditary disease in which the muscle action has a prolonged contraction phase and slow relaxation.

Myringa The eardrum or tympanic membrane.

Myringitis Inflammation of the tympanic membrane.

Myringoplasty A plastic operation to repair the tympanic membrane; Tympanoplasty.

Myringotome An instrument for puncturing the tympanic membrane in myringotomy.

Myringotomy Incision of the tympanic membrane to drain fluid from an infected middle ear.

Mythophobia Abnormal fear of making an incorrect statement.

Myxoedema A condition, caused by hypothyroidism, which is marked by mucoid infiltration of the skin. There is oedematous swelling of the face, limbs and hands, dry and rough skin, loss of hair, slow pulse, subnormal temperature, slowed metabolism and mental dullness.

Congenital myxoedema Cretinism.

Myxoma A benign mucous tumor of connective tissue.

Myxosarcoma A sarcoma containing mucoid tissue.

Myxovirus The group name of a number of related viruses, including the causal viruses of influenza, para-influenza, mumps and Newcastle disease (of fowl).

M

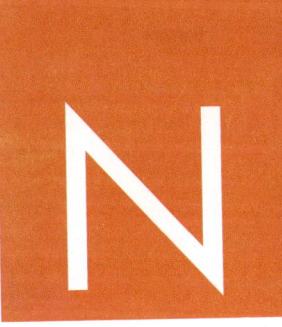

N Symbol for nitrogen and newton.

Na Symbol for sodium.

Naboth's follicle or cyst *M. Naboth. German anatomist, 1675–1721.* Cystic swelling of a cervical gland, the duct of which has become blocked by regenerating squamous epithelium.

NAAC National Assessment and Accreditation Commission.

Nabumetone Anti-inflammatory pain killer.

Nadir The lowest out of a series of measurements, e.g., the lowest level to which the viral load falls after starting antiretroviral treatment. The opposite is Zenith.

Nadolol A betablocker, used in hypertension.

Nadroparin Factor Xa inhibitor anticoagulant.

Naegele *German obstetrician (1777-1851).*

   Naegele obliquity Anterior parietal presentation of fetal head in labor.

   Naegle pelvis An obliquely contracted pelvis.

   Naegele rule The method of counting expected date of delivery by counting 90 days backwards from LMP and adding 7 days to that date.

Naevus A birthmark; a circumscribed area of pigmentation of the skin due to dilated blood vessels. A hemangioma.

   Naevus flammeus A flat bluish-red area, usually on the neck or face; popularly known as 'portwine stain'.

   Naevus pilosus A hairy naevus.

   Spider naevus A small red area surrounded by dilated capillaries.

   Strawberry naevus A raised tumor-like structure of connective tissue containing spaces filled with blood.

Nafcillin A semisynthetic penicillinase resistant penicillin.

Nafoxidin Antiestrogen.

Naftidrofuryl An agent used in the treatment of peripheral and cerebral vascular disorders.

Nägele's rule Rule for calculating the estimated date of labor; add one year, subtract 3 months and add 7 days to the first day of the last menstrual period.

NAI Non-accidental injury.

Nail The keratinized portion of epidermis covering the dorsal extremity of the fingers and toes.

   Hang nail A strip of epidermis hanging at one side or at the root of a nail.

   Ingrowing nail A condition in which the flesh overhangs the edge of the nail, a sharp corner of which may pierce the skin, causing a wound which may become septic.

   Intermedullary nail Surgical rod inserted into the intermedullary canal to fix the fracture.

   Nail bed The skin underlying a nail.

   Smith – Peterson nail A three flanged nail used to fix fracture neck of femur.

   Spoon nail A nail with a depression in the center and raised edges. Koilonychia.

Naked Exposed to view, without cloth.

Nalbuphine Opioid receptor antagonist.

Nalidixic acid An antibacterial agent used in the treatment of urinary infections.

Nalorphine Narcotic antagonist.

Naloxone A narcotic antagonist used as an antidote to narcotic overdosage and as an antagonist for pentazocine over dosage.

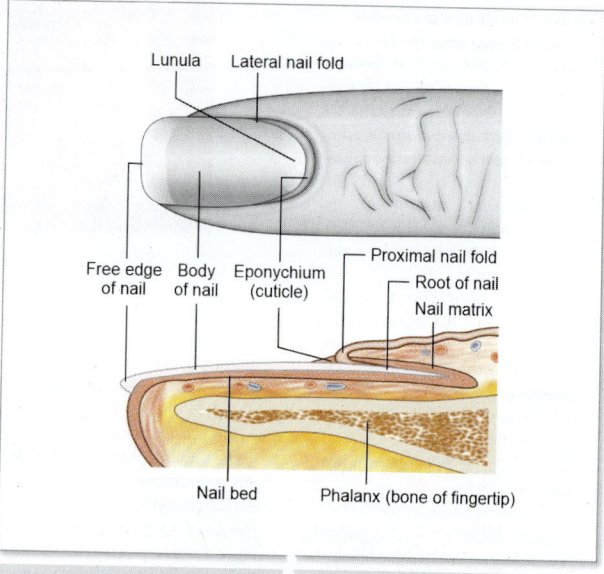

Lunula   Lateral nail fold

Free edge   Body   Eponychium
of nail   of nail   (cuticle)

Proximal nail fold
Root of nail
Nail matrix

Nail bed   Phalanx (bone of fingertip)

Structure of Nail

Naltrexone Narcotic antagonist.

NANDA North American Nursing Diagnosis Association.

Nandrolone An anabolic steroid that promotes protein metabolism and skeletal growth.

Nanism Dwarf-like body build.

Nano 10^{-9} or one billionth part.

Nanometer Symbol nm. A unit of measurement equal to one billionth (10^{-9}) of a meter, or more commonly used to describe a measure equal to one thousandth (10^{-3}) of micrometer (um). Nanometers are used to describe the smallest particles in nature, e.g., atoms, small molecules, viruses, electromagnetic radiation). A nanometer is approximately the length of three to six atoms placed side by side, or the width of a single strand of DNA; the thickness of a human hair is between 50,000 and 1,00,000 mm and represents the smallest feature an unaided human eye can see.

Nape The back of the neck.

Naphazoline hydrochloride Topical vasoconstrictor; ingredient of nasal and eye drops.

Naphthalene A coaltar derivative, used as antimoth agent.

Nappy rash An erythematous rash that may occur in infants in the napkin area. Many causes include the passage of frequent loose stools, thrush and ammoniacal dermatitis.

Naproxen Anti-inflammatory pain killer.

Narcissism The stage of infant development when children are mainly interested in themselves and their own bodily needs. In adults it may be a symptom of mental disorder. The term is derived from the Greek legend of *Narcissus*.

Narcoanalysis A form of psycho therapy in which an injection of a narcotic drug produces a drowsy relaxed state during which a patient will talk more freely, and in this way much repressed material may be brought to consciousness.

Narcolepsy A condition in which there is an uncontrollable desire for sleep.

Narcosis A state of unconsciousness produced by a narcotic drug.
Basal narcosis A state of unconsciousness produced prior to surgical anesthesia.

Narcosynthesis The inducement of a hypnotic state by means of drugs. An aid to psychotherapy.

Narcotic A drug that produces narcosis or unnatural sleep.

Nares The nostrils.
Posterior nares The opening of the nares into the nasopharynx.

Nasal Pertaining to the nose.

Nasal feeding Feeding through a tube passing through nose.

Nasal index The greater width of nasal aperture in relation to line from the lower edge of nasal aperture to the nasion.

Nasal obstruction Blockage of nasal passage.

Nasal reflex Inducible sneezing from irritation of nasal mucosa.

Nasal septum deviation (NSD) Is a deformity of the nasal septum from midline, and the resulting nasal obstruction may lead to hypoxia.

Nascent 1. At the time of birth. 2. Incipient.

Naseptin Trade name for a combination preparation containing chlorhexidine and neomycin, a nasal cream for the treatment of staphylococcal infections.

Nasion The point where sagittal plane intersects frontonasal suture (root of nose).

Nasmyth's membrane Epithelial membrane that envelops the enamel of a tooth after birth.

Nasoduodenal Related to the nose and duodenum.
N. tube A fine-bore tube passed through the nose into the duodenum and used for enteral nutrition.

Nasogastric Referring to the nose and stomach.
Nasogastric tube One passed into the stomach via the nose.

Nasojejunal feeding A method in which a silicone-coated catheter is passed through the nose into the jejunum to provide sufficient nutrition to a sick baby on a ventilator or receiving continuous inflating pressure (CIP) by mask or nasal tube. It is used to prevent the dangers of aspiration with a nasogastric tube feed.

Nasolacrimal Concerning both the nose and lacrimal apparatus.
Nasolacrimal duct The duct draining the tears from the inner aspect of the eye to the inferior meatus of the nose.

Nasomental reflex Percussion on side of nose causing contraction of mentalis muscle with elevation of lower lip and wrinkling of skin of the chin.

Nasopharyngitis Inflammation of nasopharynx.

Nasopharynx The upper part of the pharynx; that above the soft palate.

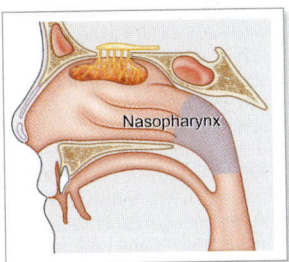

Nasopharynx

Nasosinusitis Inflammation of the nose and adjacent sinuses.

Natal Relating to birth.

Natality See birth rate.

Natamycin Topical antibiotic.

Nateglinide Antidiabetic.

Nates Gluteal region *SYN* – buttocks.

National Audit office (NAO) This is an independent Parliamentary body in the UK, responsible for scrutinizing public spending by auditing the financial statements of all central government departments, agencies and other public bodies. The NAO reports to the Comptroller and Auditor General in Parliament. Audit Scotland performs a similar role in Scotland. The Wales Audit Office is responsible for auditing the Welsh Assembly Government, its public bodies and local government in Wales. The Northern Ireland Audit Office performs similar functions in Northern Ireland.

National Boards The National Boards for Nursing, Midwifery and Health Visiting were originally set up in England, Wales, Scotland and Northern Ireland by the 1979 Nurses, Midwives and Health Visitors Act. The key role of the Boards is to approve institutions in relation to the provision of courses. In fulfilling this role, the Boards are required to ensure that the courses so approved meet the standards of the United Kingdom Central Council for Nursing, Midwifery and Health Visiting (UKCC). Each National Board has an important relationship with the UKCC and its respective functions are defined in law.

National confidential Enquiry into Patient Outcome and Death (NCEPOD) Is the system for reviewing the management of patients by undertaking confidential surveys and research. Mothers and Babies: Reducing Risk through Audits and Confidential Enquiries (MBRRACE) runs the national program of work conducting investigations into maternal deaths, stillbirths and infant deaths. The national confidential inquiry into suicide and homicide by people with mental illness (NCISH) delivers the mental health outcome review program. *(See Confidential Enquiry).*

National Institute for health and care Excellence Abbreviated NICE. An executive non-departmental public body serving England and Wales, providing formal advice for the NHS and social care through the publication of guidelines in four areas: 1. Use of new technologies within the NHS e.g., use of new and existing medicines, treatments and procedures. 2. Clinical practice focused on care and treatment of people with specific diseases and conditions. 3. Guidance for public sector workers on health promotion. 4. Guidance for social care services and users.

National Vocational Qualifications Abbreviated NVQs. Nationally recognized work-related qualifications that are coordinated by the National Council for Vocational Qualifications. NVQs are based on a system of credits earned after a work-based assessment of skills and the level of competence attained.

Native Born with, inherent.

Natriuresis Excess excretion of sodium in urine.

Natural childbirth A term used to describe an approach to labor and delivery in which the parents are prepared for the event so that the mother is awake and cooperative and the father is able to assume an active and supportive role during the birth of their child. The underlying concept for all methods of natural childbirth is avoidance of medical interference and analgesia in labor, and education of the parents so that they can actively participate in and share the experience of childbirth.

Natural family planning A method of family planning in which a woman keeps records of her menstrual cycle and tracks her fertile time. It does not require any pill or device for family planning.

Natural killer cells Large T-lymphocytes that bind to cells infected with viruses and kill them and often kill tumor cells; the most natural defence against tumor/viral infection.

Nature-nurture debate The debate surrounding the issue of to what extent human behavior is the result of hereditary or innate influences (nature) or is determined by the environment and learning (nurture).

Naturopathy A drugless system of healing by a combination of diet, fasting, exercise, hydrotherapy and positive thinking.

Nausea A sensation of sickness with an inclination to vomit.

Nausea gravidarum Morning sickness of pregnancy.

Nauseant Provoking nausea.

Navel The umbilicus.

Navicular Boat-shaped.

Navicular bone One of the tarsal bones of the foot.

Near point Closest point of near vision with maximum accommodation. It is 3 at 2 years and recedes to 40 at 60 years.

Nearsighted Only able to see clearly the near objects; *SYN* – myopia, corrected by concave lens.

Nabivolol A beta blocker for hypertension.

Nebula A slight opacity or cloudiness of the cornea, caused by injury or by corneal ulceration.

Nebulizer An apparatus for reducing a liquid to a fine spray. An atomizer.

NEC Necrotizing enterocolitis.

Necator A genus of nematode hookworms, includes *N. americanus.*

Neck 1. The narrow part of an organ or bone. 2. The part of the body which connects the head and the trunk.

Derbyshire neck Simple goiter.

Femoral neck The thick compact portion of femur joining head with the shaft.

Neck of mandible The narrow area below the articular condyle where are attached the lateral pterygoid muscle and the articular capsule.

Surgical neck of humerus The narrowed portion of humerus below the tuberosity; more prone for fracture.

Wry neck Torticollis.

Necklace of Casal Ring of pigmented reddened skin around the neck in pellagra.

Necrobiosis Localized death of a part as a result of degeneration.

Necromimesis A delusion in which one believes to be dead.

Necrophilia Sexual intercourse with dead; abnormal interest in corpses.

Necropsy Autopsy; a postmortem examination of a body.

Necrosis Death of a portion of tissue.

Necrosis coagulation Necrosis where the necrosed area is converted to a homogeneous mass.

Necrotizing Causing necrosis.

Necrotizing enterocolitis Abbreviated NEC. A condition of neonates in which there is severe diarrhea and blood in the stools. It occurs in preterm or low birth weight neonates. Exact cause is not known but is often associated with infection.

Necrotizing fascilitis A bacterial infection of Streptococcus type A underneath the skin in the fascia layer; produces necrosis and toxins, resulting in shock and organ failure. Urgent treatment is required with antibiotics and surgical excision of the infected tissues.

N

Need analysis Exercise often undertaken by NHS Trusts, service organizations and agencies of a target population to assess a service or situation with a view to change, e.g., alteration in clinic times. Multiple research methods and techniques for data collection and analysis may be used in the process.

Needle holder Forceps used for holding surgical needle.

Needle stick injury An accidental injury with a needle that is contaminated with blood or body fluids. The term is also used sometimes to include other sharp injuries. The injuries have been reported as a means of infecting the nurse or health-care professional with hepatitis or human immunodeficiency virus (HIV).

Needling Discission, the operation for cataract of lacerating and splitting up the lens so that it may be absorbed.

Needs (See Joint Strategic Needs Assessment and Maslow's Hierarchy of Needs).

Nefopam Pain killer.

Negative The opposite of positive. The absence of some quality or substance.

Negativism A symptom of mental illness in which the patient does the opposite of what is required and so presents an uncooperative attitude. Common in schizophrenia.

Negligence In law, the failure to do something that a reasonable person of ordinary prudence would do in a certain situation or the doing of something that such a person would not do. Negligence may provide the basis for a lawsuit when there is a legal duty, as in the duty of a doctor or nurse to provide reasonable care to patients, and when the negligence results in damage to the patient.

Negri bodies Aggregation in nerve cells as in rabies.

Neisseria ALS Neisser, German acteriologist, 1855–1916. A genus of paired, spherical Gram-negative bacteria.
Neisseria gonorrhoeae The causative organism of gonorrhea.
Neisseria meningitides The cause of meningococcal meningitis.

Nelfinavir Anti-HIV agent.

Nelton's line Line from anterior superior iliac spine to tuberosity of ischium.

Nematoda A phylum of worms, including the *Ascaris* or roundworm and the *Enterobius* or threadworm.

Neoadjuvant therapy Chemotherapy given prior to radiation treatment or surgery to reduce the size of a tumor.

Neocerebellum The posterior lobe of cerebellum that develops last and is concerned with integrations of voluntary movements.

Neocortex The cerebral cortex, excluding the hippocampal formation and piriform area.

Neodymium A silvery rare earth metal used in LASER.

Neogenesis Regeneration of tissue.

Neoglycogenesis The formation of liver glycogen from non-carbohydrate sources. Glyconeogenesis.

Neologism The formation of new words, either completely new ones or ones formed by contraction of two separate words. This is done particularly by schizophrenic patients.

Neomycin An antibiotic drug used against a wide range of bacteria, frequently those affecting the skin or the eyes. Also given orally to sterilize the bowel before surgery.

Neon A rare inert gas.

Neonatal Referring to the first month of life.
Neonatal mortality rate The number of deaths of infants up to 4 weeks old per 1000 live births in any 1 year.
Neonatal period The interval from the birth to 28 days of age and the period of greatest risk to the infant.

Neonate Newborn; specifically pertaining to a baby under 1 month old.

Neonatologist A medically qualified person specializing in the management, assessment, diseases and intensive care of newborn babies, especially those of low birthweight and those with congenital abnormalities.

Neonatology The branch of medicine dealing with disorders of the newborn infant.

Neoplasia The development of neoplasms.

Neoplasm A morbid new growth; a tumor. It may be benign or malignant.

Benign neoplasm Growth having a definite capsule and non-infiltrating.

Malignant neoplasm Growth that lacks a capsule, infiltrates surrounding structures or has distant metastasis, or recurs after surgery.

Neostigmine A synthetic preparation akin to physostigmine used in the treatment of myasthenia gravis and as an antidote to some muscle relaxant drugs, and as eye drops in the treatment of glaucoma.

Neostriatum Caudate nucleus and putamen together.

Neothalamus The lateral and dorsomedial parts of thalamus.

Nepenthe Trade name for a preparation containing opium alkaloids, used as an analgesic.

Nephralgic Relating to pain arising from the kidney.

Nephralgic crises Spasms of pain in the lumbar region in tabes dorsalis.

Nephrectomy Excision of a kidney.

Nephritis Inflammation of the kidney; a focal or diffuse proliferative or destructive disease that may involve the glomerulus, tubule or interstitial renal tissue. Also called Bright's disease. The most usual form is glomerulonephritis.

Nephritogenic Causing nephritis.

Nephroblastoma A rapidly developing malignant mixed tumor of the kidneys, made up of embryonic cells, and occurring chiefly in children before the fifth year; Wilm's tumor.

Nephrocalcinosis A condition in which there is deposition of calcium in the renal tubules, resulting in calculi formation and renal insufficiency.

Nephrocapsulectomy An operation for removal of the capsule of the kidney.

Nephrogram A radiograph of the kidney with contrast medium in the renal tubules. Usually the immediate film in an excretion urogram.

Nephroid Resembling kidney.

Nephrolith Stone in the kidney; renal calculus.

Nephrolithiasis The presence of a calculus or a gravel in the kidney.

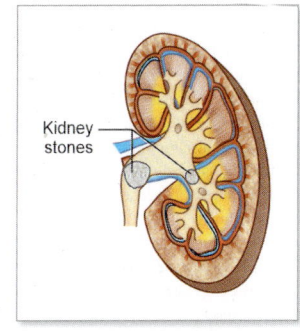

Kidney stones

Nephrolithiasis

Nephrolithotomy Removal of a renal calculus by incising the kidney or by extra corporeal shock wave lithotripsy.

Nephrology Study of structure and function of kidneys and diseases related to them.

Nephroma Tumor of the kidney.

Nephromere The intermediate mesoderm of embryo from which kidney develops.

Nephron The functional unit of the kidney, comprising Bowman's capsule, the proximal and distal tubules, the loop of Henle and the collecting duct, which conveys urine to the renal pelvis.

Nephropathy Any diseased condition of kidney including inflammatory, degenerative, arteriosclerotic lesions. For example, analgesic nephropathy, membranous nephropathy, etc.

Nephropexy The fixation of a floating (mobile) kidney, usually by sutures to neighboring muscle.

Nephroptosis Downward displacement, or undue mobility, of a kidney.

Nephropyeloplasty A plastic operation on the pelvis of the kidney, performed in cases of hydronephrosis.

Nephropyosis Suppuration in the kidney.

Nephrosclerosis Constriction of the arterioles of the kidney. Seen in benign and malignant hypertension and in arteriosclerosis in old age.

Nephrosis Any disease of the kidney, especially that characterized by edema, albuminuria and a low-plasma albumin. Caused by non-inflammatory degenerative lesions of the tubules.

Nephrostomy Creation of a permanent opening into the renal pelvis.

Nephrotic Referring to or caused by nephrosis.

Nephrotic syndrome A clinical syndrome in which there is albuminuria, low plasma protein and gross edema. The result of increased capillary permeability in the glomeruli. It may occur as a result of acute glomerulonephritis, in subacute nephritis, diabetes mellitus, amyloid disease, systemic lupus erythematosus and renal vein thrombosis.

Nephrotomogram A tomogram of the kidney obtained by nephrotomography.

Nephrotomography Radiological visualization of the kidney by tomography after introduction of a contrast medium.

Nephrotomy Incision of the kidney.

Nephrotoxic Poisonous or destructive to the cells of the kidney.

Nephroureterectomy Surgical removal of the kidney and the ureter.

Nerve A bundle of conducting fibers enclosed in a sheath called the epineurium. Its function is to transmit impulses between any part of the body and a nerve center. Cranial nerve (s) -12, (mnemonic – ooottafagvah), 1. Olfactory, 2. Optic, 3. Oculomotor, 4. Trochlear, 5. Trigeminal, 6. Abducens, 7. Facial, 8. Vestibulocochlear, 9. Glossopharyngeal, 10. Vagus, 11. Accessory, 12. Hypoglossal.

Motor (efferent) nerve One that conveys impulses causing activity from a nerve center to a muscle or gland.

Nerve block A method of producing regional anesthesia by injecting a local anesthetic into the nerves supplying the area to be operated on.

Nerve fiber The prolongation of the nerve cell, which conveys impulses. Each fiber has a sheath. Medullated nerve fibers have an insulating myelin sheath.

Nerve gas A gas that interferes with the functioning of the nerves and muscles. Such gases may cause death from respiratory paralysis; some of them act through the skin and cannot be avoided by the use of gas masks.

Sensory (afferent) nerve One that conveys sensation from an area to a nerve center.

Nervous 1. Pertaining to, or composed of, nerves. 2. Apprehensive.

Nervous breakdown A popular and misleading term for any type of mental illness that interferes with a person's normal activities.

A so-called 'nervous breakdown' can include any of the mental disorders, including neurosis, psychosis or depression, but is usually used to describe neurosis.

Nervousness Excitability of the nervous system, characterized by a state of mental and physical unrest.

Nesiblastoma Islet tumor of pancreas.

Nettle rash An allergic skin condition; urticaria.

Nesting The provision of an enclosed space bounded by a small blanket roll encircling the sick or preterm infant in a cot or incubator. This helps to provide a supportive, calming environment for the infant.

Netilmicin Aminoglycoside antibiotic.

Network 1. An interconnected group or system of voluntary organizations or of colleagues with similar interests. 2. A system of interconnected computer terminals in which the user has access to others using the system for sharing data, etc.

Networking 1. Forming and maintaining professional connections and contacts through informal social meetings. 2. The interconnection of two or more computer networks in different places.

Neural Pertaining to the nerves.

Neural arch The bony arch on each vertebra, which encloses the spinal cord.

Neural crest A band of cells along the neural tube of embryo from which cells forming cranial, spinal and autonomic ganglia arise.

Neural fold One of two longitudinal elevations of the neural plate of embryo that unite to form the neural tube.

Neural plate A thickened band of ectoderm along the dorsal surface of an embryo.

Neural tube Tube formed from fusion of neural folds.

Neural tube defect Any of a group of congenital malformations involving the neural tube, including anencephaly, hypocephalus and spina bifida.

Neuralgia A sharp stabbing pain, usually along the course of a nerve, owing to neuritis or functional disturbance.

Glossopharyngeal neuralgia Severe pain in the back of throat, tonsils and middle ear along the distribution of glossopharyngeal nerve.

Trigeminal neuralgia Neuralgia involving the gasserian ganglion or one or more branches of trigeminal nerve.

Neurapraxia An injury to a nerve resulting in temporary loss of function and paralysis. It is usually caused by compression of the nerve, and there is no lasting damage.

Neurasthenia A neurosis in which there is much mental and physical fatigue, inability to concentrate, loss of appetite, and a failure of memory.

Neurectomy Excision of part of a nerve.

Neurilemma The membranous sheath surrounding a nerve fiber.

Neurillemmoma Firm encapsulated tumor of peripheral nerve.

Neurinoma A benign tumor arising in the neurilemma of a nerve fiber.

Neuritis Inflammation of a nerve, with pain, tenderness and loss of function.

Multiple neuritis That involving several nerves; polyneuritis.

Nutritional (alcoholic) neuritis That which may be caused by alcoholism or lack of vitamin B complex.

Optic neuritis That affecting the optic disc or nerve.

Peripheral neuritis That involving the terminations of nerves.

Sciatic neuritis Sciatica.

Tabetic neuritis A type occurring in tabes dorsalis.

Traumatic neuritis That which results from an injury to a nerve.

Neuroblast An embryonic nerve cell.

Neuroablation The act of destroying nerve tissue by surgery, cautery, injection of sclerosing agents, lasers or cryotherapy.

Neuroblastoma A malignant tumor of immature nerve cells, most often arising in the very young.

Neurocirculatory asthenia Functional circulatory and nervous disturbance with precordial pain and fatigue.

Neurodermatitis A localized prurigo of somatic and psychogenic origin. It irritates, and rubbing causes thickening and pigmentation of the skin.

Neurodevelopmental therapy (NDT) A non-invasive approach to the rehabilitation of patients with neurological problems based on current research findings into motor development and neurophysiology.

Neuroepithelioma A malignant tumor of the retina of the eye, which may spread into the brain.

Neuroepithelium Specialized epithelial structure forming the gustatory cells, olfactory cells, hair cells of inner ear, rods and cones of retina.

Neurofibril Tiny fibrils in the cytoplasm of nerve cell body.

Neurofibroma A benign tumor of nerve and fibrous tissue.

Neurofibromatosis von Reckling Hausen's disease. A generalized hereditary disease in which there are numerous fibromas of the skin and nervous system.

Neurogenesis Growth and development of nerve tissues.

Neurogenic Derived from or caused by nerve stimulation.

Neurogenic bladder A disorder of the urinary bladder caused by a lesion of the nervous system.

Neurogenic shock Shock originating in the nervous system.

Neuroglia The special form of connective tissue supporting nerve tissues.

Neurohypophysis The posterior lobe of the pituitary gland.

Neuroleptic A drug which acts on the nervous system.

Neurolinguistic programming (NLP) An approach to communication based on the notion of a connection between neurological processes, language and behavior patterns learned through experience.

Neurological assessment Evaluation of the health status of a patient with a nervous system disorder or dysfunction. Purposes of the assessment include establishing nursing goals to guide the nurse in planning and implementing nursing measures to help the patient cope effectively with daily living activities. Nursing assessment of a patient's neurological status is concerned with identifying functional disabilities that interfere with the person's ability to provide self-care and lead an active life. A functionally oriented nursing assessment includes: (a) Consciousness; (b) Mental functions; (c) Motor function; and (d) Sensory function. Evaluation of these functions gives the nurse information about the patient's ability to perform everyday activities such as thinking, remembering, seeing, eating, speaking, moving, smelling, feeling and hearing. A patient with an acute and life threatening alteration in neurological function is evaluated and monitored in four general areas: (a) Level of consciousness; (b) Sensory and motor function; (c) Pupillary changes; and (d) Vital signs and pattern of respiration.

Neurologist A medical practitioner specializing in neurology.

Neurology 1. The scientific study of the nervous system. 2. The branch of medicine concerned with diseases of the nervous system.

Neurolysis Stretching of a nerve to relieve tension; release of a nerve from fibrous tissue.

Neuroma A tumor consisting of nervous tissue.

Neuromatosis Multiple tumors of nerve tissue.

Neuromuscular Pertaining to nerves and muscles.

Neuromuscular junction The small gap between the end of the motor nerve and the motor end-plate of the muscle fiber supplied. This gap is bridged by the release of acetylcholine whenever a nerve impulse arrives.

Neuromyasthenia Muscular weakness consequent to emotional disorder.

Neuromyelitis Neuritis associated with myelitis. It is a condition a kin to multiple sclerosis.

Neuromyelitis optica A disease in which there is bilateral optic neuritis and paraplegia.

Neuron A nerve cell.

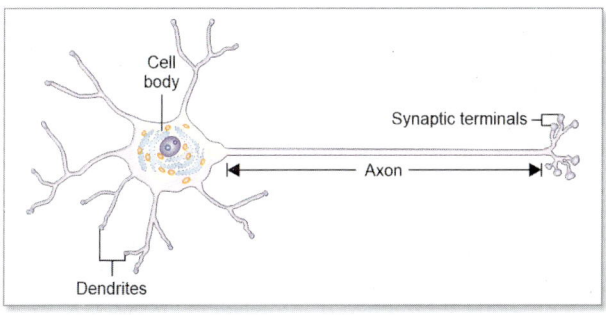

Neuron

Lower motor neuron The anterior horn cell and its neuron which convey impulses to the appropriate muscles.

Afferent neuron Neuron conducting impulses to the brain and spinal cord.

Associative neuron Neuron coordinating impulses between sensory and motor neurons.

Efferent neuron Neurons conducting impulses away from brain and spinal cord.

Preganglionic neuron Neuron of autonomic nervous system whose cell body lies in central nervous system and axon terminates in peripheral ganglia.

Postganglionic neuron Neuron whose cell body lies in an autonomic ganglion and its axon terminates in effect or organ.

Upper motor neuron That in which the cell is in the cerebral cortex and the fibers conduct impulses to associated cells in the spinal cord.

Neuronitis Inflammation of nerve cell.

Neuroparalysis Paralysis due to disease of a nerve or nerves.

Neuropathy A disease process of nerve degeneration and loss of function.

Alcoholic neuropathy Neuropathy due to thiamine deficiency in chronic alcoholism.

Diabetic neuropathy That associated with diabetes.

Entrapment neuropathy Any of a group of neuropathies, e.g., carpal tunnel syndrome, due to mechanical pressure on a peripheral nerve.

Ischemic neuropathy That caused by a lack of blood supply.

Neurophysin Proteins that bind oxytocin and ADH, secreted by posterior pituitary.

Neuroplasticity The capacity for nerve cells to regenerate and recover function.

Neuroplasty The surgical repair of a damaged nerve.

Neuropraxia Trauma to a nerve followed by loss of conduction even though anatomical integrity is maintained.

Neuropsychiatry The medical specialization concerned with the effects on mind and behavior of organic disorders of the nervous system, combining both neurology and psychiatry.

Neuroradiology Branch of medical science utilizing radiography for diagnosis of neurological diseases.

Neurorrhaphy The operation of suturing a divided nerve.

Neurosis A mental disorder, which does not affect the whole personality, characterized by exaggerated anxiety and tension.

Anxiety neurosis Persistent anxiety and the accompanying symptoms of fear, rapid pulse, sweating, trembling, loss of appetite and insomnia.

Obsessive-compulsive neurosis One characterized by compulsions and obsessional rumination.

Neurosurgery That branch of surgery dealing with the brain, spinal cord and nerves.

Neurosyphilis A manifestation of third stage syphilis in which the nervous system is involved. The three most common forms are: (a) Meningovascular syphilis, affecting the blood vessels to the meninges; (b) Tabes dorsalis *(See Ataxia)*; and (c) General paralysis of the Insane.

Neurotensin Tridecapeptide from hypophysis stimulating pituitary.

Neurotic A loosely applied adjective denoting association with neurosis.

Neurotmesis Nerve injury with complete loss of function in absence of anatomical disruption.

Neurotoxic Poisonous or destructive to nervous tissue.

Neurotransmitter A substance, e.g., noradrenaline, acetylcholine, dopamine, that is released from the axon terminal to produce activity in other nerves.

Neurotripsy The surgical bruising or crushing of a nerve.

Neurotropic Having an affinity for nerve tissue.

Neurotropic viruses Those that particularly attack the nervous system.

Neutral Neither alkaline nor acidic, indifferent.

Neutralization The process of counteracting the effects of any harmful agent/substance.

Neutral point A pH of 7.0 which is neither acid nor alkaline.

Neutral red An indicator dye.

Neutron Electrically neutral particle equal in mass to proton.

Neutropenia A decrease in the number of neutrophils in the blood.

Neutrophil A polymorphonuclear leukocyte which has a neutral reaction to acid and alkaline dyes.

Never events Serious events that are entirely preventable and have the potential to cause harm or death to a serious patient.

Nevirapine Anti-HIV agent.

Nevus Congenitally discolored localized area of skin; vascular skin tumor due to hyperplastic blood vessels.

Junctional nevus Nevus in the basal layer of epidermis appearing as a non hairy pigmented area, with high malignancy potential.

Newborn blood spot screening A blood test offered to all babies of 5 days old for the screening of a number of diseases, which are amenable to healthcare interventions if they are identified early. Blood is taken from the baby's heel.

Next of kin Technically a person's closest living relative, whose name is often required for health care information. Patients should be asked whom they wish to nominate as their 'next-of-kin' of 'significant other' in accordance with their own personal situation.

NHS 111/NHS 24 (services in Scotland) A telephone health advice service providing 24-hour access to health care assessment and health information. The service (a) is a private, confidential, reliable and consistent source of professional advice; (b) is speedy with simple access to a comprehensive range of the latest health and health-related information; (c) improves quality, increases cost effectiveness and reduces demands on other NHS services; and (d) allows professionals to develop their role in enabling patients to be partners in self-care.

NHS Blood and Transplant (NHSBT) Special Health Authority for England and Wales set up for the purpose of providing a reliable and efficient supply of blood, tissues, stem cells and organs for transplantation throughout the NHS. *(See also Blood)*.

NHS Improvement (NHSI) An organization, which aims to support NHS Trusts to provide consistent high quality care through the provision of resources and innovations, and by holding providers to account.

NHS Number Ten-digit number used as a unique identifier for every patient.

Niacin Nicotinic acid.

Niche A depression or recess on a smooth surface e.g., ulcer niche.

Nicergoline Cerebral activator.

Nicking Compression of retinal vein at the site crossed by artery.

Niclosamide An antihelmintic used as a single dose in tapeworm infestations.

Nicorandil Vasodilator for angina.

Nicotinamide adenine diphosphate (NADP) An enzyme that accepts electrons.

Nicotine A poisonous alkaloid in tobacco.

Nicotinic acid Niacin. A water-soluble vitamin in the B complex. A deficiency of this vitamin causes pellagra.

Nidation Implantation of the fertilized ovum in the uterus.

Nidus 1. A nest. 2. A place in which an organism finds conditions suitable for its growth and development. 3. The focus of an infection.

Niemann-Pick disease *A. Niemann, German pediatrician, 1880–1921; F Pick, German physician, 1868–1935.* A rare inherited disease occurring primarily in Jewish children and resulting in learning difficulties. There is lipoid storage abnormality and wide spread deposition of lecithin in the tissues.

Nifedipine A calcium channel blocker used as a coronary vasodilator in the treatment of angina pectoris, and in the treatment of hypertension.

Night blindness Nyctalopia; difficulty in seeing in the dark. This may be a congenital defect or be caused by a vitamin A deficiency. Also occurs as a result of retinal degeneration.

Nightmare A bad dream accompanied by fear.

Night sweat Profuse perspiration during sleep, associated usually with an acute feverish illness.

Night terror An unpleasant experience in which the subject, usually a young child, screams while asleep and seems terrified. On waking the individual is unable to remember the cause of the fear.

Nigrostrial Bundle of nerve fiber connecting corpus striatum with substantia nigra.

N

Nihilism In psychiatry, a term used to describe feelings of not existing and hopelessness, that all is lost or destroyed.

Nikethamide A cardiac and respiratory stimulant given intravenously in cases of respiratory failure.

Nikolsky's sign Spreading of pemphigus bleb by application of mild pressure due to easy epidermal separation.

Nimesulide Analgesic anti-inflammatory agent.

Nimodipine Calcium channel blocker.

Nipple The small conical projection at the tip of the breast, through which, in the female, milk can be withdrawn. *Accessory nipple* A rudimentary nipple anywhere in a line from the breast to the groin.

Depressed nipple One that does not protrude.

Nipple shield A shield fitted with a rubber teat which covers the areola of a nursing mother when her nipple is sore or not sufficiently protractile for the baby to suck.

Retracted nipple One that is drawn inwards. It may be a sign of cancer of the breast.

Niridazole Antihelmintic used for guinea worm and schistosomiasis.

Nissl granules *F. Nissl. Germanneuropathologist, 1860–1919.* RNA-containing units found in the cytoplasm of cells. Probably associated with protein synthesis.

Nit The egg of the head louse, attached to the hair near the scalp.

Nitazoxanide Anti-amoebic agent.

Nitrate drugs A group of coronary vasodilator drugs used to treat angina pectoris, e.g., glyceryl trinitrate and isosorbide. These drugs provide rapid relief of symptoms and improve exercise tolerance. They may be given as tablets to be chewed or dissolved sublingually, as skin patches, gel or sublingual sprays.

Nitrate Salt of nitric acid.

Nitrazepam A hypnotic and sedative drug used to treat insomnia with early morning wakening.

Nitrendipine Calcium channel blocker.

Nitric oxide A potent vasodilator, released from vascular endothelium, synthesized from arginine.

Nitrite Salt of nitrous acid, an antispasmodic and smooth muscle dilator.

Nitrobluetetrazolium test A test of ability of leukocytes to transform nitrobluetetrazolium from a colorless state to deep blue, a test of leukocyte bacterial killing ability.

Nitrofurantoin A urinary antiseptic which is bactericidal and is effective against a wide range of organisms.

Nitrofurazone Topically used antibacterial agent.

Nitrogen Symbol N. A gaseous element. Air is largely composed of nitrogen, and it is one of the essential constituents of all protein foods.

Nitrogen balance The state of the body in regard to the rate of protein intake and protein utilization. A negative nitrogen balance occurs when more protein is utilized by the body than is taken in. A positive nitrogen balance implies a net gain of protein in the body. Negative nitrogen balance can be caused by such factors as malnutrition, debilitating disease, blood loss and glucocorticoids. A positive balance can be caused by exercise, growth hormone and testosterone.

Nitrogen mustards A group of toxic, blistering alkylating agents, including nitrogen mustard itself (mechlorethamine hydro *nitrogen* chloride) and related compounds; some have been used as anti neoplastics in certain forms of cancer.

Nitroglycerin Glyceryltrinitrate. A drug which causes dilatation of the coronary arteries. In angina pectoris a tablet should be dissolved sublingually before exertion.

Nitromersol Topically used mercurial antiseptic.

Nitrous oxide (N_2O) Laughing gas. An inhalation anesthetic ensuring a brief spell of unconsciousness.

Nitrosourea Anti-neoplastic agents including carmustine, lomustine, semustine and streptozocin.

Nitroxazepine Antidepressant.

NK *(See Natural Killer Cells).*

NMC *(See Nursing and Midwifery Council).*

NNT *(See Numbers Needed to Treat).*

Nocardiosis Infection with gram positive aerobic bacteria (often acid fast to be confused with tubercle bacillus), causing pulmonary infection or foot infection (maduramycosis).

Nociassociation The discharge of nervous energy which occurs unconsciously in trauma, as in surgical shock *(See Anociassociation).*

Nociceptive reflex Reflex initiated by painful stimuli.

Noctambulation Sleep walking; somnambulism.

Nocturia The production of large quantities of urine at night.

Nocturnal Referring to the night.

Nocturnal enuresis Bed wetting; incontinence of urine during sleep.

Nocturnal penile tumescence Penile erection during sleep, a normal phenomenon, when present excludes organic causes of impotency.

Nodal points A pair of points situated on the axis of optical system.

Nodal rhythm Cardiac rhythm originating at AV node.

Nodding Falling forward of the head.

Node A swelling or protruberance.

Atrioventricular node The specialized tissue between the right atrium and the ventricle, at the point where the coronary vein enters the atrium, from which is initiated the impulse of contraction down the atrioventricular bundle.

Node of Ranvier A constriction occurring at intervals in a nerve fiber to enable the neurilemma with its blood supply to reach and nourish the axon of the nerve.

Sinoatrial node The pacemaker of the heart. The specialized neuro muscular tissue at the junction of the superior vena cava and the right atrium, which, stimulated by the right vagus nerve, controls the rhythm of contraction in the heart.

Nodule A small swelling or protuberance.

Noma A gangrenous condition of the mouth; cancrum oris.

Nominal The level of measurement that simply assigns data into categories that are mutually exclusive.

Nomogram A graph with several scales arranged so that a ruler laid on the graph intersects the scales at related values of the variables; the values of any two variables can be used to find the values of the others. Increasingly used in the determination of drug therapy dosage, e.g., in pediatrics.

Non-compos mentis [L.] Not of sound mind. Applied to people whose mental state is such that they are unable to manage their own affairs.

Non-accidental injury Abbreviated NAI. Injuries inflicted upon children or infants by those looking after them, usually the parents. The injuries are usually physical (beating, burnings, biting) but the term includes the giving of poisons and dangerous drugs, sexual abuse, starvation and any other form of physical assault.

Non-allergic rhinitis Inflammation in the inside of the nose not caused by allergy leading to a blocked, runny nose and sneezing.

Non-compliance Describes the decision made by a patient not to comply with a drug regimen, even though fully understanding the rationale for such therapy.

N

Non-experimental research design A research design in which an investigator observes a phenomenon without manipulating the independent variable(s).

Non-invasive Any medical procedure that does not penetrate the skin or organ of the body, e.g., CT scanning or blood pressure monitoring. The term may also be used to describe non-cancerous tumours that do not metastasize.

Non-maleficence The concept in the health care services of the duty to avoid harm to the interests of others.

Nonoxynol A spermicide.

Non-shivering thermogenesis The use of brown adipose tissue by the neonate to produce heat in times of stress. Brown fat is stored in the mediastinum, around the nape of the neck, between the scapulae and around the kidneys and suprarenal glands.

Non-specific 1. Not due to any single known cause. 2. Not directed against a particular agent, but rather having a general effect.

N. urethritis Abbreviated NSU. A common, sexually transmitted disease, which may be due to a variety of agents, e.g., Chlamydia trachomatis that causes 40% of cases. Also called non-gonococcal urethritis.

Non-steroidal anti-inflammatory drugs Abbreviated NSAIDs. A group of drugs with analgesic, antipyretic and anti-inflammatory activity due to their ability to inhibit the synthesis of prostaglandins. It includes aspirin, phenylbutazone, indomethacin, tolmetic, ibuprofen and related drugs.

Non-union In a fracture, failure of the two pieces of bone to unite.

Noonan's syndrome Congenital pulmonary stenosis with skeletal abnormalities.

Noradrenaline A hormone present in extracts of the suprarenal medulla and at synapses in the peripheral sympathetic nervous system. It causes vasoconstriction and raises both the systolic and the diastolic blood pressure.

Norepinephrine Vasopressor hormone secreted by adrenal medulla.

Norethandrolone An anabolic steroid.

Norethindrone Progestational agent.

Norethisterone An anabolic steroid similar in action to progesterone. Used in the treatment of amenorrhea. Also used in the combined contraceptive pill.

Norfloxacin A quinolone with broad spectrum antibacterial activity.

Norgestrel A progestational agent.

Norm A fixed standard or value against which values are measured.

Normal Conforming to a standard; regular or usual.

Normal flora Bacteria which normally live on body tissues and have a beneficial effect.

Normals aline Isotonic solution of sodium chloride. Physiological solution.

Normetanephrine A metabolite of epinephrine.

Normoblast A nucleated precursor red blood cell in bone marrow *(See Erythrocyte).*

Normochromic Normal in color. Applied to the blood when the hemoglobin level is within normal limits.

Normochromasia Normal staining capacity of tissue.

Normocyte A red blood cell that is normal in size, shape and color.

Normoglycemia Normal blood sugar level.

Normosthenuria Urine of normal amount and specific gravity.

Normotension Normal tone, tension or pressure. Usually used in relation to blood pressure.

Norovirus Common cause of vomiting and diarrhea transmitted through fecal contamination of food and water. Also known as the winter vomiting bug.

Norplant Implantable contraceptive system containing levogestrel.

Norrie's disease Sex-linked blindness with retinal malformation, vitreous opacity, often with hearing loss and mental retardation.

North American Nursing Diagnosis Association Abbreviated NANDA. Formed as a professional organization of registered nurses in 1982. The purpose of NANDA is to develop, refine and promote a taxonomy of nursing diagnostic terminology of general use to the professional. Meets at regular intervals to review previously approved nursing diagnoses and to further develop the classification systems.

Norton score A pressure sore risk assessment scale devised by *Norton, McLaren and Exton Smith in 1987.* Used primarily in the care of elderly patients and reviewed on a weekly basis. It comprises five health state components, each with a four-point descending scale. Maximum points are 20 and the minimum five; a 'score' of 14 and below indicates that the patient is at risk of developing pressure sores and needs 1–2-hourly changes of posture and the use of pressure-relieving aids.

Nortriptyline A tricyclic antidepressant drug used for the relief of various types of depression.

Norwalk agent A virus implicated in gastroenteritis.

Noscapine Antitussive opium alkaloid.

Nose The organ of smell and the airway for respiration.

Nosocomial Pertaining to, or acquired in hospital.

Nosocomial disease For the patient a new disorder, not related to the original disease, that is caused or precipitated during hospitalization.

Nosocomial infection An infection acquired in hospital at least 72 hours after admission. Also called hospital acquired infection (HAI). Contact transmitted infection is the most important and frequent mode of transmission of nosocomial infections and may be either direct or indirect.

Direct contact transmitted infections involve direct 'body surface-to-body surface' contact, such as occurs in patient care activities, e.g., bathing a patient. Direct contact can also occur between two patients, with one serving as the source of infectious micro-organisms, the other being a susceptible host.

Indirect contact transmitted infections involve contact of a susceptible host with a contaminated intermediate object, usually inanimate *(See Fomites)*, e.g., contaminated instruments, needles, dressings or gloves that are not changed between patients. Unwashed, contaminated hands may also be a source of nosocomial infection.

Nosology The classification of disease into groups by criteria, based on (expert) agreement of the boundaries of the groups, e.g., by the Delphi technique.

Nosophilia An abnormal desire to be ill.

Nostalgia Homesickness.

Nostril One of the anterior orifices of the nose.

Notch Depression, narrow gap.

Acetabular notch Notch on the inferior border of acetabulum.

Aortic notch Notch of aortic valve closure in pulse tracing.

Sciatic notch Two in number, greater and lesser sciatic notches on hip bone.

Notifiable Applied to such diseases as must by law be reported to the health authorities. These include measles, scarlet fever, typhus and typhoid fever, cholera, diphtheria, tuberculosis, dysentery and food poisoning.

Notochord The axial skeleton of embryo, its remnant in adult is nucleus pulposus of intervertebral disc.

Novocain Procaine hydrochloride.

Noxious Harmful.

NPF Nurse Prescribers' Formulary.

NREM sleep Non-rapid eye movement sleep.

NRHM National Rural Health Mission.

NSAIDs Non-steroidal anti-inflammatory drugs.

NSU Non-specific urethritis.

Nuck's canal A peritoneal pouch extending into labium in female, homologous to processus vaginalis of male.

Nuclear Pertaining to a nucleus.

Nuclear medicine That branch of medicine concerned with the use of radionuclides in the diagnosis and treatment of disease.

Nuclear magnetic resonance Abbreviated NMR. A phenomenon exhibited by atomic nuclei having a magnetic momentum, i.e., those nuclei that behave as if they are tiny bar magnets. In the absence of a magnetic field these magnets are arranged randomly but when a strong magnetic field is applied they align with the field. These signals can be analysed and used for chemical analysis (NMR spectroscopy) or for imaging (magnetic resonance imaging).

Nuclease An enzyme which breaks down nucleic acids.

Nucleic acids Deoxyribonucleic acid (abbreviated DNA) and ribonucleic acid (abbreviated RNA), both of which are found in cell nuclei; RNA is also found in the cytoplasm. They are composed of series of nucleotides.

Nucleolus A small dense body in the cell nucleus which contains ribonucleic acid. It disappears during mitosis.

Nucleoprotein A compound of nucleic acid and protein.

Nucleosidase Enzyme causing hydrolysis of nucleoside.

Nucleoside Glycoside formed by union of pentose sugar with purine or pyrimidine.

Nucleotide A compound formed from pentose sugar, phosphoric acid and a nitrogen-containing base (a purine or a pyrimidine).

Nucleotoxic Applied to drugs, toxins, viruses and other agents that are toxic to cell nuclei.

Nucleus 1. The essential part of a cell, governing nutrition and reproduction, its division being essential for the formation of new cells. 2. The positively charged center portion of an atom. 3. A group of nerve cells in the central nervous system. *Caudate nucleus* and *lenticular nucleus* Part of the basal ganglia.

Nucleus pulposus The jelly-like center of an intervertebral disc.

NUHM National Urban Health Mission.

Null hypothesis The hypothesis that the observed difference between two groups of patients studied is accidental.

Nullipara A woman who has never given birth to a child.

Numb Dead, insensible.

Numbers needed to treat Abbreviated NNT. A measure of clinical significance in medicine and pharmacology used to communicate the effectiveness of a healthcare intervention. It refers to the average number of patients who need to be treated with a specific intervention to prevent one additional bad outcome. It is used in pharmacology to make decisions between treatment options being based upon the number of subjects receiving the medication before one subject has a positive outcome.

Nurse Prescriber's Formulary For Community Practitioners abbreviated NPF. A formulary which community nurses who are appropriately qualified may prescribe for patients.

Numular Shaped-like a coin.

Nurse 1. A person who is qualified in the art and science of nursing and meets certain prescribed standards of education and clinical competence. Is registered with the respective councils of the country. The person so registered is entitled legally to use the title of nurse. 2. To provide services that are essential to or helpful in the promotion, maintenance and restoration of health and well-being. 3. to nourish at the breast *(See also Breast (Feeding)).*

Nurse practitioner A qualified nurse who works with general medical practitioner in the clinic, surgery or health center in the community or in an acute care setting, e.g., accident and emergency services, orthopedic clinics and minor injuries departments. The patients have a choice of seeing either the doctor or the nurse when they attend.

Practice nurse A qualified nurse who works with a general practitioner (GP), or with a group of GPs, in a health center or surgery.

Primary nurse A named nurse who is responsible for the overall coordination of the patient's care.

Registered nurse In India, one whose name is on the register held by the INC.

Wet nurse A woman who breastfeeds the infant of another.

Nursery Newborn care center.

Nursing and midwifery council (NMC) The statutory regulatory body for nursing and midwifery in England, Wales, Scotland and Northern Ireland. Its prime purpose is to protect the public through establishing and monitoring professional standards, setting the standard for education and training, conduct and performance. The council replaced the former UKCC and National Boards. It (a) maintains a register of qualified staff; (b) sets standards for professional education, practice and conduct; (c) provides advice for nurses, midwives and health visitors on professional standards; (d) considers allegations of misconduct or unfitness to practice because of illness; and (e) publishes professional conduct rules and other documents to guide professional practice.

Nursing The profession of performing the functions of a nurse.

Nursing assessment The systematic collection and analysis of patient data pertaining to the individual's health status, abilities and preferences for care and treatment. The first step of the nursing process leading to a clinical nursing judgement *(See Assessment).*

Nursing audit A systematic procedure for assessing the quality of nursing care rendered to a specific patient population.

Nursing care plan Devised by a nurse and based upon a nursing assessment and nursing diagnosis for an individual patient. The plan has four essential components: (a) Identification of the nursing care problems; (b) An outline of the means/methods of solving these; (c) A statement of the anticipated benefit to the patient; and (d) An account of the specific actions used to achieve the goals specified.

Nursing diagnosis A statement of a health problem or of a potential health problem in the patient's or client's health status that a nurse is professionally competent to treat.

Nursing goal The objective that the nurse hopes to achieve through nursing interventions and activities related to the patient's health status, needs and abilities, e.g., the development of self-care skills.

Nursing history A written record providing data for assessing the nursing care needs of a patient.

Nursing models A conceptual frame work of nursing practice based on knowledge, ideas and beliefs. A model or theory of nursing clarifies the meaning of nursing, provides criteria for policy and gives direction to team nursing, thereby obviating conflicts in approach and giving the framework for continuity of care. It identifies the nurse's role, highlights areas of practice where research is needed and can be a basis for the nursing curriculum.

Nursing practice The performance or compensation of any act in the observation, care and counsel of the ill, injured or infirm, or in the maintenance of health or prevention of illness of others, or in the supervision and teaching of other personnel, or in the administration of medication and treatment as prescribed by a doctor or dentist. This requires substantial specialized judgement and skill and is based on knowledge and application of the principles of biological, physical and social sciences.

Nursing process A systematic approach to nursing care derived from many occupational groups. The system itself is not specific to nursing. It has been used as a framework for nursing care by American nurses and subsequently its principles have been adapted by all nurses. It is an organized approach to the identification of a patient's nursing care problems and the utilization of nursing actions that effectively alleviate, minimize or prevent the problems being presented or from developing.

Theories of nursing Proposed explanations of the way in which nursing achieves its aims. They require a definition of the nurse's perception of the patient's needs, the nurse's own role and the context in which nursing care is being performed. The understanding of the relationship of these variables enables nursing care to be planned in such a way that the outcome maybe predicted and set goals achieved.

Nutation Uncontrollable nodding of the head.

Nutrient Food; any substance that nourishes. The six classes of nutrient are fats, carbohydrates, proteins, vitamins, minerals and water.

Nutrition 1. The sum of the processes involved in taking in nutriments and assimilating and utilizing them. 2. Nutriment.

Enteral nutrition The provision of nutrients in fluid form to the alimentary tract by mouth, nasogastric tube or via an opening into the tract such as through a gastrostomy.

Nutritional disease One that is due to the continued absence of a necessary food factor.

Parenteral nutrition A technique for meeting a patient's nutritional needs by means of intravenous feedings; sometimes called hyper alimentation.

Nutritous Providing nutrition.

Nutritional status The condition of the body as a result of its receiving and using nutrients.

Nux vomica Poisonous seed containing strychnine.

Nyctalopia Night blindness *(See Hemeralopia).*

Nyctamblyopia Poor night vision without any other eye changes.

Nyctaphonia Hysterical loss of voice only at night.

Nyctophilia Abnormal preference for darkness.

Nyctophobia Abnormal fear of darkness.

Nylidrin Peripheral vasodilator.

Nymph Wingless immature stage in development cycle of insects.

Nympha Labia minora.

Nymphomania Excessive sexual desire in a woman.

Nystagmograph Apparatus for recording nystagmus.

Nystagmus An involuntary, rapid movement of the eyeball. It may be hereditary or result from disease of the semicircular canals or of the central nervous system. It can occur from visual defect or be associated with other muscle spasms.

Nystatin An antibiotic drug effective against fungi. Used in the treatment of fungal infections of the ear.

Nysten's law The law that states that rigor mortis begins with muscles of mastication and then progresses down.

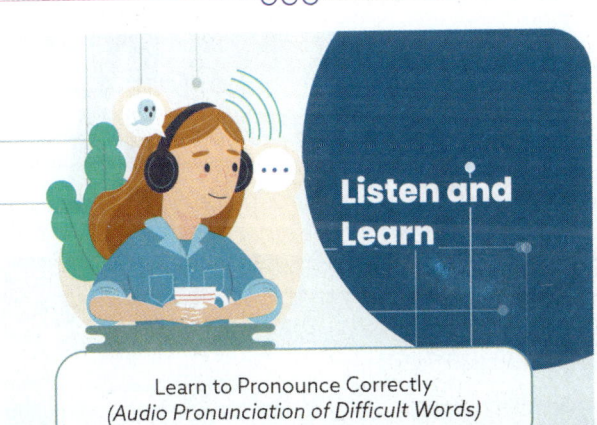

N

Dil Mange More Content

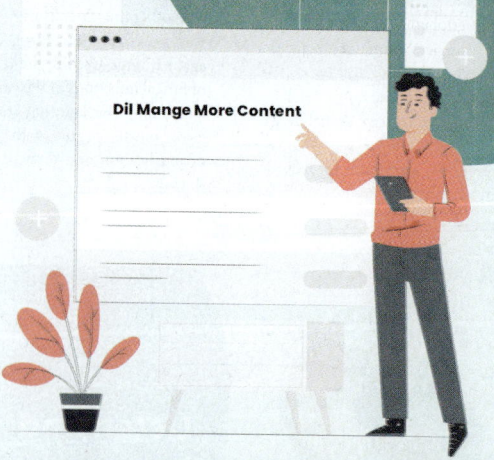

- Get additional explanations of Important Terminologies
- Word Quiz on Day-To-Day Basis on Scientific and General Terminology (One New Word Every Day with example)
- **50+** Animated & Interactive Videos on various important Topics and Concepts on nursing students' day-to-day interactions/daily needs.
- 4 Hybrid Updates (Every Quarter) covering New Words, Recent Topics & Interactive Videos

O Symbol for oxygen.

Oat A cereal used as food.

Oat meal Porridge of oat.

Obduction Autopsy.

Obese Very fat; corpulent.

Obesity Corpulence; excessive development of fat throughout the body. A body mass index (BMI) of over 30 kg/m².

Object Anything visible to senses.

Objective 1. In microscopy, the lens nearest the object being looked at. 2. A purpose; a desired end-result. 3. Concerning matters outside oneself.

Objective signs Signs that the observer notes, as distinct from symptoms of which the patient complains (subjective).

Objective symptoms Symptoms apparent to physical means of diagnosis.

Obligate Necessary.

Oblique Slanting.

Oblique muscles 1. A pair of muscles, the inferior and the superior, which turn the eye upwards and downwards, and inwards and outwards. 2. Muscles found in the wall of the abdomen.

Obliquity The state of slanting.

Litzmann's obliquity Inclining of fetal head with posterior parietal bone presenting.

Naegele's obliquity Inclining fetal head with oblique biparietal diameter in relation to pelvic brim.

Oblongata Oblong. e.g., medulla oblongata.

Obscure Hidden, indistinct.

Observation The act or faculty of closely noticing and paying attention to someone or something. In nursing, this is an active process whereby the nurse uses the senses for the purpose of collecting patient data for developing a nursing diagnosis or care plan.

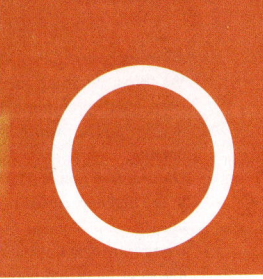

Observation register A register of children whose development may be adversely affected by problems occurring during the fetal or neonatal period. They should be carefully followed up by the health visitor, general practitioner, social worker and special pediatric department.

Observational study A research methodology in which the researcher is a non-participant observer and records behavior without influencing it.

Obsession An idea which persistently recurs to an individual, although resisted and regarded as being senseless. A compulsive thought *(See Compulsion)*.

Obsessive compulsive disorder A psychiatric disorder in which a person repeats same action or behavior for many hours which effects daily living.

Obstetrician One who is trained and specializes in obstetrics.

Obstetrics The branch of medicine and surgery dealing with pregnancy, labor and the puerperium.

Obstipation Intractable constipation.

Obstruction The act of blocking or clogging; the state of being clogged.

Intestinal obstruction Any hindrance to the passage of feces.

Obstructive lung disease A group of diseases which cause increased resistance to passage of air in and out of the lungs, e.g., asthma, chronic bronchitis, etc.

Obstructive sleep apnea The walls of the throat relax and narrow during sleep, interrupting normal breathing.

Obturator That which closes an opening.

Obturator foramen The large hole in the hipbone, closed by fascia and muscle.

Obturator sign Inward rotation of hip so as to stretch obturator internus, causes pain in acute appendicitis.

Obtusion Weakening or blunting of normal sensations, a condition produced by certain diseases.

Occipital Relating to the occiput.

Occipital bone The bone forming the back and part of the base of the skull.

Occipital lobe Posterior lobe of cerebral hemisphere shaped like a three sided pyramid.

Occipitoanterior Referring to the position of the fetal occiput when it is to the front of the maternal pelvis as it comes through the birth canal. The opposite of occipito-posterior.

Occipitoposterior Referring to the position of the fetal occiput when it is to the back of the maternal pelvis as it comes through the birth canal. The opposite of occipitoanterior.

Occiput The back of the head.

Occlusion Closure, applied particularly to alignment of the teeth in the jaws.

Coronary occlusion Obstruction of the lumen of a coronary artery.

Occlusion of the eye Covering a good eye to improve the visual acuity of the other, lazy eye.

Occlusion of the pupil May be congenital or occur in iridocyclitis or after injury.

Occult Hidden, concealed.

Occult blood Blood excreted in the stools in such a small quantity as to require chemical tests to detect it.

Occupational Relating to work and working conditions.

Occupational disease One likely to occur among workers in certain trades. An industrial disease.

Occupational health nurse Provides immediate care to ill or injured workers and follows up the return to work of the sick and injured. Develops accident prevention program and promotes good health amongst the work force. Also has an educational role and a health and safety obligation.

Occupational health nursing The branch of nursing that is concerned with the health of people in the workplace.

Occupational medicine The branch of medicine concerned with people at work and the effects of work on health. Essentially a branch of preventive or environmental medicine. It is concerned with ensuring that health and safety in the workplace is maintained and legislation complied with.

Occupational neurosis Neurosis that develops in certain persons in particular occupations.

Occupational therapy Treatment by provision of interesting and congenial work within the limitations of the patient in cases of mental disability and in order to re-educate and coordinate muscles in physical defect.

Ochlesis Any disease caused by over crowding.

Ochlophobia Abnormal fear of populated places or crowds.

Ochronosis An inborn error of metabolism marked by dark pigmentation of cartilage, ligaments and skin with black coloration of homogentisic acid.

Octapeptide Peptide with eight amino acids.

Octogenerian A person in his/her eighties.

Octopanrine An adrenergic transmitter.

Octreotide Growth hormone antagonist.

Ocular Relating to the eye.

Ocular myopathy A gradual bilateral loss of mobility of the eyes.

Ocular myositis Inflammation of the orbital muscles.

Oculentum An eye ointment.

Oculocardiac reflex Slowing of pulse following pressure on eyeball.

Oculocerebrorenal syndrome A sex-linked syndrome characterized by cataract, mental retardation, amino aciduria, vitamin D resistant rickets, etc.

Oculogyric Causing movements of the eyeballs.

Oculogyric crisis Involuntary, violent movements of the eye, usually upwards.

Oculomotor Relating to movements of the eye.

Oculomotor nerve The third pair of cranial nerves, which control the eye muscles.

Odontitis Inflammation of the tooth.

Odontoblast The dentin forming cells in dental papilla or pulp chamber.

Odontocele An alveodental cyst.

Odontoclast A class of cells that bring about resorption of roots of deciduous teeth.

Odontogenesis The formation/development of teeth.

Odontograph Equipment to determine the degree of unevenness of enamel.

Odontoid Resembling a tooth.

Odontoid process A tooth-like projection from the axis vertebra upon which the head rotates.

Odontology The art and science of dentistry.

Odontoma A tumor of tooth structures.

Ameloblastic odontoma Tumor of dental tissue containing enamel, dentine and odontogenic tissue but does not form enamel.

Composite odontoma Odontoma in which epithelial and mesenchymal cells are completely differentiated producing enamel and dentin.

Odorant Anything that stimulates the sense of smell.

Odoriferous Perfumed.

Odorous Having fragrance.

Odor Any smell

Odynophagia Dysphagia.

Edema An excessive amount of fluid in the body tissues. If the finger is pressed upon an affected part, the surface pits and slowly regains its original contour.

Angioneurotic edema Temporary edema suddenly appearing in areas of skin or mucous membrane and occasionally in the viscera.

Brain edema An excessive accumulation of fluid in the brain substance (wet brain).

Cardiac edema A manifestation of congestive heart failure, due to increased venous and capillary pressures and often associated with renal sodium retention.

Dependent edema Edema affecting most severely the lowermost parts of the body.

Edema neonatorum A disease of preterm and feeble infants resembling sclerema, marked by spreading edema with cold, livid skin.

Famine edema That due to protein deficiency.

Pitting edema Edema in which pressure leaves a persistent depression in the tissues.

Pulmonary edema Diffuse extra vascular accumulation of fluid in the tissues and air spaces of the lung due to changes in hydrostatic forces in the capillaries or to increased capillary permeability.

Oedipus complex The suppressed sexual desire of a son for his mother, with hostility towards his father. It is a normal stage in the early development of the child, but may become fixed if the child can not solve the conflict during his early years or during adolescence. Named after a mythical Greek hero.

Oesophageal Pertaining to the oesophagus.

Oesophageal atresia A congenital abnormality in which the oesophagus is not continuous between the pharynx and the stomach. May be associated with a fistula into the trachea.

Oesophageal varices Varicose veins of the lower oesophagus secondary to portal hypertension.

Oesophagitis Inflammation of the oesophagus.

Reflux oesophagitis Caused by regurgitation of acid stomach contents through the cardiac sphincter.

Oesophagojejunostomy An operation to create an anastomosis of the jejunum with the oesophagus after a total gastrectomy.

Oesophagoscope An endoscope for viewing the inside of the oesophagus.

Oesophagus The canal that extends from the pharynx to the stomach. It is about 23 cm long. The gullet.

Oestradiol The chief naturally occurring female sex hormone produced by the ovary. Prepared synthetically, it is used to treat menopausal conditions and amenorrhea.

Oestrogen One of several steroid hormones, including oestradiol, all of which have similar functions. Although they are largely produced in the ovary, they can also be extracted from the placenta, the adrenal cortex and the testis. They control female sexual development.

Ogilvie syndrome Acute intestinal pseudo-obstruction.

Ohm's law The strength of an electric current expressed in amperes is equal to the electromotive force expressed on volts divided by resistance.

Ointment An external application with a greasy base in which the remedy is incorporated.

Olecranon The curved process of the ulna which forms the point of the elbow.

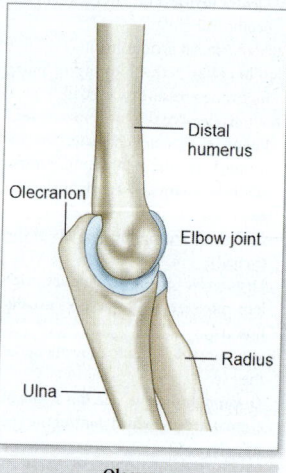

Olecranon

Oleum An oil.

Oleic acid Fatty acid.

Oleogranuloma Granuloma formation at the site of injection of oily substances.

Olfactory Relating to the sense of smell.

Olfactory nerves The first pair of cranial nerves; those of smell.

Olfactometer The apparatus for testing power of sense of smell.

Olfactory bulb Enlarged upper end of olfactory tract.

Olfactory membrane Membrane in the upper part of nasal cavity containing olfactory receptors.

Olfactory nerves Fine unmyelinated fibers arising from olfactory mucosa and ending in olfactory bulb after piercing cribi form plate.

Olfactory tract The tract that extends from olfactory bulb to the anterior perforated substance where it divides into olfactory striae.

Olfactory trigone Small triangular area between lateral and medial olfactory striae.

Oligemia A deficiency in the cellular component of the blood.

Oligocythaemia A cell deficiency in the blood.

Oligodendroglia The neuroglial cell with long slender processes which maintains the myelin sheath.

Oligodendroglioma A central nervous system tumor of the glial tissue.

Oligohydramnios A deficiency in the amount of amniotic fluid.

Oligomenorrhoea 1. A diminished flow at the menstrual period. 2. Infrequent occurrence of menstruation.

Oligosaccharide Compound made up of small number of monosaccharides.

Oligospermia A diminished output of spermatozoa.

Oligotrophy Inadequate nutrition.

Oliguria A deficient secretion of urine.

Olivary Shaped like an olive.

Olivary body A mass of gray matter situated behind the anterior pyramid of the medulla oblongata.

Ollier's disease Chondrodysplasia .

Ollier's layer The deepest layer of periosteum containing bone forming osteoblasts.

Olmesartan ACE receptor inhibitor.

Ombudsman A person appointed to receive complaints about unfair administration. The officer in the National Health Service, appointed as 'ombudsman' or Health Service Commissioner, investigates complaints about failures in the health services and issues a regular report. Is not able to pass judgement on clinical matters.

Omental bursa The cavity in greater omentum.

Omentopexy Fixation of omentum to anterior abdominal wall.

Omentum A fold of peritoneum joining the stomach to other abdominal organs.

Greater omentum The fold reflected from the greater curvature of the stomach and lying in front of the intestines.

Lesser omentum The fold reflected from the lesser curvature and attaching the stomach to the undersurface of the liver.

Omeprazole Proton pump inhibitor, used in peptic ulcer, Zollinger-Ellison syndrome.

Ommaya reservoir A mushroom-shaped reservoir with a self sealing plastic dome and attached to a catheter. The reservoir is implanted under the skin flap in skull and catheter is put into lateral ventricle useful for measuring CSF pressure and administration of drugs.

Omnivorous Eating food of both plant and animal origin.

Omohyoid Concerning scapula and the hyoid bone, the muscle attached to these two structures.

Omphalitis Inflammation of the umbilicus.

Omphalocele An umbilical hernia.

Ompholotomy Cutting of umbilical cord after birth.

Onanist Person practicing coitus interruptus.

Onanoff's reflex Contraction of bulbocavernosus muscle on pressing the glans penis.

Onchocerca A genus of filarial worms, found in tropical parts of Africa and America, which may give rise to skin and subcutaneous lesions and attack the eye.

Onchocerciasis A tropical skin disease caused by infestation with *Onchocerca.*

Oncogenesis The causation and formation of tumors.

Oncogenic Giving rise to tumor formation.

Oncology The scientific study of tumors.

Oncotic pressure The osmotic pressure exerted by proteins in plasma.

Oncovin Vincristine sulphate.

Ondine's curse Primary alveolar hypoventilation due to reduced responsiveness of respiratory centre to CO_2.

Oneirology The scientific study of dreams.

Oneiroscopy Dream analysis for study of one's emotional state.

Oniomania An irrepressible urge to spend money.

Onlay A graft applied to the surface of tissue. For example, bone graft.

Ontogeny The history of development of an individual.

Onychia Inflammation of the matrix of a nail, with suppuration, which may cause the nail to fall off.

Onychodystrophy Maldevelopment of a nail.

Onychograph Device that records capillary blood pressure under the finger nail.

Onychogryphosis Enlargement of the nails, with excessive ridging and curvature, most commonly affecting the elderly.

Onycholysis Loosening or separation of a nail from its bed.

Onychomycosis Infection of the nails by a fungus.

Oocyte The immature egg cell or ovum in the ovary.

Oogenesis The development and production of the ovum.

Oogonium The primordial cell from which an oocyte originates.

Ookinesis Mitotic phenomena taking place within an ovum during maturation and fertilization.

Ookinete Motile zygote of plasmodia.

Oophorectomy Excision of an ovary; ovariectomy.

Oophoritis Inflammation of an ovary.

Oophorocystectomy Surgical removal of an ovarian cyst.

Oophorocystosis The development of one or more ovarian cysts.

Oophoron An ovary.

Oophoropexy The surgical fixation of a displaced ovary to the pelvic wall.

Oophorosalpingectomy Removal of an ovary and its associated uterine tube.

Oophorrhaphy Suture of displaced ovary to pelvic wall.

Opacity Cloudiness, lack of transparency. Opacities occur in the lens of an eye when a cataract is forming. They also occur in the vitreous humour and appear as floating objects.

Open ended items Questions that the respondent may answer in their own words

Open heart surgery Surgery on heart or its blood vessels requiring cardiopulmonary bypass.

Open reduction Exposure of fractured ends of a bone for bringing reunion by suitable reduction.

Operant conditioning A form of behavior therapy in which a reward is given when the subject performs the action required. The reward serves to encourage repetition of the action.

Operating framework Annually sets out the business and planning arrangements for the NHS in England.

Operation A surgical procedure in which instruments or hands are used by the operator.

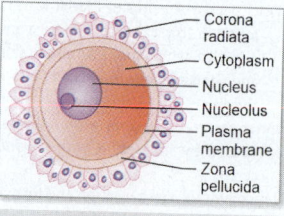

Corona radiata
Cytoplasm
Nucleus
Nucleolus
Plasma membrane
Zona pellucida

Oocyte

Operational definition The measurements used to observe or measure a variable; delineates the procedures or operations required to measure a concept.

Opercular Concerning a covering structure.

Operculitis Inflammation of gingivale over a partly erupted tooth.

Operculum Any covering.

Operon A term used in genetics to mean a group of linked genes and regulatory elements functioning as a unit for transcription.

Ophiases A form of baldness of scalp.

Ophidism Poisoning from snake bite.

Ophritis Inflammation of eyebrow.

Ophthalmia Severe inflammation of the eye or of the conjunctiva or deeper structures of the eye.

Ophthalmia neonatrum Any hyperacute purulent conjunctivitis which may be caused by the gonococcus, *Escherichia coli, staphylococci* or *Chlamydia trachomatis,* occurring within the first 21 days of life, usually contracted during birth from infected vaginal discharge of the mother. This condition is notifiable.

Sympathetic ophthalmia Granulomatous inflammation of the uveal tract of the uninjured eye following a wound involving the uveal tract of the other eye, resulting in bilateral granulomatous inflammation of the entire uveal tract. Also called sympathetic uveitis.

Ophthalmic nerve A branch of trigeminal, having only sensory function.

Ophthalmitis Inflammation of the eyeball.

Ophthalmo dynamometer Instrument for measuring pressure in ophthalmic arteries.

Ophthalmologist A specialist in diseases of the eye.

Ophthalmology The study of the eye and its diseases.

Ophthalmometer Instrument for measuring errors of refraction, size of eye and anterior curvature.

Ophthalmoplegia Paralysis of the muscles of the eye.

Ophthalmoscope An instrument fitted with a light and lenses by which the interior of the eye can be illuminated and examined.

Ophthalmoscopy Examination of the interior of the eye using an ophthalmoscope.

Opiate Any medicine containing opium.
Opiate receptor Specific receptors on cell surfaces to which combine the opiates, endorphins and encephalins for mediating their effects.

Opioid Synthetic narcotics or endogenous substances with opium like activity e.g., encephalins and endorphins.

Opisthotonus A muscle spasm causing the back to be arched and the head retracted, with great rigidity of the muscles of the neck and back. This condition may be present in acute cases of meningitis, tetanus and strychnine poisoning.

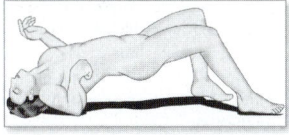

Opisthotonus

Opium A drug derived from dried poppy juice and used as a narcotic. It produces deep sleep, slows the pulse and respiration, contracts the pupils and checks all secretions of the body except sweat. It is a highly addictive drug. Opium derivatives include apomorphine, codeine, morphine and papaverine.

Oppenheim's disease *SYN-* myotonia congenital characterized by poor muscular development in the limbs.

Opponens Opposing. A term applied to certain muscles controlling the movements of the fingers.

Opponens pollicis A muscle that adducts the thumb so that it can be brought together with the little finger.

Opportunistic 1. Denoting a micro-organism which does not ordinarily cause disease but becomes pathogenic under certain circumstances.
2. Denoting a disease or infection caused by such an organism.

Opsin One of the colorless proteins in rods and cone.

Opsonic index A measurement of the bactericidal power of the phagocytes in the blood of an individual.

Opsonin An antibody, present in the blood, which renders bacteria more easily destroyed by the phagocytes. Each kind of bacterium has its specific opsonin.

Optic Relating to vision.

Optic atrophy Degeneration of the optic nerve.

Optic axis The imaginary line passing through center of cornea and posterior pole of retina.

Optic canal The groove at the apex of orbit through which pass the optic nerve and ophthalmic artery.

Optic chiasma The crossing of the fibers of the optic nerves at the base of the brain.

Optic disc The point where the optic nerve enters the eyeball.

Optic foramen The opening in the posterior part of the orbit through which passes the optic nerve and the ophthalmic artery.

Optic nerve A bundle of nerve fibers running from the optic chiasma in the brain to the optic disc on the eyeball.

Optic neuritis Involvement of optic nerve due to inflammation, degeneration, demyelination resulting in visual loss.

Optic radiation The geniculo-calcarine tract connecting lateral geniculate body with area 17 and 19 of calcarine cortex.

Optic tract The visual path from optic chiasma to lateral geniculate body.

Optical Pertaining to sight.

Optical center The point where the secondary axes of a refractory system meet and cross the principal axis.

Optical density The refractive power of the transparent tissues through which light rays pass, changing the direction of the ray.

Optical index A constant applied to objectives for purpose of comparison taking into account the focal length.

Optical isomerism Substances having similar structural formula but differing rotation of polarized light.

Optics Branch of science relating to properties of light, its refraction, reflection and relation to vision.

Optician A professional trained in the detection of refractive errors and the dispensing of appropriate spectacles or contact lenses.

Optimum The best and most favorable.

Optokinetic Relating to eye movements in relation to movements of objects in visual field.

Optokinetic nystagmus Nystagmus occurring when moving objects traverse the field of vision or vice versa.

Optometer Instrument for measuring refractive errors of eye.

Optometry The measuring of visual acuity and the fitting of glasses to correct visual defects.

OPV Oral Polio Vaccine

Ora [L.] A margin.

Ora serrata The jagged edge of the retina.

Oral 1. Pertaining to the mouth; taken through or applied in the mouth, as an oral medication or an oral thermometer. 2. Denoting that aspect of the teeth which faces the oral cavity or tongue.

O

Orbicularis oculi The ring muscle of eye, causing its closure.

Orbicularis oris The ring muscle of mouth, causing pursing of lips.

Orbit 1. The bony cavity containing the eyeball. 2. The path of an object moving around another object.

Orchic Testis.

Orchidectomy Excision of a testicle.
Bilateral orchidectomy The operation of castration.

Orchidopexy An operation to free an undescended testicle and place it in the scrotum.

Orchiepididymitis Inflammation of a testicle and its epididymis.

Orchitis Inflammation of a testicle.

Orf A virus infection transmitted from sheep to humans. It may give rise to a boil-like lesion on the hands of meat handlers.

Organ A part of the body designed to perform a particular function.

Organelle A structure within a cell which has specialized functions, e.g., nucleus, endoplasmic reticulum, mitochondrion, etc.

Organic 1. Pertaining to the organs. 2. Pertaining to chemicals containing carbon.
Organic acid Any acid containing carboxyl group.
Organic brain syndrome Diffuse impairment of brain function.
Organic disease Disease of an organ, accompanied by structural changes.
Organic murmur Murmur due to structural changes in heart valves.

Organism An individual living being, animal or vegetable.

Orgasm The climax of sexual excitement with pelvic throbbing, contraction of levator ani and anal sphincters to culminate in seminal ejaculation.

Orientation A sense of direction. 1. The ability of a person to estimate position in regard to time, place and persons. 2. The imparting of relevant information at the onset of a course or conference so that its content and objects may be understood.
Reality orientation The way in which older people who may be confused or mentally ill are assisted in keeping in touch with the world around them on a day-to-day basis. This may be achieved in a variety of ways, with large clocks, calendar boards, signs on doors and daily newspapers.

Orifice Any opening in the body.

Origin The starting point. In anatomy: 1. The point of attachment of a muscle. 2. The point at which a nerve or a blood vessel branches from the main stem.

Ormeloxifine Selective estrogen receptor modulator.

Ornidazole Antiamoebic agent.

Ornithine An amino acid in the urea cycle.

Ornithosis A virus disease of birds, usually pigeons, which may be transmitted to humans in a form resembling bronchopneumonia.

Orogenital Pertaining to the mouth and external genitalia.

Oropharynx The lower portion of the pharynx behind the mouth and above the esophagus and larynx.

Orosomucoid An acidic muco -protein from nephritic urine.

Orotic acid A pyrimidine precursor.

Oroya fever Bartonellosis.

Orphan A child whose parents are dead.
O. drugs Those that have been found to be useful in the treatment of rare diseases but which are not commercially produced usually because of high costs involved in manufacture and minimal demand.
O. viruses Those that have been isolated in the laboratory but which do not appear to be associated with any particular.

O

Orphenadrine A drug used to treat Parkinsonism, especially when accompanied by depression.

Orthochromatic Having normal staining characteristics.

Orthodontics Dentistry that deals with the prevention and correction of malocclusion and irregularities of the teeth.

Orthodox sleep *(See Sleep)*

Orthodontics Branch of dentistry that deals with the prevention and correction of malocclusion and irregularities of the teeth.

Orthograde Walking or standing in upright position.

Orthomyxovirus RNA viruses belonging to the family of orthomyxoviridae, which cause influenza in humans and other mammals, e.g., birds and swine. *(See Avian Flu and Swine Flu)*. These viruses originated in aquatic birds and crossed the species barrier *(See Zoonosis)* about 10,000 years ago to infect humans.

Orthopaedics The science dealing with deformities, injuries and diseases of the bones and joints.

Orthophoria Normal balance of eye muscles i.e., parallel.

Orthopnoea Difficulty in breathing unless in an upright position, e.g., sitting up in bed.

Orthoptics The practice of treating by non-surgical methods (usually eye exercises) abnormalities of vision such as strabismus (squint) .

Orthoscopy Examination of eye using orthoscope.

Orthostat Device for straightening curvatures of long bones.

Orthostatic Pertaining to or caused by standing erect.

Orthostatic albuminuria (See Albuminuria).

Orthostatic hypotension Low blood pressure, occurring when the person stands up.

Orthotic Serving to protect or to restore or improve function; pertaining to the use or application of an orthosis (a supportive appliance that can be applied to or around the body in the care/treatment of physical impairment or disability).

Orthotist A person skilled in orthotics and practising its application in individual cases.

Ortolani's sign *M Ortolani, 20th century Italian orthopedic surgeon.* A test performed soon after birth to detect possible congenital dislocation of the hip. A 'click' is felt on reversing the movements of abduction and rotation of the hip while the child is lying with knees flexed.

Orthotonus Tetanic spasm that causes a rigid straightness of the body.

Orthotopic In the natural or normal position.

Orthotopic transplantation Transplantation of an organ from a donor into its normal anatomical position in recipient.

Os [L.] 1. (pl. ora) Any body orifice. 2. (pl. ora) The mouth. 3. (pl. ossa) A bone.

Oscillation 1. A backward and forward motion. 2. Vibration.

Ossilopsia A form of visual aberration where stationary objects appear to move to and fro leading to blurred vision.

Oscilloscope An apparatus using a cathode-ray tube to depict visibly, data fed into it electronically, e.g., the way in which the heart is performing.

Osgood-Schlatter disease Osteochondritis of tibial tubercle.

Osler's disease Polycythemia vera.

Osler's nodes *Sir W. Osler, Canadian physician, 1849–1919.* Small painful swellings which occur in or beneath the skin, especially of the extremities in subacute bacterial endocarditis, caused by minute emboli. They usually disappear in 1–3 days.

Osler-Weber-Rendu syndrome Also known as hereditary hemorrhagic telangiectasia, it is a genetic disorder in which some blood vessels are underdeveloped

Osmole The quantity of a solute existing in solution as molecules, commonly stated in grams, that is osmotically equivalent to one mole of an ideally behaving electrolyte.

Osmometer Instrument for measuring osmotic pressure.

Osmophobia Abnormal fear of odors.

Osmoreceptor One of a group of specialized nerve cells which monitor the osmotic pressure of the blood and the extracellular fluid. Impulses from these receptors are relayed to the hypothalamus.

Osmosis The passage of fluid from a low concentration solution to one of a higher concentration through a semipermeable membrane.

Osmotic Pertaining to osmosis.
Osmotic fragility The susceptibility of RBC's to lyse in hypotonic solutions.
Osmotic pressure The pressure exerted by large molecules in the blood, e.g., albumin and globulin proteins, which draws fluid into the bloodstream from the surrounding tissues.

Osseous Bony.

Ossicle A small bone.
Auditory ossicle One of the three bones in the middle ear: the malleus, incus and stapes.

Ossification The process by which bone is developed; osteogenesis.

Ossifying fibroma A benign tumor from connective tissue of bone.

Osteitis Inflammation of bone.
Osteitis deformans (See Facet's disease).
Osteitis fibrosa cystica or *parathyroid osteitis* Defects of ossification, with fibrous tissue production,

leading to weakening and deformity. It affects children chiefly, and is associated with parathyroid tumor, removal of which checks it.

Osteoarthritis *(See Arthritis).*

Osteoarthrosis Degenerative joint disease.

Osteoarthrotomy Surgical excision of the jointed end of a bone.

Osteoblast A cell which develops into an osteocyte and turns into bone.

Osteoblastoma Malignant tumor of osteoblasts. *SYN*-Osteosarcoma.

Osteocarcinoma A condition of cancer of bone.

Osteochondritis Inflammation of bone and cartilage, particularly a degenerative disease of an epiphysis, causing pain and deformity.
Osteochondritis of the hip Perthes' disease.
Osteochondritis of the tarsal scaphoid bone Kohler's disease.
Osteo chondritis of the tibial tuberosity Osgood-Schlatter disease.

Osteochondroma A tumor consisting of both bone and cartilage.

Osteochondrosis A process involving ossification centers with avascular necrosis followed by slow regeneration.

Osteoclasis 1. The surgical fracture of bones to correct a deformity such as bowleg. 2. The restructuring of bone by osteoclasts during growth or the repair of damaged bone.

Osteoclast 1. A large cell that breaks down and absorbs bone and callus. 2. An instrument designed for surgical fracture of bone.

Osteoclastoma Giant cell tumor.

Osteocyte A bone cell.

Osteodystrophy A metabolic disease of bone.

Osteofibroma A benign bone tumor with fibrous tissue component.

Osteogenesis The formation of bone.

O

O. imperfecta A congenital disorder of the bones, which are very brittle and fracture easily. Fragilitas ossium.

Osteogenic sarcoma A malignant tumor composed of mesenchymal anaplastic cells with varying elements of osteogenesis, osteolysis, telangiectasis and bone cyst formation.

Osteoid The young hyaline matrix of true bone in which calcium is deposited.

Osteoma A benign tumor arising from bone.

Osteolysis Bone resorption/degeneration.

Osteoma Benign bony tumor arising from membranous bone.

Osteomalacia A disease characterized by painful softening of bones due to vitamin D deficiency.

Osteomatosis Presence of multiple osteomas.

Osteometry The study of proportions and measurement of skeleton.

Osteomyelitis Inflammation of bone, localized or generalized, due to pyogenic infection. It may result in bone destruction, stiffening of joints, and, in extreme cases occurring before the end of the growth period, in the shortening of a limb if the growth center is destroyed. Acute osteomyelitis is caused by bacteria that enter the body through a wound, spread from an infection near the bone, or come from a skin or throat infection. The infection usually affects the long bones of the arms and legs and causes acute pain and fever. It most often occurs in children and adolescents.

Osteopath One who practices osteopathy.

Osteopathy A system of treatment of disease by bone manipulation. Osteopathic treatment is manipulative and is aimed at freeing and loosening joints and re-establishing proper relationships of the spinal column, its component bones with the pelvis and limb bones.

Osteopenia Less bone tissue than normal.

Osteoperiostitis Inflammation of bone and periosteum.

Osteopetrosis A rare congenital disease in which the bones become abnormally dense. Albers-Schonberg disease.

Osteophyte A small outgrowth of bone, usually in a joint damaged by osteoarthritis.

Osteopoikilosis Disease of unknown etiology with ellipsoidal dense foci in all bones of body.

Osteoporosis Abnormal rarefaction of bone which may be idiopathic or secondary to other conditions. The disorder leads to thinning of the skeleton and decreased precipitation of lime salts. There may also be inadequate calcium absorption into the bone and excessive bone resorption. The principal causes are lack of physical activity, lack of oestrogens or androgens, and nutritional deficiency. There is almost always some degree of osteoporosis that occurs with ageing. Symptoms include pathological fractures and collapse of the vertebrae without compression of the spinal cord.

Osteosarcoma An osteogenic sarcoma malignant bone tumor.

Osteosclerosis An increase in density and hardening of bone.

Osteosclerosis congenital Achondroplasia.

Osteosclerosis fragilis Osteopetrosis.

Osteotome An instrument for cutting bone.

Osteotomy The cutting into or through a bone, sometimes performed to correct deformity.

Osteotomy of the hip A method of treating osteoarthritis by cutting the bone and altering the line of weight-bearing.

Ostium A mouth or aperture.

Abdominal ostium The opening at the end of the uterine tube into the peritoneal cavity.

Otic Relating to the ear.

Otic capsule The cartilage capsule that surrounds the developing auditory vesicle and later fuses with the sphenoid and occipital cartilage.

Otic ganglion The nerve ganglion immediately below foramen ovale of sphenoid bone giving rise to prostaglionic parasympathetic fibers to parotid gland.

Otitic hydrocephalus Hydrocephalus associated with chronic ear infection, especially mastoiditis.

Otitis Inflammation of the ear.

Aviation otitis A symptom complex resulting from fluctuations between atmospheric pressure and air pressure in the middle ear; also called barotitis media.

Furuncular otitis The formation of furuncles in the external ear.

Otitis externa Inflammation of the external ear.

Otitis interna, Otitis labyrinthica Labyrinthitis.

Otitis mastoidea Inflammation of the mastoid spaces.

Otitis media Inflammation of the middle ear, occurring most often in infants and young children, and classified as serous, secretory and suppurative.

Otoacoustic emission (OAE) A computer linked hearing test used for screening infants in the first few weeks of life to ascertain hearing levels.

Otogenic Originating or arising within the ear.

Otolith 1. A calculus in the middle ear. 2. One of a number of small calcareous concretions of the inner ear, at the base of the semicircular canals.

Otology The science of ear and its diseases.

Otomycosis A fungal infection of the auditory canal.

Otorhinolaryngology The branch of medical science dealing with functions and diseases of ear, nose and larynx.

Otorrhoea Discharge from the ear, especially of pus.

Otosclerosis The formation of spongy bone in the labyrinth of the ear, causing the auditory ossicles to become fixed and less able to pass on vibrations when sound enters the ear. The cause of otosclerosis is still unknown. It may be hereditary, or perhaps related to vitamin deficiency or otitis media. An early symptom is ringing in the ears, but the most noticeable symptom is progressive loss of hearing.

Otoscope An auriscope; an instrument for examining the ear.

Otosporin Trade name for a combination preparation of ear drops containing hydrocortisone, neomycin and polymyxin.

Ototoxic Anything which has a deleterious effect on the eighth cranial nerve or on the organs of hearing.

Ouabain A cardiac glycoside; its effect is similar to that of digitalis, but digitalization is achieved more rapidly.

Ounce A unit of measurement equivalent to 28 grams.

Outgrowth Growth or development from a pre-existing structure or state.

Outbreak An epidemic of an infectious disease limited to a localized increase in the incidence of the disease, e.g., in a village, town or institution. *(See Epidemic).*

Outcome A consequence or objective for a health care intervention, e.g., a patient goal. The implications are that the outcome is (a) measurable and that (b) can be expected as a result of the planned intervention.

O. framework High level indicators, which set out the expected priority outcomes the NHS will deliver.

O indicator Measurement of the success of a clinical treatment /intervention in terms of the impact on the health of the individual.

Outlet A means or route of exit or egress.

Pelvic o. The inferior opening of the pelvis; laterally bounded by the ischial spine, lower border of the symphysis pubis and the sacrococcygeal joint.

Out-of-the-body experience A sensation of leaving one's body and travelling through tunnels and lights onto another plane of experience. The condition has been attributed to anoxia of the brain following anesthesia or severe illness.

Outpatient A patient who has a medical consultation or receives treatment at a hospital but who does not require to stay overnight in a hospital bed.

Output The yield or total of something produced by a system.

Cardiac o. The effective volume of blood expelled by either ventricle of the heart per unit of time (usually volume per minute); it is equal to the stroke output multiplied by the number of beats per the time unit used in the computation.

Fluid o. The amount or urine passed, usually measured in comparison to oral fluid intake.

Outreach Health care services provided in an alternative setting such as within a community setting, e.g., a specialized clinic held in a general practitioner's surgery , sports center or other public building enabling patients and /or clients to access care more conveniently and avoid long or difficult journeys. An example of outreach in an acute setting might be staff from ICU providing care for patients and support for staff on general wards.

Ovalocyte Elliptocyte.

Ovarian Relating to an ovary.

Ovarian agenesis Failure of development of ovaries.

Ovarian cyst A tumor of the ovary containing fluid.

Ovarian follicle An ovum and the granulosa cells surrounding it occupying the cortex of ovary.

Ovarian graft A portion of ovary implanted commonly to abdominal wall to preserve hormone secretion.

Ovarian hormones 1. Follicular hormones—estradiol, estrone, estriol. 2. Luteal hormone— progesterone.

Ovarian ligament The terminal portion of genital ridge uniting the caudal end of embryonic ovary with the uterus.

Ovarian plexus A network of veins in the broad ligament or nerve plexus around the ovary.

Ovariectomy Oophorectomy; excision of an ovary.

Ovariotomy 1. Surgical removal of an ovary. 2. Excision of an ovarian tumor.

Ovary One of a pair of glandular organs in the female pelvis. They produce ova, which pass through the uterine tubes into the uterus, and steroid hormones which control the menstrual cycle.

Over-the-counter drugs Abbreviated OTC drugs. Drugs that can be purchased from a pharmacy without a prescription from a doctor. The list of derestricted drugs available to the public is growing and includes corticosteroid ointments, antihistamines, acyclovir, ibuprofen and nicotine patches.

Overuse injury Injury due to the repetitive movement of a joint or part of the body. *(See Repetitive Strain Injury).*

Overbite An overlapping of the lower teeth by the upper teeth.

Overcompensation A mental mechanism by which people try to assert themselves by aggressive behavior or by talking or acting 'big' to compensate for a feeling of inadequacy.

Overriding The extent of overlapping of broken ends in a fracture.

Overweight Excessive weight of an individual by more than 10% than permissible for gender and age.

Oviduct A uterine tube.

Oviparous Producing eggs.

Ovoid Egg shaped.

Ovotestis Ovarian and testicular tissue combined in the same gonad.

Ovulation The process of rupture of the mature Graafian follicle when the ovum is shed from the ovary.

Ovum [L.] An egg. The reproductive cell of the female.

Oxalate Any ester or salt of oxalic acid.

Oxalic acid An acid found in plants and vegetables, used as reagent.

Oxaluria Presence of oxalic acid or oxalates in urine.

Oxazepam A benzodiazepine tranquilizer.

Oxcarbazepine Antiepileptic drug.

Oxidase Enzyme that promotes an oxidation reaction.

Oxidization Oxidation. The process by which combustion occurs and breaking up of matter takes place, e.g., oxidization of carbohydrates gives carbon dioxide and water. The opposite of reduction.

Oximeter A photoelectric cell used to determine the oxygen saturation of blood.

Ear oximeter One attached to the ear by which the oxygen content of blood flowing through the ear can be measured.

Oximetholone Anabolic steroid.

Oxprenolol A beta-blocking drug used in the treatment of angina, hypertension and cardiac arrhythmias.

Oxybutynin Urinary antispasmodic.

Oxycephaly A condition where head is conical in shape.

Oxygen Symbol O. A colorless, odorless gas constituting one-fifth of the atmosphere. It is stored in cylinders at high pressure or as liquid oxygen. It is used medicinally to enrich the air when either respiration or circulation is impaired.

Oxygen deficit A physiological state that exists in cells during episodes of temporary oxygen bound to hemoglobin in the blood.

Oxygen hyperbaric Oxygen given at 1½ – 3 times of atmospheric pressure in gangrene, cyanide poisoning, burns, smoke inhalation, crush injury, etc.

Oxygen tent A large plastic canopy that encloses the patient in a controlled environment; used for oxygen therapy, humidity therapy or aerosol therapy. Not widely used now, but still used for children with severe breathing difficulties.

Oxygen therapy Supplementary oxygen administered for the purpose of relieving hypoxemia and preventing damage to the tissue cells as a result of oxygen lack.

Oxygen radicals Hydrogen peroxide, superoxide produced by incomplete reduction of oxygen that cause membrane damage.

Oxygen saturation The amount of oxygen bound to hemoglobin in the blood.

Oxygenation Saturation with oxygen; a process which occurs in the lungs to the hemoglobin of blood, which is saturated with oxygen to form oxyhemoglobin.

Oxygenator A machine through which the blood is passed to oxygenate it during open heart surgery.

Oxygenator pump A machine which pumps oxygenated blood through the body during heart surgery.

O

Oxyhemoglobin Hemoglobin that has been oxygenated, as in arterial blood.

Oxymetazoline A vasoconstrictor used topically to reduce nasal congestion.

Oxyntic Acid-forming.

Oxyntic cell A parietal cell of the gastric glands which secretes hydrochloric acid.

Oxyopia Unusual acuity of vision.

Oxypertine An anti-psychotic tranquilizing drug used in the treatment of schizophrenia and related psychoses, and of mania and hyperactivity.

Oxyphenonium bromide An anticholinergic agent used in peptic ulcer and gastrointestinal hyper- motility or spasm.

Oxypurinol A xanthine oxidase inhibitor, used in gout.

Oxytetracycline A broad-spectrum antibiotic, chiefly used against infections caused by *Chlamydia, Rickettsia* and *Brucella.*

Oxytocic Any drug that stimulates uterine contractions and may be used to hasten delivery.

Oxytocin A pituitary hormone which stimulates uterine contractions and the ejection of milk. Synthetically prepared, it is used to induce labor and to control postpartum hemorrhage.

Oxyuriasis Infestation by threadworms of the genus *Enterobius.*

Ozena A severe form of rhinitis in which the mucus membrane of the nose atrophies. This is associated with a thick offensive nasal discharge that crusts and often results in severe halitosis.

Ozone An intensified form of oxygen containing three O atoms to the molecule (O_3) and often discharged by electrical machines, such as X-ray apparatus. In medicine, it is employed as an antiseptic and oxidizing agent.

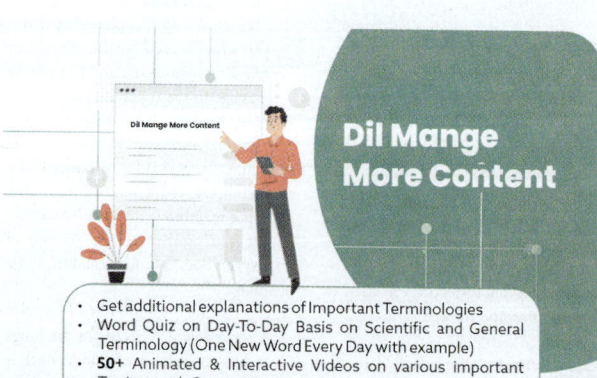

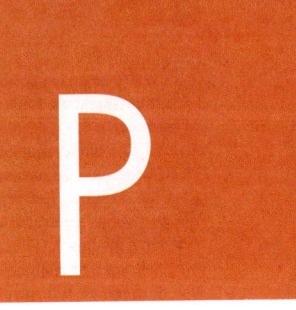

P Symbol for phosphorus

P value The symbol used to denote the probability of test results occurring by chance.

Pa Symbol for pascal.

Pachhionian bodies Pedunculated fibrous tissue growths along longitudinal fissure of cerebrum.

Pacemaker An object or substance that controls the rate at which a certain phenomenon occurs. The natural pacemaker of the heart is the sinoatrial node.

Electronic cardiac pacemaker An electrically operated mechanical device which stimulates the myocardium to contract. It consists of an energy source, usually batteries and electrical circuitry connected to an electrode which is in direct contact with the myocardium. Pacemakers may be temporary or permanent. Temporary ones usually have an external energy source, whereas permanent ones have a subcutaneously implanted one. The rate at which the pacemaker delivers pulses may be either fixed or on demand. Fixed pacing means that pulses are delivered to the heart at a predetermined rate irrespective of any cardiac activity. A demand pacemaker is programmed to deliver pulses only in the absence of spontaneous cardiac activity. The need for replacement of batteries is usually indicated when the rate of the pulse slows by five beats or more.

Pachydactyly Abnormal thickening of the fingers or toes.

Pachydermia An abnormal thickening of the skin.

Pachydermia laryngis Chronic hypertrophy of the vocal cords.

Pachymeningitis Inflammation of dura mater.

Pachyonychia Abnormal thickening of the nails.

Pachysomia Abnormal thickening of parts of the body, as in acromegaly.

Pacing code A three letter code for describing pacemaker type and function. The first letter indicates the heart chamber paced (V = ventricle, A = atrium, D = dual), the second letter indicates the chamber from which electrical activity is sensed and the third letter indicates the response to sensed electrical activity.

Pacini's corpuscles *F Pacini, Italian anatomist, 1812–1883.* Specialized-end-organs, situated in the subcutaneous tissue of the extremities and near joints, which react to firm pressure.

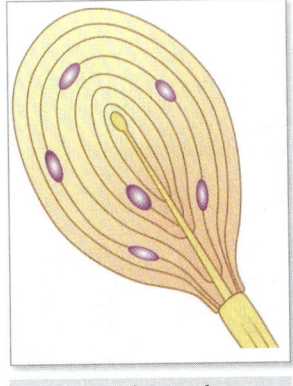

Pacini's Corpuscle

Pack A dry or moist; hot or cold blanket or sheet used for therapeutic purpose.

Packed cell Blood containing cellular elements only, devoid of plasma.

Paclitaxel Antineoplastic agent.

PaCO$_2$ Partial pressure of CO$_2$ in arterial blood.

PACT Prescribing analysis and cost.

Pad Cushion of soft material used to apply pressure, or support on an organ.

Paediatrician A medically qualified person specializing in the diseases of children.

Paediatrics The branch of medicine dealing with the care and development of children and with the treatment of diseases that affect them.

Paedophilia A sexual attraction towards young children.

Paget's disease *Sir J Paget, British surgeon, 1814–1899.* 1. A chronic disease of bone in which over-activity of the osteoblasts and osteoclasts leads to dense bone formation with areas of rarefaction. Osteitis deformans. 2. An inflammation of the nipple caused by cancer of the milk ducts of the breast.

Paget's disease of breast Carcinoma of mammary ducts.

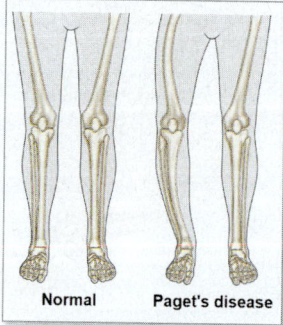

Normal   **Paget's disease**

Paget's Disease

Pagophagia A form of pica where patient loves eating ice.

Pain A feeling of distress, suffering or agony, caused by stimulation of specialized nerve endings. Its purpose is chiefly protective; it acts as a warning that tissues are being damaged and induces the sufferer to remove or withdraw from the source. Pain is a subjective experience and one person's pain cannot be compared to another's experience.

Bearing down pain Pain accompanying uterine contractions during the second stage of labor.

False pains Ineffective pains during pregnancy which resemble labor pains, but not accompanied by cervical dilatation; also called false labor *(See also Braxton Hicks contractions).*

Gas pain Pain caused by distension of the stomach or intestine by accumulations of air or other gases.

Hunger pain Pain coming on at the time of feeling hunger for a meal; a symptom of gastric disorder.

Intermenstrual pain Pain accompanying ovulation, occurring during the period between the menses, usually about midway. Also called mittelschmerz.

Labour pains The rhythmic pains of increasing severity and frequency due to contraction of the uterus at child birth *(See also Labor).*

Lancinating pain Sharp, darting pain.

Phantom pain Pain felt as if it were arising in an absent (amputated) limb *(See also Amputation).*

Referred pain Pain in a part other than that in which the cause that produced it is situated. Referred pain usually originates in one of the visceral organs but is felt in the skin or sometimes in another area deep inside the body. Referred pain probably occurs because pain signals from the skin. The person perceives the pain but interprets it as having originated in the skin rather than in a deep-seated visceral organ.

Rest pain A continuous burning pain due to ischemia of the lower leg, which begins or is aggravated after reclining and is relieved by sitting or standing.

Painful arc syndrome A condition in which pain occurs when the arm is raised from the side between 45 and 160 degrees. The most usual cause is an inflamed tendon or bursa around the shoulder joint that is being squeezed between the scapula and humerus on movement. *(See Frozen Shoulder and Shoulder Impingement Syndrome).*

Paint Castellani's A germicide containing phenol, resorcinol, boric acid, etc.

Palatal reflex Soft palate contraction during attempt of swallowing.

Palate The roof of the mouth.

Artificial palate A plate made to close a cleft palate.

Cleft palate A congenital deformity where there is lack of fusion of the two bones forming the palate.

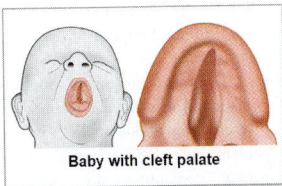

Baby with cleft palate

Cleft Palate

Hard palate The bony part at the front.

Soft palate A fold of mucous membrane that continues from the hard palate to the uvula.

Palatine arches Two arch like folds of mucous membrane (glossopalatine and pharyngopalatine) that form the lateral margin of faucial and pharyngeal isthmus.

Palatine artery Branch of maxillary artery, supplying palate and pharynx.

Palatine bone One of a pair of bones which form a part of the nasal cavity and the hard palate.

Palatoglossus Muscle that arises from sides and under surface of tongue and inserted to palatine aponeurosis. It acts as a constrictor of faucial isthmus by raising the root of tongue.

Palatography Recording of movement of palate during speech.

Palatopharyngeus Muscle that arises from thyroid cartilage and pharyngeal wall and inserted into aponeurosis of soft palate. It constricts pharyngeal isthmus and raises larynx.

Palatorrhaphy Operation for cleft palate.

Paleocerebellum The oldest portion of cerebellum that includes flocculi, and part of vermis concerned with equilibrium, and locomotion.

Paleothalamus Medial older parts of thalamus.

Palilalia Rapid repetition of same words and phrases.

Palliative Treatment that relieves, but does not cure disease.

Pallidotomy An operation performed to decrease the activity of the globus pallidus, the medial part of the lentiform nucleus in the base of the cerebrum. It has brought about a marked improvement in severely agitated cases of Parkinsonism.

Pallor Abnormal paleness of the skin.

Palm Anterior surface of hand from wrist to fingers.

Palmar Relating to the palm of the hand.

Deep palmar arches The deep and superficial palmar arches are the chief arterial blood supply to the hand, formed by the junction of the ulnar and radial arteries.

P

Palmar fascia The arrangement of tendons in the palm of the hand.

Superficial palmar arches (See Deep palmar arches above).

Palmitic acid A long chain fatty acid found in palm oil.

Palpable Perceptible to touch.

Palpation The examination of the organs by touch or pressure of the hand over the part.

Palpebral Referring to the eyelids.

Palpebral commissure The union of the eyelids at each end of palpebral fissure.

Palpebral fissure Opening between the eyelids.

Palpebral ligaments A band of ligaments which stretches from the junction of the upper and lower lid to the orbital bones, both medially and laterally.

Palpitation Rapid and forceful contraction of the heart of which the patient is conscious.

Palsy A historical term for paralysis.

Bell's palsy Paralysis of the facial muscles on one side, supplied by the seventh cranial nerve.

Crutch palsy Paralysis due to pressure of a crutch on the radial nerve, and a cause of 'dropped wrist'.

Shaking palsy Parkinsonism; paralysis agitans.

Pamidronate A biphosphonate for osteoporosis.

Panitumumab Monoclonal antibody for colon cancer.

Pampiniform Convoluted like a tendril.

Pampinocele SYN – varicocele; swollen dilated veins of pampiniform plexus of spermatic cord.

Panacea A remedy for all diseases.

Panangitis Inflammation of all the three layers of blood vessels.

Panarteritis Inflammation of all the three coats of an artery.

Panarthritis Inflammation of all the joints or of all the structures of a joint.

Pancarditis Inflammation of all the three layers of heart, i.e., pericardium, myocardium and endocardium.

Pancoast's tumor HK Pancoast, American radiologist, 1875–1939. Pain, wasting and weakness of the arm, which occur as secondary features of carcinoma of the bronchus as a result of neurological involvement. The tumor is at the apex of the lung.

Pancolectomy Surgical excision of entire colon.

Pancreas An elongated, racemose gland about 15 cm long, lying behind the stomach, with its head in the curve of the duodenum and its tail in contact with the spleen. It secretes a digestive fluid (pancreatic juice) containing ferments which act on all classes of food. The fluid enters the duodenum by the pancreatic duct, which joins the common bile duct. The pancreas also secretes the hormones insulin and glucagon.

Pancreatectomy Surgical excision of the whole or a part of the pancreas.

Pancreatic juice 500–800 mL of alkaline pancreatic secretion per day containing enzymes like trypsinogen, amylopsin, lipase, etc. Secretin and cholecystokinin secreted by duodenum stimulate pancreatic secretion.

Pancreaticoduodenostomy Surgical creation of an artificial tract between pancreas and duodenum.

Pancreatin An extract from the pancreas containing the digestive enzymes. Used to treat deficiency, as in cystic fibrosis, and after pancreatectomy.

Pancreatitis Inflammation of the pancreas.

Acute pancreatitis A severe condition in which the patient experiences sudden pain in the upper abdomen and back. The patient often becomes severely shocked.

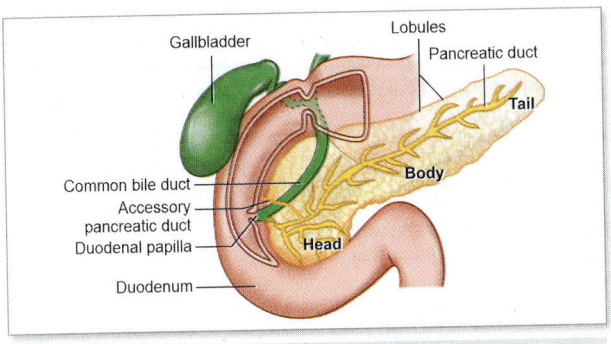

Gallbladder

Lobules

Pancreatic duct

Tail

Body

Common bile duct
Accessory
pancreatic duct
Duodenal papilla

Head

Duodenum

Pancreas

Chronic pancreatitis Chronic inflammation occurring after acute attacks. Pancreatic failure may lead to diabetes mellitus.

Pancreatolith Calculus within pancreas.

Pancreozymin A hormone of the duodenal mucosa that stimulates the external secretory activity of the pancreas, especially its production of amylase.

Pancuronium A neuromuscular blocking agent of the nerve depolarizing type, used as a muscle relaxant during surgery. It has a relatively long duration of action, a single intravenous dose lasting 45–60 minutes. It is often used in poor-risk patients.

Pancytopenia A reduction in number of all types of blood cell due to failure of bone marrow formation.

Pandemic An epidemic spreading over a wide area, sometimes all over the world.

Pandiculation Yawning and stretching of limbs as on awakening from sleep.

Panencephalitis A diffuse inflammation of brain.
Subacute sclerosing panencephalitis A cerebral degenerative disease which is common in childhood and is due to chronic measles.

Paneth cells Secretory cells in the intestinal crypts.

Panic An unreasoning and overwhelming fear or terror. It may occur in anxiety states and acute schizophrenia.

Panniculitis Inflammation of the subcutaneous fat causing tender nodules on the abdomen and thorax and on the thighs.

Pannus Increased vascularity of the cornea leading to granulation tissue formation and impaired vision. It occurs in trachoma after inflammation of the cornea.

Panophthalmia Panophthalmitis; inflammation of all the tissues of the eyeball.

Pansinusitis Inflammation of all paranasal sinuses, i.e., maxillary frontal, ethmoidal

Panting Shallow rapid breathing.

Pantograph A device that reproduces figures or drawings.

Pantopaque Iophendylate, a radiographic contrast for myelography.

Pantoprazole Proton pump inhibitor.

Pantothenic acid One of the vitamins in the B complex.

PaO$_2$ Partial pressure of oxygen in arterial blood.

Papain Proteolytic enzyme from papaya.

Papanicolaou test (Pap test) *GN Papanicolaou, Greek physician, anatomist and cytologist, 1883–1962.* A smear test to detect diseases of the uterine cervix and endometrium.

Papaveretum A preparation of the alkaloids of opium with an action similar to morphine. It is used to counteract severe pain.

Papaverine Smooth muscle relaxant.

Papilla A small nipple-shaped protuberance.

Circumvallate papilla One surrounded by a ridge. A number are found at the back of the tongue arranged in a V-shape, and containing taste buds.

Filiform papilla One of the fine, slender filaments on the main part of the tongue which give it velvety appearance.

Fungiform papilla A mushroom-shaped papilla of the tongue.

Optic papilla The optic disk, where the optic nerve leaves the eyeball.

Tactile papilla A projection on the true skin which contains nerve endings responsible for relaying sensations of pressure to the brain. A touch corpuscle.

Papillary muscle The two muscle groups in each ventricle of heart connecting to free margin of A-V valves.

Papillitis 1. Inflammation of the optic disk. 2. Inflammation of a papilla.

Papilledema Edema and hyperaemia of the optic disk, usually associated with increased intracranial pressure; also called choked disk.

Papilliform Resembling papilla.

Papillitis Inflammatain of optic nerve head.

Papilloma A benign growth of epithelial tissue, e.g., a wart.

Papillomatosis The occurrence of multiple papillomas.

Papovavirus A family of DNA-producing viruses which cause tumors, usually benign, such as warts.

Pappataci fever *(See Phlebotoms).*

Pappus The fine downy beard hair appearing at puberty.

Papule A pimple, or small solid elevation of the skin.

Papulopustular Descriptive of skin eruptions of both papules and pustules.

Papulosquamous Descriptive of skin eruptions that are both papular and scaly. They include such conditions as lichen planus, pityriasis and psoriasis.

Para-aminobenzoic acid A member of the B group of vitamins. It is used in creams and lotions to prevent sunburn.

Para-aminohippuric acid Derivative of amino benzoic acid used for testing renal excretory function.

Para-aminosalicylic acid Abbreviated PAS. An acid, the salts of which were used together with other drugs, usually isoniazid (INH) or streptomycin, in the treatment of tuberculosis.

Paracentesis Puncture of the wall of a cavity with a hollow needle in order to draw off excess fluid or to obtain diagnostic material.

Paracentral Near to center.

Paracentral lobule Cerebral convolution on medial surface serving as motor area of leg.

Paracetamol A mild analgesic drug used to treat headaches, toothache and rheumatic pains, and also to treat pyrexia.

Parachromatism Defective color perception.

Paracoccidioidomycosis Chronic granulomatous fungal disease of skin.

Paracrine Hormone secretion from nonendocrine cells.

Paracusis A perverted sense of hearing.

Paracusis of Willis An improvement in hearing when surrounded by noise.

P

Paradoxical respiration 1. Seen in open pneumothorax where lungs fill during expiration. 2. Moving up of diaphragm during inspiration in diaphragmatic palsy.

Paradigm Any example or representative instance of a concept or theoretical approach.

Paradoxical sleep Rapid eye movement (REM) sleep.

Paraesthesia An abnormal tingling sensation. 'Pins and needles'.

Paraffin Any saturated hydrocarbon obtained from petroleum.

Liquid paraffin A mineral oil which is used as a laxative

Paraffin wax A hard paraffin that can be used for wax treatment for chronic inflammation of joints.

Soft paraffin Petroleum jelly. Used as a barrier agent to protect the skin.

Paraganglia Sympathetic ganglia akin to adrenal medulla.

Paraganglioma Tumor of adrenal medulla and paraganglia.

Paragonimus A genus of trematode parasites. The flukes infest the lungs and are found mainly in tropical countries.

Paragranuloma Benign form of Hodgkin's disease only limited to lymphatic system.

Parainfluenza virus A group of viruses causing actue upper respiratory infection.

Parakeratosis A partial keratinization process where keratinocytes still contain nuclei.

Paraldehyde A sedative, hypnotic and anticonvulsant that has an unpleasant taste and imparts an unpleasant odour to the breath. It is now less used.

Paralexia Difficulty in comprehension of vocal/printed matter with substitution of meaningless words.

Parallax Displacement of objects change in observer's position.

Paralysis Loss or impairment of motor function in a part owing to a lesion of the neural or muscular mechanism; also, by analogy, impairment of sensory function (sensory paralysis). Paralysis is a symptom of a wide variety of physical and emotional disorders rather than a disease in itself. Palsy.

Paralysis agitans Parkinsonism.

Bulbar paralysis (labioglossopharyngeal paralysis) Paralysis due to changes in the motor center of the medulla oblongata. It affects the muscles of the mouth, tongue and pharynx.

Facial paralysis (Bell's palsy) Paralysis that affects the muscles of the face and is due to injury or to inflammation of the facial nerve.

Flaccid paralysis Loss of tone and absence of reflexes in the paralyzed muscles.

General paralysis of the insane Abbreviated GPI. Paralytic dementia occurring in the late stages of syphilis.

Infantile paralysis The major form of polio myelitis.

Spastic paralysis Paralysis characterized by rigidity of affected muscles.

Paralytic Affected by or relating to paralysis.

Paralytic ileus Obstruction of the ileum due to absence of peristalsis in a portion of the intestine.

Paramagnetic Anything attracted by a magnet.

Paramedian Situated on the side of the median line.

Paramedic A trained person to assist doctor.

Paramedical Associated with the medical profession and the delivery of health care. The paramedical services include trained ambulance personnel, occupational and speech therapy, physiotherapy, lab technology, radiography and social work.

Paramedical Associated with the medical profession and the delivery of health care. The paramedical services include trained ambulance personnel, occupational and speech therapy, physiotherapy, radiography and social work.

Paramethidione Anticonvulsant.

Parametritis Inflammation of the parametrium; pelvic cellulitis.

Parametrium The connective tissue surrounding the uterus.

Paramnesia A defect of memory in which there is a false recollection. The patient may fill in the forgotten period with imaginary events, which are often described in great detail.

Paramyotonia Increased muscle tone and poor relaxation after contraction.

Paramyxoviruses Includes measles, mumps, parainfluenza and respiratory syncytial virus.

Paranasal sinuses Frontal, maxillary, ethmoidal and sphenoidal sinuses.

Paraneoplastic syndrome Symptoms of multiple organ dysfunction in a patient of cancer (lung, kidney) without actual metastasis.

Paranoia A mental disorder characterized by delusions of grandeur or persecution which may be fully systematized in logical form, with the personality remaining fairly well preserved.

Paranoid Resembling paranoia. Refers to a condition that can occur in many forms of mental disease. Delusions of persecution are a marked feature. *Paranoid schizophrenia (See Schizophrenia).*

Paraparesis An incomplete paralysis affecting the lower limbs.

Paraphasia A speech disorder involving the substitution of a similar sound or word for that intended, thereby producing a nonsensical utterance.

Paraphilia A psychosexual disorder that includes fetishism, transvestism, pedophilia, voyeurism which mean bizarre acts for sexual excitation.

Paraphimosis Retraction of the prepuce behind the glans penis, within ability to replace it, resulting in a painful constriction.

Paraphrenia Schizophrenia occurring for the first time in later life and not accompanied by deterioration of the personality.

Paraphrasia Unintelligible speech due to incorrect and jumbling up of words used.

Paraplegia Paralysis of the lower extremities and lower trunk. All parts below the point of lesion in the spinal cord are affected. It may be of sudden onset from injury to the cord or may develop slowly as the result of disease.

Paraprofessional 1. A person who is specially trained in a particular field or occupation to assist a professional. 2. An allied health professional. 3. Pertaining to a paraprofessional.

Paraprotein Abnormal plasma protein like macroglobulin, myeloma protein.

Parapsychology The branch of psychology dealing with psychical effects and experiences that appear to fall outside the scope of physical law, e.g., telepathy and clairvoyance.

Paraquat A poisonous compound used as a contact herbicide. Contact with concentrated solutions causes irritation of the skin, cracking and shedding of the nails, and delayed healing of cuts and wounds. After ingestion renal and hepatic failure may develop, followed by pulmonary insufficiency and death.

Parasite Any animal or vegetable organism living upon or within another, from which it derives its nourishment.

Parasitemia Presence of parasite in the blood.

Parasiticide A drug that kills parasites.

Parasitize To infest with a parasite.

Parasternal Adjacent to sternum.

Parasuicide A suicidal action such as self-mutilation or the taking of a drug overdose which is motivated by a need to attract attention and seek help rather than commit suicide.

Parasympathetic nervous system The agent that opposes the effects of the parasympathetic nervous system.

Parasympathetic system The craniosacral part of the autonomic nervous system.

Parasympatholytic Anticholinergic; an agent that opposes the effects of the parasympathetic nervous system.

Parasympathomimetic Agent that produces actions similar to parasympathetic stimulation.

Parasystole Ectopic rhythm from ventricle.

Parathion Insecticide, toxic to humans.

Parathormone The endocrine secretion of the parathyroid glands.

Parathyroid gland One of four small endocrine glands, two of which are associated with each lobe of the thyroid gland, and sometimes embedded in it. The secretion from these has some control over calcium metabolism, and lack of it is a cause of tetany.

Parathyroidectomy The surgical removal of the parathyroid glands.

Paratrychosis Abnormality of hair or its growth pattern.

Paratyphoid A notifiable infection caused by *Salmonella* of all groups except *S. typhi*. The disease is usually milder and has a shorter incubation period, more abrupt onset and lower mortality rate than does typhoid. Clinically and pathologically, the two diseases cannot be distinguished. Also called paratyphoid fever.

Paravertebral Near or alongside the vertebral or spinal column.

P. block Anesthesia induced by the infiltration of a local anesthetic around the spinal nerve roots emerging from the intervertebral foramina.

P. injection An injection of local anesthetic into the sympathetic chain. May be used as a test in ischemic limbs to ascertain if a sympathectomy would be a useful treatment.

Parazoon An animal that lives as parasite on another animal.

Parecoxib Anti-inflammatory, analgesic.

Paregoric 1. Soothing. 2. Tincture opium used for diarrhea.

Parenchyma The essential active cells of an organ, as distinguished from its vascular and connective tissue.

Parent A father or mother.

Parenteral Apart from the alimentary canal. Applied to the introduction into the body of drugs or fluids by routes other than the mouth or rectum: For instance, intravenously or subcutaneously.

Parent-infant relationship The unique relationship that develops between parents and their infant(s), sometimes referred to as 'bonding', which endures throughout life. Promoted by early touching, fondling, speech, with eye-to-eye contact and breast feeding.

Paresis Partial paralysis.

Paresthesia Sensation of numbness, pricking, needling, tingling due to irritation of a nerve or its central connections.

Parietal Relating to the walls of any cavity. *Parietal bones* The two bones forming part of the roof and sides of the skull.

Parietal cells The oxyntic cells in the gastric mucosa that secrete hydrochloric acid.

Parietal pleura The pleura attached to the chest wall.

Parieto-occipital Relating to parietal and occipital bones or lobes.

484

Perinaud's syndrome Paralysis of vertical gaze due to subthalamic bleed.

Parai passu Side by side, occurring at the same time/rate.

Parity The classification of a woman with regard to the number of children that have been born live to her.

Parkinson's disease *J Parkinson, British physician, 1755–1824.* Parkinsonism; paralysis agitans. A slowly progressive disease usually occurring in later life, characterized pathologically by degeneration within the nuclear masses of the extrapyramidal system, and clinically by mask-like fades *(See Facies (Parkinson))*, a characteristic tremor of resting muscles, a slowing of voluntary movements, a festinating gait, peculiar posture and muscular weakness. When this symptom complex occurs secondarily to another disorder, the condition is called Parkinsonism.

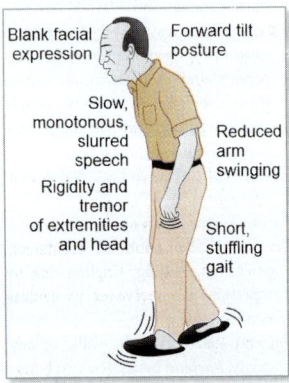

Blank facial expression
Forward tilt posture
Slow, monotonous, slurred speech
Reduced arm swinging
Rigidity and tremor of extremities and head
Short, stuffling gait

Symptoms of Parkinson's Disease

Paromomycin Aminoglycoside antibiotic used to treat amebiasis.

Paronychia An abscess near the fingernail; a whitlow or felon.

Paronychia tendinosa A pyogenic infection that involves the tendon sheath.

Paronychosis Growth of nail in an abnormal position.

Paroophoron Vestigial structure consisting of minute tubules, the remains of caudal group of mesonephric tubules, homologous to paradidymis of male.

Parosmia Perversion of sense of smell where agreeable odors are considered offensive and vice versa.

Parosteal Connected to or arising from outer layer of periosteum.

Parotid Situated near the ear.

Parotid duct The duct of parotid gland 2" long opening into mouth opposite second upper molar.

Parotid glands Two salivary glands, one in front of each ear.

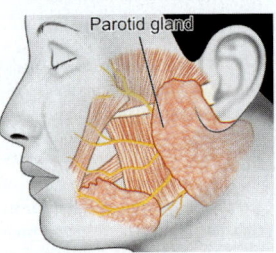

Parotid gland

Parotid Gland

Parotitis Inflammation of a parotid gland. Caused usually by ascending infection via its duct, when hygiene of the mouth is neglected or when the natural secretions are lessened, especially in severe illness or after operation.

Epidemic parotitis Mumps.

Parous Having borne one or more children.

Parovarium Vestigial remains of mesonephric tubules located in mesosalpinx between the ovary and fallopian tubes.

Paroxysm 1. A sudden attack or recurrence of a symptom of a disease. 2. A convulsion.

Paroxysmal Occurring in paroxysms.

Paroxysmal cardiac dyspnea Cardiac asthma. Recurrent attacks of dyspnea associated with pulmonary edema and left-sided heart failure.

Paroxysmal tachycardia Recurrent attacks of rapid heartbeats that may occur without heart disease.

Parrot disease *(See Psittacosis).*

Parrot's node Bony outgrowths on the skull of infants with congenital syphilis.

Pars flaccida A portion of ear drum that is not taut. *SYN*-Sharpnell's membrane.

Pars tensa Tightly stretched larger portion of tympanic membrane.

Parthenogenesis A sexual reproduction by means of an egg that has not been fertilized.

Particle A minute piece of substance.

Alpha particle A charged radioactive particle of low penetrability.

Beta particle A high speed electron emitted during decay of an atom.

Dane particle HBsAg, serum hepatitis capsular antigen.

Partnership working The relationship between Central government, NHS Trusts, NHS Foundation Trusts, Clinical Commissioning Groups, local authorities and patient representatives that has been developed to provide coordinated health care and social services to those in need. One of the core NHS values, this approach aims to achieve improved health for all with the coordinated and collaborative working between all involved agencies.

Parturient Giving birth; relating to childbirth.

Parturition The act of giving birth to a child.

Parvovirus A group of viruses pathogenic to humans and animals. *P. V. B19* – causes benign rash (fifth disease) but in immunocompromised can cause aplastic anemia. Intrauterine infection can cause fetal hydrops.

Parvovirus B19 *(See Fifth Disease).*

PAS Para-aminosalicylic acid.

Pascal Symbol Pa. The SI unit of pressure.

Passion Great emotion or zeal usually concerning sexual excitement.

Passive Not active.

Passive immunity (See Immunity).

Passive movements In massage, manipulation by a physiotherapist without the help of the patient.

Passive smoking Inhaling tobacco smoke exhaled by others; associated with a significant risk of increase in lung cancer.

Passivity In psychiatry, a delusional feeling that a person is under some outside control and must, therefore, be inactive.

Pasteurella *L Pasteur, French chemist and bacteriologist, 1833–1895.* A genus of short Gram-negative bacilli.

Pasteurella pestis The causative organism of plague transmitted by rat fleas to humans.

Pasteurization The process of checking fermentation in milk and other fluids by heating them to a temperature of 72°C for 15–20 minutes or 63°C for 30 minutes and then rapidly cooling. This kills most pathogenic bacteria.

Patau's syndrome A rare and serious genetic disorder caused by having an additional copy of chromosome 13. Also known as trisomy 13. Development is severely disrupted and in many cases leads to death in utero or shortly after birth.

Past pointing Inability to place fingers at a selected point in space, a feature of cerebellar disorder.

Patch test A test of skin sensitivity in which a number of possible allergens are applied to the skin under plaster. The causal agent of the allergy will produce an inflammation.

Patella The small, circular, sesamoid bone forming the knee-cap.

Patellar Belonging to the patella.

Patellar ligament The extension of quadriceps femoris tendon beyond inferior pole of patella to be attached to tuberosity of tibia.

Patellar reflex A knee jerk obtained by tapping the tendon below the patella.

Patellectomy Excision of the patella.

Patency The state of being open.

Patent Open.

Patent ductus arteriosus Failure of the ductus arteriosus to close, causing a shunt of blood from the aorta into the pulmonary artery and producing a continuous heart murmur.

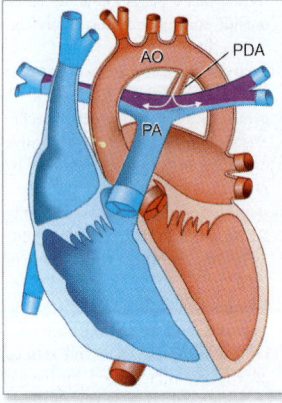

Patent Ductus Arteriosus

Paternity test Group of tests (blood group, HLA, and gene analysis) done to determine if a particular individual has fathered the specific child in question.

Paternity testing The use of blood samples to assist in establishing the paternity of child. Blood taken from the suspected father, the child and sometimes the mother is tested to ascertain similarities in DNA.

Pathetism Winning over and exploring some one's mind by suggestion.

Pathogen A microorganism that can cause disease, e.g., *Clostridium tetani* can cause tetanus.

Pathogenicity The ability of a micro organism to cause disease.

Pathognomonic Specifically characteristic of a disease. A sign or symptom by which a pathological condition can positively be identified.

Pathological 1. Pertaining to pathology. 2. Causing or arising from disease.

Pathological fracture A fracture occurring in diseased bone where there has been little or no external trauma.

Pathology The branch of medicine that deals with the essential nature of disease, especially of the structural and functional changes in tissues and organs of the body, which cause or are caused by disease.

Pathophobia An exaggerated dread of disease.

Pathophysiology Study of changes in physiology by the diseased process.

Patient A person who is ill or is under going treatment for disease.

Patient Advice and Liaison Service Abbreviated PALS. An advice service for patients in NHS Trusts and Foundation Trusts providing on-the-spot help and information about the health services to patients, their families and carers. PALS also monitors trends, highlighting gaps within the service and provides reports for action to the trust managers. It also represents patients concerns to the trust management and board.

Patient–controlled analgesia A system of controlling pain by drugs whose delivery is controlled by the patient himself; usually helpful in obstetric pain of labor by epidural catheter drug delivery.

Patients' right Basic rights of patients set out for example in the NHS Constitution for England and the Patient Rights (Scotland) Act 2011.

Patient's rights Patients have three basic rights: Namely, the right to know, the right to privacy and the right to treatment. The first two are moral rights while the third is both a moral and legal right.

Patulous Open, spread apart.

Paul-Bunnell test *JR Paul, American physician, 1893–1971; WW, Bunnell, American physician, 1902–1966.* An agglutination test which, if positive, confirms the diagnosis of glandular fever.

Pavlov's method *IP Pavlov, Russian-physiologist, 1849–1936.* A method for the study of the conditioned reflexes. Pavlov noticed that his experimental dogs salivated in anticipation of food when they heard a bell ring.

Pb Symbol for lead.

PDSA *(See Plan, Do, Study, Act)*

Peau d'orange (Fr.) A dimpled appearance of the overlying skin. Blockage of the skin lymphatics causes dimpling of the hair follicle openings which resembles orange skin. Particularly associated with breast cancer.

Pecten pubis 1. The middle third of the anal canal. 2. A ridge on the pubic crest to which the inguinal ligament is attached.

Pectineal line The ride of pubis bone.

Pectineus The quadrangular muscle at upper and inner thigh acting as a flexor and adductor of thigh.

Pectoral Relating to the chest.

    Pectoral muscles Two pairs of muscles, pectoralis major and pectoralis minor, which control the movements of the shoulder and upper arm.

Pectoral Relating to the chest.

    P. muscles Two pairs of muscles, pectoralis minor, which control the movements of the shoulder and upper arm.

Pectoriloquy The distinct transmission of vocal sounds to ear through the chest wall as in consolidation.

Pectus The chest.

    Pectus carinatum Abnormal prominence of sternum as in rickets *SYN* – Pigeon chest.

    Pectus excavatum Abnormal depression of sternum.

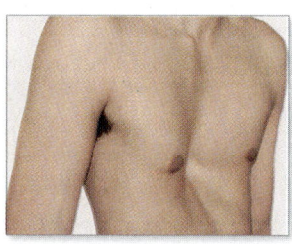

Pectus Excavatum

Pedesis Brownian movement of particles in a system, may be liquid or gas.

Pediatric advanced life support (PALS) *(See Annexure 2 and Advanced Life Support).*

Pediatrics Medical science dealing with children below 14 years of age.

Pedicle The stem or neck of a tumor.

    Pedicle graft A tissue graft that is partially detached and inserted in its new position while temporarily still obtaining its blood supply from the original source.

Pediculosis The condition of being infested with lice.

Pediculus A genus of lice.

    Pediculus humanus A species that feeds on human blood and is an important vector of relapsing fever, typhus and trench fever. Two subspecies are recognized:

    Pediculus humanus var. capitis (head louse), Found on the scalp hair and *Pediculus humanus var. corporis* (body or clothes louse), found elsewhere on the body.

Pedigree The tree or chart involving one's ancestors as used for genetic analysis.

Pedodontis Dentist practicing pediatric dentistry.

Pedograph Imprint of foot on paper.

Peduncle A narrow part of a structure acting as a support.

Cerebellar peduncle One of the collections of nerve fibers connecting the cerebellum with the medulla oblongata.

PEEP Positive end-expiratory pressure.

Peer review A basic component of a quality assurance *(See Quality)* program in which the results of health and/or nursing care given to a specific patient, population are evaluated according to defined criteria established by the peers of the professionals delivering the care. Peer review is focused on the patient and on the results of care given by a group of professionals rather than on individual professional practitioners.

Pegrete The downward extension of thickened epidermis between the dermal papillae.

Pel-Ebstein syndrome P.K. Pel, Dutch physician, 1852-1919; W. Ebstein, German physician, 1836-1912. A recurrent pyrexia, having a cycle of 15-21 days, which is a rare occurrence in people with Hodgkin's lymphoma.

Pelger – Huet anomaly A congenital inherited anomaly of neutrophils which have coarse chromatin in the nuclei but function in normal manner.

Peliosis Purple patches on skin and mucous membrane. *SYN* – purpura.

Pellagra A syndrome caused by a diet seriously deficient in niacin (or by failure to convert tryptophan to niacin). Most persons with pellagra also suffer from deficiencies of vitamin B; (riboflavin) and other essential vitamins and minerals. The disease also occurs in persons suffering from alcoholism and drug addiction. Characterized by debility, digestive disorders, peripheral neuritis, ataxia, mental disturbance and erythema with exfoliation of the skin.

Pellet A small ball of medicine or food.

Pelotherapy Therapeutic use of mud or hay to treat disease by application on body.

Pelvic Pertaining to the pelvis.

Pelvic exenteration Removal of all the pelvic organs.

Pelvic girdle The ring of bone to which the lower limbs are joined. It consists of the two hip bones and the sacrum and coccyx.

Pelvic inflammatory disease Persistent infection of the internal reproductive organs of the female, often resulting in infertility.

Pelvic inlet Upper pelvic entry, i.e., space between sacral promontory and upper aspect of symphysis pubis.

Pelvic outlet Lower pelvic outlet outlined by tip of coccyx, ischial tuberosities and lower margin of symphysis pubis.

Pelvimetry Measurement of the pelvis.

Pelvis (pl. pelves) A basin-shaped cavity.

Bony pelvis the pelvic girdle, formed of the hip bones and the sacrum and coccyx.

Contracted pelvis Narrowing of the diameter of the pelvis. It may be of the true conjugate or the diagonal. Effective antenatal care will recognize this condition, and cesarean section may be necessary.

False pelvis The part formed by the concavity of the iliac bones above the ileopectineal line.

Renal pelvis The dilatation of the ureter which, by enclosing the hilum, surrounds the pyramids of the kidney substance.

True pelvis The basin-like cavity below the false pelvis, its upper limit being the pelvic brim.

P

Pemphigoid 1. Resembling pemphigus. 2. A bullous disease of the elderly with the blisters arising beneath the epidermis. The skin and the mucosa are affected, and sometimes the conjunctiva.

Pemphigus A distinctive group of rare but serious diseases characterized by successive crops of large bullae ('water blisters'); the name is derived from the Greek word for blister, pemphix. Clusters of blisters usually appear first near the nose and mouth (sometimes inside them) and then gradually spread over the skin of the rest of the body. When the blisters burst, they leave round patches of raw and tender skin. Pemphigus is considered to be an autoimmune disorder.

Pendulous Hanging down.

Pendulous abdomen The hanging down of the abdomen over the pelvis, due to weakness and laxity of the abdominal muscles.

Penetrance The frequency of manifestation of a hereditary disease in individuals who have the dominant or double recessive gene.

Penfluridol Antipsychotic agent.

Penicillamine A chelating agent that is used in heavy metal poisoning to aid excretion of the metal and in the treatment of hepatolenticular degeneration (Wilson's disease). Also used in the treatment of severe rheumatoid arthritis.

Penicillin An antibiotic cultured from certain molds of the genus Penicillium. The drug is used in various forms to treat a wide variety of bacterial infections. Disk overed by Fleming in 1929, it was first used therapeutically in 1941. Varieties of the drug include: benethamine penicillin, benzylpenicillin, benzathine penicillin, procaine penicillin, cloxacillin, ampicillin and amoxycillin.

Penicillinase An enzyme that inactivates penicillin. Many bacteria, particularly staphylococci, produce this enzyme.

Penicillium A genus or mold-like fungi, from some of which the penicillins are derived. Some species are pathogenic to humans.

Penicilloyl-polylysine A substance of a person to pencillins by intradermal skin test or instillation to conjunctival sac.

Penile prosthesis Implantable device in the penis to achieve erection, the device is in form of inflatable plastic cylinders implanted to corpora cavernosa attached to a pump embedded in scrotal pouch. The fluid reservoir to fill the cylinders is implanted behind the rectus.

Penile reflex Contraction of bulbo-cavernous muscle on percussion of dorsum of penis or compression of glans penis.

Penis ring A malleable ring that by preventing venous return from penis helps to maintain erection and delaying orgasm.

Penis The male organ of copulation and urination.

Pentaerythritol tetranitrate Organic nitrate for angina pectoris.

Pentagastrin A synthetic hormone with a similar structure to gastrin. It has largely replaced histamine in gastric secretion tests as it has no apparent side effects.

Pentamidine An anti-protozoal drug used mainly in the treatment of *Pneumocystis carinii* infections.

Pentavalent Having valency of five.

Pentazocine An analgesic similar to morphine and used in the treatment of moderate to severe pain.

Pentobarbital A hypnotic sedative agent.

Pentolinium Ganglion blocking agent.

Pentose A monosaccharide containing five carbon atoms in a molecule.

Pentosuria A benign inborn error of metabolism due to a defect in the activity of the enzyme L-xylulose dehydrogenase, resulting in pentose in the urine.

Pentothal sodium Thiopental sodium, used for induction of anesthesia.

Pentoxifylline Vasodilator, improve hemorheology.

Penumbra In radiology, an area of blurring around the edge of structure
Penumbra ischemic An area of moderately ischemic zone around a more severely ischemic zone.

PEP Post-exposure prophylaxis.

Pepsin An enzyme found in gastric juice. It partially digests proteins in an acid solution.

Pepsinogen The precursor of pepsin, activated by hydrochloric acid.

Peptic Relating to pepsin or the action of the gastric juices in promoting digestion.
Peptic ulcer An ulcer, usually in the stomach or the duodenum, caused by an erosion of the surface to expose the muscle wall by the stomach acid and digestive enzymes. It is often precipitated by *Helicobacter pylori* organisms.

Peptide Any of a class of compounds of low molecular weight which yield two or more amino acids on hydrolysis. Peptides form the constituent parts of proteins.

Peptidoglycan The material making the cell wall of most micro-organisms.

Peptidyl dipeptidase An enzyme of hydrolase class that converts angiotensin I to angiotensin II, hence called angiotensin convering enzyme (ACE).

Peptococcus Anaerobic gram postive cocci present in oral, intestine and urinary tract.

Peptone A substance produced by the action of pepsin on protein.

Peptonuria The presence of peptones in the urine.

Per anum Through anus.

Per os [L.] By the mouth.

Percentile A term used in statistics to show how common some characteristic is. The line represents the percentage of the population who have this characteristic. The 90th percentile (or centile) for height means that 90% of the population will be no taller than the figure. The 50th percentile is the median or average.

Percept, Perception An awareness and understanding of an impression that has been presented to the senses. The mental process by which we perceive.

Percolate To filter, to strain.

Percolator Apparatus used for extraction of a drug with a liquid solvent.

Percussion A method of diagnosis by tapping with the fingers or with a light hammer upon any part of the body. Information can thus, be gained as to the condition of underlying organs.

Percutaneous Through the skin, particularly in relation to ointments that are applied to unbroken skin.

Percutaneous transluminal coronary angioplasty (PTCA) A non-operative balloon dilatation of partially occluded coronary vessels.

Percutaneous ultrasonic lithotripter Device using ultrasound applied externally to break up kidney stone.

Perforation A hole or break in the containing walls or membranes of an organ or structure of the body. Perforation occurs when erosion, infection or other factors create a weak spot in the organ and internal pressure causes a rupture. It may also result from a deep penetrating wound.

Performance indicators A 'package' of routine statistics derived nationally by the Department of Health and

P

visually presented in ways that highlight the relative efficiency of health services. Performance indicators are intended to compare services and identify aspects that merit further scrutiny locally with a view to changes in organization or practice.

Perfusion The passage of liquid through a tissue or an organ, particularly the passage of blood through the lung tissue.

Periactin Cypro heptadine hydrochloride, antiserotonin.

Periadenitis Inflammation of tissue surrounding a lymphnode.

Perianal Surrounding or located around the anus.

Perianal abscess A small subcutaneous pocket of pus near the anal margin.

Periarteritis Inflammation of the outer coat and surrounding tissues of an artery.

Periarthritis Inflammation of the tissues surrounding a joint.

Peribronchial Surrounding the bronchus.

Pericardial rub Friction between the inflamed layers of pericardium.

Pericardiectomy Surgical removal of the pericardium; pericardectomy. Used in the treatment of chronic constrictive pericarditis.

Pericardiocentesis Drainage of pericardial sac.

Pericardiopexy Increasing blood supply to heart by joining pericardium to adjacent tissue.

Pericarditis Inflammation of the pericardium.

Adhesive pericarditis The presence of adhesions between the two layers of pericardium owing to a thick fibrinous exudate.

Bacterial pericarditis Inflammation of the pericardium due to bacterial infection.

Chronic constrictive pericarditis Thickening and sometimes calcification of the pericardium, which inhibits the action of the heart.

Rheumatic pericarditis Pericarditis due to rheumatic fever.

Pericardium The smooth membranous sac enveloping the heart, consisting of an outer fibrous and an inner serous coat. The sac contains a small amount of serous fluid.

Pericholangitis Inflammation of tissue surrounding bile duct.

Perichondritis Inflamed perichondrium.

Perichondrium The membrane covering cartilaginous surfaces.

Pericranium The periosteum of the cranial bones.

Pericyazine A phenothiazine stronger than chlorpromazine; used in behavioral disturbances, schizophrenia and related psychoses.

Perilymph The fluid that separates the bony and the membranous labyrinths of the ear.

Perimenopause The phase before menopause in which pattern of regular menstrual cycle changes to irregular cycles with increased period of amenorrhea.

Perimeter 1. The line marking the boundary of any area or geometrical figure; the circumference. 2. An instrument for measuring the field of vision.

Perimetrium The peritoneal covering of the uterus.

Perinatal Relating to the period shortly before and 7 days after birth.

Perinatal mortality rate The number of stillbirths plus deaths of babies under 7 days old per 1000 total births in any one year.

Perinatologist A medically qualified person specializing in perinatology.

Perinatology The branch of medicine (obstetrics and pediatrics) dealing with the fetus and infant during the perinatal period.

Perindopril ACE inhibitor.

P

Perineal Relating to the perineum.

Perieoraphy Repair of perineal tear caused during parturition

Perineotomy Incision into perineum to facilitate delivery as in rigid perineum of primi.

Perineorrhaphy Suture of the perineum to repair a laceration caused during childbirth.

Perinephric Around the kidney.

Perineum The tissues between the anus and external genitals.

Lacerated perineum A torn perineum, which may result from childbirth but is often forestalled by performing an episiotomy. Treatment is by perineorrhaphy.

Perineural Around the nerve.

Perineurium Connective tissue sheath around bundle of nerve fibers.

Periodic Recurring at regular or irregular intervals.

Periodic apnea of the newborn Occurring in the normal full-term infant, periodic episodes of rapid breathing followed by a brief period of apnea which is associated with rapid eye movements.

Periodic syndrome Recurrent head, limb or abdominal pains in children for which no organic cause can be found. It often leads to migraine in adult life.

Periodic table The chart depicting chemical elements arranged by their atomic numbers.

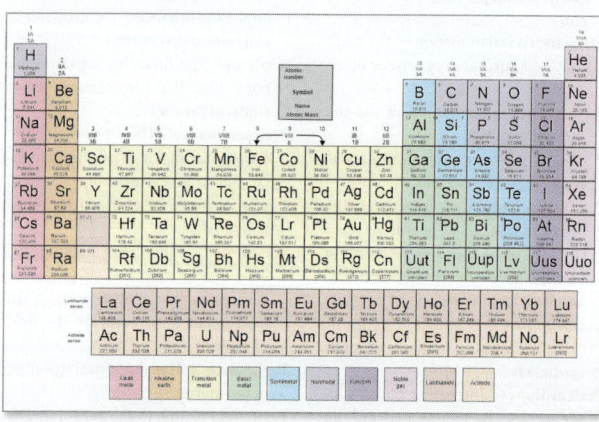

Periodic Table

Periodicity Recurring at more or less regular intervals.

Periodontal abscess Abscess formation in gingival periodontal pockets.

Periodontal disease Disease of supporting structure of teeth with bleeding gum loosening of teeth, etc.

Periodontal ligament The fibrous bundles attaching tooth to a alveolar bone.

Periodontics The branch of dentistry dealing with study and treatment of periodontal disease.

Periodontitis Inflammation of the periodontium.

Periodontium The connective tissue between the teeth and their bony sockets.

Periodoscope Pregnancy table for knowing expected date of delivery.

Perionychia Inflammation around a nail.

Perioperative Pertaining or relating to the period immediately before or after an operation, as in perioperative care.

Perioral Around the mouth.

Periosteal Pertaining to or composed of periosteum.

Periosteal elevator An instrument for separating the periosteum from the bone.

Periosteum The fibrous membrane covering the surface of bone. It consists of two layers: the inner or osteogenetic layer, which is closely adherent and forms new cells (by which the bone grows in girth); and in close contact with it, the fibrous layer richly supplied with blood vessels.

Periostitis Inflammation of the periosteum, usually as a result of injury.

Peripheral Relating to the periphery.

Peripheral iridectomy Excision of a small piece of iris from its peripheral edge.

Peripheral nervous system Those parts of the nervous system lying outside the central nervous system.

Peripheral neuritis Inflammation of terminal nerves.

Peripheral resistance The resistance in the walls of the arterioles, which is a major factor in the control of blood pressure.

Periphlebitis Inflammation of outer coat of vein or tissue around the vein.

Periphery The outer surface or circumference.

Peristalsis A wave-like contraction, preceded by a wave of dilatation, which travels along the walls of a tubular organ, tending to press its contents onwards. It occurs in the muscle coat of the alimentary canal.

Reversed peristalsis A wave of contraction in the alimentary canal which passes towards the mouth.

Visible peristalsis A wave of contraction in the alimentary canal that is visible on the surface of the abdomen.

Peristasis A temporary decrease in blood flow in early inflammation.

Peritomy Incision around cornea to treat pannus.

Peritoneal Referring to the peritoneum.

Peritoneal cavity The cavity between the parietal and the visceral peritoneum.

Peritoneal dialysis A method of removing waste products from the blood by passing a cannula into the peritoneal cavity, running in a dialysing fluid, and after an interval, draining it off.

Peritoneopexy Fixation of uterus by way of vagina.

Peritoneoscopy Visual examination of the peritoneum by means of a peritoneoscope.

Peritoneum The serous membrane lining the abdominal cavity and forming a covering for the abdominal organs.

Parietal peritoneum That which lines the abdominal cavity.

Visceral peritoneum The inner layer which closely covers the abdominal organs and includes the mesenteries.

Peritonitis Inflammation of the peritoneum.

Acute peritonitis This may be produced by inflammation of abdominal organs, by irritating substances from a perforated gallbladder or gastric ulcer, by rupture of a cyst, or by irritation from blood, as in cases of internal bleeding.

Chronic peritonitis This is comparatively rare, and is often associated with tuberculosis. Less frequently, it may result from long standing irritation caused by the presence in the abdomen of a foreign body, such as gunshot, or by chronic peritoneal dialysis.

Peritonsillar Around the tonsil.

Peritonsillar abscess Quinsy.

Peritrichous Organism with cilia/flagella covering its entire body.

Periurethral Around the urethra.

Perlèche (Fr.) Inflammation with fissuring at the angles of the mouth; often due to vitamin B deficiency, poorly fitting dentures or thrush infection.

Permeability The degree to which fluid can pass from one structure through a wall or membrane to another.

Pernicious Highly destructive; fatal.

Pernicious anaemia An anemia due to lack of absorption of vitamin B_{12} for the formation of red blood cells.

Pernio Swelling of skin due to cold.

Perniosis A condition, resulting from persistent exposure to cold, which produces vascular spasm in the superficial arterioles of the hands and feet, causing thrombosis and necrosis. Perniosis includes chill blains and Raynaud's disease.

Per oral By the mouth.

Peroneal Concerning fibula.

Peroneal sign In tetany tapping over peroneal nerve causes dorsiflexion and eversion of foot.

Peroral Through the mouth.

Peroxidase An enzyme essential for oxygen transfer, hence important in cellular respiration.

Peroxisome Granules in cell cytoplasm that contain a variety of enzymes.

Perphenazine An antiemetic and tranquillizing drug similar to chlorpromazine. Used in the treatment of nausea and vomiting, and of schizophrenia and other psychoses.

Perseveration The constant recurrence of an idea or the tendency to keep repeating the same words or actions.

Persistent vegetative state A long term dependent state that may last for weeks, months or years. Caused by damage to the cerebral cortex of the brain that controls higher mental functions, while the brainstem controlling respiration and circulation remains undamaged. The individual appears awake but is totally dependent on others for all care and remains unresponsive.

Personal development plan A planned process whereby an individual develops skills and knowledge that are beneficial to themselves and their career. This is part of a life-long learning commitment for nurses and other health professionals.

Personality The sum total of heredity and inborn tendencies, with influences from environment and education, which forms the mental make-up of a person and influences attitude to life.

Antisocial personality A personality disorder in which repetitive antisocial behavior is associated with ego eccentricity, lack of guilt or anxiety, and imperviousness to punishment. Also called sociopathic (psychopathic) personality.

Cyclothymic personality A personality marked by alternate moods of elation and dejection.

Double personality, dual personality Multiple personality.

Multiple personality A dissociative reaction in which an individual adopts two or more personalities alternatively, in none of which is their awareness of the experiences of the other (s).

Psychopathic personality Antisocial personality, sociopathic personality.

Schizoid personality A personality disorder marked by timidity, self-consciousness, introversion, feelings of isolation and loneliness, and failure to form close interpersonal relationships; the individual is frequently ambitious, meticulous and a perfectionist.

Perspiration Sweat or the act of sweating.

Insensible perspiration Water evaporation from the moist surfaces of the body, such as the respiratory tract and skin, that is not due to the activity of the sweat glands. It occurs at a constant rate of about 500 mL/day. When treating dehydration this loss must be taken into account.

Sensible perspiration Sweat that is visible as droplets on the skin. Part of the mechanism for regulation of body temperature.

Perthes' disease *GC Perthes, German surgeon, 1869–1927*. Osteochondritis of the head of the femur. Pseudocoxalgia (Legg Calve-Perthes disease).

Perturbation Agitated, uneasiness of mind.

Pertussis Whooping cough.

Pertussis immunoglobulin Globulin derived from patients immunized with pertussis vaccine, used for passive immunization.

Pertussis vaccine Killed pertussis bacilli used for active immunization.

Perversion Morbid diversion from a normal course.

Sexual perversion Abnormal sexual desires and behavior. A deviation.

Pervert One who has deviated from normal path.

Pervious Capable of being permeated.

Pes The foot, or any foot-like structure.

Pes cavus A foot with an abnormally high arch. Claw foot.

Pes malleus valgus Hammer toe.

Pes planus Flat foot.

Pessary 1. A plastic or metal ring shaped device which is inserted in the vagina to support a prolapsed uterus. 2. A medicated suppository inserted into the vagina for antiseptic or contraceptive purposes.

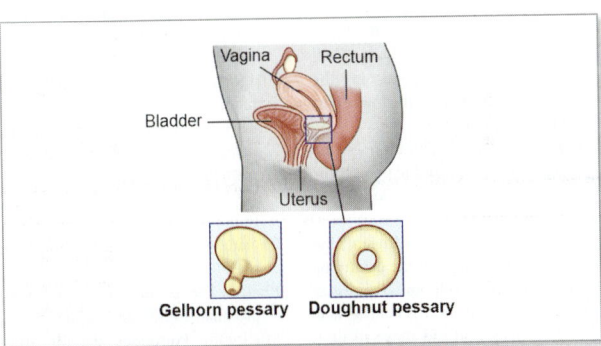

Pessary

Pessimism A state of mind where one feels dejected, hopeless and gloomy.

Pest Destructive insect.

Pesticide Chemicals used to kill pests.

PET Positron emission tomography.

Petechia A small spot due to an effusion of blood under the skin, as in purpura.

Pethidine A synthetic narcotic analgesic, less potent than morphine with quicker onset but shorter duration of action; used in obstetrics and pre-and postoperative medication. Particularly useful, because it relaxes smooth muscle, in patients with ureteric and biliary colic and as an analgesic in patients with asthma.

Petit's ligament Uterosacral ligament.

Petit's triangle An area on lateral abdominal wall bounded by iliac crest, posterior margin of external oblique and lateral margin of latissimus dorsi.

Petit mal A mild form of epilepsy common in children and characterized by a sudden and brief loss of consciousness.

Petridish A shallow dish with a cover to hold solid media for culture.

Petrifaction Process of hardening.

Petrissage A kneading action used in massage.

Petrositis Inflammation of the petrous portion of the temporal bone, usually spread from a middle ear infection.

Petrous Resembling a stone.

Petrous bone Part of the two temporal bones that forms the base of the skull and contains the middle and inner ear.

Peutz-Jegher's syndrome Small intestinal polyposis with hypermelanosis of skin and mucous membrane.

Peyer's glands or **patches** *JC Peyer, Swiss anatomist, 1653–1712.* Small lymph nodules situated in the mucous membrane of the lower part of the small intestine.

Peyronie's disease Induration of the corpora cavernosa of the penis, producing a fibrous chordae leading to painful erection.

pH A measure of the hydrogen ion-concentration, and so the acidity or alkalinity of a solution. Expressed numerically 1 to 14; 7 is neutral, and below this is acid and above alkaline *(See Hydrogen (Ion concentration))*.

Phacoemulsification A method of cataract removal by disintegrating it, followed by aspiration.

Phaeochromocytoma A tumor of the adrenal medulla which gives rise to paroxysmal hypertension.

Phacomatosis A group of hereditary diseases manifesting with cutaneous and neurological symptoms. Included in this group are von-Recklinghausen's disease, Hippel-Lindau disease, Sturge-Weber syndrome, tuberous sclerosis and incontinentia pigmenti.

Phage Bacteriophage, a virus that lives on bacteria but is confined to a particular strain.

Phage typing The identification of certain bacterial strains by determining the presence of strain-specific phages. Used in detecting the causative organisms of epidemics, especially food poisoning.

Phagocyte A blood cell that has the power of ingesting bacteria, protozoa and foreign bodies in the blood.

Phagocytic index Average number of bacteria ingested by each leukocyte.

Phagocytosis The engulfing and destruction of microorganisms and foreign bodies by phagocytes in the blood.

Phagolysosome The body formed when membrane bound phagosome inside a macrophage fuses with lysosome.

Phagomania Abnormal craving for food.

Phagosome A membrane bound vacuole inside a phagocyte containing matters to be digested.

Phakoma Microscopic gray white tumor of retina in tuberous sclerosis.

Phalanges The bones of the fingers or toes.

Phalanx Bones on finger and toes; proximal, middle and distal.

Phalloidin Poisonous peptide from mushroom *Amanita phalloides.*

Phallus The penis.

Phaneromania Abnormal tendency to bite nails, pull or play with hair, beard or moustache.

Phantasy *(See Fantasy).*

Phantom 1. An image or impression not evoked by actual stimuli. 2. A model of the body or of a specific part there of. 3. A device for simulating the in vivo interaction of radiation with tissues.

Phantom pain Pain felt as if it were arising in an absent (amputated) limb.

Phantom pregnancy (See Pseudocyesis).

Phantom tumor A tumor-like swelling of the abdomen caused by contraction of the muscles or by localized gas.

Pharmaceutics Science of dispensing medicines.

Pharmacist A person professionally qualified to carry out pharmacy. The traditional role of giving advice, dispensing prescriptions, providing vaccinations and selling over –the-counter medicines. More than 10,000 community pharmacies in England has been supplemented by the appointment of pharmacy advisers to the NHS at national and local level together with an expanded role associated with community health. *(See Annexure 4).*

Pharmacodynamics Study of drugs and their action on living organisms.

Pharmacogenetics The study of genetically determined variations in drug metabolism and the response of the individual.

Pharmacognosy The science of natural drugs and their properties.

Pharmacokinetics Branch of pharmacology dealing with the fate of drug substances.

Pharmacology The science of the nature and preparation of drugs and particularly of their effects on the body.

Pharmacopoeia An authoritative publication that gives the standard formulae and preparations of drugs used in a given country.

Pharmacy 1. The art of preparing, compounding and dispensing medicines. 2. The place where drugs are stored and dispensed.

Pharyngeal Relating to the pharynx.

Pharyngeal bursa A small blind sac occasionally present in lower portion of pharyngeal tonsils.

Pharyngeal pouch Dilatation of the lower part of the pharynx.

Pharyngeal reflex Contraction of pharyngeal musculature following its stimulation of contact.

Pharyngectomy Excision of a section of the pharynx.

Pharyngismus Spasm of pharyngeal muscles.

Pharyngitis Inflammation of the pharynx.

Pharyngocele Hernia through pharyngeal wall.

Pharyngoconjunctival fever An adenovirus infection.

Pharyngolaryngeal Referring to both the pharynx and larynx.

Pharyngotympanic tube The tube that joins the middle ear to the pharynx; the Eustachian tube.

Pharynx The muscular tube, lined with mucous membrane, situated at the back of the mouth. It leads into the esophagus, and also communicates with the nose through the posterior nares, with the ears through the pharyngotympanic (Eustachian) tubes, and with the larynx *(See Laryngopharynx nasopharynx and Oropharynx).*

Phase A stage of development.

Phenacemide Anticonvulsant agent, rarely used because of serious side effects.

Phenacetin An analgesic and antipyretic agent.

Phenanthrene A coal tar derivative with high carcinogenic potential.

Phenazocine An analgesic drug used to relieve severe pain. It is a drug of addiction.

Phenazopyridine Urinary analgesic causing red urine.

Phencyclidine A hallucinogen, also used as anesthetic in veterinary medicine (angel dust).

Phenelzine A monoamine oxidase inhibitor used in the treatment of depressive illness.

Phenergan Promethazine hydrochloride.

Phenformin An oral hypoglycemic agent, having propensity to cause lactic acidosis.

Phenindione An anticoagulant drug used in the treatment of deep vein thrombosis.

Pheniramine maleate An antihistaminic agent.

Phenmetrazine A sympathomimetic often used to treat obesity.

Phenobarbital Phenylethyl barbituric acid used as a hypnotic and anti convulsant.

Phenobarbitone A long-lasting barbiturate drug used to treat severe insomnia and also as an anticonvulsant drug in the treatment of epilepsy.

Phenol Carbolic acid. A disinfectant derived from coal tar.

Phenolphthalein A cathartic. Its use should be avoided because it may cause rashes, albuminuria and hemoglobinuria. Its laxative effects may continue for several days.

Phenomenology An approach in research, as the study of the living experience of people or a way of thinking about what life experiences are like for people.

Phenomenon 1. An objective sign or symptom. 2. A noteworthy occurrence.

Phenoperidine A synthetic narcotic analgesic used intraoperatively to supplement general anesthesia. Also used in the intensive care unit to facilitate patients acceptance of mechanical ventilation.

Phenothiazine One of a group of drugs used in the treatment of severe psychiatric disorder. The first to be used was chlorpromazine.

Phenotype The characteristics of an individual that are due to the environment and genetic makeup.

Phenoxy acetic acid A fungicide.

Phenoxybenzamine A vasodilator drug used in the treatment of peripheral conditions such as Raynaud's disease.

Phenoxymethylpenicillin A penicillinase sensitive antibiotic similar in action to benzyl penicillin. Used mainly against streptococcal infections in children. It is taken orally. Penicillin V.

Phenozygous A developmental anomaly where the skull is much narrower than the face.

Phensuximide An anticonvulsant used in the treatment of petit mal epilepsy; administered orally.

Phentermine An appetite-suppressant drug used in the treatment of obesity.

Phentolamine A vasodilator, used to reduce blood pressure in treating pheochromocytoma.

Phenylalanine An essential amino acid which cannot be properly metabolized in persons suffering from phenylketonuria.

Phenylbutazone An analgesic antipyretic drug used in the treatment of gout and rheumatic disorders.

Phenylephrine Adrenergic agent used as nasal decongestant.

Phenylethyl alcohol An antibacterial agent used as a preservative.

Phenylhydrazine Used as a test reagent for detecting sugar in urine.

Phenylketonuria Abbreviated PKU. A congenital disease due to a defect in the metabolism of the amino acid phenylalanine. The condition is hereditary. It results from lack of an enzyme, phenylalanine hydroxylase, necessary for the conversion of phenylalanine into tyrosine. Thus, there is accumulation of phenylalanine in the blood, with eventual excretion of phenylpyruvic acid in

P

the urine. If untreated, the condition results in learning difficulties and other abnormalities. The condition can be detected soon after birth, and screening of newborns for PKU entails a simple blood test. A sample of blood is taken from infants' heels at approximately 2 weeks and phenylalanine levels are assessed (Guthrie test). Treatment is with a diet low in phenylalanine.

Phenylpyruvic acid An abnormal constituent of the urine present in phenylketonuria.

Phenylmercuric nitrate A bacteriostatic agent employed for wound dressing and preservation of IV solutions.

Phenylproparolamine Nasal decongestant.

Phenylpyruvic acid A metabolic derivative of phenylalanine.

Phenytoin An anticonvulsant drug used in the treatment of major epileptic fits.

Pheochromocyte The chromaffin cells of adrenal medulla giving yellowish reaction with chrome salts.

Pheochromocytoma A benign chromaffin cell tumor of adrenal medulla producing adrenaline and noradrenaline.

Pheromone A chemical substance which acts as a means of communication between species insects through its smell.

Philadelphia chromosome Dislocation of long arm of chromosome 21 to chromosome 9, seen in 90% patients of chronic myelocytic leukemia.

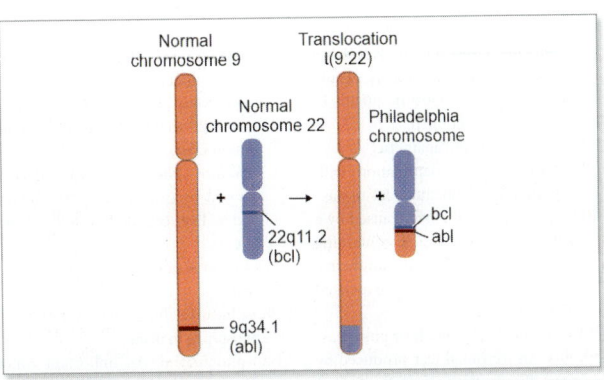

Philadelphia Chromosome

Philtrum The median groove on upper lip.

Phimosis Constriction of the prepuce so that it cannot be drawn back over the glans penis. The usual treatment is circumcision.

Phlebectomy Excision of a vein or a portion of a vein.

Phlebitis Inflammation of a vein, usually in the leg, which tends to lead

to the formation of a thrombus. The symptoms are pain and swelling, and redness along the course of the vein, which is felt later as a hard, tender cord.

Phelebogram A venous pulse tracing.

Phlebography 1. Radiographic examination of a vein containing a contrast medium. 2. The graphic representation of the venous pulse.

Phlebolith A stone formed in a vein by calcification of a blood clot.

Phlebotom Lancet used in incising vein.

Phlebothrombosis Obstruction of a vein by a blood clot, without local inflammation. It is usually in the deep veins of the calf of the leg, causing tenderness and swelling. The clot may break away and cause an embolism.

Phlebotomus A genus of sand flies, the various species of which transmit leishmaniasis in its many forms, and also sand fly fever.

Phlebotomy The puncture of a vein for the withdrawal of blood. Venesection.

Phlegm Mucus secreted by the lining of the air passages.

Phlegmasia An inflammation.

Phlegmasia albadolens Acute edema in a leg due to lymphatic blockage. 'White leg'. Rarely occurs now but was seen most frequently in women after childbirth.

Phlegmatic Dull and apathetic.

Phelgmon Acute inflammation with suppuration of subcutaneous tissue.

Phlycten 1. A small blister caused by a burn. 2. A small vesicle containing lymph occurring in the conjunctiva or cornea of the eye. Often associated with tuberculosis.

Phlyctenula A tiny vesicle or pustule.

Phobia An irrational fear produced by a specific situation which the patient attempts to avoid.

Phocomelia A rare congenital deformity in which the long bones of the limbs are minimal or absent and the individual has hands or feet resembling the flippers of seals, or stump-like limbs of various lengths. The drug thalidomide, taken by the mother early in pregnancy, has produced this deformity.

Pholcodine A linctus for the suppression of a dry or painful cough.

Phonation The art of uttering meaningful vocal sounds.

Phonetics Science of pronunciation and speech.

Phonocardiogram A record of the heart sounds made by a phonocardiograph.

Phonocardiograph An instrument that graphically records heart sounds and murmurs.

Phonology The study of speech sounds, their production and the relationship between sounds as elements of language.

Phonophobia Morbid fear of sound or noise.

Phonophoresis Use of ultrasound to introduce drugs into tissue.

Phosgene A poisonous gas used in production of pharmaceutical and chemical products.

Phosphatase One of a group of enzymes involved in the metabolism of phosphate.

Acid phosphate Present in semen, prostatic secretion, osteoclasts and odontoclasts.

Alkaline phosphate An enzyme formed by osteoblasts in the bones and by liver cells and excreted in the bile.

Phosphate A salt or ester of phosphoric acid.

Phosphaturia Increased excretion of phosphate in urine.

Phosphocreatine An important compound in muscle metabolism.

Phosphofructokinase A glycolytic enzyme.

Phospholipid A lipid of glycerol fats found in cells, especially those of the nervous system.

Phosphorescence The emission of light without heat.

Phosphoric acid Principally used to etch enamel of teeth during restoration work.

Phosphorus Symbol P. Phosphorus is an essential element in the diet.

It is a major component of bone, is involved in almost all metabolic processes and also plays an important role in cell metabolism. It is obtained by the body from milk products, cereals, meat and fish. Its use by the body is controlled by vitamin D and calcium. Phosphorus is very inflammable and exceedingly poisonous. Inhalation of its vapour by workers in chemical industries may cause necrosis of the mandible (phosphonecrosis or phossy jaw). Free phosphorus causes fatty degeneration of the liver and other viscera.

Phosphorylase An enzyme, found in the liver and kidneys, which catalyses the breakdown of glycogenin to glucose-1-phosphate.

Phosphorylation The reaction of phosphate with an organic compound.

Photic epilepsy Convulsion following light stimulation.

Photocoagulation The use of a powerful light source to induce inflammation of the retina and choroid to treat retinal detachment.

Photodermatitis Skin allergy due to ultraviolet light.

Photometer Device for measuring the intensity of light.

Photomicrograph Photograph of an object under microscope.

Photon Unit of energy of light ray.

Photophobia Intolerance of light. It can occur in many eye conditions, including conjunctivitis, corneal ulceration, iritis and keratitis.

Photophone Instrument for production of sound by action of light.

Photophthalmia Inflammation of the eye due to overexposure to bright light, especially to ultraviolet light.

Photopic Pertaining to bright light.
Photopic vision Vision in bright light when the cones of the retina provide the visual appreciation of color and shape.

Photopsia A sensation of flashes of light sometimes occurring in the early stages of retinal detachment.

Photoptometer Instrument determining the smallest amount of light required to make an object visible.

Photoptometry Measurement of light perception.

Photoreceptor Sensory nerve endings or cells capable of being stimulated by light, e.g., rods and cones.

Photoretinitis Macular burn on exposure to intense light.

Photosensitizer Substance that compounds abnormal reaction of skin to light.

Photosensitivity An abnormal degree of sensitivity of the skin to sunlight.

Photosynthesis The process by which plants combine water and trapped carbon dioxide to produce carbohydrates.

Phototherapy Treatment using fluorescent light, containing a high output of blue light, to reduce the amount of unconjugated bilirubin in the skin of a mildly jaundiced neonate.

Phototropism Tendency of plants and some microorganisms to grow towards light.

Phrenic 1. Relating to the mind. 2. Pertaining to the diaphragm.
Phrenic avulsion The surgical extraction of a part of the phrenic nerve.
Phrenic nerve One of a pair of nerves controlling the muscles of the diaphragm.

Phrenicotomy Severing the phrenic nerve to produce paralysis of diaphragm in order to provide rest to that lung.

Phthalylsulfathiazole An insoluble sulphonamide, poorly absorbed in the intestine and so used to kill intestinal bacteria before surgery.

Phthirus pubis The crab louse.

Phthisic Concerning pulmonary tuberculosis.

Phthisis Pulmonary tuberculosis.

Phthisis bulbi A shrinking of the eyeball following inflammation or injury.

Phycomycosis A fungal disease caused by inhalation of spores.

Phylogeny Growth and development of a race.

Phylum One of the primary divisions of animal or plant kingdom.

Physical In medicine, relating to the body as opposed to the mental processes.

Physical examination Examination of the bodily state of a patient by ordinary physical means, such as inspection, palpation, percussion and auscultation.

Physical handicap A term used when a physical disadvantage is due to impairment of physiological or anatomical structure of function.

Physical medicine The treatment and rehabilitation of patients with physical disabilities. It includes physiotherapy and manipulation.

Physical signs Those observed by inspection, percussion, etc.

Physician A medically qualified person who practices medicine as opposed to surgery.

Community physician A doctor who practices community medicine (See Medicine).

Consultant Physician Senior doctor whois overall in charge of patients within a specialist medical field, and responsible for directing junior medical staff working for the same firm.

House physician A junior doctor, resident in hospital while on duty, acting under the orders of a consultant physician.

Physicist A specialist in physics.

Physics The science of laws of matter, their properties and various forms of energy.

Physiological Relating to physiology. Normal as opposed to pathological.

Physiological jaundice (See Jaundice).

Physiological solutions Those of the same salt composition and same osmotic pressure as blood plasma.

Physiology The science of the functioning of living organisms.

Physiotherapy Treatment and rehabilitation by natural forces, e.g., heat, light, electricity, massage, manipulation and remedial exercises.

Physometra Distention of uterine cavity with gas.

Physique The structure of the body.

Physostigmine Eserine, an alkaloid from the calabar bean. It is an antidote to curare; it constricts the pupils and is used with pilocarpine in the treatment of glaucoma.

Phytin Calcium or magnesium salt of inositol and hexaphosphoric acid, present in cereals.

Phytobezoar An accumulated mass of vegetable matter found in the stomach.

Phytogenesis The origin and development of plants.

Phytohemagglutinin A plant lectin agglutinating red blood cells.

Phytomenadione An intravenous preparation of vitamin K, effective in treating hemorrhage occurring during anticoagulant therapy.

Phytophotodermatitis Dermatitis produced from exposure to certain plants and then to sunlight.

Phytosis Disease caused by vegetable parasite.

Phytotoxin Plant toxin.

Pia mater [L.] The innermost membrane enveloping the brain and spinal cord, consisting of a network of small blood vessels connected by areolar tissue. This dips down in to all the folds of the nerve substance.

Pica An unnatural craving for strange foods and for things not fit to be eaten. It may occur in pregnancy, and sometimes in children with learning disabilities.

Pick's disease *A. Pick Czechoslovakian physician, 1851–1924.* A form of presenile brain failure (dementia) with an age of onset between 50 and 60 years. There is shrinkage of the brain and loss of cortical cells.

Pickwickian syndrome (named after the fat boy 'Joe' in Pickwick Papers). A condition in which extreme obesity is associated with severe congestive cardiac failure.

Pico = 10^{-12}

Picornavirus A family of small RNA containing viruses including echoviruses and rhinoviruses.

PID Prolapse of an intervertebral disk.

Picrotoxin A CNS stimulant, a shrub derivative not in use now.

PICU Pediatric intensive care unit.

Pie chart A circular graph divided into sectors proportional to the magnitudes of the quantities represented.

Pierre Robin syndrome Small jaw, cleft palate and absent gag reflex.

Piezo electricity Production of electricity by application of pressure to certain crystals like mica, quartz, etc.

Pigeon breast A deformity in which the sternum is unduly prominent.

Pigeon breeder's lung A form of hypersensitive pneumonitis due to exposure to excreta of pigeons and parakeets.

Pigeon toed *SYN* – Pes varus; walking with feet turned inward.

Pigment Coloring matter.
  Bile pigments Bilirubin and biliverdin.
  Blood pigments Hemoglobin.
  Melanotic pigment Melanin.

Pigmentation The deposition in the tissues of an abnormal amount of pigment.

Pigmentophore A cell that carries pigment.

Pile A hemorrhoid.
  Sentinel pile Thickened anal mucous membrane at the lower end of an anal fissure.

Pili Hairs.

Piliation Formation and development of hair.

Piliform Hair like.

Pill A rounded mass of one or more drugs, sometimes coated with sugar. Taken orally.

Pillar An upright support/column.

Pilobezoar Trichobezoar, hairball concretion in GI tract.

Pilocarpine An alkaloid prepared from jaborandi leaves. It is used to constrict the pupils in the treatment of glaucoma.

Piloerection Standing out of body hairs due to contraction of arrector pili muscles.

Pilomotor Capable of moving the hair.
  Pilomotor nerves Sympathetic nerves which control muscles in the skin connected with hair follicles. Stimulation causes the hair to be erected, and also the condition of gooseflesh of the skin.

Pilonidal Having a growth of hair.
  Pilonidal cyst A congenital infolding of hair bearing skin over the coccyx. It may become infected and lead to sinus formation.

Pilot study A small scale version of a planned experiment or observation used to test the design of the larger study. A pilot study is helpful to see if any difficulties or problems arise in order that they can be clarified before embarking on the larger study, thus saving time and resources. A pilot study may also indicate possible extensions to the study or suggest restrictions of those aspects likely to be unhelpful.

Pimozide Antipsychotic agent.

Pimple A small papule or pustule.

Pindolol A betablocker antihypertensive agent.

Pineal Shaped like a pine cone. *Pineal body* A small cone shaped structure attached by a stalk to the posterior wall of the third ventricle of the brain and composed of glandular substance.

Pinealoma Encapsulated tumor of pineal body usually causing precocious puberty.

Pinguecula [L.] A small, benign, yellowish spot on the bulbar conjunctiva, seen usually in the elderly. Caused by degeneration of the elastic tissue of the conjunctiva.

Pinhole pupil Extremely contracted pupil as in opium poisoning and pontine hemorrhage.

Pink disease Acrodynia.

Pink eye Acute contagious conjunctivitis.

Pinna (pina) The projecting part of the external ear; the auricle.

Pinocytosis A process by which cells absorb and ingest nutrients.

Pinosome The fluid filled vacuole formed during pinocytosis.

Pin's sign The disappearance of symptoms of pleurisy and pain in a patient of pericarditis when he leans forward in knee-chest position.

Pinta A nonveneral skin infection caused by *Treponema carateum* which is similar to the causative agent of syphilis. It is prevalent in the West Indies and Central America.

Pinworm A thread worm; *Enterobius vermicularis.*

Pioglitazone Antidiebetic agent.

Piperacillin A broad-spectrum semisynthetic penicillin active against a wide variety of Gram-negative, Gram-positive and anaerobic bacteria.

Piperazine An anthelmintic drug used in the treatment of thread worms and roundworms.

Piracetam Cerebral activator.

Pirenzepine A drug which inhibits gastric acid secretion and promotes ulcer-healing in the stomach.

Piriformis syndrome Pain in buttock, thigh and lower back due to sciatic nerve entrapment in piriformis muscle, common to women.

Piriton Trade name for chlorpheniramine maleate; a preparation used for the relief of allergy and the emergency treatment of anaphylactic reactions.

Piroxicam A nonsteroidal anti-inflammatory drug used for the treatment of rheumatic diseases.

Pisiform The smaller pea-shaped carpal bone in proximal row of wrist.

Pitch The quality of sound dependent upon frequency.

Pithiatry Treatment of disease by suggestion or persuasion.

Pitressin Vasopressin secreted from posterior pituitary (contains ADH + pressor agent).

Pitting Removal of senescent RBC by spleen.

Pituitary An endocrine gland suspended from the base of the brain and protected by the sella turcica in the sphenoid bone. It consists of two lobes: (a) The anterior, which secretes a number of different hormones, including adrenocorticotrophic hormone (ACTH), gonadotrophin, thyroid stimulating hormone (TSH) and prolactin; (b) The posterior, which secretes oxytocin and vasopressin.
Pituitary dwarfism A stunting of growth in the early years of life due to a deficiency of pituitary growth hormone.

Pituitrin Posterior pituitary extract.

Pityriasis A skin disease characterized by fine scaly desquamation.
Pityriasis alba A condition, common in children, in which white scaly patches appear on the face.
Pityriasis capitis Dandruff.
Pityriasis rosea An inflammatory form, in which the affected areas are macular and ring shaped.

PKU Phenylketonuria.

Place of safety order A court order whereby a child is arbitrarily removed from the care of its parents in the interests of the child's safety.

Placebo (pla'seeboh) [L.] A substance given to a patient as medicine or a procedure performed on a patient that has no intrinsic therapeutic value and relieves symptoms or helps the patient in some way only because the patient believes or expects that it will. A placebo may be prescribed to satisfy a patient's psychological need for drug therapy and may also be given during controlled experiments.

Placebo effect After the administration of a drug or treatment, a change (usually temporary) in a patient's physical or emotional condition following publicity or media interest in the drug or treatment. The placebo response is due more to the patient's expectations or to the expectations of the person giving the drug or treatment than to the result of any direct physiological or pharmacological substance response.

Placenta The afterbirth. A vascular structure inside the pregnant uterus, supplying the fetus with nourishment through the connecting umbilical cord. The placenta develops in about the third month of pregnancy and is expelled after the birth of the child.

Battledore placenta One in which the cord is attached to the margin and not the center.

Placenta praevia One attached to the lower part of the uterine wall. It may cause severe antepartum hemorrhage.

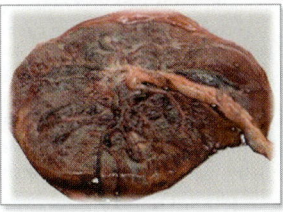

Placenta

Placental soufflé Auscultatory sound of placental blood flow.

Placido's disk A disk with black and white lines used to measure corneal astigmatism.

Plagiocephaly Asymmetry of the head resulting from the irregular closing of the sutures.

Plague An acute, febrile, infectious, highly fatal disease caused by the bacillus *Yersinia pestis*. It is a notifiable disease. Transmitted to humans by the bites of fleas that have derived the infection from diseased rats.

Bubonic plague A type in which the lymph glands are infected and buboes form in the groins and armpits. Known in medieval times as 'The Black Death'.

Pneumonic plague A type in which the infection attacks chiefly the lung tissues. A fatal form.

Septicaemic plague A very severe and fatal form when the infection enters the bloodstream.

Plan, do, study, act A widely used method used in service improvement methodology to test out small changes.

Plane A smooth surface; imaginary cut through a body part.

Planes Used in the description of location and movement of parts of the body. Three planes are perpendicular to each other passing through the middle of the body. These are defined: sagittal, vertical, front-to-back; frontal, vertical, side-to-side; transverse, horizontal. See Axis.

Coronal plane Vertical plane at right angles to sagittal plane so that body is divided into anterior and posterior halves.

Median plane Anteroposterior plane dividing body or organ into two equal parts.

Sagittal plane Plane dividing body into equal right and left halves.

P

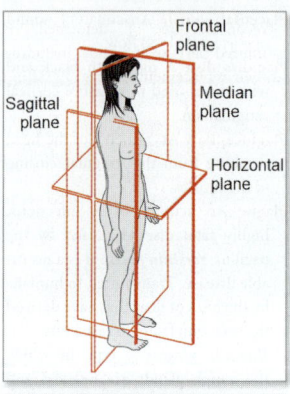

Different Planes of Body

Planned parenthood The concept of choosing the time to have children.

Planning The stage of the nursing process in which the nurse and the patient together plan how to manage identified needs and problems and consider the measurable goals to achieve and produce an evidence-based, patient-focused care plan. A forward date is also set for evaluation of whether or not the goals have been achieved.

Planoconcave An optical lens concave on one side but plane on the other side.

Planoconvex An optical lens convex on one side but plane on the other side.

Planorbis The genus of fresh water snails that serve as intermediate hosts for *Schistosoma*.

Plantar Relating to the sole of the foot.

Plantar arch The arch made by anastomosis of the plantar arteries.

Plantar flexion Bending of the toes downwards and so arching the foot.

Plantar reflex Contraction of the toes on stroking the sole of the foot.

Plantar wart A common wart located on the sole of the foot. Plantar warts are epidermal tumors caused by a virus which may be picked up by going barefoot. Also called verruca plantaris.

Plantaris A slim muscle in the calf.

Plantigrade The type of foot where the entire sole of foot touches the ground while walking.

Plaque 1. A flat patch on the skin. 2. A deposit of food and bacteria on the enamel of teeth which may produce tartar and caries.

Plasma The fluid portion of the blood in which corpuscles are suspended. Plasma is to be distinguished from serum, which is plasma from which the fibrinogen has been separated in the process of clotting.

Plasma proteins Those present in the blood plasma: albumin, globulin and fibrinogen.

Plasma volume expander A solution transfused instead of blood to increase the volume of fluid circulating in the blood vessels. Also called artificial plasma extender.

Reconstituted plasma Dried plasma when again made liquid by addition of distilled water.

Plasmacyte The plasma cell as found in connective tissue with eccentric muscles.

Plasmacytoma Meyloma arising from marrow.

Plasma exchange Removal of patient's plasma with replacement by colloid solution. This removes the immune complexes, excess antibodies or drugs and poisons.

Plasmapheresis A method of removing a portion of the plasma from circulation. Venesection is performed, the blood is allowed to settle, the plasma is removed, and the red blood cells are returned to the circulation. Used in the treatment of those diseases caused by antibodies circulating in the patient's plasma.

Plasmid Extranuclear cell inclusion having genetic function; commonly seen in bacteria and used in DNA cloning and recombinant DNA technology.

Plasmin A fibrinolytic, found in blood plasma, which can dissolve fibrin clots.

Plasminogen The inactive precursor of plasmin.

Plasmodium A genus of protozoan parasites in the red blood cells of animals and humans. Four species, *P. falciparrum, P. malariae, P. ovale* and *P. vivax,* cause the four specific types of human malaria.

Plaster 1. A mixture of materials that hardens; used for immobilizing or making impressions of body parts. 2. An adhesive substance spread on fabric or other suitable backing material for application to the skin.

Bohler's plaster Plaster for Pott's fracture. A leg splint of plaster of Paris, in which is embedded an iron stirrup extending below the foot which enables the patient to walk without putting weight on the joint.

Corn plaster An adhesive strip or patch impregnated with salicyclic acid and applied to corns on the feet.

Frog plaster A plaster of Paris splint used to maintain the position after correction of the deformity due to congenital dislocation of the hip.

Plaster of Paris Calcium sulphate or gypsum which sets hard when water is added to it; it is used to form a plaster cast to immobilize apart, and in dentistry for making dental impressions.

Plastic 1. Constructive; tissue-forming. 2. Capable of being molded; pliable.

Plastic bronchitis Brochitis with fibrin casts of bronchi.

Plastic lymph The exudate which, in wounds and inflamed serous tissues, is organized into fibrous tissue and promotes healing.

Plastic surgery The branch of surgery that deals with the repair and reconstruction of deformed or injured parts of the body, including their replacement, by tissue grafting or other means.

Plate 1. A flattened part or portion. 2. Disk holding culture medium.

Bite plate In dentistry used for getting dental impression of bites.

Epiphyseal plate The cartilage between diaphysis and epiphysis on which depends the longitudinal growth of bone.

Plateau Elevated and flat area or steady and consistent phase of disease or fever.

Platelet A disk-shaped structure present in the blood and concerned in the process of clotting. A thrombocyte.

Play An occupation, for either children or adults, which is voluntary and may be a spontaneous or an organized activity providing enjoyment, entertainment, amusement or a diversion. Play is important in childhood as a necessary part of psychological and physical development.

Play group A session of care and activities for preschool children. It can be organized by any interested person at home or in other premises, but it must be registered by the social services department.

Play specialist A person who is qualified to use play constructively to help children come to terms with illness and hospitalization.

Play therapist One trained in the skills of play therapy.

Play therapy A technique used in child psychotherapy in which play is used to reveal unconscious material. Play is the natural way in which children express and work through unconscious conflicts; thus play therapy is analogous to the technique of free association used in adult psychotherapy.

Platinum A bard heavy silver white metal.

Platybasia A developmental defect where the floor of posterior fossa of skull protrudes upward often causing hydrocephalus and high cervical cord compression.

Platycephaly Flattening of the skull.

Platysma A thin aponeurotic muscle of neck which on contraction causes wrinkling of skin of neck and depression of jaw.

Platysmal reflex Dilatation of pupil on pinching platysma muscle of neck.

Plegia Suffix meaning paralysis.

Pleocytosis Increased number of lymphocytes if CSF.

Pleomorphism Having many shapes or forms.

Pleoptics An orthoptic method of improving the sight in cases of strabismus by stimulating the use of the macular part of the retina.

Plethora A general term denoting a red, florid complexion or, specifically, an excessive amount of blood.

Plethysmography The measurement of changes in the volume of organs or limbs due to alterations in blood pressure, using an oncometer.

Pleura The serous membrane lining the thorax and enveloping each lung.

Parietal pleura The layer that lines the chest wall.

Pleural fibrosis Thickening of pleura from inflammation, irritation.

Visceral pleura The inner layer which is in close contact with the lung.

Pleurisy, Pleuritis Inflammation of the pleura; it may be caused by infection, injury or tumor. It may be a complication of lung diseases, particularly of pneumonia, or sometimes of tuberculosis, lung abscess or influenza. The symptoms are cough, fever, chills, sharp, sticking pain that is worse on inspiration, and rapid shallow breathing.

Dry pleurisy, fibrinous pleurisy Pleurisy in which the membrane is inflamed and roughened, but no fluid is formed.

Pleurisy with effusion Wet pleurisy. A type that is characterized by inflammation and exudation of serous fluid into the pleural cavity.

Purulent pleurisy Empyema. The formation of pus in the pleural cavity. An operation for drainage is usually necessary.

Wet pleurisy Pleurisy with effusion.

Pleurodesis Production of adhesion between visceral and parital pleura.

Pleurodynia Pain in the intercostals muscles, probably rheumatic in origin.

Pleurolysis Loosening of pleural adhesions.

Plexiform Resembling a network.

Pleximeter The one that receives the percussion.

Plexus A network of nerves, lymphatics or blood vessels.

Auerbach's plexus The nerve ganglion situated between the longitudinal and circular muscle fibers of the intestine. The nerves are motor nerves.

Brachial plexus The network of nerves of the neck and axilla.

Choroid plexus A capillary network situated in the ventricles of the brain which forms the cerebrospinal fluid.

Coeliac plexus Solar plexus.

Enteric plexus One of the two plexuses of nerve fibers and ganglion cells lying in the wall of alimentary canal namely Auerbach's plexus and submucosal Meissner's plexus.

Meissner's plexus The sensory nerve ganglion situated in the submucous layer of the intestinal wall.

Pampiniform plexus A network of veins draining the testis in male or ovary in the female.

Rectal plexus The network of veins which surrounds the rectum and forms a direct communication between the systemic and portal circulations.

Solar plexus Celiac plexus. The network of nerves and ganglia at the back of the stomach, which supply the abdominal viscera.

Plica A fold.

Plicate Folded.

Plication The taking of tucks in a structure to shorten it; a folding to decrease the size of a structure or organ during a surgical procedure.

Ploidy the number of chromosome sets in a cell.

Plototoxin A toxic substance present in cat fish.

Plug A mass closing or intending to close a hole.

Dittrich's plug A putrid mass of bacteria and fatty acids crystals in bronchiectasis.

Plumbism Lead poisoning.

Plummer-Vinson syndrome Iron deficiency anemia with dysphagia, achlorhydria, koilonychia and esophageal web, occurring commonly in women.

Pluripotent An embryonic cell having power to differentiate into different kinds of cells.

Plutomania Delusion of richness.

Plutonium A fissile material derived from uranium.

Pneodynamics The dynamics of breathing.

Pneumarthrogram X-ray of joint after air injection.

Pneumatics Branch of physics dealing with properties of gases.

Pneumatization Formation of airfilled cavities especially of mastoid.

Pneumatocele A swelling containing gas or air.

Pneumatosis Presence of air or gas in abnormal location of body.

Pneumaturia The passing of flatus with the urine owing to a vesicointestinal fistula and air from the bowel entering the bladder.

Pneumococcal vaccine polyvalent A vaccine containing 23 of the known 83 pneumococcal capsular polysaccharides; providing immunity for 3–5 years. The vaccine is particularly useful to patients with sickle cell disease, immunodeficiency and post-spleenectomy.

Pneumocephalus The presence of air in the ventricles of the brain caused usually by an anterior fracture of the base of the skull.

Pneumococcus The causative agent of lobar and bronchopneumonia and of other bronchial diseases. A Gram-positive, ovoid diplococcus, *Streptococcus pneumoniae*.

Pneumoconiosis An industrial disease of the lung due to inhalation of dust particles over a period of time *(See Anthracosis, Asbestosis and Silicosis)*.

Pneumocystis A genus of microorganism of uncertain status, but usually considered to be protozoans.

Pneumocystis carinii Abbreviated PCP. The causative organism of interstitial plasma cell pneumonia, particularly in immunosuppressed patients, people with human immunodeficiency virus (HIV) infection or small children.

Pneumocystis jirovecii (carinii) Is a yeast-like fungus acquired by the airborne route, which frequently causes pneumonia in people with human immunodeficiency virus (HIV) infection and in other immunosuppressed persons. Previously known as Pneumocystis carinii.

Pneumocystography Cystogram after injection of air into bladder.

Pneumodynamics The mechanics of respiration.

Pneumoencephalogram X-ray for subarachnoid cisterns and ventricles of brain after injection of air into subarachnoid space via lumbar puncture.

Pneumoencephalography *(See Encephalography).*

Pneumogastric Pertaining to lungs and stomach.

Pneumogastric nerve The tenth cranial nerve to the lungs, stomach, etc. The vagus nerve.

Pneumohemopericardium Presence of air and blood in the peritoneal cavity.

Pneumomediastinum Presence of gas in the mediastinum.

Pneumomelanosis Pigmentation of lung as seen in pneumoconiosis.

Pneumomycosis Infection of the lung by microfungi *(See Bronchomycosis).*

Pneumonectomy Partial or total removal of a lung.

Pneumonia Inflammation of the lung with consolidation and exudation.

Aspiration pneumonia An acute condition caused by the aspiration of infected material into the lungs.

Hypostatic pneumonia A form which occurs in weak, bedridden patients.

Lobar pneumonia An acute infectious disease caused by a pneumococcus and affecting whole lobes of either or both lungs.

Virus pneumonia Inflammation of the lung occurring during some virus disease and secondary to it.

Pneumonitis hypersensitive Diffuse granulomatous disease due to inhalation of organic dusts.

Pneumonitis An imprecise term denoting any inflammatory condition of the lung.

Pneumoperitoneum The presence of air or gas in the peritoneal cavity, occurring pathologically or introduced intentionally for diagnostic or therapeutic purposes.

Pneumoradiography Radiographic examination of a cavity or part after air or a gas has been injected into it.

Pneumorrhachis Presence of gas in the spinal canal.

Pneumotaxic Regulating the rate of respiration.

Pneumotaxic centre The center in the pons that influences inspiratory effort during respiration.

Pneumothorax Accumulation of air or gas in the pleural cavity, resulting in collapse of the lung on the affected side. The condition may occur spontaneously, as in the course of a pulmonary disease, or it may follow trauma to, and perforation of, the chest wall.

Artificial pneumothorax A surgical procedure sometimes used in the treatment of tuberculosis or after pneumonectomy.

Spontaneous pneumothorax Sometimes occurs when there is an opening on the surface of the lung allowing leakage of air from the bronchi into the pleural cavity.

Tension pneumothorax A particularly dangerous form of pneumothorax that occurs when air escapes into the pleural cavity from a bronchus but cannot regain entry into the bronchus. As a result, continuously increasing air pressure in the pleural cavity causes progressive collapse of the lung tissue.

Podagra Gout, particularly of the big toe.

Podalic Relating to the feet.

Podalic version A method of changing the lie of a fetus so that its feet will present.

Podarthritis Inflammation of any of the joints of the foot.

Podiatry Chiropody; a specialty concerned with the care of the feet and the treatment of minor foot complaints.

Podocyte A special type of epithelial cell lining the glomeruli.

Podology The study of anatomy and physiology of foot.

Podophyllum Preparation from roots of Podophyllum pellatum to treat warts.

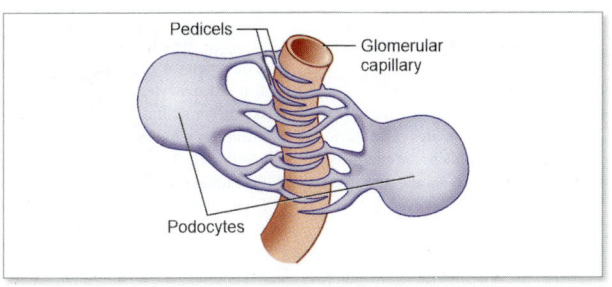

Podocyte

Poikilocyte Red blood cells of abnormal shape.

Poikiloderma A skin disorder characterized by pigmentation, telangiectasia, purpura, pruritus and atrophy.

Poikilothermy The condition of having same temperature as that of the environment.

Point A minute spot, sharp end of any object.

   Boa's point A tender spot on left of 12th thoracic vertebra in patients of gastric ulcer.

   Far point Point (20 feet or more) at which normal eye does not use a accommodation. The far point is less than 20' in myopia and there is no far point for hypermetropic eye.

   McBurney's point Point 4–5 cm above the right anterior superior iliac spine on the line joining it to umbilicus, the point of tenderness in appendicitis.

Pointillage A method of massage using the tips of the fingers.

Poison Any substance which, applied to the body externally or taken internally, can cause injury to any part or cause death.

   Ivy poison A climbing vine which on contact produces severe dermatitis.

   Oak poison A climbing vine producing dermatitis similar to ivy.

Poisoning The morbid condition produced by a poison. The poison may be swallowed, inhaled, *(See Carbon (Monoxide))*, injected by a stinging insect as in a bee sting, or spilled or otherwise brought into contact with the skin.

Policosanol Mixture of plant alcohols for hyperlopridemia.

Polioencephalitis Acute inflammation of the cortex of the brain.

Poliomyelitis An acute, notifiable, infectious viral disease that attacks the central nervous system, injuring or destroying the nerve cells that control the muscles and sometimes causing paralysis; also called polio or infantile paralysis. Paralysis most often affects the limbs but can involve any muscles, including those that control breathing and swallowing. Since the development and the use of vaccines against poliomyelitis, the disease has been virtually eliminated in developed, wealthy countries, where vaccination rates are high, but is still common in many other parts of the world.

Poliosis Whiteness of hair.

Polio vaccine Available as oral live attenuated vaccine or injectable killed vaccine prepared from types I, II, III polioviruses, given in 3 doses starting at 1 ½ months of age and then repeated for 2 more doses at 4–6 weeks interval.

Poliovirus A small RNA-containing virus which causes poliomyelitis.

Politzer Rubber bag used for inflating middle ear.

Pollen The microspores of a seed plant constituting the male gametocyte. Many airborne pollens are allergens.

Pollinosis Hay fever; an allergy caused by various kinds of pollen. Pollenosis.

Pollution The act of destroying the purity of or contaminating something.

Poly Implant Prostheses (PIP) A type of breast implant withdrawn from the UK in 2010 after discovery that they were prone to splitting.

Polyandry Having more than one husband.

Polyarteritis Inflammatory changes in the walls of the small arteries.

Polyarteritis nodosa (PAN) Inflammatory changes in the walls of the small arteries.

Polyarthralgia Pain in several joints.

Polyarthritis Inflammation of several joints at the same time, as seen in rheumatoid arthritis.

Polychromasia Having many colors.

Polychromatophilia The quality of a cell being stainable with more than one stain.

Polyclinic A clinic catering for many variety of ailments.

Polycoria A congenital abnormality in which there are one or more holes in the iris in addition to the pupil.

Polycystic Containing many cysts.
Polycystic ovary disease Stein-Leventhal syndrome.
Polycystic renal disease A hereditary disease in which there is massive enlargement of the kidney with the formation of many cysts. Severe bleeding into cysts can occur. End-stage renal disease can affect many members of one family.

Polycythemia An abnormal increase in the number of red cells in the blood. Erythrocythemia.

Polycythemia vera A rare disease in which there is a greatly increased production of red blood cells and also of leucocytes and platelets. The skin becomes flushed, with cyanosis, thrombosis and splenomegaly.

Polycythemia An abnormal increase in the number of red cells in the blood. Erythrocythemia.
P. Vera A rare disease in which there is a greatly increased production of red blood cells and also of leukocytes and platelets. The skin becomes flushed, with cyanosis, thrombosis and splenomegaly.

Polydactylism The condition of having more than the normal number of fingers or toes.

Polydipsia Abnormal thirst. It may be a symptom of diabetes.

Polydystrophy Condition of having multiple congenital anomaly of connective tissue.

Polyendocrine deficiency syndrome Hypofunction of many endocrine glands, may be type I or type II; Type I – hypoparathyroidism, adrenal insufficiency, mucocutaneous candidiasis. Type II: IDDM, thyroid deficiency and adrenal insufficiency.

Polyethylene A polymer used in production of IV tubing.

Polyethylene glycol Used as ointment base.

Polygamy Practice of having several wives or husbands.

Polygraph Machine that records arterial and venous pulse.

Polyhydramnios Excess of amniotic fluid.

Polymenorrhea Menses occurring at rapid frequency.

Polymer A synthetic substance made of two or more molecules.

Polymerase An enzyme catalyzing polymerization of nucleosides to form DNA.

Polymerization The process of changing a simple chemical substance into another of higher molecular weight.

Polymorphonuclear 1. Having nuclei of many different shapes. 2. A polymorphonuclear leucocyte.

Polymorph A polymorphonuclear leucocyte.

Polymorphism Appearing in many forms.

Polymorphous Occurring in several or many different forms.

Polymyalgia rheumatica Persistent aching pain in the muscles, often involving the shoulder or the pelvic girdle.

Polymyoclonus Muscular contraction proceeding in wave form to involve many muscle groups.

Polymyositis A generalized inflammation of the muscles with weakness and joint stiffness, particularly around the hips and shoulders.

Polymyxin An antibiotic drug used in the treatment of Gram-negative bacteria, particularly *Pseudomonas*.

Polyneuritis Inflammation of many nerves at the same time.

Polyneuropathy A number of disease conditions of the nervous system.

Polyneuroradiculitis Inflammation of nerve roots, peripheral nerves and spinal ganglia.

Polynucleotide Nucleic acid composed of one or more nucleotides.

Polyomavirus A papovavirus family causing malignancy in lower animals.

Polyopia The perception of two or more images of the same object. Multiple vision.

Polyorchidism Condition of having more than two testicles.

Polyostotic Concerning many bones.

Polyp A pedunculated tumor of mucous membrane. A polypus.

Polypeptide Union of two or more amino acids.

Polyphagia Frequent and excess eating.

Polypharmacy 1. The administration of many drugs together. This increases the likelihood of side effects from drug interactions and of noncompliance by the patient. 2. The administration of excessive medication.

Polyphenon E Tea extract for warts.

Polyphrasia Talkativeness.

Polyploidy Condition characterized by twice or more number of normal haploid chromosome numbers of gametes.

Polyposis The presence of many polyps in an organ.
  Familial polyposis A hereditary condition in which large numbers of polyps develop in the colon, which may become malignant.

Polysaccharide Complex sugars which on hydrolysis yield more than 2 molecules of simple sugar.

Polyserositis Inflammation of many serous cavities, e.g., pleural effusion, ascites, pericardial effusion.

Polystyrene A synthetic resin.

Polythiazide A mercurial thiazide diuretic.

Polyunsaturated Pertains to fatty acids having many carbon atoms joined by double or triple bonds.

Polyuria An abnormally large output of urine due either to an excessive intake of liquid or to disease, often diabetes.

Polyvalent Substance with combining power of more than two atoms of hydrogen.

Polyvinyl alcohol A water soluble synthetic resin used for preparation of ophthalmic solutions.

Polyvinyl pyrrolidine Povidone.

Pompe's disease Glycogen storage disease type II.

Pompholyx An intensely pruritic skin condition in which vesicles appear on the hands and feet, particularly on the palms and soles. Typically occurring in repeated, self-limiting attacks.

Ponderal index Height in inches/cube root of weight in pounds.

514

Pons A bridge of tissue connecting two parts of an organ.

Pons varolii The part of the brain that connects the cerebrum, cerebellum and medulla oblongata.

Pontiac fever An influenza-like illness with little or no pulmonary involvement, caused by *Legionella pneumophila*. It is not life-threatening, as is the pulmonary form known as legionnaires' disease. The name Pontiac fever comes from an out break of the disease in Pontiac, Michigan.

Pontic An artificial tooth set in a bridge.

Pontocaine hydrochloride Topical or spinal anesthetic.

Popliteal Relating to the posterior part of the knee joint.

Popliteus Muscle that flex the knee.

Poppers A street name for nitrite inhalants generally, or amyl nitrite in particular, taken in substance, misused to achieve an 'elevated mood' or 'high'.

Poppy Any plant of genus Papaver; opium is obtained from juice of unripe pods.

Population 1. The total number of persons inhabiting a given geographical area or location. 2. In statistics the aggregate of individuals or items from which a sample for a study is drawn. 3. Any group that is distinguished by a particular trait or situation.

Porcine Pig like, obtained from porks.

Pore A minute circular opening on a surface.

Sweat pore An opening of a sweat gland on the skin surface.

Porencephaly A congenital brain anomaly where ventricles extend up to subarachnoid space.

Pornography Sex stimulating photographs or literature.

Purphobilinogen An intermediate product in heme biosynthesis, often present in urine in patients of porphyria, when exposed to air for long time changes to porphobilin imparting red color to urine.

Porphyria An inborn error in the metabolism of porphyrins, resulting in porphyrinuria. Two general types of porphyria are known: erythropoietic porphyrias, which are concerned with the formation of erythrocytes in the bone marrow; and hepatic porphyrias, which are responsible for liver dysfunction. The manifestations of porphyria include gastrointestinal, neurological and psychological symptoms, cutaneous photosensitivity, pigmentation of the face (and later of the bones) and anemia, with enlargement of the spleen.

Porphyrin One of a number of pigments used in the production of the heme portion of hemoglobin.

Porphyrinuria The presence of an excess of porphyrin in the urine.

Port wine stain position *(See Naevus Flammeus).*

Porta An opening in an organ through which pass the main vessels.

Portacath A catheter to provide a central venous line; attached to it is an injectable depot which is placed under the skin.

Portacaval Pertaining to the portal vein and the inferior vena cava.

Portacaval anastomosis The joining of the portal vein to the inferior vena cava so that much of the blood by passes the liver. It is used in the treatment of portal hypertension.

Porta hepatis The transverse fissure on visceral surface for entry of hepatic artery and portal vein and exit of hepatic ducts.

Portal circulation The circulation of blood in liver via portal vein and hepatic vein.

Portal hypertension Increased pressure in portal vein due to obstruction to portal blood flow in liver.

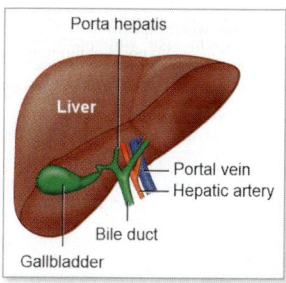

Porta Hepatis

Portal vein The vein formed from union of superior and inferior mesenteric, splenic, gastric and cystic veins.

Portage system A method of behavior modification taught to family members to enable them to assist a handicapped child in development and acquiring skills for everyday living.

Portfolio A collection of competency evidence assembled by the practitioner/student which demonstrates the owner's professional development. The portfolio may include such material as journals, marked assessments, evidence of reflective practice or other examples that document the acquisition of newskills, knowledge, understanding and achievements relevant to professional practice *(See Profile)*.

Portography X-ray of portal vein after injection of contrast.

Portwine mark Superficial purple red birthmark.

Position Attitude or posture.
Dorsal position Lying flat on the back.
Genupectoral or *knee-chest position* Resting on the knees and chest with alms crossed above the head.
Lithotomy position Lying on the back with thighs raised and knees supported and held widely apart.
Prone position Face down.

Sims' position or *semiprone position* Lying on the left side with the right knee well flexed and the left arm drawn back over the edge of the bed.
Trendelenburg position Lying down on a tilted plane (usually an operating table at an angle of 30°–45° to the floor), with the head lowermost, the shoulders supported and the legs hanging over the raised end of the table.

Positive Having a value greater than zero; indicating existence or presence, as chromatin positive or Wassermann positive; characterized by affirmation or cooperation. The opposite of negative.

Positive end-expiratory pressure Abbreviated PEEP. In mechanical ventilation, a positive airway pressure maintained until the end of expiration. A PEEP higher than the critical closing pressure holds alveoli open until the end of expiration and can markedly improve the arterial PO_2 in patients with a lowered functional residual capacity (FRC), as in acute respiratory failure.

Posseting Regurgitation of a small amount of milk by an infant immediately after a feed.

Positron Positively charged particle.
Positron emission tomography A method of demonstrating brain image by use of positron emitting radionuclide.

Possum Patient-operated selector mechanism; a machine that can be operated with a very slight degree of pressure, or suction, using the mouth, if no other muscle movement is possible. It may transmit messages from a light panel or be adapted for typing, telephoning or working certain machinery.

Postcibal After meals.
Postclimacteric After menopause.
Postcoital After sexual intercourse.
Postconnubial After marriage.

Postexposure prophylaxis Abbreviated PEP. The administration of antibiotics, antiviral agents, or active and/ or passive vaccination following exposure to an infectious agent, e.g., antiretroviral drugs after exposure (usually occupationally, but may include sexual exposure) to human immunodeficiency virus (HIV).

Post-exposure prophylaxis Abbreviated PEP. The administration of antibiotics, antiviral agents, or active and/or passive vaccination following exposure to an infectious agent, e.g., antiretroviral drugs after exposure (usually occupationally, but may include sexual exposure) to human immunodeficiency virus (HIV).

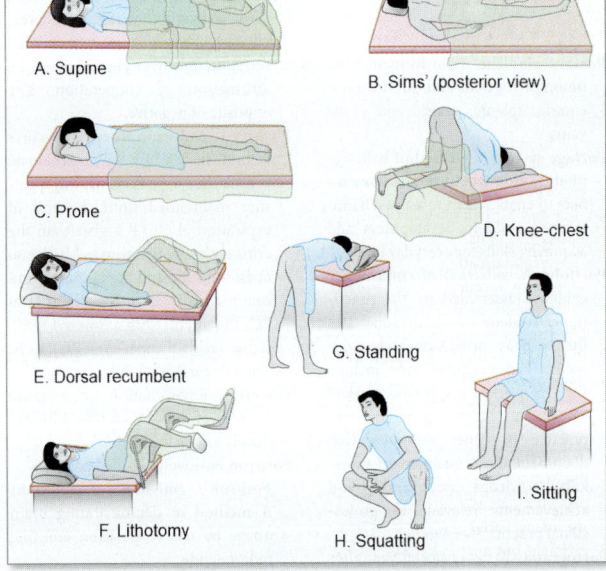

A. Supine

B. Sims' (posterior view)

C. Prone

D. Knee-chest

E. Dorsal recumbent

G. Standing

F. Lithotomy

H. Squatting

I. Sitting

Different Position in Patients

Post-traumatic stress disorder Following the experience of a major incident personal, such as injury, rape or drowning, or other serious event, such as a natural disaster the person may experience insomnia, acute anxiety, nightmares and 'flashbacks' resulting in depression, loss of concentration, apathy and guilt. This reaction may be immediate or delayed, and may last for a variable time. Support and counseling are needed.

Postconcussional syndrome Constant headaches with mental fatigue, difficulty in concentration and insomnia that may persist after head injury.

Posterior Behind a part. Dorsal. The opposite of anterior.

Posterior chamber Part of the aqueous chamber that lies behind the iris, but in front of the lens.

P

Posterior drawer sign A test for posterior cruciate ligament tear of knee.

Posteroanterior From the back to the front.

Posteroanterior Movement from back to front.

Posteromedial On the back towards midline.

Postfebrile After fever.

Postganglionic Situated posterior or distal to a ganglion.

Postganglionic fibre A nerve fiber posterior to a ganglion of the autonomic nervous system.

Postgastrectomy syndrome *(See Dumping).*

Posthemorrhagic Occurring after a bleeding episode.

Post-herpetic neuralgia Persistent nerve pain following shingles.

Posthetomy Circumcision, removal of fore skin of pinis.

Posthitis Inflammation of prepuce.

Posthumous Occurring after death.

Posthumous birth One occurring after the death of the father, or by cesarean section after the death of the mother.

Postictal Following an attack of epileptic fit.

Postmature A state in which the pregnancy is prolonged after the expected date of delivery. Owing to the many variables it is difficult to estimate, but may exist when a pregnancy has lasted 41–42 weeks from the last menstrual period. There is a danger of hypoxia to the fetus.

Postmenopausal Relating to or occurring in the period following menopause. *(See Menopause).*

P. bleeding That happens at least 12 months after menstruation has ceased.

Postmortem After death.

Postmortem examination Autopsy.

Postnasal Located behind the nose.

Postnatal After childbirth.

Postnatal care Includes the care of the mother for at least 6 weeks after delivery.

Postnatal clinic An examination center where the patient can be examined (postnatally), preferably 6 weeks after childbirth: (a) Regarding her general health; (b) Specifically, to find out the state of the uterus, pelvic floor and vagina.

Postnatal depression A low mood experienced by some mothers for a few days after the birth of their baby. Sometimes called 'baby blues'.

Postnatal period Defined in law as a period of not less than 10 days and not more than 28 days after the end of labor, during which the continued attendance of a midwife on the mother and baby is requisite.

Postpalatine Behind the palate.

Postpaludal After an attack of malaria.

Postpartum Occurring after labor.

Postpartum depression Depression occurring in puerperium.

Postpartum hemorrhage Bleeding after childbirth in excess of 500 mL usually due to uterine atony, or cervical laceration.

Postpartum psychosis Psychosis occurring within the six months following childbirth. The symptoms and sign are hallucination, delusion, preoccupation with death, etc.

Postprandial Occurring after a meal.

Postpubescent Following puberty.

Poststenotic Distal to a stenosed site.

Post-term pregnancy Pregnancy which has continued beyond 42 weeks from the onset of last menstrual period or 40 completed weeks from conception.

Posttransfusion syndrome Fever, splenomegaly, a typical lymphocytosis that follow blood transfusion.

Postulate Supposition.

Postural Relating to a position or posture.

P

Postural drainage Drainage of secretions from specific lobes or segments of the lung, aided by careful positioning of the patient.

Postural hypotension Severe drop in blood pressure on assuming erect posture.

Posture Attitude or position of body.

Postviral fatigue syndrome Muscle fatigue unrelieved by rest after attack of viral fever.

Post-void residual Amount of urine that remains in the bladder after urination.

Postable Water free from impurities and hence fit for drinking.

Potash Potassium carbonate.

Caustic potash Potassium hydroxide.

Potassium Symbol K. A metallic alkaline element which is a constituent of all plants and animals. Its salts are widely used in medicine.

Potassium chloride A compound used orally or intravenously as an electrolyte replenisher.

Potassium citrate A diuretic, expectorant and systemic alkalizer.

Potassium gluconate An electrolyte replenisher used in the prophylaxis and treatment of hypokalemia.

Potassium iodide An expectorant and antithyroid agent.

Potassium permaganate A topical anti-infective, oxidizing agent and antidote for many poisons.

Potassium sodium tartrate A compound used as a saline cathartic and also in combination with sodium bicarbonate and tartaric acid.

Potency Strength, power, ability to perform sexual intercourse in case of male.

Potent Powerful, highly effective.

Potentiate To augment or increase the potency.

Potion Liquid medicine.

Pott's disease *P Pott, British surgeon, 1714–1788.* Tuberculosis of the spine.

Pott's fracture A fracture dislocation of the ankle, involving fracture of the lower end of the tibia, displacement of the talus and sometimes fracture of the medial malleolus.

Pouch A pocket-like space or cavity.

Morison's pouch A fold of peritoneum below the liver.

Pouch of Douglas The lowest fold of the peritoneum between the uterus and rectum.

Poultice A soft, moist mass of about the consistency of cooked cereal, spread between layers of muslin, linen, gauze or towels and applied hot to a given area in order to create moist local heat or to counterirritation.

Poupart's ligament *F Poupart, French anatomist, 1616–1708.* The inguinal ligament. The tendinous lower border of the external oblique muscle of the abdominal wall, which passes from the anterior spine of the ilium to the os pubis.

Poverty The lack of sufficient material, economic and cultural resources to sustain an existence compatible with wellbeing.

Absolute p. The situation of not having sufficient resources to maintain nutrition for good health or to provide shelter and living accommodation.

P. of speech Marked deficit in spontaneous speech; replies to questions are perfunctory, monosyllabic or unforthcoming.

P. Trap A situation whereby an increase in a person's income results in a loss of state benefits leaving them no better off.

Relative p. Where a person's living standards are below those of the community in which the person lives.

Povidone-iodine A complex of iodine with the polymer povidone; used as a topical anti-infective and in preoperative skin preparation.

P

Power calculation A measure of statistical power used in research. The likelihood of a study to produce statistically significant results.

Powerlessness Without power or ability, leading to a feeling of being without influence upon their personal situation. People may feel powerless in their dealings with health services and health care professionals.

PPS Pelvic Pain Syndrome.

Pox Pustular lesion.

Practice The exercise of a profession.

Family practice The medical specialty concerned with the planning and provision of comprehensive primary health care, regardless of age or sex, on a continuing basis.

Practitioner A person who practices a profession *(See Nurse (Practitioner))*.

Practolol A drug used in the treatment of tachycardia and irregular heart rhythms. It is a beta blocker and can only be given by injection.

Prader-Willi syndrome A genetic disorder due to loss of function of specific genes. Symptoms include poor feeding in babies, weak muscles and delayed development. In childhood, there is constant hunger leading to obesity and type 2 diabetics, and mild to moderate learning disability.

Praecox Early.

Praevia Going before in time or place.

Pragmatagnosia Inablity to recognize even familiar object.

Pragmatic Pertains to practical aspect of anything.

Pralidoxime A cholinesterase reactivator used in organoph-osphorus poisoning.

Pramipexole Dopamine receptor agonist for parkinsonism.

Pramoxine A topical anesthetic.

Prandial Related to meal.

Prausnitz-Kustner reaction Intracutaneous transfer of antibody to a healthy person followed by application of suspected allergen to produce wheal and flare. Not recommended nowadays because of fear of AIDS and viral hepatitis.

Praxiology Study of behavior

Praxis Planning and execution of co-ordinated movements.

Prazepam Antianxiety medicine.

Praziquantel Broad spectrum antihelminth and antischistosomal drug.

Prazosin Alpha-adrenergic receptor blocker; antihypertensive agent.

Precancerous Any growth or lesion that will probably become cancerous.

Precentralconvolution The frontal convolution or motor area.

Pre-eclampsia A condition occurring in late pregnancy. The symptoms include proteinuria, hypertension and edema.

Precancerous Applied to conditions or histological changes that may precede cancer.

Preceptor 1. A teacher, an instructor. 2. A first-level nurse, midwife or health visitor, with at least 12 months (or equivalent) experience in the relevant clinical field, who provides newly registered practitioners with support and guidance in making the transition from student to registered practitioner. Preceptors should be provided with specific preparation for their role.

Preceptorship A period of support, given by a preceptor, of at least the first 4 months of registered practice for the newly registered nurse, midwife or health visitor practitioner or for those returning to nursing after a break of more than 5 years.

Precipitate A deposit of solid matter which was previously in solution.

Precipitate labor Unusually rapid labor with extremely quick delivery. There is danger to the mother of severe perineal lacerations, and to the child of intracranial trauma as a result of the rapid passage through the birth canal.

Precipitin An antibody in animal, due to soluble protein antigen.

Precipitin test The formation of precipitate in a solution containing soluble antigen or addition of antibody.

Precocious Developed in advance of the norm, either mentally or physically or both.

Precognition A direct perception of a future event which is beyond the reach of inference.

Preconception Before pregnancy. Ensuring the mother is in optimum health before becoming pregnant.

Precordium The area lying over the heart.

Precornu Anterior horn of lateral ventricle of brain.

Precursor A substance that precedes another substance, e.g., angiotensinogen is a precursor substance of angiotensin.

Prediabetes A state which precedes diabetes mellitus, in which the disease is not yet clinically manifested. In pregnancy the diabetes may become evident, or the patient may remain well but give birth to an unusually large child. Screening by urine testing can detect the condition.

Predisposing A susceptibility to disease.

Predisposition Susceptibility to a specific disease.

Prednisolone A synthetic corticosteroid used in the treatment of inflammatory and rheumatic conditions and of asthma and allergic skin diseases.

Prednisone A synthetic drug with an action and usage similar to prednisolone.

Preeclampsia Toxemia of pregnancy with albuminuria, hypertension and edema.

Preeruptive Before eruption in exanthema.

Preexcitation Premature excitation of the ventricle by an impulse by passing A-V node.

Preganglionic fibres Fibers transmitting autonomic impulse from CNS to peripheral autonomic ganglia.

Pregnancy Being with child; the condition from conception to the expulsion of the fetus. The normal period is 280 days or 40 weeks. *Ectopic* or *extrauterine pregnancy* Pregnancy occurring outside the uterus, in the uterine tube (tubal p.) or very rarely in the abdominal cavity.

Pregnancy tests Tests used to demonstrate whether conception has occurred. These detect the human chorionic gonadotrophin (hCG) produced by the embryo 8 days after the first missed period. Immunological laboratory tests are more accurate and less likely to give a false positive result than an over the counter kit.

Pregnanediol Progesterone metabolite (end product) in urine.

Pregnanetriol An intermediate metabolite of progesterone.

Pregnenolone A synthetic corticosteroid.

Prehension The primary functions of hand that includes pinching, grasping, etc.

Prejudice Preconceived opinion, which can be used negatively or positively

Preleukemia Some blood changes that may be fore warners of leukemic process, i.e., unexplained anemia, purpura, mucositis.

Preload In cardiac physiology it is ventricular wall stretch at end diastole.

Premarin Conjugated estrogen.

Premature Occurring before the anticipated time.

Premature contraction A form of cardiac irregularity in which the ventricle contracts before its anticipated time *(See Systole).*

Premature ejaculation Emission of semen before or at the beginning of sexual intercourse.

Premature infant Preterm infant. A child born before the 37th completed week of gestation.

Premature rupture of membrane Rupture of amniotic membranes during pregnancy before 37 weeks of gestation.

Premedication Drugs given pre operatively in order to reduce fear and anxiety and to facilitate the induction and maintenance of, and recovery from, anesthesia.

Premenstrual Preceding menstruation.

Premenstrual endometrium The hypertrophied and vascular mucous lining of the uterus immediately before the menstrual flow starts.

Premenstrual tension Feelings of nervousness, depression and irritability experienced by some women in the days before their menstrual periods. Emotional and physical symptoms usually disappear with the onset of menstruation.

Premolar A bicuspid tooth in front of the molars on each side of the upper and lower jaws.

Premolar teeth A bicuspid tooth in front of the molars on each side of the upper and lower jaws. *(See Dentition).*

Premonition A feeling of an impending event.

Premorbid Prior to onset of disease.

Prenatal Preceding birth; antenatal.

Prenatal care Care of the pregnant woman before delivery of the infant.

Prenatal diagnosis Diagnosis of developmental defects and diseases while the baby is *in utero* by use of chemical tests, ultrasound, amnioscopy and amniocentesis.

Preoperative care Care preceding an operation like preparation of operation site, sedation, bowel wash, breathing exercise, etc.

Preoptic area The anterior portion of hypothalamus.

Prepatellar bursitis Inflammataion of bursa in front of patella. *SYN* – Housemaid's knee.

Preprandial Before a meal.

Prepubescent Just prior to puberty.

Prepuce Foreskin; the loose fold of skin covering the glans penis.

Prepucial glands Sebaceous glands at corona or penis secreting smegma. *SYN* – Tyson's glands.

Prepyloric Preceding the pylorus of stomach.

Prerenal 1. In front of kidney. 2. Uremia or any condition occurring prior to defects or changes affecting the kidney.

Presbycusis Progressive bilateral deafness in the higher frequencies in old age.

Presbyopia Diminution of accommodation of the lens of the eye, due to a loss of elasticity, occurring normally with ageing and usually resulting in hyperopia, or farsightedness.

Prescribe To advise or indicate medicines/treatment to be taken.

Prescribed diseases A group of occupational diseases on an annually reviewed official listing, e.g., pneumoconiosis or occupational deafness, that give the sufferers legal entitlement to financial benefits.

Prescribing analysis and cost tabulation Abbreviated PACT. Data on the prescribing of drugs in primary care.

Prescription A formula written by a medically qualified doctor, and in some instances a specially qualified nurse directing the pharmacist to supply the medication. Also contains instructions to the patient indicating how the medication is to be taken.

Prescription-only medicines Drugs and medicines that are not available 'over the counter' and can only be obtained by prescription from the pharmacist.

Presenile Prematurely aged in mind and body *(See Dementia).*

Presenium Prior to onset of senility.

Presentation In obstetrics, the portion of the fetus that appears in the centre of the neck of the uterus.

P

Preservative A chemical additive to drug preparations and food stuffs that prevents growth of molds and fungi.

Pressure Stress or strain. The force exerted by one object upon another.

Pressure areas Areas of the body where the tissues may be compressed between the bed and the underlying bone, especially the sacrum, greater trochanters and heels; the tissues become ischemic.

Pressure point The point at which an artery can be compressed against a bone in order to stop bleeding.

Pressure sore A decubitus ulcer; a bedsore. Ulceration of the skin due to pressure, which causes interference with the blood supply to the area.

Pressure palsy Temporary palsy due to pressure on a nerve, e.g., Saturday night palsy.

Presystole The period in the cardiac cycle just before systole.

Preterm infant One with a gestational age of less than 37 weeks.

Preterm Before term, i.e., before the 37th completed week of pregnancy. P. Infant Baby born before 37 weeks of gestation. The baby will be of low birth weight, but may also be small for gestational age. Gestational age is assessed using the Dubowitz score. Preterm infants are prone to respiratory distress syndrome, feeding problems due to immature sucking, swallowing and coughing reflexes, hypothermia, jaundice and infection.

P. Labor Labor that occurs before 37 weeks of gestation. It may occur spontaneously as a result of changing hormone levels, an overstretched uterus or weak cervix or due to infection; the obstetrician may attempt to arrest labor by the administration of tocolytic drugs until conditions are more favorable for the baby to be born. Labor may be induced before term because of poor maternal or fetal health, and thus the extrauterine environment will be less hazardous for the infant.

Prevalence The number of cases of a disease present in a specified population at a given time.

Preventative Serving to avert the occurrence of; prophylactic.

Preventive medicine The branch of medicine concerned with prevention of mental and physical illness and disease.

Prevertebral In front of vertebra.

Prevesical In front of bladder.

Priapism Persistent erection of the penis, usually without sexual desire. It may be caused by local or spinal cord injury.

Prickle cell A cell with rod shaped processes.

Prickly heat Miliaria; heat rash. A skin eruption characterized by minute red spots with central vesicles.

Primaquine A drug used in the treatment of benign tertian malaria after initial treatment with other antimalarial drugs.

Primary care The level of care in the health care system that consists of initial care outside institutions.

Primary care groups Abbreviated PCGs. A grouping of general practitioners and their services within a defined area agreed with the health authority and encompassing a natural community of about 1,00,000 people. PCGs provide a direct means by which general practitioners (and their primary care teams) and community nurses working in cooperation with other health and social care professionals will lead the process of securing appropriate, high quality care for local people. Responsible also for the commissioning of health services as well as the promotion of good health to combat inequalities in health in partnership with other agencies, develop primary care services and integrate primary and community services.

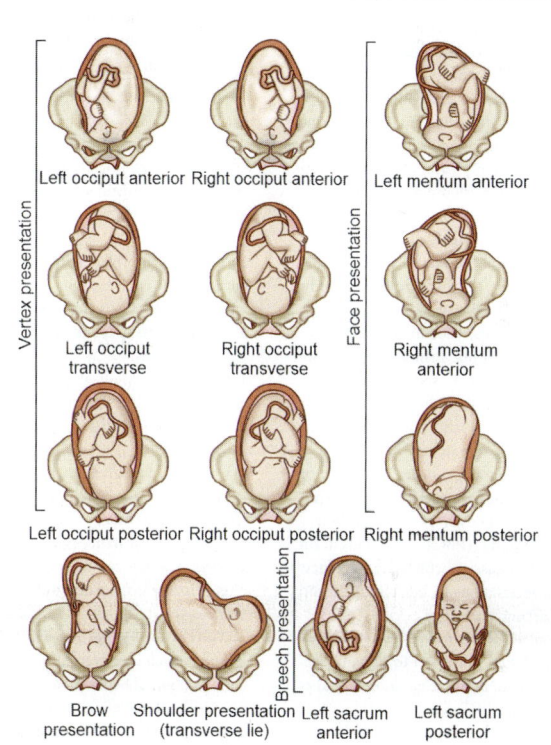

Presentation of Fetus

Primary health care The care given to individuals in the community at the first point of contact with the primary health care team. First contact may be the general practitioner, a health visitor, paramedic or a district nurse.

Primary health care team Usually made up of a general practitioner, district nurse, health visitors and possibly paramedical staff, such as a physiotherapist. They may serve a geographical area and be based in a health center or a general practice area.

Primary nurse A nurse who is responsible for the planning, implementation and evaluation of nursing care for assigned patients and their families for the duration of the patient's stay in hospital. The primary nurse delegates to an associate nurse when off duty but the primary nurse remains responsible and accountable for the patient's nursing care.

Primary nursing Manthey (1980) described a system for delivering nursing care that consists of four design elements: (a) Allocation and acceptance of individual responsibility for decision-making to/by one individual; (b) Individual assignment of daily care; (c) Direct communication channels: and (d) One person responsible for the quality of care administered to patients on a unit 24 hours a day, 7 days a week.

Primary source In a research study, the original source of data, e.g., manuscripts, documents or first-hand accounts. Primary sources are preferred over secondary sources because of the reduced potential for bias and distortion beyond the control of the researcher.

Primary First in order of time or importance. Primary biliary cirrhosis, also known as primary biliary cholangitis (PBC), is a long-term liver disease in which the bile ducts become damaged, bile builds up and scarring of the liver occurs.

Primates An order of vertebrates highly developed in respect to nervous system and brain, e.g., monkey, apes and man.

Prime Period of the greatest health and strength.

Primidone An anticonvulsant drug used in the treatment of major epilepsy.

Primigravida A woman who is pregnant for the first time.

Primipara A woman who has given birth to her first child.

Primitive Early in point of time.

Prinzmetal's angina Angina of coronary spasm with ST elevation.

Prion The proteinaceous infectious agent, without any detectable nucleic acid and immune response causing degenerative neurological diseases.

Prism A transparent solid, three sides of which are parallelograms. Light rays passing through a prism are split into primary colors.

Maddox prism Two base together prisms used in testing cyclophoria or torsion of eyeball.

Privacy Right of the patient to revelation of a data concerning illness.

Private Finance Initiative Abbreviated PFI. An agreement between the private and public sector whereby a health care facility, e.g., a hospital, is built using private funding. The facility is then leased to the NHS Trust. The lease agreement may also contain provision for the delivery of on-site services.

Private practice Medical practice not under external policy control other than professional ethics.

Privileged communication Confidential information given by patient to treating doctor which is not to be divulged by the latter.

Proactivator A substance that contains a portion which can be split off and then it is able to activate another substance.

Proantithrombin The substance of plasma which is converted to thrombin by action of heparin.

Probability A statistical term meaning the likelihood of an association between variables being due to chance.

Proband The initial person with disease who serves as nucleus to study the same disease in his family and subsequent generations.

Probang A device to apply medicines in larynx.

Probanthine Propantheline bromide, an anticholinergic agent.

Probe An instrument for knowing depth and direction of sinus and wound.

Probenecid A drug which increases the excretion of uric acids and is used between attacks of gout to prevent their occurrence.

Probiotic Bacteria having health promoting effect on living organisms.

Problematic internet use Addiction or excessive use of the internet.

Problem-oriented record A multi professional approach to patient care record-keeping that focuses on the patient's specific health problems requiring immediate attention, and the structuring of a health care plan designed to cope with the identified problems.

Probucol An antihyperlipidemic drug.

Procainamide A cardiac depressant drug used in the treatment of abnormal heart rhythms.

Procaine A local anesthetic used by filtration.

Pricaine penicillin A long-acting antibiotic drug, chiefly used in the treatment of venereal diseases.

Procarbazine A monoamine oxidase inhibitor used in the treatment of some malignant conditions, such as lymphadenoma.

Procedure A way of accomplishing a task to obtain desired result.

Proceious Concave anteriorly.

Procerus muscle A muscle that arises in the skin over the nose and is connected to forehead.

Process In anatomy, a prominence or outgrowth of any part. *Process of nursing (See Nursing (Process)).*

Prochlorperazine A tranquillizing drug used in the treatment of schizophrenia and other psychoses and also of vertigo, nausea and vomiting.

Procidentia Complete prolapse of an organ, particularly the uterus so that the cervix extrudes through the vagina.

Procollagen Precursor of collagen.

Proconvertin Coagulation factor VIII.

Proctalgia Pain in the rectum and anus; proctodynia.

proctectomy Surgical removal of the rectum.

Proctitis Inflammation of the rectum.

Proctoclysis Infusion into rectum and anus.

Proctocolitis Inflammation of rectum and colon.

Proctology Branch of medicine dealing with diseases of rectum, colon and anus.

Proctoscope An instrument for examination of the rectum.

Tuttle's protoscope A speculum illuminated by an electric bulb, combined with an arrangement by which the rectum can be dilated with air.

Proctosigmoiditis Inflammation of the rectum and sigmoid colon.

Proctosigmoidoscopy Visual examination of rectum and sigmoid colon by sigmoidoscope.

Procyclidine A drug used in the treatment of Parkinsonism because it reduces muscle tremor and rigidity.

Prodromal Initial stage of disease before appearance of distinguished features.

Prodrome A symptom which appears before the true diagnostic signs of a disease.

Prodrug A compound that, on administration, must undergo chemical conversion by metabolic processes before becoming an active pharmacological agent, thus avoiding gastrointestinal side effects.

Proenzyme Inactive form of an enzyme.

Proerythroblast The earliest bone marrow precursor of erythrocyte.

Proestrus The period before menstruation.

Profession 1. An avowed, public declaration or statement of intention or purpose. 2. A calling or vocation requiring specialized knowledge, methods and skills, as well as preparation, in an institution of higher learning, in the scholarly, scientific and historical principles underlying such methods and skills. Members of a profession are committed to continuing study, to enlarging their body of knowledge, to placing service above personal gain and to providing practical services vital to human and social welfare. A profession functions autonomously and is committed to higher standards of achievement and conduct.

Professional 1. Pertaining to one's profession or occupation. 2. One who is a specialist in a particular field or occupation.

Allied health professional A person with special training, and licensed when necessary, who works closely with health professionals with responsibilities bearing on patient care.

Profile 1. A simple outline, as of the side view of the head or face; by extension, a graph representing quantitatively a set of characteristics determined by tests. 2. A record of achievements developed during a course of study, or subsequently.

Profunda Deep seated especially blood vessel.

Progenitor An ancestor.

Progeny Issue. Descendants.

Progeria Premature senility, the signs of which appear in childhood.

Progestational Concerned with luteal phase of menstrual cycle; action of hormone progesterone.

Progesterone A hormone of the corpus luteum which plays an important part in the regulation of the menstrual cycle and in pregnancy.

Progestin Group of synthetic drugs having progesterone like effect on uterus.

Progestogen One of a group of steroid hormones having an action similar to that of progesterone.

Proglottid A segment of tapeworm containing both male and female reproductive organis.

Prognathism Enlargement and protrusion of one or both jaws.

Prognosis A forecast of the probable course and outcome of an attack of disease and the prospects of recovery, as indicated by the nature of the disease and the symptoms of the case.

Nursing prognosis The application of information obtained during a nursing assessment in order to determine the prospect for altering, through nursing intervention, a client's/patient's response to illness or injury. The prognosis provides a rationale for setting priorities for meeting a particular client's/patient's nursing care needs and enhances continuity of nursing care by clearly indicating agreed priorities.

Prognosticate To state about outcome of a disease.

Progranulocyte Promyelocyte.

Progress notes Notes endorsed by doctors and nurses during course of treatment.

Progressive Advancing bad to worse.

Progressive muscular atrophy Gradually advancing muscle atrophy due to disease of spinal cord.

Progressive supranuclear palsy A rare and progressive condition caused by damage to brain cells over time due to a build-up of the tau protein. Symptoms include problems with balance, movement, speech and swallowing.

Proguanil A widely used drug taken daily to prevent malarial infection.

Prohormone Precursor of hormone.

Proinsulin Insulin precursor produced in pancreas.

Projectile vomiting Vomiting where the stomach content is ejected with great force.

Projection In psychology, an unconscious process by which painful thoughts or impulses are made acceptable by transferring them on to another person or object in the environment.

Prokaryote Organism with a single circular chromosome without mitochondria and lysosomes, e.g., bacteria and algae.

Prolabium Central portion of upper lip.

Prolactin A milk-producing hormone of the anterior lobe of the pituitary body which stimulates the mammary gland.

Prolapse The downward displacement of an organ or part of one.

Prolapse of the cord Expulsion of the umbilical cord before the fetus presents.

Prolapse of an intervertebral disk Abbreviated PID. Displacement of part of an intervertebral disk; 'slipped disk'.

Prolapse of the iris Protrusion of a part of their is through a wound in the cornea.

Prolapse of the rectum Protrusion of the mucous membrane through the anal canal to the exterior.

Prolapse of the uterus Descent of the cervix or of the whole uterus into the vagina owing to a weakening of its supporting ligaments.

Proliferation Rapid multiplication of cells, as may occur in a malignant growth and during wound healing.

Proliferous cyst Cyst with epithelial lining which proliferates and protrudes from its inner surface.

Proline An amino acid.

Promazine A tranquilizing drug used to treat confusion and anxiety in elderly patients.

Promegakaryocytes A precursor cell for a megakaryocytes arising from a mega karyoblast.

Promethazine A powerful long-acting antihistamine drug used in conditions of hypersensitivity, e.g., hay fever, contact dermatitis, drug rashes, etc.

Promine A tissue extract that promotes growth of certain tumors in mice.

Prominence In anatomy, a projection, usually on a bone.

Promonocyte Precursor of monocyte.

Promontory A projecting surface or part.

Promontory of sacrum The anterior projecting surface of sacrum.

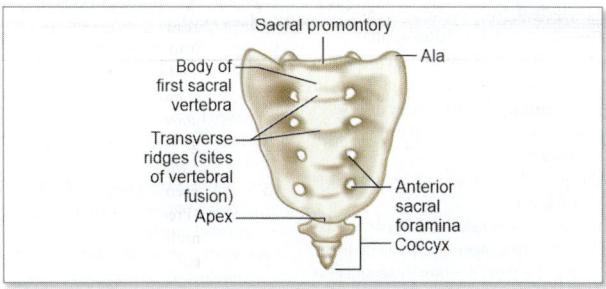

Sacral promontory
Body of first sacral vertebra
Transverse ridges (sites of vertebral fusion)
Apex
Ala
Anterior sacral foramina
Coccyx

Promontory of Sacrum

Pronation Turning the palm of the hand downwards.

Pronator syndrome Syndrome of median nerve entrapment at elbow with paresthesia, thumb weakness, and tenderness in thenar muscles.

Prone Lying with face downwards *(See Supine)*.

Pronephric duct Duct that connects posteriorly to cloaca and to which pronephric tubules are connected.

Pronephric tubulus Tubules that open into cranial portion of pronephric duct and communicate with celom.

Pronephros The earliest and simplest type of excretory organ in vertebrates.

Pronestyl Procainamide hydrochloride.

Pronormoblast An early precursor of red blood cells.

Pronucleus Nucleus of ovum or spermatozoa after fertilization.

Propantheline An antispasmodic drug that blocks the impulses from the vagus nerve to the stomach and is used in the treatment of peptic ulcer and spastic colon.

Propafenone Anti-arrhythmic agent.

Proparacine Topical anesthetic.

Properdin A serum protein with some bactericidal property.

Prophase First stage of mitotic cell division.

Prophylactic 1. Relating to prophylaxis. 2. A drug used to prevent a disease developing.

Prophylaxis Measures taken to prevent a disease.

Propiolactone A disinfectant used in preparing certain viral and bacterial vaccines.

Propiomazine A sedative agent.

Propionic acid A constituent of sweat.

Propositus Index case or proband in investigation of hereditary disease.

Propoxycaine hydrochloride Local anesthetic agent.

Propoxyphene hydrochloride Analgesic agent.

Propranolol A beta-blocking drug used in the treatment of cardiac arrhythmias, angina, thyrotoxicosis and also of anxiety states.

Proprietary medicine Any preparation used in treatment of diseases and has patent and copyright.

Proprietary name The name assigned to a drug by the firm that first made it. A drug may have several different proprietary names.

Proprioception Knowledge of body position, movement.

Proprioceptor One of the sensory end organs that provide information about movements and position of the body. They occur chiefly in the muscles, tendons, joint capsules and labyrinth.

Proptometer Instrument for measuring degree of exophthalmos.

Proptosis Forward displacement of the eyeball; exophthalmus.

Propylene glycol A demulcent agent used as solvent.

Propylhexedrine A sympathomimetic used as inhalation for nasal congestion.

Propyliodone Radiopaque dye used in bronchography.

Propylparaben An antifungal agent used as preservative.

Propylthiouracil A thyroid inhibitor used in the treatment of thyrotoxicosis.

Prosection Dissection for demonstrating anatomic structures.

Prosector One who dissects body for demonstration.

Prosencephalon Embryonic fore brain giving rise to telencephalon and diencephalon.

Prosody The normal rhythm, melody and articulation of speech.

Prosopagnosia Inability to recognize a person from face.

Prosopectasia Abnormal enlargement of face.

Prosoplasia Progressive development of cells to produce cells with higher degree of function.

Prospective study A clinical or epidemiological investigation over a period of time.

Prostacyclin An intermediate in the metabolic pathway of arachidonic acid, formed from prostaglandin endoperoxides in the walls of arteries and veins; it is a potent vasodilator and a potent inhibitor of platelet aggregation.

P

Prostaglandin One of several hormone substances produced in many body tissues, including the brain, lungs, uterus and semen. They are active in many ways, having cardiac, gastric and respiratory effects and causing uterine contractions. They are sometimes used for the induction of abortion. Chemically they are fatty acids.

Prostate The gland surrounding the male urethra at its junction with the bladder; during ejaculation it produces a fluid which forms part of semen. It often becomes enlarged after middle age and may require removal if it causes obstruction to the outflow of urine.

Prostate screening Routine examination and blood testing for prostate-specific antigen (PSA) in older men, as a means to detect cancer of the prostate at an early stage.

Prostate cancer Malignant tumor of prostate gland.

Prostatic plexus Plexus of nerves and veins that lie in the capsule of prostate.

Prostatic urethra That portion of urethra surrounded by prostate.

Prostatectomy Surgical removal of the whole or a part of the prostate gland.

Retropubic prostatectomy Removal of the gland by incising the capsule of the prostate after making a suprapubic abdominal incision.

Transurethral prostatectomy Resection of the gland through the urethra using a resectoscope.

Transvesical prostatectomy Removal of the gland by incising the bladder after making a low abdominal incision.

Prostatism Symptoms of nocturia, increased frequency and dribbling of any cause.

Prostatitis Inflammation of the prostate gland.

Prostatorrhea A thin urethral discharge from the prostate gland occurring in prostatitis.

Prosthesis [Gr.] 1. The replacement of an absent part by an artificial substitute. 2. An artificial substitute for a missing part.

Prosthetics Branch of surgery dealing with prosthesis.

Prostitute Woman who sells herself for sexual exploitation, the major cause of spread of AIDS and other venereal diseases.

Prostration A condition of extreme exhaustion.

Protal Existing before birth, i.e., congenital.

Protamine One of a number of proteins occurring only in fish sperm.

Protamine sulphate A drug used to neutralize circulating heparin, should hemorrhage arise during anticoagulant therapy.

Protanopia Red color blindness.

Protean Variable.

Protease A proteolytic enzyme in the digestive juices that causes the breakdown of protein.

Protective isolation A type of isolation designed to prevent contact between potentially pathogenic microorganisms and uninfected persons who have seriously impaired resistance. Also called reverse isolation.

Protein One of a group of complex organic nitrogenous compounds formed from amino acids and occurring in every living cell of animal and vegetable tissue.

Bence Jones protein An abnormal protein found in the urine of patients suffering from multiple myeloma.

First class protein One that provides the essential amino acids. Sources are meat, poultry, fish, cheese, eggs and milk.

Protein-bound iodine The iodine in the plasma which is combined with protein. Measurement of this is made when assessing thyroid function.

Protein losing enteropathy A condition in which protein is lost from the lumen of the intestine. This causes hypoproteinemia and edema.

Protein–calorie malnutrition Symptoms complex due to deficiency of protein and calorie in small children.

Protein hydrolysate A solution of amino acids and short chain peptides.

Second-class protein One that comes from a vegetable source (e.g., peas, beans and wholecereal) that cannot supply all the body's needs.

Proteinosis Accumulation of excess proteins in tissues.

Proteinuria An excess of serum proteins in the urine.

Proteolysis The processes by which proteins are reduced to an absorbable form by digestive enzyme in the stomach and intestines.

Proteolytic Pertaining to, characterized by or promoting proteolysis, e.g., a proteolytic enzyme.

Proteose An intermediate product of proteolysis.

Proteus A genus of Gram-negative bacteria common in the intestines of humans and animals and in decaying matter. They are frequently to be found in secondary infections of wounds and in the urinary tract.

Prothrombia A constituent of blood plasma, the precursor of thrombin, which is formed in the presence of calcium salts and thrombokinase when blood is shed.

Prothrombia time A test to measure the activity of clotting factors. Deficiency of any of these factors leads to a prolongation of clotting time. This test is widely used for the establishment and maintenance of anticoagulant therapy.

Prothrombinase An enzyme that catalyzes conversion of prothrombin into thrombin in presence of calcium and platelets.

Protocol Description of steps to be taken in an experiment.

Protodiastole The first phase of diastole occurring immediately after closure of aortic and pulmonary valves.

Protoduodenum The upper half of duodenum.

Proton A positively charged particle in the atom.

Protoplasm The essential chemical compound of which living cells are made.

Protoporphyrin A tetra pyrole, derivative of hemoglobin.

Protoporphyrinuria Protoporphyrin in urine.

Prototype The original from which all other forms are derived.

Protozoa A phylum comprising the unicellular eukaryotic organisms;- most are free-living but some lead commensalistic, mutualistic or parasitic existences. Pathogenic protozoa include *Entamoeba histolytica* (cause of amoebic dysentery) and *Plasmodium vivax* (cause of malaria) *(See Metazoa).*

Protractor Instrument for removing foreign bodies from bodies.

Protriptyline An antidepressant drug used in the treatment of extreme apathy and withdrawal.

Protrude To project.

Protuberance In anatomy, a rounded projecting part.

Proud flesh Excessive granulation tissue in a wound or ulcer.

Provider In the health services, a person, group of people or organization supplying a service.

Provitamin A precursor of a vitamin. *Provitamin 'A'* Carotene. *Provitamin 'D'* Ergosterol.

Proxemics The study of how the use of personal space and other spatial aspects affects human behavior and interactions.

Proximal In anatomy, nearest that point which is considered the center of a system; the opposite to distal.

Prurigo A chronic skin disease with an irritating papular eruption.

Pruritus Great irritation of the skin. It may affect the whole surface of the body, as in certain skin diseases and nervous disorders, or it may be limited in area, especially involving the anus and vulva.

Prussak's space Tiny space in middle ear between Sharpnell's membrane laterally and neck of malleus medially.

Prussic acid Hydrocyanic acid, a potent poison.

Psammoma A small tumor of choroid plexus and other areas of brain containing sand like calcareous particles.

Psammoma bodies Sarcoma with psammoma bodies.

Psammo therapy Use of sand baths as therapy.

Psammous Sandy – gritty.

Pseudacusis Hearing of false sounds.

Pseudarthrosis A false joint formed when the two parts of a fractured bone have failed to unite together.

Pseudoangina False angina. Precordial pain occurring in anxious individuals without evidence of organic heart disease.

Pseudoarthrosis A false joint formed when the two parts of fractured bone have failed to unite together.

Pseudoacanthosis nigricans Velvety pigmented thickening of flexure surfaces as occurring in obese persons.

Pseudoaneurysm Dilatation of vessel giving impression of aneurysm.

Pseudocoxalgia Osteochondritis of the head of the femur. Perthes' disease.

Pseudocrisis A false crisis which is sometimes accompanied by the symptoms of true crisis, but in which the temperature rises again almost at once, and there is continuation of the disease.

Pseudocyesis False pregnancy; development of all the signs of pregnancy without the presence of an embryo.

Pseudocyst A dilatation resembling cyst.

Pseudodementia Social withdrawal but without mental deterioration.

Pseudoephedrine Vasoconstrictor, nasal decongestant.

Pseudofracture A line of decalcification as seen in osteomalacia.

Pseudogeusia A subjective sensation of taste in absence of any stimulus to taste buds.

Pseudoganglion Local thickening of nerve resembling ganglion.

Pseudogout Joint pain resembling gout but caused by calcium pyrophosphate dehydrate crystals.

Pseudogynecomastia The deposition of adipose tissue in the male breast, which may give the appearance of enlarged mammary glands.

Pseudohermaphrodite Individual with sex chromatin and sex organs of one sex but with some of the physical appearance of opposite sex.

Pseudohermaphrodite male Genetically male with a small rudimentary penis and a scrotum without testis resembling labia, usually occurs due to disease of adrenals or feminizing tumors of undecescended testis.

Pseudohermaphrodite female A genetically female with large clitoris resembling penis and hypertrophied labia mimicking scrotum.

Pseudohermaphroditism A congenital abnormality in which the external genitalia are characteristic of the opposite sex and confusion may arise as to the true sex of the individual.

Pseudohypoparathyroidism Features of hypoparathyroidism due to tissue resistance to parathormone. Features are short stature, cataract, tetany, etc.

Pseudoisochromatic chart A chart of colored dots for testing color blindness. Ishihara color chart.

Pseudojaundice Yellow coloration of skin due to carotinemia.

P

Pseudomania Pathological lying or a form of psychosis where patient falsely accuses himself for crimes which he has not committed.

Pseudomembrane A false membrane as in diphtheria.

Pseudomenstruation Bleeding from uterus without menstrual changes of endometrium.

Pseudomonas A genus of Gram-negative motile bacilli commonly found in decaying organic matter. *Pseudomonas aeruginosa. Pseudomonas pyocyanea.* One found in pus from, wounds ('blue pus') and also in urinary tract infections.

Pseudomyopia Spasm of the ciliary muscle causing the same focusing defect as in myopia.

Pseudomyxoma A peritoneal tumor containing a thick viscid fluid resembling myxoma.

Pseudoneuroma A tumor forming at the end of amputation stump.

Pseudopapilledema Optic neuritis causing swelling of optic nerve head

Pseudoparalysis Apparent loss of muscular power without real paralysis. *Arthritic general pseudoparalysis* A condition resembling dementia paralytica, dependent on intracranial atheroma in arthritic patients. Also called Klippel's disease.

Parrot's pseudoparalysis, syphilitic pseudoparalysis Pseudoparalysis of one or more extremities in infants, due to syphilitic osteochrondritis of an epiphysis.

Pseudoparesis Hysterical palsy.

Pseudopodium Any temporary out pouching of cell membrane in protozoa for locomotion.

Pseudopolyp Hypertrophied area of mucous membrane resembling polyp.

Pseudotuberculosis A group of diseases resembling clinically tuberculosis but caused by Gram-negative organism, Yersinia pseudotuberculosis.

Pseudotumor cerebri Benign intracranial hypertension of unknown cause, most patients recover spontaneously.

Pseudoxanthoma elastium Chronic degenerative skin disease with angioid streaks in retina, degeneration of vessel walls.

Psilocybin A hallucinogen obtained from mushrooms.

Psiphenomena Events without explanation, e.g., telepathy.

Psittacosis A disease of parrots and-budgerigars due to *Chlamydia psittaci,* communicable to humans. The symptoms resemble paratyphoid fever with bronchopneumonia.

Psoas A long muscle originating from the lumbar spine and inserting into the lesser trochanter of the femur. It flexes the hip joint. *Psoas abscess* One that arises in the lumbar region and is due to spinal caries as a result of tuberculous infection.

Psoralen Plant derivatives causing phototoxic dermatitis; used in psoriasis and vitiligo.

Psoriasis A chronic, recurrent skin disease characterized by reddish marginated patches with profuse silvery scaling on extensor surfaces, such as the knees and elbow, but which may be more widespread. It is non-infectious and the cause is unknown. It tends to occur in families; about one-third of cases are believed to be related to a hereditary factor.

Psyche The mind, both conscious and unconscious.

Psychedelic Mind altering; a term applied to hallucinatory or psychotomimetic drugs capable of profound effects upon the nature of the perception and conscious experience *(See also Hallucinogen).*

Psychiatrist A medically qualified doctor who specializes in psychiatry.

Psychiatry The branch of medicine that deals with the study, treatment and prevention of mental illness.

Psychoanalysis 1. A method of investigating mental processes, deve loped by Sigmund Freud, which uses the techniques of free association, interpretation and dream analysis. 2. A system of theoretical psychology, formulated by Freud, based on the recognition of unconscious mental processes, such as resistance, repression and transference, and of the importance of infantile experience as a determinant of adult behavior. 3. A method of psychotherapy based on the psychoanalytical method and psychoanalytical psychology.

Psychoanalyst One who specializes in psychoanalysis.

Psychodrama Group psychotherapy in which patients dramatize their individual conflicting situations of daily life.

Psychodynamics The understanding and interpretation of psychiatric symptoms or abnormal behavior in terms of unconscious mental mechanisms.

Psychogenesis The origin and development of mind.

Psychogenic Originating in the mind.

Psychogenic illness A disorder that has a psychological as opposed to an organic origin.

Psychogeriatrics The study and treatment of the psychological and psychiatric problems of the aged.

Psychograph A chart that lists personality traits.

Psychokinesis Impulsive maniacal behavior caused by defective inhibition.

Psycholepsy Sudden alteration of mood.

Psychologist One who studies normal and abnormal mental processes, development and behavior.

Psychology The study of the mind and mental processes.

Psychometry The measurement of psychological variables like intelligence, aptitude, behavior and emotion.

Psychometrics The measurement of mental characteristics by means of a series of tests.

Psychomotor Related to the motor effects of mental activity. The term is applied to those mental disorders that affect muscular activity.

Psychomotor epilepsy Temporal lobe epilepsy.

Psychomotor retardation Genralized slowing of physical and mental reactions.

Psychoneurosis A mental disorder characterized by an abnormal mental response to a normal stimulus. The psychoneuroses include anxiety states, depression, hysteria and obsessive-compulsive neurosis.

Psychopath *(See Sociopath).*

Psychopathic disorder A persistent disorder or disability of the mind (whether or not including significant impairment of intelligence) which results in abnormally aggressive or seriously irresponsible conduct on the part of the patient (Mental Health Act, 1983).

Psychopathology The study of the causes and processes of mental disorders.

Psychopharmacology The study of drugs that have an action on the mind, and how such action is produced.

Psychoplegic Drug reducing excitability.

Psychoprophylaxis 1. A psychological technique used to prevent emotional disturbances. 2. A technique involving breathing control and exercises used to relieve pain during childbirth.

Psychosexual Relating to the mental aspects of sex.

Psychosexual development The stages through which an individual passes from birth to full maturity, especially in regard to sexual urges, in the total development of the person.

Psychosexual disorders Disorder of sexual function not due to organic causes, e.g., paraphilias, transvestism, pedophilia, etc.

Psychosis Any major mental disorder of organic or emotional origin, marked by derangement of the personality and loss of contact with reality, often with delusions, hallucinations or illusions. Psychoses are usually classified as functional psychoses, those for which no physical cause has been discovered, and organic psychoses, which are the result of organic damage to the brain.

Psychosomatic Relating to the mind and the body.

Psychosomatic disorders Those illnesses in some individuals in which emotional factors (either causative or aggravating) have a profound influence, including anorexia nervosa and asthma, respectively.

Psychotherapy Any of a number of related techniques for treating mental illness by psychological methods. These techniques are similar in that they all mainly rely on establishing communication between the therapist and the patient as a means of understanding and modifying the patient's behavior. On occasion, drugs may be used, but only in order to make this communication easier.

Psychotropic Pertaining to drugs that have an effect on the psyche. These include antidepressants, stimulants, sedatives and tranquilizers.

Psyllium seeds Used as mild laxative.

Pterygium Triangular thickening of bulbar conjunctiva with apex towards pupil.

Pterygoid Wing shaped.

Pterygoid process Downward projection from sphenoid bone at junction of body and greater wings.

Pthirus pubis The crab louse.

Ptomaine A nitrogenous putrefactive product from bacterial action on proteins.

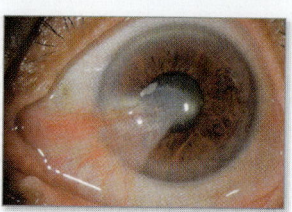

Pterygium

Ptosis 1. Drooping of the upper eyelid due to paralysis of the third cranial nerve. It may be congenital or acquired. 2. Prolapse of an organ, e.g., gastroptosis.

Ptyalagogue Agent that stimulates secretion of saliva.

Ptyalin An enzyme (amylase) in saliva which metabolizes starches.

Ptylism Excessive secretion of saliva.

Ptyalography X-ray of salivary glands and ducts.

Puberty The period during which secondary sexual characteristics develop and the reproductive organs become functional. Generally between 12 to 17 years.

Pubescence Puberty.

Pubes Pubic hair or the area on which it grows.

Pubic Pertaining to the pubis.

Pubiotomy Surgical division of a pubic bone during labor to increase the pelvic diameter.

Pubis The anterior part of a hip bone. The left and right pubic bones meet at the front of the pelvis at the pubic symphysis.

Public domain Intellectual property, e.g., published documents, programs or files, usually from government sources and other organizations that have been released for unconditional access and use by the public.

Public health The field of medicine that is concerned with safeguarding and improving the physical, mental and social well-being of the community as a whole. Environmental aspects are the responsibility of the district local authority, whereas communicable disease control is supervised by the Medical Officer for Environmental Health, from the District Health Authority. Central government formulates national policy andis responsible for international aspects.

Public health laboratory service A central service that provides the necessary resources for investigation, diagnosis and testing in suspected cases or in outbreaks of infectious disease.

Pudendal block A form of local analgesia induced by injecting a solution of 0.5 or 1% lignocaine around the pudendal nerve. Used mainly for episiotomy and forceps delivery.

Pudendum The external genitalia, especially those of a woman.

Pucrile Concerning puerperium.

Puerperal Pertaining to childbirth. *Puerperal fever* or *sepsis* Infection of the genital tract following childbirth.

Puerperium A period of about 6 weeks following childbirth when the reproductive organs are returning to their normal state.

Pulex A genus of fleas. *Pulex irritans* Those parasitic on humans. The type that infests rats may transmit plague to humans.

Pulmometer Spirometer. An instrument to measure lung capacity.

Pulmometry Determination of lung capacity.

Pulmonary Pertaining to or affecting the lungs.
Pulmonary embolism Obstruction of the pulmonary artery or one of its branches by an embolus.
Pulmonary hypertension An increase of blood pressure in the lungs, usually as a result of disease of the lung.
Pulmonary edema An excess of fluid in the lungs.

Pulmonarystenosis Narrowing of the passage between the right ventricle of the hemi and the pulmonary artery. The condition is frequently congenital.
Pulmonary tuberculosis (See Tuberculosis).
Pulmonary valve The valve at the point where the pulmonary artery leaves the heart.

Pulp Any soft juicy animal or vegetable tissue.
Pulp capping Covering and protecting the exposed or infected pulp by metal cap thus allowing it to heal and be protected by formation of secondary dentin.
Digital pulp The soft pads at the ends of the fingers and toes.
Pulp cavity The center of a tooth containing blood tissue and nerves.
Splenic pulp The reddish brown tissue of the spleen.

Pulpectomy Extirpation of dental pulp.

Pulpitis Inflammation of pulp.

Pulsate To throb, or beat.

Pulsation A beating or throbbing.

Pulse The local rhythmic expansion of an artery, which can be felt with the fingers, corresponding to each contraction of the left ventricle of the heart. It may be felt in any artery sufficiently near the surface of the body, which passes over a bone, and the normal adult rate is about 72 beats/min. In childhood it is more rapid, varying from 130 in infants to 80 in older children.
Alternating pulse Alternate strong and weak beats; pulsus alternans.
Bigeminal pulse Pulse where every third beat is irregular.
Collapsing pulse Pulse striking the finger with force, then abruptly subsiding.
High-tension pulse Cordy pulse. The duration of the impulse in the artery is long, and the artery feels firm and like a cord between the beats.

Low-tension pulse One easily obliterated by pressure.

Paradoxical pulse Pulsus paradoxus; the pulse rate slows on inspiration and quickens on expiration. It may occur in constrictive pericarditis.

Pulse deficit A sign of atrial fibrillation; the pulse rate is slower than the apex beat.

Running pulse There is little distinction between the beats. It occurs in hemorrhage.

Thready pulse Thin and almost imperceptible pressure.

Venous pulse That felt in a vein; it is usually taken in the right jugular vein.

Waterhammer pulse Sudden jerky pulse with immediate collapse.

Pulse generator The component of cardiac pacemakers that provides electrical discharge.

Pulseless disease Progressive obliteration of the vessels arising from the aortic arch, leading to loss of the pulse in both arms and carotids and to symptoms associated with ischemia of the brain, eyes, face and arms.

Pulse pressure Difference between systolic and diastolic pressure. Pulse pressure above 50 and below 30 are considered abnormal.

Pulverization To crush any hard substance into powder form.

Punch drunk Boxers with repeated head trauma leading to multiple scars and intellectual deterioration and Parkinsonian features.

Punched out Small clearly defined hole like appearance.

Punctate Dotted.

Punctate erythema A rash of very fine spots.

Punctate rash Minute rash.

Punctum A point or small spot. *Punctum lacrimalis* One of the two openings of the lacrimal ducts at the inner canthus of the eye.

Puncture 1. The act of piercing with a sharp object. 2. The wound so produced.

Cisternal puncture The with drawal of fluid from the cistern magna.

Lumbar puncture The removal of cerebrospinal fluid by puncture between the third and fourth lumbar vertebrae.

Sternal puncture The withdrawal of bone marrow from the manubrium of the sternum.

Ventricular puncture The withdrawal of cerebrospinal fluid from a cerebral ventricle.

Pupil The circular aperture in the center of the iris, through which light passes into the eye.

Argyll Robertson pupil Absence of response to light but not to accommodation; characteristic of syphilis of the central nervous system.

Artificial pupil One made by cutting a piece out of the iris when the center part of the cornea or the lens is opaque.

Fixed pupil One that fails to respond to light or convergence.

Multiple pupil Two or more openings of the iris.

Tonic pupil One that reacts slowly to light or to convergence or both.

Pupillary Referring to the pupil.

Pupillary reflex Constriction of pupil upon stimulation of retina by light.

Pupilometer Instrument for measuring diameter of pupil.

Purchaser In the health services, a budget-holder who agrees to buy a service from a provider.

Purgative A laxative; an aperient drug. Purgatives may be: (a) Irritants, like cascara, senna, and castor oil; (b) Lubricants, like liquid paraffin; (c) Mechanical agents that increase bulk, like bran and agar preparations.

Purge To evacuate the bowel.

Purine A heterocyclic compound that is the nucleus of the purine bases such as adenine and guanine, which occur in DNA and RNA *(See Pyrimidine)*.

Purine free diet Diet devoid of meat, liver, kidney, poultry fish, condiments, alcohol, sweets, pastries, fried foods.

Purine low diet Diet that excludes foods like meat, fish, fowl, spinach, lentils, mushrooms, peas, aspargus.

Purkinje Anatomist and physiologist.

Purkinje cells Large neurons that have dendrites extending from cortex to deep white matter.

Purkinje fibers A type of muscle fibers which conduct electrical impulse to ventricular muscle.

Purkinje network Fibrous network of large muscle cells beneath the endocardium.

Purkinje phenomenon The maximum papillary movement while dark adaptation occurs in green rather than yellow light.

Purpura A condition characterized by extravasation of blood in the skin and mucous membranes, causing purple spots and patches. There are two general types of purpura: primary or idiopathic (usually auto immune) thrombocytopenic purpura, in which the cause is unknown; and secondary or symptomatic thrombocytopenic purpura, which may be associated with exposure to drugs or other chemical agents, systemic diseases such as systemic lupus erythematosus, diseases affecting the bone marrow, such as leukemia, and infections such as septicaemia and viral infections.

Allergic purpura, anaphylactic purpura Schönlein-Henoch purpura; also called Henoch-Schönlein.

Idiopathic thrombocytopenic purpura Abbreviated ITP. An acquired thrombocytopenia which may be acute or chronic in its course. Acute ITP is common in young children. The disorder is usually self-limiting and rarely fatal. Chronic ITP is more insidious in onset, and is more common in young adult women.

Purpura senilis Dark purplish red ecchymoses occurring on the fore arms and backs of the hands in the elderly; the platelet count is normal.

Schönlein-Henoch purpura Non-thrombocytopenic purpura of unknown cause, most often seen in children; associated with various clinical symptoms, such as urticaria and erythema, arthropathy and arthritis, gastrointestinal symptoms and renal involvement.

Steroid purpura Purpura secondary to prolonged use of steroids. The platelet count is normal, the basic defect being the loss of supporting connective tissue.

Thrombocytopenic purpura Purpura associated with a decrease in the number of platelets in the blood.

Purpurin An acid dye used to stain nuclei, a red pigment often present in urine.

Purulent Containing or resembling pus.

Pus A thick, yellow semiliquid substance consisting of dead leukocytes and bacteria, debris of cells, and tissue fluids. It results from inflammation caused by invading bacteria, mainly *Staphylococcus aureus* and *Streptococcus haemolyticus,* which have destroyed the phagocytes and set up local suppuration.

Blue pus That produced by infection with *Pseudomonas pyocyanea.*

Pus cells Dead and degenerated leukocytes.

Pustule A small pimple or elevation of the skin containing pus.

Malignant pustule (See Anthrax).

Putative Supposed, reputed.

Putative father The man believed to be the father of an illegitimate child.

Putrefaction Decomposition of animal or vegetable matter under the influence of microorganisms, usually accompanied by an offensive odor due to gas formation.

Putrefy To undergo putrefaction.

Putrescence Decay, rottenness.

Putrescine A poisonous polyamine formed by bacterial action on arginine.

Pyaemia A condition resulting from the circulation of pyogenic microorganisms from some focus of infection. Multiple abscesses occur, the development of which causes rigor and high fever.

Portal pyaemia Pylephlebitis.

Pyarthrosis Suppuration in a joint.

Pyelitis Inflammation of the renal pelvis. Pyelitis is a fairly common disease, particularly among young children, affecting girls more often than boys. The most common presentation includes urgency of micturition, frequency and dysuria. Pyuria is present.

Pyelography *(See Urography)*.

Pyelolithotomy The surgical removal of a stone from the renal pelvis.

Pyelonephritis Inflammation of the renal pelvis and renal substance, characterized by fever, acute loin pain and increased frequency of micturition, with the presence of pus and albumin in the urine.

Pyeloplasty Plastic repair of the renal pelvis.

Pygmy A very small person or dwarf.

Pygodidymus Conjoined twins with fusion of chest and head but free abdomen and limbs.

Pyknocyte A form of speculated red cell.

Pyknodysostosis A form of osteopetrosis, but without hematologic and neurologic abnormalities.

Pyknosis Shrinking of cell through degeneration and becoming thick.

Pylephlebitis Inflammation of the portal vein, which gives rise to severe symptoms of septicemia or pyemia.

Pyopoiesis formation of pus Also known as pyesis, suppuration and pyosis.

Pyosalpingitis This refers to the suppurative inflammation of the fallopian tube.

Pyosalpinx Distension of uterine tube due to collection of pus.

Pyosis (*See pyopoiesis*).

Pyliphlebitis Inflammation of the portal vein which gives rise to severe symptoms of septicemia or pyemia.

Pylethrombosis Thrombosis of the portal vein.

Pylon A temporary artificial leg.

Pyloric Relating to the pylorus.

Pyloric stenosis Stricture of the pyloric orifice. It may be: (a) Hypertrophic, when there is thickening of normal tissue; this is congenital and occurs in infants from 4–7 weeks old, usually males and first babies; (b) Cicatricial, when there is ulceration or a malignant growth near the pylorus.

Pyloromyotomy Ramstedt's operation; an incision of the pylorus performed to relieve congenital pyloric stenosis.

Pyloroplasty Plastic operation on the pylorus to enlarge the outlet. A longitudinal incision is made and it is resutured transversely.

Pylorospasm Forceful muscle contraction of the pylorus which delays emptying of the stomach and causes vomiting.

Pylorotomy Incision into pyloric submucosa to relieve hypertrophic stenosis.

Pylorus The opening into the duodenum at the lower end of the stomach. It is surrounded by a circular muscle, the pyloric sphincter, which contracts to close the opening.

Pyocele Any cavity distended with pus.

Pyoderma Any purulent skin disease.

Pyoderma gangrenosum A rapidly evolving cutaneous ulcer or ulcers, with undermining of the border. Once regarded as a complication peculiar to ulcerative colitis, it is now known to occur in other wasting diseases.

Pyogenic Producing pus.

Pyometra Pus in the uterus.

Pyovarium Pus in the ovary.

Pyopneumothorax Pus and gas present in pleural cavity.

Pyorrhea A disk harge of pus.

Pyorrhea alveolaris Pus in the sockets of the teeth; suppurative periodontitis.

Pyramid An object whose three triangular sides meet at an apex.

Pyramid of medulla A pair of elongated prominences on the anterior surface of medulla oblongata representing descending corticospinal tract.

Renal pyramid Cone shaped structures making the medulla of the kidney, the apex those projects as renal papilla into the renal sinus.

Pyramidal Of pyramid shape.

Pyramidal cells Cortical cells shaped like a pyramid from which originate nerve impulses to voluntary muscle.

Pyramidal tract The nerve fibers that transmit impulses from pyramidal cells through the cerebral cortex to the spinal cord.

Pyrantel pamoate Drug used in helminthiasis especially ascariasis and enterobiasis.

Pyrazinamide A drug used in the treatment of tuberculosis, especially tuberculous meningitis.

Pyrethrum Compounds having antipeduculosis property and insecticidal.

Pyrexia Fever; a rise of body temperature to any point between 37° and 40°C; above this is hyperpyrexia.

Pyrexin A substance isolated from inflammatory exudates that produces fever.

Pyridium Urinary antiseptic and soothing agent.

Pyridostigmine A drug that prevents destruction of acetylcholine at the neuromuscular junction and is used in treating myasthenia gravis. It is less powerful than neostigmine but has a more prolonged action.

Pyridoxal – 5 phosphate A derivative of pyridoxine acting as a coenzyme.

Pyridoxamine One of the vitamin B_6 group.

Pyridoxine Vitamin B_6 that includes pyridoxal and pyridoxamine.

Pyriform shaped like a pear.

Pyrilaminemaleate Antihistaminic agent.

Pyrimethamine A folic acid antagonist used as an antimalarial, especially for suppressive prophylaxis, and also used concomitantly with a sulphonamide in the treatment of toxoplasmosis.

Pyrimidine A nitrogen-containing organic compound. Thymine and cytosine are essential constituents of DNA, and uracil and cytosine of RNA *(See Purine).*

Pyritinol Cerebral activator.

Pyridoxine Vitamin B_6. This vitamin is concerned with protein metabolism and blood formation. It is found in many types of food and deficiency is rare.

Pyrogen A substance that can produce fever.

Pyromania An irresistible desire to set things on fire.

Pyrophosphatase An enzyme that catalyzes splitting of phosphoric groups.

Pyrophosphate Any salt of phosphoric acid.

Pyrosis Heartburn; a symptom of indigestion marked by a burning sensation in the stomach and esophagus with eructation of acid fluid.

Pyrrobutamine phosphate An antihistaminic agent.

P

Pyrrole A heterocyclic substance acting as a building block for hemoglobin and others.

Pyrrolidine Substance obtained from pyrole or tobacco.

Pyruvate Ester of pyruvic acid.

Pyruvic acid An intermediate product in metabolism of carbohydrates and fats. Its blood level increases in thiamine deficiency.

Pyrvinium pamoate A drug for pinworms.

Pyuria The presence of pus in the urine; more than three leucocytes per high power field on microscopic examination.

⊙ ⊙ ⊙

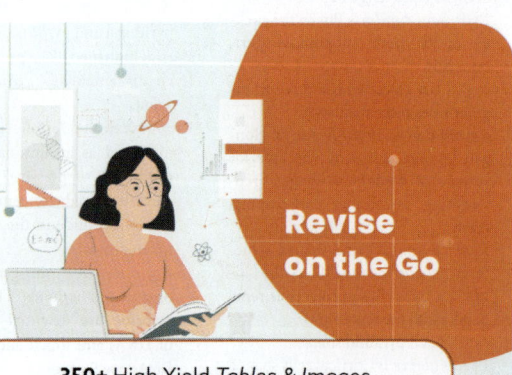

Revise on the Go

350+ High Yield *Tables & Images* covered (Print + Digital) for Quick Reference

CBS Digital Dictionary *for* Nurses

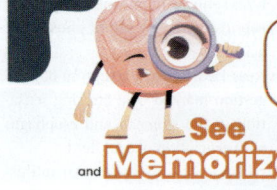

See and Memorize

15+ Annexures *Related to Nursing Procedures in PDF form*

CBS Digital Dictionary *for* Nurses

Q fever An acute infectious disease of cattle which is transmitted to humans, usually by infected milk. It is caused by a rickettsia, *Coxiella-burnetii,* and has symptoms resembling pneumonia.

QNST (Quick neurological screening test) An assessment tool for neurological functions that evaluates attention, balance, motor planning, coordination and spatial organization in people of age 5 years and older.

QRS complex A group of waves depicted on an electrocardiogram; also called the QRS wave. It actually consists of three distinct waves created by the passage of the cardiac electrical impulse through the ventricles and occurs at the beginning of each contraction of the ventricles.

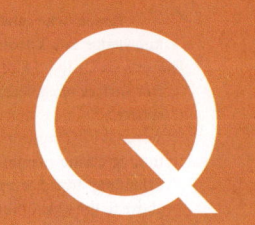

In a normal electrocardiogram the R wave is the most prominent of the three; the Q and S waves may be extremely weak and are sometimes absent.

QT segment In ECG, the period from beginning of Q wave to the end of T wave.

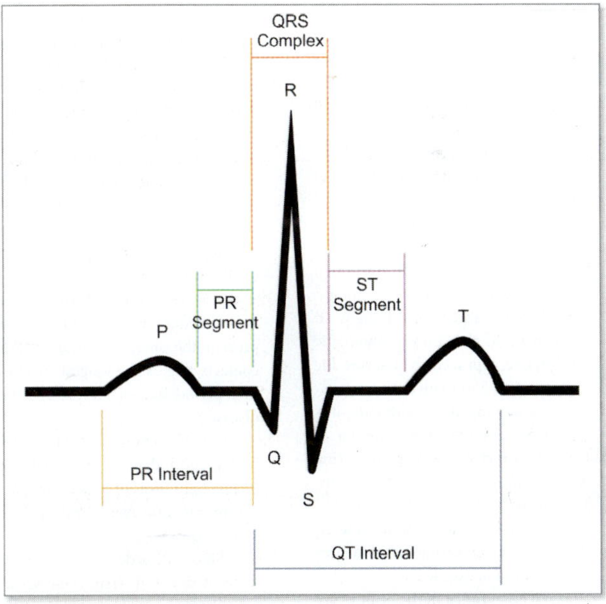

QRS Complex

Quack Person who pretends to have knowledge and skill of medicine.

Quadrangular lobe A region on superior surface of each cerebellar hemisphere.

Quadrangular membrane Upper portion of elastic membrane of larynx extending from aryepiglottic folds above to the level of ventricular folds below.

Quadrantanopia Diminished vision or blindness on one quadrant of visual field.

Quadrate lobe A small lobe of liver on the visceral surface lying in contact with pylorus and duodenum.

Quadrates Four-sided. The term is used to describe a number of four-sided muscles.

Quadriceps Four-headed muscle of thigh consisting of rectus femoris, vastus lateralis, vastus medialis and vastus intermedius.

Quadriceps reflex Extension of leg following contraction of quadriceps muscle.

Quadriplegia Paralysis in which all four limbs are affected; tetraplegia.

Quadruped Four footed animal.

Quadruplet Giving birth to 4 babies at a time.

Quadruplets Four children born at the same labor.

Qualitative research A research method widely used in sociology, psychology and anthropology. It is a method that uses a systematic subjective approach to describe life experiences and to give them meaning. In nursing and health care, it is used to promote understanding of human experiences of pain, caring and comfort. *(See also Quantitative Research)*.

Quality 1. A distinguishing characteristic, property or attribute. 2. A degree or standard of excellence.

Quality assurance In the health-care field, a pledge to the public by those within the various health disciplines that they will work towards the goal of an optimal achievable degree of excellence in the services rendered to every patient *(See Cost effectiveness and Performance indicators)*.

Quality indicator A defined, measurable variable used to monitor the quality or appropriateness of an important aspect of care. Indicators may be activities, events, occurrences or outcomes.

Quango A form of government agency used to provide services or to carry out other duties determined by government. Originally an acronym for 'quasi-autonomous non-governmental organization,' which initially comprised voluntary and non-profit organizations but became increasingly dependent upon government grants.

Quantitative research A formal objective systematic approach to research in which numerical data are utilized to obtain information. It is used to describe variables, examine relationships among variables and to determine cause and effect interactions between variables. Some researchers believe this form of research provides a sound knowledge base to nursing and midwifery practice than qualitative research.

Quarantine The period of isolation of an infectious or suspected case, to prevent the spread of disease. For contacts, this is the longest incubation period known for the specific disease.

Quartan 1. Recurring in 4-day cycles (every third day). 2. A variety of intermittent fever of which the paroxysms recur on every third day *(See Malaria)*.

Quartz Silicon dioxide.

Queckenstedt's test *HHG Queckenstedt, German physician, 1876–1918.* A test, carried out during lumbar puncture, by compression of the jugular veins. When normal there is a sharp rise in pressure, followed by a fall as the compression is released. Blockage of the spinal canal or thrombosis of the jugular vein will result in an absence of rise, or only a sluggish rise and fall.

Quickening The first perceptible fetal movement, felt by the mother usually between the fourth and fifth months of pregnancy.

Quick lime Calcium oxide.

Quick's test A liver function test for measuring hippuric acid after a dose of sodium benzoate.

Quiescent Inactive or at rest. Descriptive of a time when the symptoms of a disease are not evident.

Quinalbarbitone An intermediate acting barbiturate drug used in the treatment of severe insomnia.

Quincke's disease Giant urticaria.

Quincke's pulse Capillary pulsation in finger nails, a sign of aortic incompetence.

Quinestrol A synthetic estrogen used for the suppression of lactation after childbirth.

Quinethazone A diuretic.

Quingestanol Aprogestational agent.

Quinidine An alkaloid obtained from cinchona. It is used in the treatment of cardiac arrhythmias.

Quinine An alkaloid obtained from cinchona. Formerly used in the prevention and treatment of malaria. Still used to treat malignant tertian malaria.

Quinoline An amine from coaltar whose salts are used as analgesic, antipyretic and in amoebiasis.

Quinolone A class of compounds whose well known derivatives are norfloxacin, ciprofloxacin, pfloxacin and of loaxacin.

Quinquad's disease Purulent folliculitis of scalp with cicatrization of the skin.

Quinsy A peritonsillar abscess; acute inflammation of the tonsil and surrounding cellular tissue with suppuration.

Quintan Occurring every fifth day.

Quintuplet Birth of 5 children at the same time to a mother.

Quintuplets Five children born at the same labor.

Quotidian Recurring every day.

Quotidian fever A variety of malaria in which the fever recurs daily.

Quotient A number obtained by dividing one number by another.

Qwerty The standard typewriter keyboard layout that is also used for computers with some additions.

Intelligence quotient Abbreviated IQ. The degree of intelligence estimated by dividing the mental age, reckoned from standard tests, by the age in years.

Respiratory quotient The ratio between the carbon dioxide expired and the oxygen inspired during a specified time. Normal value – 0. 9.

Q Wave The downward defection before R wave in ECG. Prominent Q waves indicate myocardial necrosis.

QALY Quality adjusted life year.

Qi energy In Chinese medicine, the energy believed to be present in all living things. Qi energy is considered to flow through 12 meridian channels in the body mainly connected to the internal organs, and considered essential to good health and wellbeing. This concept is used in a variety of complementary therapies, e.g., reflexology and acupuncture. Complementary therapy practitioners consider that any disturbance or blockage to the flow of Qi energy results in illness or bodily and mental disturbances but that can be manipulated, e.g., through acupuncture, the Qi flow can be increased. Also called chi, prana and aura.

Q

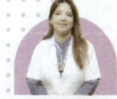
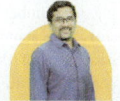
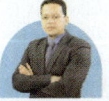
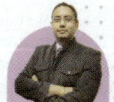
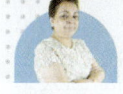
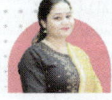
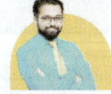
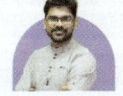
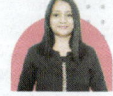
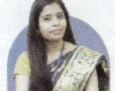
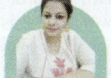
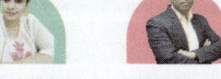
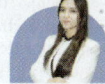

R Symbol for the roentgen unit.

Ra Symbol for radium.

Rabeprazole A proton pump inhibitor for hyper acidity.

Rabid Infected with rabies.

Rabies Hydrophobia; an acute notifiable infectious disease of the central nervous system of animals, especially dogs, foxes, wolves and bats. The virus is found in the saliva of infected animals and is usually transmitted by a bite. Symptoms include fever, muscle spasms and intense excitement, followed by convulsions and paralysis, and death usually occurs. Vaccines are available.

Rabies immune globulin Antibodies against rabies isolated from plasma of those immunized with rabies vaccine. It is used for imparting passive immunity.

Race A distinct ethnic group who originated from a common ancestor, or a taxonomic classification of individuals within the same species who exhibit distinct genetic characteristics.

Racemose Grape-like

Racemose gland A compound gland composed of a number of small sacs, e.g., the salivary gland.

Rachi graph Device for outlining the spinal curvature.

Rachial Concerning spine.

Rachilysis Mechanical treatment of scoliosis by traction and pressure.

Rachiometer Device for measuring curvature of spine.

Rachischisis Spina bifida.

Rachitis Rickets.

Rachitome Instrument for opening spinal canal.

Racism The belief that races are inherently different from one another. A belief that is usually associated with the view that one race has an intrinsic superiority over others, leaning to stereotyping, prejudice and discrimination. Also called racialism.

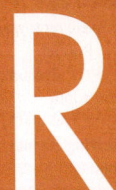

Radial reflex Flexon of forearm on percussion on lower end of radius.

Radiant Emitting rays.

Radiation The emanation of energy in the form of electromagnetic waves, including gamma rays, X-rays, infra-red and ultraviolet rays, and visible light rays. Radiation may cause damage to living tissues, e.g., in sunburn.

Radiation pneumonitis Inflammatory changes in the alveoli and interstitial tissue caused by radiation and which may lead to fibrosis later.

Radiation sickness A toxic reaction of the body to radiation. Any or all of the following maybe present: anorexia, nausea, vomiting and diarrhea.

Radiation absorbed dose The quantity of ionizing radiation absorbed by any material per unit mass measured as ergs per gram.

Radiation carcinoma Squamous cell carcinoma of skin attributed to radiation injury.

Radiation injury Injury to cells by ionizing radiation which can lead to cell death or malignancy.

Radiation protection Preventive measures against radiation like shielding of source, keeping appropriate distance, use of protective clothing, dosimeter, lead apron and limiting the dose and duration of exposure.

Radical Dealing with the root or cause of a disease.

Radical cure One which cures by complete removal of the cause.

Radicle Rootlet.

Radiculitis Inflammation of spinal nerve roots.

Radiculomyelopathy Any disease involving spinal cord and nerve roots.

Radiculopathy Disease of nerve roots.

Radioactive Capable of emitting radiant energy.

Radioactive decay The decrease in number of radioactive atoms in a substance with passage of time.

Radioactive patient A patient who was treated with radioactive substance or was accidentally contaminated with radioactive material and hence remains radioactive to be a source of radiation injury to family and friends.

Radioactivity Disintegration of certain elements to ones of lower atomic weight, with the emission of alpha and beta particles and gamma rays.

Induced radioactivity That brought about by bombarding the nuclei of certain elements with neutrons.

Radioallergosorbent test A test to measure the quantities of IgE.

Radioautograph Photograph of tissue section to show distribution of radioactive substances.

Radiobiology The branch of medical science that studies the effect of radiation on live animal and human tissues.

Radiocolloid A radioactive isotope, in the form of a large molecule solution, which can be instilled into the body cavities to treat malignant ascites.

Radiode The metal container for radium.

Radiodermatitis A late skin complication of radiotherapy in which there is atrophy, scarring, pigmentation and telangiectases of the skin.

Radiograph Skiagram; the picture obtained, on specially sensitized film, by passing X-rays through the body.

Radiographer A professional health care worker in a diagnostic X-ray department (diagnostic radiographer) or in a radiotherapy department (therapy radiographer).

Radiography The making of film records (radiographs) of internal structures of the body by exposure of film specially sensitized to X-rays or gamma rays.

Body-section radiography A special technique to show in detail images and structures lying in a predetermined plane of tissue, while blurring or eliminating detail in images in other planes; various mechanisms and methods for such radiography have been given various names, e.g., laminagraphy, tomography, etc.

Double-contrast radiography A technique for revealing an abnormality of the intestinal mucosa; it involves injection and evacuation of a barium enema, followed by inflation of the intestine with air under light pressure.

Neutron radiography That in which a narrow beam of neutrons from a nuclear reactor is passed through tissues; especially useful in visualizing bony tissue.

Serial radiography The making of several exposures of a particular area at arbitrary intervals.

Radioimmunoassay A method for determining concentration of substances particularly protein- bound hormones to the range of pictograms.

Radial immunodiffusion Study of antigen-antibody interaction by use of radioisotope labeled antigens or antibodies diffused through a gel.

Radioiodine Radioactive isotope of iodine 131 used in diagnosis of thyroid disorders.

Radioisotope An isotope of an element that emits radioactivity. These isotopes may occur naturally or be produced artificially by bombardment with neutrons.

Radiologist A medically qualified doctor who specializes in the science of radiology.

Radiology The science of radiation. In medicine the term refers to its use in the diagnosis and treatment of disease.

Radiolucent Permitting the X-rays to pass through.

Radiometer Equipment for measuring the intensity of radiation.

Radiomimetic Producing effects similar to those of ionizing radiations.

Radionecrosis Tissue destruction on exposure to radiant energy.

Radionuclide A radioactive substance which is inherently unstable. It is used in both radiodiagnosis and in radiotherapy.

Radiopaque Impermeable to X-ray or other form of radiation.

Radiopelvimetry Measurement of pelvis by use of X-rays.

Radiopharmaceuticals Radioactive chemicals or their combination with carriers. Used for determining size and function of body organs.

Radioresistant Tumors that cannot be destroyed by radiation, and hence are radioresistant.

Radioscopy The examination of X-ray images on a fluorescent screen.

Radiosensitive Pertaining to those structures that respond readily to radiotherapy.

Radiotelemetry Transmission of data via radio from a patient to a remote monitor for analysis.

Radiotherapist A medically qualified doctor specializing in radiotherapy. Radiotherapy treatment of disease by X-rays or radioactive isotopes.

Radiotherapy The treatment of disease by application of X-rays, radium, ultraviolet or other forms of radiations.

Radium Symbol Ra. A radioactive element, obtained from uranium ores, which gives off emanations of great radioactive power. Used in the treatment of some malignant diseases.

Radium needles Metallic needle shaped containers which contain radium and are inserted to tissue to destroy malignant growths.

Radon A radioactive gaseous element resulting from disintegration of radium. It occurs in nature and is estimated to cause 5–10% of lung cancers occurring in general population.

Raffinose A trisaccharide which on hydrolysis yields fructose and melibiose.

RAI Relatives assessment interview.

RAID Rapid access interface and discharge team. RAID teams are specialist mental health professionals working in acute settings to ensure that patients with mental health needs are properly managed.

Raimiste's phenomenon In hemiplegia resistance to hip abduction or adduction in the non-involved extremity evokes same response in involved limb.

Raised intracranial pressure Abbreviated ICP. Maybe associated with a variety of conditions, e.g., hemorrhage, edema, brain tumor, head injury or disturbance to the flow of cerebrospinal fluid.

Rale An abnormal rattling sound, heard on auscultation of the chest during respiration when there is fluid in the bronchi.

Raloxifene Selective estrogen receptor modulator.

Ramipril ACE inhibitor.

Ramsay Hunt syndrome A complication of shingles.

Ramstedt's operation *WC Ramstedt, German surgeon, 1867–1963.* Operation for congenital stricture of the pylorus in which the fibers of the

R

sphincter muscle are divided, leaving the mucous lining intact.

Ramus A branch or division of a forked structure.

Rancid Disagreeable smell or taste from decomposition of fatty substances.

Random controlled trial An experimental study for testing the effectiveness of a drug or treatment regime in which subjects are divided at random into two groups experimental and control.

Randomization *SYN* – Double blind technique, a method used to assign subjects into treatment or nontreatment group by procedures like tossing a coin or use of numbers.

Random sample A sample from a population, obtained by ensuring that each member of that population has an equal chance of being selected. The sample selected should then demonstrate the same profile as the parent population.

Ranitidine H_2 receptor blocker, used in peptic ulcer.

Ranula A retention cyst, usually under the tongue when blockage occurs in a submaxillary or sublingual duct, or in a mucous gland.

Ranvier's nodes Constriction in myelin sheath of nerve fibers at regular intervals.

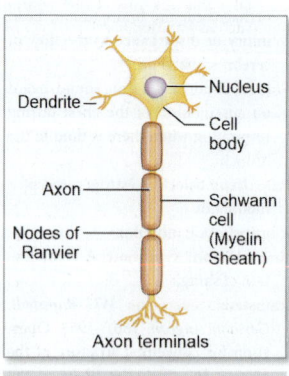

Ranvier's Nodes

Rape Sexual assault or abuse; criminal forcible sexual intercourse (e.g., penetration) without the consent of the adult or child. Many cases are not reported because of feelings of shame, guilt, embarrassment or fear. Although rape can occur between men, it is usually associated with victims who are women.

Raphe A seam or ridge of tissue indicating the junction of two parts.

Rapport In psychiatry, a satisfactory relationship between two persons, either the doctor and patient or nurse and patient, or the patient with any significant other.

Rarefaction The process of becoming less dense.

Rash A superficial eruption on the skin, frequently characteristic of some specific fever.

Rashkind catheter *WJ Rashkind, American pediatric cardiologist, b. 1922.* A balloon catheter used to increase the size of the atrial septal defect in children who have transposition of the great vessels.

Rat A rodent of genus *Rattus* that serve as reservoirs of many infections and infestations, e.g., rat bite fever.

Rate The speed or frequency with which an event or circumstance occurs per unit of time, population, or other standard of comparison.

Basal metabolic rate Abbreviated BMR. An expression of the rate at which oxygen is utilized in a fasting subject at complete rest as a percentage of a value established as normal for such a subject.

Birth rate The number of live births in a population in a specified period of time (crude birth rate), for the female population (refined birth rate), or for the female population of child-bearing age (true birth rate), usually expressed per year per 1,000 of the estimated mid-year population.

Death rate The number of deaths per stated number of persons (1000, 10,000 or 100,000) in a certain region in a certain time (crude death rate). The death rate calculated with allowances made for age and sex distribution in the population is termed the standardized death rate. Also called mortality rate.

Glomerular filtration rate An expression of the quantity of glomerular filtrate formed each minute in the nephrons of both kidneys, calculated by measuring the clearance of specific substances, e.g., insulin or creatinine.

Rathke's pouch A depression in the embryo giving origin to anterior lobe of pituitary.

Ratio An expression of the quantity of one substance or entity in relation to that of another; the relationship between two quantities expressed as the quotient of one divided by the other.

Albumin-globulin ratio Ratio of albumin to globulin in blood; usually 1.3:1 or 1.4:1.

Arm ratio In chromosome the ratio of long arm to short arm.

Lecithin sphingomyelin ratio The ratio of lecithin to sphingomyelin in amniotic fluid.

Ratio odd's In epidemiological and case control studies a relative measure of disease occurrence.

Therapeutic ratio A ratio of effective therapeutic dose to minimum lethal dose.

Ration Fixed food and drink per day/month.

Rational Logical.

Rationale The reasoning for course of action.

Rationalization In psychiatry, the mental process by which individuals explain their behavior, giving reasons that are advantageous to themselves or are socially acceptable.

It maybe a conscious or an unconscious act.

Rattle A gurgling sound.

Death rattle The crepitant rale heard due to fluid accumulation in trachea in a dying person.

Rattle snake A poisonous snake that produces a characteristic rattle.

Raucous Hoarse or harsh.

Rauwolfia A genus of tropical trees and shrubs. The dried root of *Rauwolfia serpentine* is sometimes used as an antihypertensive and sedative, e.g., reserpine.

Rave Irrational talk, as in delirium.

Ray Any narrow beam of light, the line of propagation of any radiant energy.

Alpha ray The less penetrative rays composed of positively charged particles of helium having powerful fluorescent, photographic and ionizing properties.

Beta ray Negatively charged electrons of disintegrating radioactive elements.

Gamma ray High velocity and penetrating rays coming from nucleus of radioactive elements with wavelength of 1.4 to 0.001 AU.

Raynaud's phenomenon or **disease** *M Raynaud, French physician, 1834–1881.* Raynaud's phenomenon is characterized by episodic digital ischaemia provoked by stimuli such as emotion, cold, trauma, hormones and drugs. It includes both Raynaud's disease, where no underlying cause can be found, and Raynaud's syndrome, where there is an associated underlying disorder. These disorders include scleroderma, mixed connective tissue disease, systemic lupus erythematosus (SLE), polymyositis, rheumatoid arthritis, neuro vascular entrapment syndromes and occlusive arterial disease.

Re-education The education and training of the physically handicapped or those with learning difficulties

R

to enable them to develop their potential.

React To respond to stimulus, to participate in chemical reaction.

Reaction Counteraction; a response to the application of a stimulus.

Reaction time The interval between the stimulus and the response.

Reactive In psychiatry, used to describe a mental condition brought about by adverse external circumstances.

Reactive depression One that arises in this way and is not endogenous.

Reading lip Interpretation of one's speech from movement of his lips.

Read only memory The part of computer's memory that contains permanent instructions in contrast to random access memory which holds only a temporary memory (program).

Reagent A substance employed to produce a chemical reaction.

Reagin IgE antibody.

Reality Agreed as an absolute by members of the same culture as the total of all things related to perception, meaning and behavior. Not imaginary, fictitious or pretended.

Reality orientation (See Orientation).

Reamer Instrument of dentists for enlargement of root canal.

Reanimate To revive, resuscitate.

Rebound phenomenon When a limb or part is moved against resistance and the resistance is suddenly withdrawn, the limb moves abruptly in the direction of effort, feature of cerebellar disease.

Recall To bring back to consciousness.

Receptaculum chyli Inferior pear shaped expanded portion of lower end of thoracic duct in abdomen.

Receptor 1. A sensory nerve ending that receives stimuli for transmission through the sensory nervous system. 2. A molecule on the surface or within a cell that recognizes

and binds with specific molecules, producing some effect in the cell.

Recess A small depression or indentation.

Recession In dentistry, the atrophy of gingival tissue leading to exposure of the roots.

Recessive Tending to recede. The opposite to dominant.

Recessive gene A gene that will produce its characteristics only when present in a homozygous state; both parents need to possess the particular gene, and there is a 1 in 4 chance of a child inheriting it homozygously.

Recidivism Habitual criminality; repetition of criminal act.

Recidivity Tendency to relapse or to return to a former position/condition.

Recipe A medicine formula.

Recipient One who receives, as a blood transfusion, or a tissue or organ graft.

Universal recipient A person thought to be able to receive blood of any type without agglutination of the donor cells.

Reciprocal Mutual, complementary.

Recklinghausen disease Multiple neurofibromata of nerve sheath, arising from cranial and spinal nerve roots and peripheral nerves.

Recline To lie down; to be a recumbent position.

Reclus' disease Multiple benign cystic growth in the breast.

Recombinant DNA Insertion of DNA segment from one organism into DNA of another organism.

Recombination In genetics, the joining together of gene combinations in the offspring that were not present in the parents.

Recon In genetics, the smallest unit that can enter into recombination.

Recover To regain lost health after the illness.

Recovery The process of becoming well after ill health.

Recovery room The room where patients are kept to recover from effects of anesthesia after the surgery.

Recrudescence Renewed aggravation of symptoms after an interval of abatement.

Recruitment 1. In audiology, an increase in the perceived intensity of sound out of proportion to the actual increase in the sound level, failure of recruitment indicates lesion. 2. Increase in the intensity of a reflex by activation of greater number of motor neurons by a reflex action even though strength of stimulus remains unchanged, e.g., patellar reflex augmented by clasping/pulling the hands apart.

Rectal Relating to the rectum.

Rectal crisis Rectal pain and tenesmus in CNS disorders.

Rectal examination Inspection of rectum by insertion of a glove-covered finger or with the aid of a proctoscope.

Rectal reflex Desire to defecate when rectum is filled with stool.

Rectified Made pure or set right.

Rectifier In electricity, a device for transforming alternating current into direct current.

Rectocele Prolapse of posterior vaginal wall along with anterior wall of rectum.

Rectoclysis Slow introduction of fluid into rectum.

Rectopexy The operation for fixation of a prolapsed rectum.

Rectosigmoid Upper portion of rectum and adjoining sigmoid colon.

Rectourethral Concerning rectum and urethra.

Rectouterine Concerning rectum and uterus.

Rectovaginal Concerning the rectum and vagina.

Rectovesical Concerning the rectum and bladder.

Rectum The lower end of the large intestine from the sigmoid flexure to the anus.

Rectus muscle 1. The short muscles of eye. 2. Two long midline muscles of abdominal wall stretching of abdominal wall stretching from pubic bone to ensiform cartilage and 5th, 6th and 7th ribs.

Recumbent Lying down in the dorsal position.

Recuperation Convalescence; recovery of health and strength.

Recurrence Return of symptoms after a period of quiescence or relapse.

Recurrent Liable to recur.

Recurrent fever Relapsing fever.

Red cross Internationally recognized sign of medical installation or a medical personnel bearing impunity against attack in war.

Redia A stage in life cycle of trematode following sporocyst which develop into infecting cercaria.

Redivac drainage tube A proprietary closed drainage system used mainly postoperatively for abdominal wounds.

Red nucleus Gray matter in the tegmentum of midbrain.

Redox Combined form to indicate oxidation reduction reaction.

Reduce 1. To restore to normal apposition as in fracture. 2. In chemistry, a type of reaction in which a substance gains electrons.

Reducing agent A substance that loses electrons easily, e.g., hydrogen sulfide, sulphur dioxide.

Reductase An enzyme accelerating the process of reduction in a chemical reaction.

Reduction 1. The correction of a fracture, dislocation or hernia. 2. The addition of hydrogen to a substance or, more generally, the gain of electrons; the opposite of oxidization.

Closed reduction The manipulative reduction of a fracture without incision.

R

Open reduction Reduction of a fracture after incision into the fracture site.

Reduction division Cell division occurring in gametogenesis so that the chromosome number is reduced to half.

Redundant Superfluous, more than necessary.

Reed-Sternberg cells Giant connective tissue cells with large nuclei (owl eye), characteristic of Hodgkin's disease.

Reentry In electrophysiology of heart, a mechanism to explain tachyarrhythmias where a stimulus passing down the conduction system is blocked in one pathway but travels down in an alternative pathway and again ascends up in previously blocked pathway to give rise to a circus movement.

Reference man A concept employed in nutritional investigation and surveys where a man weighing 70 kg of 22 years of age engaged in light physical activity consumes 2800 kcal/day.

Reference woman Woman of around 22 years of age weighing 58 kg and consuming 2000 kcal/day.

Referred pain That which occurs at a distance from the place of origin due to the sensory nerves entering the cord at the same level, e.g., the phrenic nerve supplying the diaphragm enters the cord in the cervical region, as do the nerves from the shoulder, and so an abscess on the diaphragm may cause pain in the shoulder. Synalgia.

Reflection 1. A turning or bending back, as in the folds produced when a membrane passes over the surface of an organ and then passes back to the body wall that it lines. 2. In nursing and health care practice, conscious and systematic thinking about one's actions; the review, analysis and evaluation of those situations that have occurred, usually after but maybe during an event. An active process by which the practitioner learns from situations with a view to improving future practice.

Reflective practice An active process by which the health care professional is able to review, analyse and evaluate events or situations. This conscious monitoring process can be based on any conceptual model, and may utilize supervision of peers in the process. The aim is to facilitate and enhance professional practice.

Reflex Reflected or thrown back.

Accommodation reflex The alteration in the shape of the lens according to the distance of the image viewed.

Conditioned reflex That which is not natural, but is developed by association and frequent repetition until it appears natural.

Corneal reflex The automatic reaction of closing the eyelids after exertion of light pressure on the cornea. This is a test for unconsciousness which is absolute when there is no response.

Deep reflex A muscle reflex elicited by tapping the tendon or bone of attachment.

Light reflex Alteration of the size of the pupil in response to exposure to light.

Reflex action An involuntary action following immediately upon some stimulus, e.g., the knee jerk, or the withdrawal of a limb from a pinprick.

Reflex arc The sensory and motor neurones, together with the connector neurone, which carry out a reflex action.

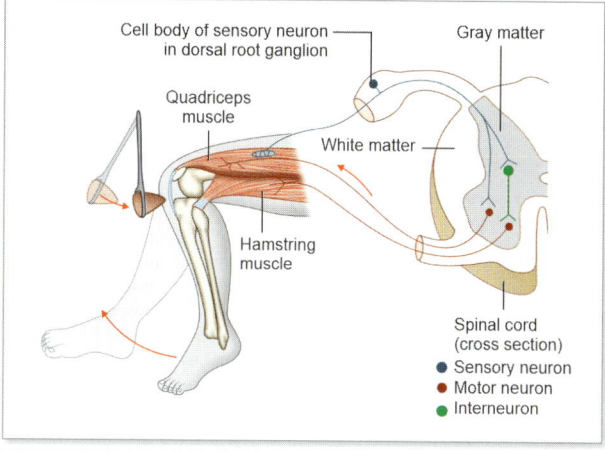

Cell body of sensory neuron in dorsal root ganglion

Gray matter

Quadriceps muscle

White matter

Hamstring muscle

Spinal cord (cross section)
- ● Sensory neuron
- ● Motor neuron
- ● Interneuron

Reflex arc

Reflex zone therapy A system of complementary therapy, similar to reflexology, in which it is believed the body is divided into ten longitudinal and three transverse zones, with corresponding divisions in the feet. Reflex zone therapy can be used to identify areas of disorder or disease in the body and a sophisticated grip technique is used to massage the feet and so treat the problem. The therapy can also be performed on the hands, which correspond closely to the feet, the tongue, the face and the back.

Reflex center An area in the brain or spinal cord where afferent input initiates impulses in the efferent pathway.

Reflexology A technique of deep massage to the soles of the feet, and occasionally the palms of the hands, to relieve somatic symptoms, and promote health and well-being.

Reflux A backward flow; regurgitation.

Refraction 1. The bending or deviation of rays of light as they pass obliquely through one transparent medium and penetrate another of different density.

2. In ophthalmology, the testing of the eyes to ascertain the amount and variety of refractive error that maybe present in each of them.

Refraction errors Pathological condition where parallel rays of light are not brought to focus on retina because of defect in refractive media, e.g., cornea and lens.

Refractive power The degree to which a transparent object deflects a ray of light from its straight path.

Refractometer Instrument for measuring refractive power.

Refractometry Measurement of refractive power of lenses.

Refractory Not yielding to, or resistant to, treatment.

Refractory period The period immediately after some activity during which a nerve or muscle is unable to react to a fresh impulse.

Refrigerant Agent producing cooling.

Refrigeration Cooling.

Refsum disease Hereditary disorder of phytanic acid metabolism manifesting with ataxia, neuropathy, visual disturbances (night blindness) and heart disease.

Regeneration Renewal, as in new growth of tissue in its specific form after injury.

Regimen A systematic plan of therapy.

Region A body part of area.

Regression Return to a former state.

Register An epidemiological term meaning an index or file of all cases with a particular disease or condition in a defined population.

Registered Nurse A qualified practitioner whose name appears on the central register of the Nursing and Midwifery Council. The title is protected by law in the UK and other countries too. *(See Nurse)*.

Registrar 1. An official keeper of records. 2. In British hospitals, a doctor training to be a specialist.

Registrar of births, marriages and deaths The official recorder of births, marriages and deaths. Local registry offices are available in most towns. Births should be registered within 14 days and deaths within 7 days in India. Without a death certificate, which indicates that the death has been registered, it is illegal to dispose of a body.

Registration The act of recording; in dentistry, the making of a record of the jaw relations, present or desired, in order to transfer them to an articulator to facilitate proper construction of a dental prosthesis.

Regression 1. A return to a previous state of health. 2. In psychiatry, a tendency to return to primitive or child-like modes of behavior. Some degree of regression frequently accompanies physical illness and hospitalization. Patients who are mentally ill may exhibit regression to an extreme degree, reverting all the way back to infantile behavior (atavistic regression).

Regulation The state of being controlled.

Regulatory bodies Organizations responsible for defining and monitoring preparation and practice of a specific professional group, e.g., Nursing and Midwifery Council and the Health and Care Professions Council. *(See Annexure 5)*.

Regurgitation Backward flow, e.g., of food from the stomach into the mouth. Fluids regurgitate through the nose in paralysis affecting the soft palate.

Aortic regurgitation Backward flow of blood into the left ventricle when the aortic valve is incompetent.

Duodenal regurgitation Reflux of duodenal secretions and bile into stomach.

Mitral regurgitation Mitral incompetence *(See Mitral)*.

Pulmonary regurgitation Back flow of blood from pulmonary artery into right ventricle.

Tricuspid regurgitation Regurgitation of blood from right ventricle into right atrium.

Rehabilitation Re-education, particularly where an individual has been ill or injured, to enable them to become capable of useful activity.

Rehabilitation center One which provides for organized employment within the capacity of the patient, and with especial regard to the physical influence of the work.

Rehabilitation evaluation of Hall and Baker Abbreviated REHAB. An assessment system for identifying the patient's level of normal, everyday living and work skills, and of any disturbed behavior.

Cardiac rehabilitation A combination of psychological support, progressive exercise and patient education to achieve maximum functional ability after one has had myocardial infarction.

Rehydration Restoration of body hydration or water balance.

Rehydration therapy The treatment of dehydration by administering fluid and salts by mouth (oral rehydration) or by intravenous infusion. *(See Fluid Balance).*

Reicher's cartilage The second bronchial arch in embryo giving rise to stapes, styloid process, stylohyoid ligament, etc.

Reimplantation Replacement of a part from where it was taken out, e.g., tooth, finger, ear.

Reinfection A second infection by the same organism.

Reinforcement The increasing of force or strength. In behavioral science, the process of presenting a reinforcing stimulus to strengthen a response *(See conditioning).* A positive reinforcer is a stimulus that is added to the environment immediately after the desired response. It serves to strengthen the response: that is, to increase the likelihood of its occurring again. Examples of a positive reinforcer are food, money, a special privilege, or some other reward that is satisfying to the subject.

Reissner's membrane The thin membrane separating the cochlear canal from the scale vestibule.

Reiter's syndrome *H Reiter, German bacteriologist, 1881–1969.* A nonspecific urethritis, affecting males, in which there is also arthritis and conjunctivitis.

Rejection 1. In immunology, the formation of antibodies by the host against transplanted tissue, with eventual destruction of the transplanted tissue. 2. In psychosocial terms, the denial of acceptance or affection, or the exclusion of another person.

Relapse The return of a disease after an interval of convalescence.

Relapsing fever One of a group of similar notifiable infectious diseases transmitted to humans by the bites of ticks. Marked by alternating periods of normal temperature and periods of fever relapse. The diseases in the group are caused by several different species of spirochaetes belonging to the genus *Borrelia*. Also called recurrent fever.

Relative risk In epidemiological studies it is the ratio of incidence rate of a disease in the exposed group to that in the unexposed group.

Relatives assessment interview Abbreviated RAI. An assessment tool used by mental health nurses and other staff to identify the perceptions and coping skills of relatives of patients with mental health problems. The data obtained forms an important component in the planning and delivery of care to the patient and the family.

Relax To diminish anxiety, tension, nervousness.

Relaxant A drug or other agent that brings about muscle relaxation or relieves tension.

Relaxation A lessening of tension, which maybe observed when muscles slacken after they have contracted; it is characterized by feelings of peace and calmness.

Relaxation therapy Classes in which patients are taught breathing and other exercises to use for the relief of pain, stress and tension. Used as part of the preparation for childbirth.

Relaxin A hormone that is produced by the corpus luteum of the ovary; it softens the cervix and loosens the pelvic ligaments to aid the birth of the baby.

Releasing factor A substance, produced in the hypothalamus, which causes the anterior pituitary gland to release hormones.

R

Releasing hormone A substance, produced in the hypothalamus, which causes the anterior pituitary gland to release other hormones.

Reliability The quality of being trustworthy or dependable. In research, the consistency of a measure in a study and the likelihood of reproducing the same results, if used again in similar circumstances.

Relieve To provide relief.

Remedy Cure.

REM Rapid Eye Movement, a phase of sleep associated with dreaming and characterized by rapid movements of the eyes. Paradoxical sleep.

Reminiscence therapy Measures to stimulate long-term elderly patients with memorabilia, films and songs meaningful to their generation. Used in conjunction with objects as a prelude to reality orientation therapy. *(See Orientation)*.

Remission Subsidence of the symptoms of a disease for a long time.

Remittent Decreasing at intervals.

Remittent fever One in which a partial fall in the temperature occurs daily.

Remodelling The reshaping or reconstructing of a part or area.

Remotivation In psychiatry, a group therapy technique administered by the nursing staff in a psychiatric hospital or department, which is used to stimulate the communication skills and an interest in the environment of long-term, withdrawn patients.

Renal Relating to the kidney.

Renal calculus Stone in the kidney.

Renal clearance tests Laboratory tests that determine the ability of the kidney to remove certain substances from the blood.

Renal dialysis The application of the principles of dialysis for treatment of renal failure *(See also Haemodialysis and Peritoneal (Dialysis))*.

Renal failure Inability of the kidney to maintain normal function. It maybe acute or chronic. Acute renal failure is a sudden, severe interruption of kidney function. It is normally the complication of another disorder and is reversible. Chronic renal failure is a progressive loss of kidney function. In its early stage, renal function can remain adequate but the glomerular filtration rate (GFR) is depressed and plasma chemistry begins to show abnormalities as waste products accumulate. In the later stage, known as end-stage renal disease (ESRD), the GFR deteriorates and when uremia becomes evident and the patient becomes symptomatic, dialysis is started or the patient receives a transplant.

Renal threshold The level of the blood sugar beyond which it is excreted in the urine; normally 10 mmol/L (180 mg/100 mL).

Renal transplant Surgical implantation of donor kidney to replace a diseased host kidney.

Renal tubule The thin tubular part of a nephron. A uriniferous tubule.

Reniform Shaped like a kidney.

Renin A proteolytic enzyme released into the bloodstream when the kidneys are ischemic. It causes vasoconstriction and increases the blood pressure.

Renin substrate Alpha – 2 globulin.

Rennin An enzyme present in gastric juice of animals that coagulates milk.

Renography X-ray of kidneys.

Renshaw cells Small cells with short axons connecting motor nerve axons with each other and thereby inhibit motor neurons.

Reorganization Healing by formation of new tissue identical to that which was injured or destroyed.

Reovirus Any of a group of RNA viruses isolated from healthy children, children with febrile and afebrile upper respiratory disease, or children with diarrhea.

Repellent An agent that repels insects, ticks and mites, e.g., dimethyphthalate.

Repetitive strain injury A soft-tissue disorder produced by repetitive use of muscle, especially if the muscle activity involves an awkward or uncomfortable position of the body. Particularly affects keyboard operators, musicians, packers and machine operators.

Repletion Complete fullness or satisfied.

Replication 1. The turning back of a tissue on itself. 2. The process by which DNA duplicates itself when the cell divides.

Replogle tube A double lumen aspiration catheter attached to low pressure suction apparatus.

Repolarization Restoration of basal electrical status in muscle or nerve fiber after excitation.

Reposition Restoration of an organ or tissue to its original position.

Repositor Instrument for reposition.

Repression 1. The act of restraining, inhibiting or suppressing. 2. In psychiatry, a defence mechanism whereby a person unconsciously banishes unacceptable ideas, feelings or impulses from consciousness. A person using repression to obtain relief from mental conflict is unaware that "forgetting" unpleasant situations is a way of avoiding them (motivated forgetting).

Reproduction The process by which plants and animals give rise to offspring.

Reproduction asexual Reproduction by fission or budding without involvement of sex cells.

Reproductive system All those parts of the male and female body associated with the production of children.

Repulsion Act of driving back or use of force to cause separation.

Rescue remedy One of the Bach Flower remedies, based on homeopathic principles, and available in liquid form, which is particularly effective in reducing stress, panic, anxiety and hysteria. Useful for those who have a fear of needles for venepuncture and injections, for the transition stage of labor and at any other time when patients are especially anxious or nervous, e.g., before surgical intervention. Four drops of the remedy are given neat on the tongue or can be added to a small glass of water or applied to the temples or wrists. *(See Bach Flower Remedies)*.

Research Scientific and diligent study, investigation and experimentation to establish facts and intelligently analyze them to derive conclusion.

Resect To cut out, e.g., a part of intestine in gangrene of bowel.

Resection Surgical removal of a part.

Submucous resection Removal of part of a deflected nasal septum, from beneath a flap of mucous membrane, which is then replaced.

Transurethral resection A method of removing portions of an enlarged prostate gland via the urethra.

Wedge resection Resection of a piece of tissue in form a wedge as in polycystic ovary.

Resectoscope A telescopic instrument by which pieces of tissue can also be removed. Used for transurethral prostatectomy.

Reserpine An alkaloid from *Rauwolfia;* A drug used to reduce the blood pressure in hypertension.

Reserve That which is held back for future use.

Reserve alkali Alkali content of body available for neutralization of acid.

Reserve cardiac The ability of heart to increase cardiac output during strenuous physical work.

Reserve air Additional amount of air that can be expelled from lungs over the normal quantity.

R

Reservoir 1. A storage place or cavity. 2. The host or environment in which an organism lives and from which it is able to infect susceptible individuals, e.g., hands, skin, nose and bowel.

Resident A doctor under training after internship.

Residential care The provision of care for frail, elderly people in a variety of settings, e.g., local authority residential homes for the elderly or private residential homes.

Residual Remaining.

Residual air Residual volume. The amount of air remaining in the lungs after breathing out fully.

Residual urine Urine remaining in the bladder after voiding; seen with bladder outlet obstruction and disorders affecting nerves controlling bladder function.

Residue-free diet Diet free of cellulose or roughage.

Resin 1. Some natural substances obtained as exudation from plants. 2. A class of solids or soft organic compounds that includes most polymers like polyethylene, polystyrene and polyvinyl.

Resin ion exchange Ionizable synthetic substances either anionic or cationic, used to remove acid or basic ions from solutions.

Resistance The degree of opposition to a force. 1. In electricity, the opposition made by a instrument substance to the passage of a current. 2. In psychology, the opposition, stemming from the unconscious, to repressed ideas being brought to consciousness.

Drug resistance To the ability of a microorganism to withstand the effects of a drug that are lethal to most members of its species.

Peripheral resistance That offered to the passage of blood through small vessels and capillaries.

Resistance to infection The natural power of the body to withstand the toxins of disease.

Resolution 1. In medicine, the process of returning to normal. 2. The disappearance of inflammation without the formation of pus.

Resolve To return to normal after pathological process subsides.

Resonance In medicine, the reverberating sound obtained on percussion over a cavity or hollow organ, such as the lung.

Resonance vocal the vibrations of voice transmitted to ears during auscultation. It is increased in consolidation, and over cavities in communication with bronchus.

Resorb To absorb again or to undergo resorption.

Resorbent An agent that promotes absorption of blood and exudates.

Resorcinol A mild antiseptic, keratolytic and fungicidal agent.

Resorption Act of removal by absorption, e.g., callus following bone fracture, root of deciduous tooth, blood from hematoma.

Respiration The gaseous interchange between the tissue cells and the atmosphere.

Artificial respiration The production of respiratory movements by external effort.

External respiration Breathing, which comprises inspiration, when the external intercostal muscles and the diaphragm contract and air is drawn into the lungs, and expiration, when the air is breathed out.

Intermittent positive pressure respiration Abbreviated IPPR. Respiration produced by a ventilator.

Internal respiration Tissue respiration. The inter change of gases that occurs between tissues and blood through the walls of capillaries.

Laboured respiration That which is difficult and distressed.

R

Stertorous respiration, Snoring; a noisy breathing.

Tissue respiration Internal respiration *(See Cheyne-Stokes respiration)*.

Respirator An apparatus to qualify the air breathed through it, or a device for giving artificial respiration or to assist pulmonary ventilation *(See also Ventilator)*.

Respirator shock Circulatory shock due to interference with the flow of blood through the great vessels and chambers of the heart, causing pooling of blood in the veins and the abdominal organs and a resultant vascular collapse. The condition sometimes occurs as a result of increased intrathoracic pressure in patients who are being maintained on a mechanical ventilator.

Respiratory Pertaining to respiration.

Acute respiratory distress syndrome Abbreviated ARDS. A group of signs and symptoms resulting in acute respiratory failure; characterized clinically by tachypnea, dyspnea, tachycardia, cyanosis, and low PaO_2 that persists even with oxygen therapy.

Respiratory distress syndrome of newborn A condition occurring in preterm infants, full-term infants of diabetic mothers, and infants delivered by cesarean section, and associated with pulmonary immaturity and inability to produce sufficient lung surfactant. Also called hyaline membrane disease, idiopathic respiratory distress syndrome, infant respiratory distress syndrome (abbreviated IRDS).

Respiratory failure A life-threatening condition in which respiratory function is inadequate to maintain the body's need for oxygen supply and carbondioxide removal while at rest; also called acute ventilatory failure.

Respiratory insufficiency A condition in which respiratory function is inadequate to meet the body's needs when increased physical activity places extra demands on it.

Respiratory quotient The ratio of the volume of expired carbondioxide to the volume of oxygen absorbed by the lungs per unit of time.

Respiratory syncytial virus A virus isolated from children with bronchopneumonia and bronchitis, characteristically causing severe respiratory infection in very young children but less severe infections as the children grow older.

Respiratory therapy The technical specialty concerned with the treatment, management and care of patients with respiratory problems, including administration of medical gases.

Respite care Temporary care provided for those with disabilities or serious and terminal conditions to allow relief for the family and other carers. Provision maybe on a daily or long-term basis and in a variety of settings, e.g., in a hospice, nursing or residential home, hostel or in the family home. *(See Hospice)*.

Restiform Rope like.

Resiform body Inferior cerebellar peduncle on lateral border of 4th ventricle.

Resting potential The potential difference existing between inside and outside of a cell membrane which the cell is at rest.

Restitution Return to a former status.

Restless leg Irrepressible ache in the legs of unknown etiology compelling the patient to move the legs to bring some relief.

Restless legs syndrome Characterized by weakness and coldness in the lower limbs with an unpleasant feeling of a creeping tingling sensation, firstly in the lower legs but possibly extending to the thighs, arms and hands. Symptoms most commonly

R

occur in the patients at night on the bed, or sometimes in those sitting on chairs for prolonged periods during the day. Occurs primarily in the elderly. The cause is unknown but maybe due to a vascular disorder. Also known as Willis-Ekbom disease.

Restoration Return of anything to its previous state; in dentistry material or device that restores or replaces a tooth.

Restraint Preventing or restricting from any action.

Resuscitation Restoration to life or consciousness of one apparently dead, or whose respirations have ceased *(See also Artificial (Respiration))*.

Cardiopulmonary resuscitation An emergency technique used in cardiac arrest to re-establish heart and lung function until more advanced life support is available.

Retardation Delay; hindrance; delayed development.

Mental retardation Low general intellectual development, associated with impairment either of learning and social adjustment or of maturation, or of both.

Retching Strong, involuntary effort to vomit.

Rete A network of vessels and nerves.

Rete testes A network of tubules in mediastinum testis that receives sperms from seminiferous tubules. From rete testis efferent ducts convey sperm to epididymis.

Retention Holding back.

Retention cyst (See Cyst).

Retention defect A defect of memory. Inability to retain material in the mind so that it can be recalled when required.

Retention enema Enema retained in colon to provide medication or nutrition.

Retention of urine Inability to pass urine from the bladder, which maybe due to obstruction or be of nervous origin.

Reticular Resembling a network.

Reticular cells Phagocytic cells present in bone marrow and lymph nodes, constitute the reticular tissue.

Reticular formation Areas in the brainstem from which nerve fibers extend to the cerebral cortex.

Reticular layer Connective tissue layer in deeper portion of dermis beneath the papillary layer.

Reticulation Formation of a network.

Reticulin A proteinacious substance in the connective tissue.

Reticulocyte A red blood cell that is not fully mature: it retains strands of nuclear material.

Reticulocytosis The presence of an increased number of immature red cells in the blood, indicating over activity of the bone marrow.

Reticuloendothelial cell A phagocytic cell of reticuloendothelial system.

Reticuloendothelial system A collection of endothelial cells in the liver, spleen, bone marrow and lymph glands that produce large mononuclear cells or macrophages. They are phagocytic, destroy red blood cells and have the power of making some antibodies.

Reticulosarcoma A malignant tumor composed of large monocytic cells originating from reticuloendothelial system.

Reticulosis Reticulocytosis, a fatal lymphoma, often familial with hepatosplenomegaly, lymphadenopathy, anemia and granulocytopenia.

Retina The innermost coat of the eyeball, formed of nerve cells and fibers, from which the optic nerve leaves the eyeball and passes to the visual area of the cerebrum. The impression of the image is focused upon it.

R

Retinaculum A band or membrane holding any organ or part in its place.

Retinal Relating to the retina.

Retinal detachment Partial detachment of the retina from the underlying choroid layer, resulting in loss of vision. It may result from the presence of a tumor, from trauma or from high myopia.

Retinene Orange yellow carotenoid pigment formed by action of light on rhodopsin.

Retinitis Inflammation of the retina.

Retinitis pigmentosa A group of diseases, frequently hereditary, marked by progressive loss of retinal function, especially associated with contraction of the visual field and impairment of vision. The disorder often follows a slow course over a period of many years, but there is considerable variation in the progression of the disease.

Retinoblastoma A malignant tumor arising from retinal cells. Occurs in infancy and maybe hereditary. Treatment includes cryosurgery, irradiation and photo coagulation, but enucleation maybe required.

Retinodialysis Peripheral retinal detachment.

Retinoic acid Vitamin A breakdown product.

Retinoid Resembling a resin.

Retinol A form of vitamin A.

Retinopathy Any non-inflammatory disease of the retina.

Diabetic retinopathy A complication of diabetes. Retinal hemorrhages occur, resulting in permanent visual damage, and retinal detachment may follow.

Hypertensive retinopathy Retinal change occurring as a result of high blood pressure.

Retinoscope An instrument which illuminates the retina and is used to detect and measure refractive errors.

Retinosis Non-inflammatory degeneration of retina.

Retort Long necked glass vessel used in distillation.

Retractile Capable of being drawn back.

Retraction Shortening, state of being drawn back.

Retraction ring A ridge of uterus separating upper contractile segment from lower dilating segment.

Retractor Instrument for holding back a tissue.

Retreat Act of withdrawal.

Retrieval The process of recalling past memory.

Retro Situated behind or backward in position, e.g., retro-ocular, retrobulbar, retrocecal, etc.

Retrobulbar Pertaining to the back of the eyeball.

Retrobulbar neuritis Dimness of vision due to inflammation of the optic nerve.

Retroflexion A bending back, particularly of the uterus when it is bent backwards at an acute angle, the cervix being in its normal position *(See Retroversion)*.

Retrograde Going backwards.

Retrograde amnesia Forgetfulness of event so ccurring immediately before an illness or injury.

Retrograde ejaculation Semen discharge into bladder rather than through urethral meatus as in diabetic neuropathy.

Retrograde pyelography Pyelography by injection of dye through ureters.

Retrograde urography Radiographic examination of the kidney after the introduction of a radiopaque substance into the renal pelvis through the urethra.

Retrolental fibroplasia A fibrous condition of the anterior vitreous body which develops when a premature infant is exposed to high concentrations of oxygen. Both eyes are affected, seriously interfering with vision and leading to retinal detachment. Early treatment with a freezing probe (cryopexy) can prevent retinal detachment.

Retroperitoneal fibrosis Fibrotic tissue growth in retroperitoneal space often compressing ureters, vena cava and aorta, a sequel to mathysergide treatment of migraine. *SYN* – Ormond's syndrome.

Retroperitoneal Behind the peritoneum.

Retropharyngeal Behind the pharynx.

Retroposition Backward displacement of an organ.

Retropubic Behind the pubic bone.

Retropulsion Moving backward involuntarily as in Parkinson's disease.

Retrospection A morbid dwelling on memories.

Retrospective study A study where patient's records are analyzed after they have experienced the disease.

Retrospective Looking back on or dealing with past events.

R. study One that examines data from the past, e.g., discharged patients' records, to discover causal factors relevant to outcomes.

Retrosternal Behind the sternum.

Retroversion A lifting backward, particularly of the uterus when the whole organ is tilted backward *(See Retroflexion)*.

Retroversion of uterus Backward tilting of entire uterus including cervix so that the latter points towards symphysis pubis.

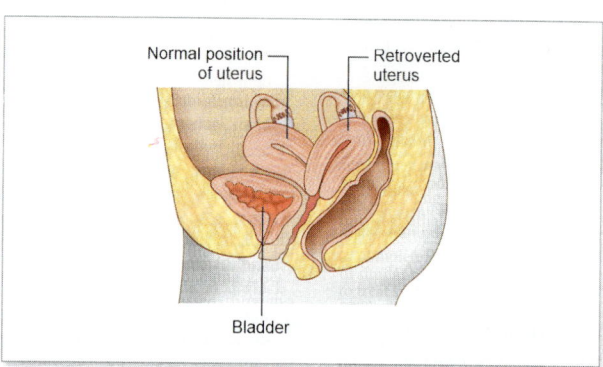

Retroversion of Uterus

Retrovirus A group of viruses belonging to the family Retroviridae, principally infecting and frequently causing diseases in animals, but also including viruses that infect and cause disease in humans, e.g., Human Immunodeficiency Virus (HIV) and human T-cell leukemia/lymphoma/lymphotropic virus type I (HTLV-I).

Rett syndrome A rare genetic disorder affecting brain development resulting in severe physical and learning disabilities caused by a mutation in the MECP2 gene.

Revalidation The requirement of registered nurses and midwives to confirm to the nursing and midwifery council (NMC) that they have the minimum requirement for practice and continuing professional development hours. They must also provide evidence of reflection and feedback *(See Annexure 12)*.

Revascularization Restoration of blood flow to a part.

Reverberation 1. Repeated echoing of a sound. 2. In neurology the process by which a single applied impulse causes continuous discharge of impulses from collaterals of the neurons.

Reverdin's graft *JL Reverdin, Swiss-surgeon, 1842–1929.* A form of skin graft; in which pieces of skin are placed as Islands over the area *(See Thiersch skin graft)*.

Reverse isolation *(See Protective Isolation; also Annexure 11)*.

Revirapine Factor Xa inhibitor, anti-coagulant.

Reye's syndrome *RDK Reye, 20th century Australian pathologist*. An acute, potentially fatal illness that may follow a virus infection occurring in children; there is fatty degeneration of the liver and the brain and raised intracranial pressure, accompanied by vomiting, convulsions and coma. The cause of Reye's syndrome is unknown but administration of salicylates in children under the age of 12 years is not recommended. This follows evidence that aspirin maybe a contributory factor in the development of Reye's syndrome.

Rh factor Rhesus factor.

Rhabdomyosarcoma A rare malignant growth of striated muscle. It grows rapidly and metastasizes early.

Rhabdomyolysis A disease with destruction of muscle cells common sequence to snake venom.

Rhabdomyoma Benign tumor of striated muscle.

Rhachischisis Congenital cleft in spinal canal.

Rhaphe A ridge.

Rhagades Cracks or fissures in the skin, especially those round the mouth.

Rhesus factor Abbreviated Rh factor. The red blood cells of most humans carry a group of genetically determined antigens and are said to be rhesus positive (Rh+). Those that do not are said to be rhesus negative (Rh–). This is of importance as a cause of anaemia and jaundice in the newly born when the infant is Rh+and the mother is Rh–. The result of this incompatibility (isoimmunization) is the formation of an antibody which causes excessive hemolysis in the child's blood *(See Antirhesus serum)*.

Rheology Study of deformation and flow of materials.

Rheumatic fever A systemic illness that follows streptococcal sore throat manifesting with carditis, fleeting polyarthritis, chorea, erythema marginatum, subcutaneous nodules, etc. believed to be an autoimmune phenomenon.

Rheumatism Any of a variety of disorders marked by inflammation, degeneration or metabolic derangement of the connective tissue structures, especially the joints and related structures, and attended by pain, stiffness or limitation of motion.

   Acute rheumatism Rheumatic fever. An acute fever associated with previous streptococcal infection and occurring most commonly in children. The onset is usually sudden, with pain, swelling and stiffness in one or more joints. There is fever, sweating and tachycardia, and carditis is present in most cases. Sometimes the symptoms are minor and ignored. This disease is the most common cause of mitral stenosis because scar tissue results from the inflammation.

Rheumatoid Resembling rheumatism.   *Rheumatoid arthritis (See Arthritis)*.

R

Rheumatoid factor An IgM auto anti-body present in up to 75% of patients suffering from rheumatoid arthritis.

Rheumatology The branch of medicine dealing with disorders of the joints, muscles, tendons and ligaments.

Rh immunoglobulin Anti-Rh gam-maglobulin, usually given to Rh –ve mothers within 72 hours of giving birth to a Rh +ve baby or following abortion.

Rhinecephalon The part of brain concerned with reception and integration of olfactory impulses.

Rhinitis Inflammation of the mucous membrane of the nose.

Rhinologist A specialist dealing with diseases of nose.

Rhinoplasty Reduction in size of nose by surgery.

Rhinophyma Hypertrophy of tissue over the nose with congestion and retention of sebum.

Rhinoplasty A plastic operation on the nose; repairing a part of or forming an entirely new nose.

Rhinorrhoea An abnormal discharge of mucus from the nose.

Rhinosalpingitis An infective disease of nose caused by *Klebsiella rhino-scleromatis* manifesting with hard nodular growth often spreading to lower respiratory tract.

Rhinoscopy Examination of the inte-rior of the nose.
Anterior rhinoscopy Examination through the nostrils with the aid of a speculum.
Posterior rhinoscopy Examination through the nasopharynx by means of a rhinoscope.

Rhinosporidiosis A fungal disease caused by Rhinosporidium seeberi characterized by growth of pedun-culated polyps in nose, larynx and genital tracts.

Rhinovirus One of a genus of small RNA-containing viruses that cause respiratory diseases, including the common cold.

Rhipicephalus A genus of ticks that can transmit the rickettsiae which cause typhus and relapsing fever.

Rhitidectomy Removal of wrinkles by plastic surgery.

Rhitiodosis Wrinkling of cornea, a feature of approaching death.

Rhizo Root.

Rhizoid Root like.

Rhisometic Concerning hip and shoulder joints.

Rhizotomy Section of nerve roots.

Rhodopsin The visual purple of the ret-ina, the formation of which is depen-dent upon vitamin A in the diet.

Rhombencephalon A primary division of embryonic brain giving rise to brain stem and cerebellum.

Rhomboid An oblique parallelogram.

Rhonchus A wheezing sound, pro-duced in the bronchial tubes, which is caused by partial obstruction and can be heard on auscultation.

Rhubarb Extract from root and stem of plant used as cathartic and astrin-gent.

Rhythm A regular recurring action.
Cardiac rhythm The smooth action of the heart when systole is followed by diastole.
Rhythm method A contraceptive technique in which intercourse is limited to the 'safe period' (avoiding the 2–3 days immediately before and after ovulation).

Rhytidectomy Commonly known as a face life, a cosmetic surgical proce-dure to remove wrinkles and excess skin to improve visible signs of aging.

Rib Anyone of the 12 pairs of long, flat curved bones of the thorax, each united by cartilage to the spinal vertebrae at the back.
Cervical rib A short extra rib, often bilateral. Pressure on this may cause impairment of nerve or vascular function *(See Scalenus (Syndrome))*.

R

False ribs The last five pairs, the upper three of which are attached by cartilage to each other.

Floating ribs The last two pairs, connected only to the vertebrae.

True ribs The seven pairs attached directly to the sternum.

Ribavirin Antiviral agent.

Riboflavin A chemical factor in the vitamin B complex.

Ribonuclease An enzyme from the pancreas which is responsible for the breakdown of nucleic acid.

Ribonucleic acid Abbreviated RNA. A complex chemical found in the cytoplasm of animal cells and concerned with protein synthesis. Certain viruses contain RNA.

Ribose A pentose sugar present in RNA and riboflavin.

Ribosome An RNA and protein containing particle which is the site of protein synthesis in the cell.

Ricin A white highly toxic protein of castor beans.

Ricinoleic acid An unsaturated fatty acid with a strong laxative action, principally found in castor oil.

Rickets A condition of infancy and childhood caused by deficiency of vitamin D, which leads to altered calcium and phosphorus metabolism and consequent disturbance of ossification of bone, resulting in deformity, such as bowing of the legs. Since the action of sunlight on the skin produces vitamin D in the human body, rickets often occurs in parts of the world where the winter is especially long, and where smoke and fog constantly intercept the sun.

Adult renal Osteomalacia; a rickets-like disease affecting adults.

Fetal renal Achondroplasia.

Late renal Osteomalacia, that occurring in older children.

Vitamin D-resistant rickets A condition almost indistinguishable from ordinary rickets clinically but resistant to unusually large doses of vitamin D; it is often familial.

Rickettsia A genus of microorganisms which are parasitic in lice and similar insects. The bite of the host is thus the means of transmitting the organisms, some of which are responsible for the typhus group of fevers.

Rickettsial pox A self-limited acute, febrile disease caused by *Rickettsia akari.*

Rider's bone Bone formation in adductor longus muscle of thigh in horse riders.

Ridge Long projecting surface or crest.

Riedel's lobe A tongue-shaped process of liver.

Rifampicin An antibiotic drug used in leprosy and, with other drugs, in the treatment of tuberculosis.

Right handedness Proneness of a person to dominantly use the right hand.

Rigidity Sustained muscle tension causing the affected part to be stiff and inflexible; maybe due to stress, injury or neurological disease.

Rigor An attack of intense shivering occurring when the heat regulation is disturbed. The temperature rises rapidly and may either stay elevated or fall rapidly as profuse sweating occurs.

Rigor mortis Stiffening of the body which occurs soon after death.

Rima A fissure or crack.

Rimiterol A beta2 agonist for use in bronchial asthma.

Rimantadine An analog of amantadine, the antiviral agent.

Ring Band around circular opening, circular form.

Abdominal ring Apertures in abdominal wall, often producing herniations, e.g., inguinal, femoral, etc.

Bandl's ring Retraction ring of uterus.

R

Lymphoid ring Lymphoid tissue in a ring fashion in pharynx consisting of palatine, pharyngeal and lingual tonsils. *SYN*-Waldeyer's ring.

Ringer's solution S *Ringer British, physiologist, 1835–1910.* A physiological solution of saline to which small amounts of calcium and potassium salts have been added. Used to replace fluids and electrolytes intravenously.

Ringworm Tinea. A contagious skin disease, characterized by circular patches, pinkish in color with a desquamating surface, and due to a parasitic fungus.

Rinne test Tuning fork test for testing bone and air conduction. The base of vibrating tuning fork is held in contact with the mastoid process till vibrations are no longer heard by the patient, then it is held close to external ear. If patient still hears the vibration it is called positive Rinne test. When the patient does not hear the vibrations once shifted from mastoid process to external ear, air conduction is tested first by placing the vibrating fork in front of external ear until the sound is no longer heard, then the stem of the fork is placed on mastoid. If vibration is still heard it is called negative Rinne test. All normal persons are Rinne positive and those with defective air conduction are Rinne negative.

Ripening 1. Softening and dilatation of cervix during labor. 2. Maturation of cataract.

Risk Hazard, or chance of developing a disease or of complications during or after treatment. This may arise because of inherent problems with the treatment itself (e.g., drug side effects) or because of the frailty of the patient. *Risk–benefit analysis* In medicare the analysis of risk and benefit from a procedure discussed between patient, doctor and relations.

Relative risk The likelihood of developing a disease after a given exposure in epidemiological terms, calculated as incidence rate of disease in an exposed group divided by incidence rate in the non-exposed group.

Risk factor A factor which, when added to others, increases the likelihood of a disease or complication (e.g., smoking and obesity are risk factors for the development of coronary artery disease).

Risperidone Antipsychotic agent.

Ristocetin An antibiotic obtained from cultures of *Nocardia lurida*.

Risus Laughter.

Risussardonicus A peculiar grin as in tetanus due to spasm of facial muscles.

Rite of passage The cultural ceremonies and rituals that may accompany the changes in status that occur in the course of a person's life. These ceremonies serve to draw attention to changes in status and social identity and also to the management of the social tensions that such changes may involve.

Ritgen's maneuver An obstetric procedure aimed to assist the delivery of the head of the fetus and protect the structure of perineum of the mother by applying an upward pressure from the coccygeal region to extend the head of the fetus.

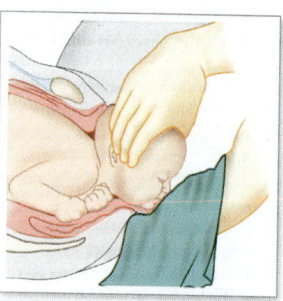

Ritgen's Maneuver

Ritodrine Beta 2 agonist for use in bronchial asthma.

Ritonavir Anti-HIV agent.

Ritualistic surgery Surgery without scientific justification performed in primitive societies.

Rivastigmine Cholinergic for brain.

Rizatriptan Antimigraine agent.

RNA Ribonucleic acid.

RNA viruses Viruses which contain ribonucleic acid as their genetic material.

Rocking A technique to increase muscle tone in hypotonic muscles through vestibular stimulation.

Rocky Mountain spotted fever A tick-borne infection caused by a Rickettsia, common in the USA, with rash, fever, muscle pain and often an enlarged liver. The disease lasts about 3 weeks.

Rod A straight thin structure.

Retinal rod One of the two types of light-sensitive end-organ of the retina, which contain rhodopsin and are responsible for night vision.

Rodent Mammals like mice, rats and squirrel.

Rodenticide Chemicals that kill rodents.

Rodent ulcer Basal cell carcinoma commonly occurring on upper face with destruction of underlying tissue and bone.

Roentgen German physicist who discovered roentgen rays, (X-rays) and won noble prize in 1901.

Rokitansky's disease Acute yellow atrophy of liver.

Role A pattern of behavior developed in response to the demands or expectations of others; the pattern of responses to the persons with who man individually interacts in a particular situation.

Role play An educational technique used in teaching interpersonal, communication and practice skills. Students are given roles (or parts) and asked to act these roles out. Some members of the group maybe given observational tasks related to the exercise. At the end of the session there is an opportunity for the group to evaluate the exercise. This technique may also be used therapeutically, usually in the psychiatric setting.

Sick role The role played by people who have defined themselves as ill. Adoption of the sick role changes the behavioral expectations of others towards the sick person, who is exempted from normal social responsibilities and is not held responsible for the condition. The patient is obliged to 'want to get well' and to seek competent medical help.

Rolando's fissure Fissure between parietal and frontal lobes.

Romberg's sign *MH Romberg, German physician, 1795–1853.* Inability to stand erect without swaying if the eyes are closed. A sign of tabes dorsalis.

Root canal The pulp cavity in root of a tooth.

Ropinirole Anti-parkinsonian agent.

Rorschach test *H Rorschach, Swiss psychiatrist, 1884–1922.* A personality trait test that consists of ten ink-blot designs, some in colors and some in black and white.

Rosacea *(See Acne (Rosacea)).*

Rosary Resembling a string of beads.

Rachiticrosary Swollen costochondral junctions in rickets.

Rosenmuller's body A rudimentary structure in mesosalpinx homologous to head of epididymis in male.

Roseola 1. A rose-colored rash. 2. Roseola infantum.

Roseola infantum A common acute viral disease that usually occurs in children under 24 months old; it attacks suddenly but disappears in a few days, leaving no permanent marks.

R

Syphilitic roseola An eruption of rose-colored spots in early secondary syphilis.

Rose's position A supine position with head and neck extended to perform a surgery within the mouth and fauces to prevent aspiration or swallowing of blood.

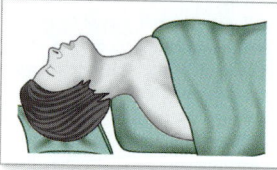

Rose's Position

Rosette Something resembling a nose.

Rosiglitazone Antidiabetic agent.

Ross bodies Copper color round bodies with dark granules seen in blood and tissue fluids of syphilis.

Rossolimo's reflex Plantar flexion of second to fifth toes in response to percussion on plantar surface of toes.

Rostellum A fleshy protrusion on anterior end of scolex of tapeworm bearing spines or hooks.

Rostral Towards cephalic end of body.

Rostrum Any hooked or beaked structure.

Rosuvastatin Lipid-lowering agent.

Rotavirus Virus causing epidemic and sporadic enteritis.

Roth's spots *M Roth, Swiss physician, 1839–1915.* Small white spots seen in the retina early in the course of subacute bacterial endocarditis.

Rotoxaminetartarate An anti-histaminic drug.

Roughage Coarse vegetable fibers and cellulose that give bulk to the diet and stimulate peristalsis.

Rouleau A rounded formation found in blood, caused by red cells piling on each other.

Round ligament Round cord like structures passing from uterus in the broad ligament and then through the inguinal canal to end in soft tissues of labia majora.

Roundworm Any of various types of parasitic nematode worm, somewhat resembling the common earthworm which sometimes invade the human intestinal tract and multiply there. Very common among them is the pinworm, or thread worm.

Rovsing's sign *NT Rovsing, Danish surgeon, 1868–1927.* A test for acute appendicitis in which pressure in the left iliac fossa causes pain in the right iliac fossa.

Roxatidine H_2 receptor blocker used in peptic ulcer.

RSI 3 Repetitive strain injury.

RTS, S/AS01 The first approved malaria vaccine. Approved for use by European regulators in July 2015.

Rub The sound of friction of one roughened surface moving on another, e.g., pleural rub, pericardial rub.

Rubefacient An agent causing redness of the skin.

Rubella German measles. An acute, notifiable virus infection of short duration, characterized by pyrexia, enlarged cervical lymph glands and a transient rash. The greatest risk from this disease is to the offspring of mothers who contract it during the early weeks of pregnancy. The child maybe born with cataract or deformities, be a deaf mute or have other congenital defects.

Rubeola *SYN* – measles.

Rubeosis iridis Vascularization of anterior surface of iris with retinal vein thrombo phlebitis often responsible for hemorrhagic glaucoma in diabetics.

Rubidium A soft silvery metal that bursts into flames spontaneously in air.

Rubin's test Carbon dioxide/air uterine insufflation to test tubal patency.

Rubor Redness caused by inflammation. The other three classical signs of inflammation are calor (heat), dolor (pain) and tumor (swelling).

Rubrospinal The descending tract from red nucleus of mid brain to gray matter of spinal cord.

Rudiment 1. Remnant of a part which was functional in earlier stage of development or in ancestors. 2. Undeveloped.

Ruffini's corpuscles Encapsulated sensory nerve endings of skin to mediate sensation of warmth.

Ruga A fold of mucous membrane, e.g., of stomach or vagina.

Ruggeri's reflex Rise in pulse rate on convergence of eyes on a near object.

Rugose, rugous Having many wrinkles or creases.

Rugosity Condition of having wrinkles or being folded.

Rule of nine Formula for estimating percentage of body surface area, where head represents 9%, front and back of trunk 18%, each lower extremity 18%, each upper extremity 9% and perineum 1%.

Rum fits Convulsion occurring within 48 hours following abstinence in habitual drinkers.

Rumination 1. Recurring thoughts. 2. Voluntary regurgitation of food, which is then chewed and swallowed again.

Obsessional rumination Thoughts which persistently recur against the patient's will.

Rump Gluteal region or buttocks.

Rumpf's symptom In neurasthenia, rise in pulse rate on pressure over a painful spot.

Rupatadine Antihistamine.

Rupia A thick cutaneous syphilitic eruption often with extensive ulceration.

Rupture 1. Tearing or bursting of a part, as in rupture of an aneurysm; of the membranes during labor; or of a tubal pregnancy. 2. A term commonly applied to hernia.

Rush The first spell of pleasure produced by a narcotic drug.

Russel bodies Small spherical hyaline bodies in cancerous and simple inflammatory growths.

Russian bath Steam bath followed by friction and plunge in cold water.

Rust's disease Tuberculosis of cervical vertebrae and their articulations.

Rutin A crystalline glucoside derived from buck wheat closely related to hesperidin, used in hemostatic preparations.

Rye A cereal used for food and beverages.

Ryle's tube *GA Ryle, British physician, 1889–1950.* A thin tube with a weighted end, introduced into the stomach. It maybe used for the withdrawal of gastric contents or for the administration of fluids.

◉◉◉

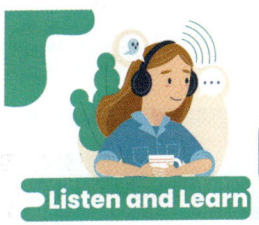

CBS Digital Dictionary
for Nurses

Learn to Pronounce Correctly
(Audio Pronunciation of Difficult Words)

▶**Listen and Learn**

Nursing Next Live
The Next Level of NURSING EDUCATION

PREPARE ANYTIME, ANYWHERE FOR
Nursing Officer/Staff Nurse/CHO/ Nursing Undergraduate & Postgraduate Exams

AIIMS NORCET 2020

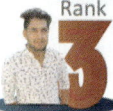

Rank **3**

Rahul Dahiya
Roll No. 9016060

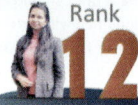

Rank **12**

Nisha Singla
Roll No. 9101820

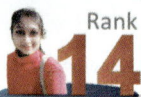

Rank **14**

Arushi Mittal
Roll No. 9079646

Rank **51**

Komal Dhull
Roll No. 9024458

Rank **72**

Shivani Bourai
Roll No. 9092877

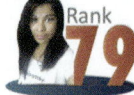

Rank **79**

Nivedita Saini
Roll No. 9004587

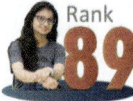

Rank **89**

Rupali Garg
Roll No. 9054544

BFUHS 2021

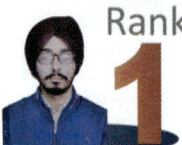

Rank **1**

Harjeet Singh
Roll No- 472478

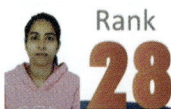

Rank **28**

Kuljit Kaur
Roll No. 473956

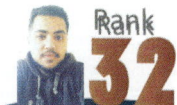

Rank **32**

Karan Sharma
Roll No. 469134

Rank **38**

Smriti Rana
Roll No. 463342

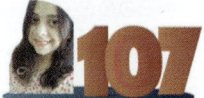

107

Harpreet Kaur
Roll No. 474125

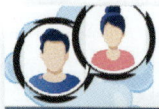

You Will Be The Next...

Follow us:

Scan the
QR Code
to download
the app

CALL US +91- 999-911-7411
w w w . n u r s i n g n e x t l i v e . c o m

S

Saber shin Convex prominent anterior border of tibia in congenital syphilis.

Sabin vaccine *AB Sabin, American-biologist, 1906–1993.* A live oral attenuated poliovirus vaccine active against poliomyelitis.

Sabulous Sandy, gritty.

Sac A cavity or pouch often containing fluid.

Sac yolk The extra-embryonic membrane that connects with midgut through long narrow yolk stalk and is the first hematopoietic organ of the embryo.

Saccades Fast involuntary movements of eyes while changing gaze from one point to another.

Saccate Enclosed in a sac.

Saccharase An enzyme catalyzing breakdown of disaccharides to monosaccharides.

Saccharic acid A dibasic acid produced by action of nitric acid on dextrose.

Saccharide One of a series of carbohydrates, including the sugars.

Saccharin A coal tar product, 300–500 times sweeter than sugar, used as artificial sweetener.

Saccharolytic Capable of splitting up sugar.

Saccharomycosis A disease due to yeasts.

Saccharose Sucrose, or cane sugar.

Saccular Resembling a sac.

Sacculation Group of sacs or formed into group of sacs.

Saccule A small sac, particularly the smaller of the two sacs within the membranous labyrinth of the ear.

Sacculus Singular of saccule.

SACH foot Solid article cushioned heel. A prosthetic foot designed to absorb shock and allow movement of the shank while walking.

Sacral Relating to the sacrum. Sacro-iliac relating to the sacrum and the ilium.

Sacralization Fusion of the sacrum and the 5th lumbar vertebra.

Sacral nerves The 5 pairs of mixed nerves emerging through sacral foramina.

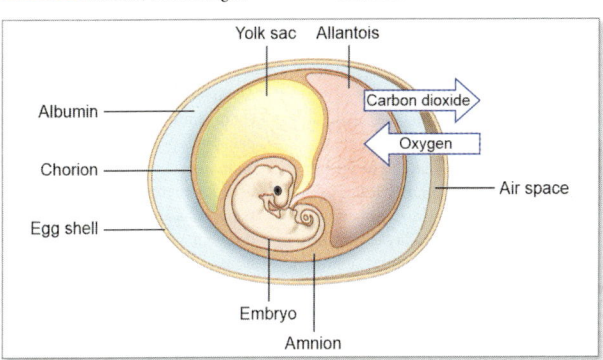

Yolk Sac

Sacral plexus Plexus of sacral nerves giving rise to sciatic nerve.

Sacrococcygeus One of the two muscles, anterior and posterior extending from sacrum to coccyx.

Sacroiliac Relating to the sacrum.

Sacroiliitis Inflammation of sacro-iliac joint.

Sacrospinalis A large muscle lying on either side of vertebral column consists of iliocostalis and longissimus.

Sacrovertebral angle Angle formed between base of sacrum and fifth lumbar vertebra.

Sacrum A triangular bone composed of five united vertebrae, situated between the lowest lumbar vertebra and the coccyx. It forms the back of the pelvis.

Saddle A seat for horse riders.

Saddle area The areas of buttocks coming in contact with the saddle during horse riding.

Saddle joint A joint where the articulating surfaces are convex and concave.

Saddle nose A depressed nasal bridge, due to congenital absence of bony or cartilaginous support or destructive disease like leprosy and syphilis.

Sadism A form of sexual perversion in which the individual takes pleasure in inflicting mental and physical pain on others.

Sadist One who practices sadism.

Sadness Feeling of dejection or melancholy.

SADS *(See Seasonal Affective Disorder Syndrome).*

Safe motherhood initiative The World Health Organization (WHO) campaigns to reduce worldwide maternal mortality and morbidity with the implementation of simple, appropriate and cost-effective strategies to enable mothers to have access to high quality, affordable care during pregnancy and childbirth. The campaign also seeks to improve the health, nutrition and the general wellbeing of girls and women of reproductive age and to the reduction of any long-term sequelae of childbirth, which often result in lifelong disabilities.

Safelight Dark room lights whose wavelength does not hamper undeveloped X-ray film.

Safer sex Preventative measures to reduce the risk of sexually transmitted infections, e.g., maintaining a monogamous sexual relationship and using a condom.

Safer staffing Ensuring that there are the right number of staff with the right skills in the right places – particularly aimed at nursing staff.

Sagittal Arrow shaped.

Sagittal plane The place that divides body into left and right halves.

Sagittal sinus The superior longitudinal sinus.

Sagittal suture The junction of the parietal bones.

Sago A starch preparation when taken as food, leaves little residue.

Saint Vitus' dance Sydenham's chorea.

Salaam spasm Infantile epilepsy with nodding of head due to spasm of sternocleidomastoids.

Salbutamol A sympathomimetic drug used in the treatment of bronchospasm.

Salacious Lustful.

Salicylate A salt of salicylic acid.

Methyl salicylate The active ingredient in ointments and lotions for joint pains and sprains.

Sodium salicylate The specific drug used for rheumatic fever. It reduces the pyrexia and relieves the pain but does not prevent cardiac complications.

Salicylic acid A drug with bacteriostatic and fungicidal properties used in the treatment of skin diseases and, in concentrated form, to remove warts and corns.

Saline A solution of sodium chloride and water.

Hypertonic saline A solution greater than normal strength.

Hypotonic saline A solution lower than normal strength.

Normal or physiological saline A 0.9% solution which is isotonic with blood.

Saline enema One teaspoon of salt dissolved in a pint of water to which is added magnesium sulfate (epson salt) to induce catharsis.

Saliva The secretion of the salivary glands. When food is taken, saliva moistens and partially digests carbohydrates by the action of its enzyme, ptyalin (amylase).

Salivant Agents that stimulate flow of saliva.

Salivary Relating to saliva.

Salivary calculus A duct.

Salivary fistula An abnormal opening on the skin of the face, leading into a salivary duct or gland.

Salivary glands The parotid, submaxillary and sublingual glands.

Salivation 1. The process of salivating. 2. Excessive salivation which may lead to soreness of mouth and gums.

Salk vaccine *JE Salk, American virologist, b. 1914.* The first poliomyelitis vaccine of killed viruses, given by injection *(See Vaccine).*

Salmeterol Beta 2 adrenergic stimulant.

Salmonella Any of the genus of Gram-negative, nonsporing, rod-like bacteria that are parasites of the intestinal tract of humans and animals. *Salmonella typhi* and *Salmonella paratyphi* Are exclusively human pathogens which cause typhoid and paratyphoid fevers.

Salmonellosis Infection with the genus *Salmonella,* usually caused by the ingestion of food containing salmonellae or their products. The organisms can be found in raw meats, raw poultry, eggs and dairy products; they multiply rapidly at temperatures between 7°C and 46°C. Symptoms of salmonellosis include violent diarrhea attended by abdominal cramps, nausea and vomiting, and fever. It is rarely fatal and can be prevented by adequate cooking.

Salmon patch Salmon colored areas of cornea in syphilitic keratitis.

Salpingectomy Excision of one or both of the uterine tubes.

Salpingitis 1. Inflammation of the uterine tubes. 2. Inflammation of the pharyngotympanic (Eustachian) tubes.

Acute salpingitis Most often a bilateral ascending infection due to a *Streptococcus* or a *Gonococcus.*

Chronic salpingitis A less acute form that maybe blood borne.

Salpingography Radiographic examination of the uterine tubes after injection of a radiopaque substance to determine their patency.

Salpingolysis Surgical procedure to free the fallopian tubes of adhesions.

Salpingo-oophorectomy Removal of a uterine tube and its ovary.

Salpingo-oophoritis Inflammation of fallopian tube and ovary.

Salpingopexy Surgical fixation of fallopian tube.

Salpingoplasty *SYN*-Tuboplasy; plastic surgery of fallopian tube to promote fertility.

Salpingorrhaphy Ligation of fallopian tube.

Salpingostomy The making of a surgical opening in a uterine tube near the uterus to restore patency.

Salpingotomy Incision on a fallopian tube.

Salpinx A tube applied to the uterine or pharyngotympanic (Eustachian) tubes.

Salt 1. Sodium chloride, common salt, used in solution as a cleansing lotion, a stimulating bath, or for infusion

S

into the blood, etc. 2. Any compound of an acid with an alkali or base. 3. A saline purgative such as Epsom salts.

Salt depletion Loss of salt from the body due to sweating or persistent diarrhea or vomiting. Common in hot climates when it maybe prevented by the taking of salt tablets.

Smelling salts Aromatic ammonium carbonate. A restorative in fainting.

Saltatory Dancing or leaping movement.

Saltatory conduction Nerve conduction where impulse skips from node to node.

Salt-free diet Diet containing <500 mg salt/day.

Saluresis Excretion of salt in urine.

Salutary Promoting health.

Salvarsan Arsenic salt previously used for syphilis.

Salve An ointment.

Sample 1. A selection of individuals made for research purposes from a larger population and intended to reflect that population in all significant aspects. 2. A small part of anything intended as representative of the whole, e.g., blood specimen.

Sampling The process of selecting a portion or part to represent the whole.

Sanatorium A place or establishment for promotion of good health or treatment of chronic ailments, e.g., tuberculosis.

Sand Fine particles from disintegration of rock.

Audiotorys sand Calcareous concretions in inner ear.

Pineal sand Calcium deposit near base of pineal gland.

Sandfly A very small fly of the genus *Phlebotomus*, common in tropical climates and the vector of most types of leishmaniasis.

Sandfly fever A fever transmitted by the bites of sandflies, and common in Mediterranean countries. Similar to dengue and sometimes known as three-day fever.

Sandhoff's disease A gangliosidosis where enzymes hexosaminidase A and B are absent.

Sane Mentally sound.

Sanfilippo's disease A form of mucopolysaccharidosis with mental retardation, dwarfism, hepatosplenomegaly and skeletal defects.

Sanguineous Pertaining to or containing blood.

Sanies Wound discharge which is thin, fetid and green.

Sanitary Clean; conditions conducive to good health.

Sanitary napkin Perineal pad used during menstruation.

Sanitation Establishment of conditions favorable to health.

Sap Any fluid essential for life.

Saphena One of two superficial veins that carry blood from the foot upwards.

Saphenous Relating to the saphena veins.

Saphenous nerve A deep branch of femoral nerve supplying innerside of foot and leg.

Saphenous veins The long saphenous vein extends from foot to saphenous opening in upper thigh whereas short saphenous vein runs up behind lateral malleolus to join popliteal vein.

Saponification 1. Conversion into soap, i.e., hydrolysis of fat by an alkali yielding glycerol and salts of fatty acid. 2. In chemistry hydrolysis of an ester into corresponding alcohol and acid.

Saponin Some plant glycosides that produce gastroenteritis.

Saporific Imparting taste or flavor.

Sapphism Female homosexuality; lesbianism.

Saprogen Any microorganism causing or produced by putrefaction.

Saprophyte Organisms living on decaying or dead organic matter.

Saquinavir Anti-HIV agent.

Saralasin Converting enzyme inhibitor for hypertension.

Sarcoblast Embryonic cell that develops into muscle cell.

Sarcocele A fleshy tumor of testicle.

Sarcocystis A genus of *Coccidian protozoan*, forms sarcocysts in human muscle.

Sarcocystosis Usually transmitted by eating undercooked pork or beef containing sporocysts or ingestion of sporocysts in the feces of animal.

Sarcoid 1. Tuberculoid; characterized by non-caseating epithelioid cell tubercles. 2. Pertaining to or resembling sarcoidosis. 3. Sarcoidosis.

Sarcoidosis A chronic, progressive, generalized disease resembling tuberculosis which may affect any part of the body but most frequently involves the lymph nodes, liver, spleen, lungs, skin, eyes and small bones of the hands and feet.

Sarcolemma A thin membrane surrounding each striated muscle fiber.

Sarcoma A malignant tumor developed from connective tissue cells and their stroma.

Kaposi's sarcoma One principally involving the skin, although visceral lesions maybe present; it usually begins on the distal parts of the extremities, most often on the toes or feet, as reddish blue or brownish soft nodules and tumors. It is viral in origin and is frequently seen in AIDS.

Melanotic sarcoma A highly malignant type, pigmented with melanin.

Round-celled sarcoma A highly malignant growth, composed of a primitive type of cell.

Sarcomere That portion of a striated muscle fibril lying between two adjacent dark lines.

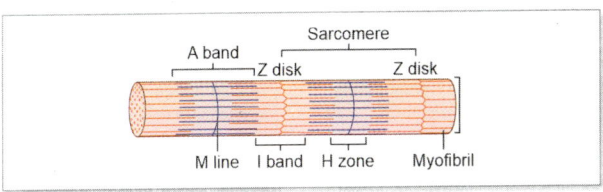

Sarcomere

Sarcomatosis Multiple sarcomatous growths in various parts of the body.

Sarcoplasm The cytoplasm inside muscle cells.

Sarcoptes A genus of mites.

Sarcoptes scabiei The cause of scabies.

SARS Severe acute respiratory syndrome.

Saprophyte A long muscle of the thigh, which flexes both the thigh and the lower leg.

Satellite A small structure attached to a larger one.

Satiety Feeling satisfied with food.

Satranidazole Antiprotozoal agent.

Saturated compound Any compound with all its carbon bonds saturated.

Saturation A state in which all of a substance, that can be dissolved in a solution. Adding more of the substance will not increase its concentration.

Saturday night palsy Paralysis of radial nerve in alcoholics from its compression against the chair.

Satyriasis Abnormally excessive sexual appetite in men.

S

Saucerization Surgical creation of a shallow area in tissue.

Sauna An enclosure where a person is exposed to high temperature and humidity for brief period and then he is given cold bath; a process to relieve aches and pains, loosen stiff joints and loose weight.

Savory Appetizing taste or odor.

Saxifragant Dissolving or breaking of bladder stones.

Scab The crust on a superficial wound consisting of dried blood, pus, etc.

Scabicide Agents effective against scabies organism, i.e., *Sarcoptes scabiei*.

Scabies "The itch"; a contagious skin disease caused by the itch mite *(Sarcoptes scabiei)*, the female of which burrows beneath the skin and deposits eggs at intervals. It is intensely irritating, and the rash is aggravated by scratching. The sites affected are chiefly between the fingers and toes, the axillae and groins. Acquired by close direct contact and may spread in institutions. All members of the family should be treated.

Scala One of the three spiral passages of cochlea; the scala media, scala tympani and scala vestibule.

Scald A burn caused by hot liquid or vapor.

Scalded skin syndrome Staphylococcal necrotizing skin infection.

Scale 1. A scheme or instrument by which something can be measured. A pair of scales is a balance for measuring weight. 2. Compact layers of dead epithelial tissue shed from the skin. 3. To scrape deposits of tartar from the teeth.

Scalenotomy Division of scalenus muscle to contain apical tuberculosis of lungs.

Scalenus One of four muscles which move the neck to either side and raise the first and second ribs during inspiration.

Scalenus syndrome Symptoms of pain and tenderness in the shoulder, with sensory loss and wasting of the medial aspect of the arm. It maybe caused by pressure on the brachial plexus, by spasm of the scalenus anterior muscle or by a cervical rib.

Scaler An instrument used for removing dental calculus.

Scaling Removal of calculus from teeth.

Scalp The hairy skin that covers the cranium.

Scalp tourniquet Tourniquet applied to scalp during IV administration of antineoplastic drugs to present alopecia.

Scalpel A small, pointed surgical knife with a convex edge to the blade.

Scan An image produced using a moving detector or a sweeping beam of radiation, as in scintiscanning, B-mode ultrasonography, scanography or computed tomography.

Scanning 1. Visual examination of an area. 2. A speech disorder that maybe present in cerebellar disease. The syllables are inappropriately separated from each other and are evenly stressed with rhythmically occurring pauses between them.

Scanning electron microscope An electron microscope that provides three-dimensional views of an object.

Scanning speech A symptom of cerebellar disease where words are pronounced by syllables, slowly and hesitantly.

Scaphoid Boat-shaped.

Scaphoid bone A boat-shaped bone of the wrist which articulates with the radius and with the trapezium and the trapezoid bones.

Scapula The large flat triangular bone forming the shoulder blade.

Scar The mark left after a wound has healed with the formation of connective tissue.

Scarlatiniform Resembling scarlet fever or its rash.

Scarlet fever Scarlatina; an acute, notifiable, rare, infectious disease of childhood. It is caused by a group A beta hemolytic *Streptococcus*. There is sore throat, high fever and a punctate rash. It is readily treated by antibiotics and the complications of nephritis and middle ear infection are less common.

Scattergram Display of data on a paper where each value is indicated by a symbol and the individual symbols are not connected by a line.

Schatzki ring A mucosal web like ring at the squamocolumnar junction of lower esophagus often causing dysphagia.

Schick test *B Schick, Austrian pediatrician, 1877–1967.* A skin test of susceptibility to diphtheria. Small amount of diphtheria toxin is injected intradermally.

Schiller's test A test to demonstrate superficial cancer cervix. Iodine is applied on the cervix. As the cancer cells do not contain glycogen, they fail to stain with iodine.

Schilling test *RF Schilling, American hematologist, b. 1919.* A test used to confirm the diagnosis of pernicious anemia by estimating the absorption of ingested radioactive vitamin B_{12}.

Schistocyte Fragmented red blood cells of various shapes and irregular surfaces.

Schistosoma A genus of minute blood flukes, some of which are parasitic in humans.
Schistosoma hematobium A species which infests the urinary bladder; widely found in Africa and the Middle East, especially in Egypt. *Schistosoma japonicum* and *Schistosoma mansoni species* Infest the large intestine, are found respectively in China, Japan and the Philippines, and in Africa, the West Indies and tropical America.

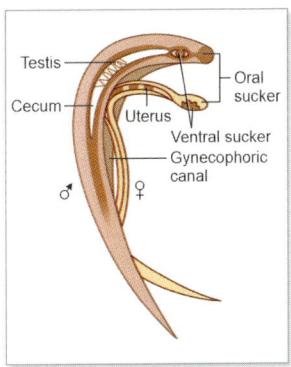

Schistosoma Hematobium

Schistosomiasis A parasitic infection of the intestinal or urinary tract by *Schistosoma*. The parasite enters the skin from contaminated water, and causes diarrhea, hematuria and anemia. The secondary hosts are freshwater snails. Bilharziasis.

Schizencephaly Deformed fetus with a longitudinal cleft in the skull.

Schizogony A sexual reproduction by binary fission as in case of malarial parasite.

Schizoid Resembling schizophrenia. *Schizoid personality* One that is marked by introspection, self-consciousness, solitariness and a failure in affection towards others. Some schizophrenics have this personality, but only a few who are schizoid become schizophrenic.

Schizont A stage in life cycle of sporozoa when it reproduces asexually to 12–24 merozoites inside RBC.

Schizophrenia A general term encompassing a large group of mental disorders (the schizophrenic disorders) characterized by mental deterioration from a previous level of functioning and characteristic disturbances of multiple psychological processes, including delusions, loosening of associations, poverty of the content of speech, auditory hallucinations, inappropriate affect, disturbed sense of self and withdrawal from the external world.

Paranoid schizophrenia Predominance of delusions of a persecutory nature.

Simple schizophrenia A progressive deterioration of the patient's efficiency with increasing social withdrawal *(See Hebephrenia and Catatonia).*

Schizotypal personality disorder A disorder characterized by severe social anxiety, paranoia and often unconventional beliefs. Individuals have great difficulty in establishing and maintaining relationships.

Schlemm's canal F *Schlemm, German anatomist, 1795–1858.* A venous channel at the junction of the cornea and sclera for the draining of aqueous humor.

Schmorl's nodes Herniation of nucleus pulposus into vertebral body producing X-ray density.

Schönlein-Henochpurpura or syndrome *JL Schönlein, German physician, 1793–1864: EH. Henoch, German pediatrician, 1820–1910 (See Purpura).*

School health service The provision of medical and dental inspection and treatment, immunization and health programs in schools.

School nurse A registered nurse who has undertaken further training to specialize in the health care of school-age children. Responsibilities include health promotion and education, monitoring growth and development, screening and caring for those with special educational needs.

Schuffner's dots Minute granules present within RBC infected by *Plasmodium vivax.*

Schwann cell Cells of ectodermal origin, form neurilemma.

Schwannoma Benign tumor of Schwann cells.

Sciatic Pertains to hip or ischium.

Sciatic nerve The largest nerve in body ($L_{4, 5}S_{1, 2, 3}$) passing from pelvis through greater sciatic for a men down the back of the thigh where it divides into tibial and peroneal nerves. Its lesion causes paralysis of hamstrings, peroneal and calf muscles and toe extensors.

Sciatica Pain down the back of the leg in the area supplied by the sciatic nerve. It is usually caused by pressure on the nerve roots by a protrusion of an intervertebral disc.

Scintigraphy A procedure in which a small amount of a radioactive chemical (radionuclide) is injected into a vein or swallowed to produce pictures (scans) of structures inside the body. Used to diagnose, stage, and monitor disease.

Science Branch of knowledge utilizing systematic study and intelligent analysis to understand, explain, quantitative and predict the phenomena of life and natural laws.

Scintiphotography Photography of scintillations emitted by radioactive substances injected into body.

Scintiscan The scintiphotography record to indicate the differential accumulation of a substance in various parts of body.

Schirrhus Hard cancerous overgrowth of fibrous tissue.

Scission To divide, split or cut.

Scissor gait Crossing of the legs while walking as in cerebral diplegia.

Scissor leg Contraction of thigh adductor causing the legs to have abnormal tendency to cross to the other side.

Scissors A cutting instrument with two opposing blades with handles held together by a pin.

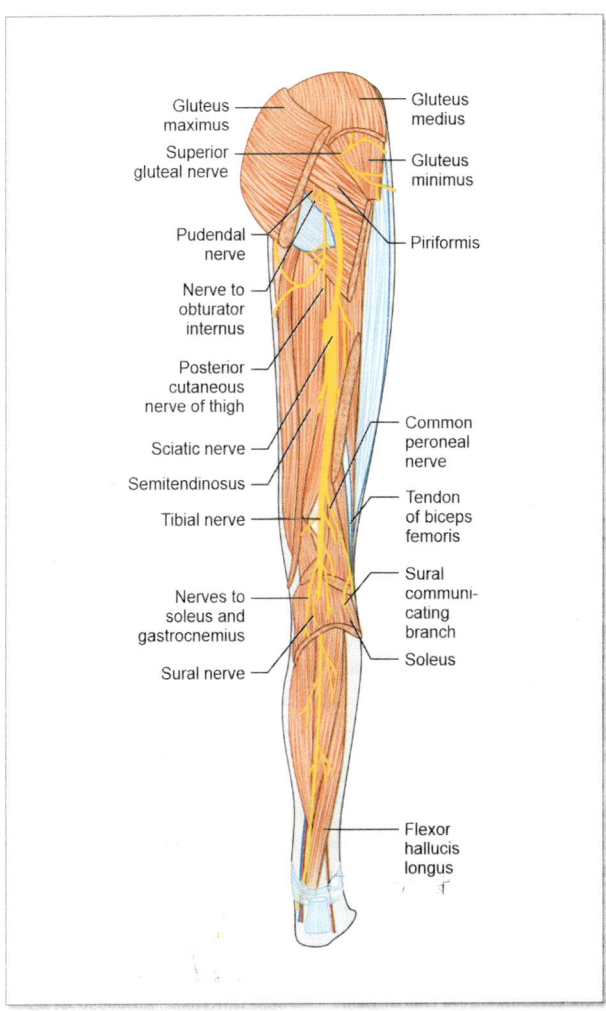

Gluteus maximus
Gluteus medius
Superior gluteal nerve
Gluteus minimus
Pudendal nerve
Piriformis
Nerve to obturator internus
Posterior cutaneous nerve of thigh
Common peroneal nerve
Sciatic nerve
Semitendinosus
Tibial nerve
Tendon of biceps femoris
Nerves to soleus and gastrocnemius
Sural communicating branch
Soleus
Sural nerve
Flexor hallucis longus

Sciatic Nerve

Sclera The fibrous coat of the eyeball, the white of the eye, which covers the posterior part and in front becomes the cornea.

Scleredema A benign self-limited disease characterized by edema and induration of skin.

Sclerema Hardening of the skin.

S

Scleritis Inflammation of sclera, can be anterior (adjacent to cornea), posterior or annular (in ring fashion around cornea).

Sclerodactyly Hardening of skin of fingers and toes.

Scleroderma A disease marked by progressive hardening of the skin in patches or diffusely, with rigidity of the underlying tissues. It is often a chronic condition *(See Raynaud's phenomenon)*.

Scleroma Circumscribed indurated area of granulation tissue in skin or mucous membrane.

Scleromalacia Softening of sclera as in late rheumatoid arthritis.

Scleropalacia Softening of sclera as in late rheumatoid arthritis.

Sclerophthalmia A congenital condition where opacity of sclera advances over the cornea.

Scleroproteins A group of insoluble proteins found in cartilage, hair, nails and skeletal tissue.

Sclerosent Any substance that produces sclerosis.

Sclerosis The hardening of any part from an overgrowth of fibrous and connective tissue, often due to chronic inflammation.

Amyotrophic lateral sclerosis Rapid degeneration of the pyramidal (motor nerves) tract and anterior horn cells in the spinal cord. Characterized by weakness and spasm of limb muscles, with wasting of the muscle, and difficulty with talking and swallowing.

Disseminated sclerosis Multiple sclerosis.

Monckeberg's sclerosis Extensive degeneration with atrophy and calcareous deposits in the middle muscle coat of arteries, especially of the small ones.

Multiple sclerosis Scattered (disseminated) patches of degeneration in the nerve sheaths in the brain and spinal cord. Characterized by relapses and remissions. Symptoms include disturbances of speech, vision, micturition and muscular weakness of a limb or limbs.

Systemic sclerosis (scleroderma) A generalized multisystem disease characterized by dense fibrosis of involved organs and a widespread vascular disorder *(See Raynaud's phenomenon)*.

Sclerosing agents Urea, alcohol, polydachonol tetradecyl sulphate.

Sclerotherapy Treatment of varicose veins and hemorrhoids by the injection of sclerosing solutions to produce fibrosis.

Sclerothrix Brittleness of hair.

Sclerotome Knife used for incision of sclera.

Sclerotic 1. Hard; indurated; affected by sclerosis. 2. Pertaining to the sclera of the eye.

Sclerotic coat The tough membrane forming the outer covering of the eyeball, except in front of the iris, where it becomes the clear horny cornea.

Sclerotomy Incision of the sclerotic coat, usually for the removal of a foreign body or for the relief of glaucoma.

Scolex The head of tapeworm possessing hooks, suckers or grooves for attachment.

Scoliosis Lateral curvature of the spine *(See Lordosis and Kyphosis)*.

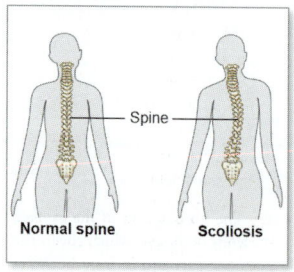

Scoliosis

Scombroid poisoning Poisoning by histamine-like toxin present in the undercooked fish of suborder scombroidea.

Scoop Spoon shaped surgical instrument.

Scopolamine Hyoscine; used in premedication as a sedative and to dry up secretions.

Scopophilia Sexual pleasure obtained from seeing nude and obscene picture.

Scorbutic Affected with or related to scurvy.

Score A rating or grade as compared to standard.

Apgar score A scoring system for evaluation of neurological maturity of newborn from pulse, respiration, reflexes, skin color, grimace, etc.

Screening 1. Fluoroscopy. 2. The carrying out of a test on a large number of people to determine the proportion of them that have a particular disease.

Scorpion sting Symptoms from scorpion bite resembling spider bite or of strychnine poisoning. The venom contains neurotoxin, hemolysins and agglutinins. Stings are fatal to children below 3 years.

Scoto Pertains to darkness.

Scotochromogen Microorganisms that produce color when grown in darkness.

Scotoma Dark or blind areas in visual field, can be annular, arcuate, central (around point of fixation), centrocecal (covering point of fixation to blindspot), peripheral.

Scintillating scotoma An irregular outline around a luminous patch in the visual field as seen in migraine.

Scotopic vision Dark adaptation.

Scotopsin The protein portion of rods of retina that combines with retinol to form visual purple, i.e., rhodopsin.

SCR Summary care record. An electronic record containing important health information of patients covering patients in England.

Scratch test An allergy test where the allergen is placed over a skin scratch. In sensitive persons wheal develops within 15 minutes.

Screen 1. A flat surface for projecting X-ray films. 2. To make fluoroscopic examinations. 3. To thoroughly examine and investigate a person for a disease. 4. Materials used to protect the body parts from ionizing radiation or X-rays.

Bjerrum screen One meter square surface which is viewed from one meter to chart blind spot, scotoma and extent of visual field.

Scrofula Tubercular cervical lymphadenopathy.

Scrotal reflex Contraction of scrotal muscle (dartos) on stroking the perineum.

Scrotum The pouch of skin and soft tissues containing the testicles.

Scrubbing Thorough washing of hands and finger nails before performing any surgical procedure.

Scrub typhus Typhus fever caused by *Rickettsia tsutsugamushi* transmitted by mites.

Scum The floating impurities in surface of a culture.

Scurf Dandruff

Scurvy Avitaminosis C. A deficiency disease caused by lack of vitamin C, which is found in raw fruits and vegetables. Clinical features include fatigue, oozing of blood from the gums and bruising. The condition rapidly improves with adequate diet.

Scybala Hard founded masses of fecal matter.

Seasonal affective disorder syndrome Abbreviated SADS. A condition in which the person notices a change in mood or feelings according to the season of the year and hence the amount of exposure to (sun) light.

Sea-sickness Akin to motion sickness with giddiness, nausea, vomiting and headache while travelling in ship.

Sebaceous Fatty, or pertaining to the sebum. *Sebaceous cyst (See Cyst).* *Sebaceous glands* Found in the communicating with the hair follicles and secreting sebum.

Seborrhea A disease of the sebaceous glands, marked by an excessive secretion of sebum which collects on the skin in oily scales.

Sebum The fatty secretion of the sebaceous glands.

Secnidazole Antiprotozoal agent.

Secobarbitol Short acting barbiturate used for its hypnotic effect.

Secondary Second in order of time or importance.
Secondary areola Pigmentation around nipple during pregnancy.
Secondary deposits (See Metastasis).
Secondary hemorrhage Hemorrhage occurring after 48 hours of injury or operation commonly due to sepsis.
Secondary intention Healing by formation of granulation tissue that fills the gap between torn or incised edges.
Secondary nursing care Nursing care aimed at early recognition and treatment of a disease.

Secretin The hormone originating in the duodenum which, in the presence of bile salts, is absorbed into the blood stream and stimulates the secretion of pancreatic juice.

Secretion A substance formed or concentrated in a gland and passed in to the alimentary tract, the blood or to the exterior. The secretions of the endocrine glands include various hormones and are important in the overall regulation of body processes.

Secretogogue Agent that stimulates secretion.

Secretomotor Nerve fibers that promote glandular secretion.

Sector The area within a circle between two radii and the arc.

Sectorial Having cutting edges like teeth.

Sedation The allaying of irritability, the relief of pain or mental distress, and the promotion of sleep, particularly by drugs.

Sedative A drug or agent that lessens excitement and relieves tension. Sedative drugs are used to induce sleep.

Sedentary Pertaining to sitting; physically inactive.

Sediment The substance settling at the bottom of a liquid.

Sedimentation The deposit of solid particles at the bottom of a liquid.
Erythrocyte sedimentation rate Abbreviated ESR *(See Erythrocyte).*

Segregation The separation during meiosis of allelic genes as the chromosomes migrate toward opposite poles of the cell.

Segment A portion.

Segmentation Division into similar parts; division of fertilized eggs into many smaller cells.

Segregation Separation.

Seizure A sudden attack of pain, disease or certain symptoms like convulsion, epilepsy.

Seldinger technique A method of introducing a catheter into a vein or artery. The vessel is punctured with a needle that contains a wire. The needle is removed and the catheter is then advanced over the wire, the latter being finally withdrawn.

Selective mutism A severe anxiety disorder where a person is unable to speak in certain situations.

Selective serotonin reuptake inhibitors (SSRIs) Widely used antidepressive medication.

Selenium sulfide Drug used in treatment of tinea versicolor and dandruff.

Self 1. A term used to denote an animals own antigenic constituents, in contrast to "not-self" denoting foreign antigenic constituents. 2. The complete being of an individual, comprising both physical and psychological characteristics, and including both conscious and unconscious components.

Self-actualization A level of psychological development in which innate potential is realized to the full, allowing transcendence of the environment.

Self-care The personal care carried out by the patient, e.g., bathing, personal grooming, eating and toilet hygiene. Maybe with assistance or instruction from a health care worker. The aim of rehabilitative care is to maximize self-care and personal independence.

Self-catheterization Men, women and older children can be taught to pass a fine catheter into the urinary bladder to evacuate urine as required.

Self-esteem A person's evaluation of their own worth as an individual.

Self-examination of breast *(See Breast).*

Self-examination of testes *(See Testicular self examination).*

Self-harm Deliberate damage to one's own body. Over half of people who die by suicide have a history of self-harm; however, the intention is more often to punish themselves, express their distress or relieve unbearable tension. Self-harm may sometimes be linked to anxiety and depression. Most often occurs in young adults and is more common in women. Also referred to as self-injury or self-mutilation.

Self-image An individual's concept of their own personality and abilities based on their own ideas and perceptions.

Self-limited A disease which without treatment pursues a definite course within a limited time.

Sella turcica A depression in the sphenoid body which protects the pituitary gland.

Sellick's maneuver Technique used during endotracheal intubation by applying pressure on the cricoids cartilage to prevent regurgitation or better visualization of the glottis by the doctor.

Selzer water Naturally occurring water with high CO_2 and mineral content.

Semen The secretion of the testicles containing spermatozoa, which is ejaculated from the penis during sexual intercourse. Seminal fluid.

Semi Prefix meaning half.

Semicircular Formed in a half-circle.

Semicircular canals Part of the labyrinth of the internal ear, consisting of three canals in the form of arches which contain fluid and are connected with the cerebellum by their nerve supply. Impressions of change of position of the body are registered in these canals by oscillation of the fluid, and are conveyed by the nerves to the cerebellum.

Semicoma Mild degree of impaired consciousness.

Semicomatose In a condition of unconsciousness from which the patient can be roused.

Semilunar Shaped like a half-moon.

Semilunar cartilages Two crescent-shaped cartilages in the knee joint.

Semilunar valve (See Valve).

Semimembranosus A large muscle at inner and back portion of thigh, a knee flexor.

Seminal vesicle Two sac like structures close to prostate in the male giving rise to ductus deferens. Act to store semen and secrete a thick viscus fluid that forms part of semen.

S

Seminiferous tubule Tubules in testes forming and conducting semen.

Seminoma A malignant tumor of the testis that is highly radiosensitive.

Semipermeable Of a membrane, permitting the passage of some molecules and hindering that of others.

Semiprone Partly prone. Applied to a position in which the patient is lying face down but the knees are turned to one side.

Semitendinosus Fusiform muscle of posterior and inner part of thigh.

Senescence The process of growing old.

Sengstaken-Blakemore tube *RW Sengstaken, American neurosurgeon, b. 1923; AH Blakemore, American surgeon, 1879–1970.* A compression tube used in the treatment of bleeding esophageal varices.

Senile Related to the involutional changes associated with old age.

Senile dementia Deterioration of mental activity in the elderly, associated with an impaired blood supply to the brain.

Senna A laxative derived from the cassia plant. Proprietary standardized preparations are available as tablets or granules.

Sensation A feeling resulting from impulses sent to the brain by the sensory nerves.

Sense The faculty by which conditions and properties of things are perceived, e.g., hunger or pain.

Sense organ One that receives a sensory stimulus, for instance, the eyes and ears.

Special sense Anyone of the faculties of sight, hearing, touch, smell, taste and muscle sense, through which the consciousness receives impressions from the environment.

Sensible 1. Capable of being perceived. 2. Sensitive.

Sensible perspiration That obvious on the skin as moisture.

Sensitive 1. Able to feel a sensation. 2. Abnormal response to substances like drugs and foreign proteins.

Sensitivity 1. The term is employed in relation to accuracy of diagnostic tests/observations. It is the proportion of people who truly have a specific disease as identified by the test. 2. Susceptibility of bacteria to antimicrobials.

Sensitization 1. The process of rendering susceptible. 2. An increase in the body's response to a certain stimulus, as in the development of an allergy.

Protein sensitization The condition occurring in an individual when a foreign protein is absorbed into the body, e.g., shell-fish causing urticaria when eaten *(See Desensitization).*

Sensitizer A substance that makes the susceptible individual react to same or another irritant.

Sensorium The sensory apparatus of body or consciousness.

Sensory Relating to sensation.

Sensory area The postcentral gyrus of cerebral cortex responsible for analysis of somatosensory input.

Sensory cortex That part of the cerebral cortex to which information is relayed by the sensory nerves.

Sensory deprivation The effecting of a major reduction of sensory information received by the body. This is damaging to the person's ability to function normally, which is dependent upon constant stimulation.

Sensory integration Skill and performance required in the development and coordination of sensory input and motor output.

Sensory nerve An afferent nerve conveying impressions from the peripheral nerve endings to the brain or spinal cord.

Sensualism State of emotions dominating one's actions.

Sensuous Affecting senses or susceptible to influence through the senses.

Sentiment An emotion directed toward some object or person. Sentiments are acquired and profoundly influence a person's actions.

Sentinel node Cancer metastasis into supraclavicular nodes.

Separation anxiety disorder Developmentally, young children experience feelings of distress at separation from home, parents or carers to whom they have formed an attachment. If hospitalized at this time without a 'live-in' parent or carer, the child may regress to a former stage of development with food refusal and incontinence. Separation anxiety usually diminishes by the age of 3 or 4 years but occasionally may occur in older children resulting in nightmares, complaints of somatic symptoms (e.g., headaches, nausea or vomiting) and refusal to attend school. It maybe associated with depression.

Separator Any device or instrument used for separating two substances, e.g., cell separators.

Sepsis An infection of the body by pus forming bacteria.

Focal sepsis A local focus of infection which produces general symptoms.

Oral sepsis Infection of the mouth which causes general ill-health by absorption of toxins.

Puerperal sepsis Infection of the uterus occurring after labor.

Septa Partition

Septate Having a partition or wall.

Septic Infected.

Septicemia The presence in the blood of large numbers of bacteria and their toxins. The symptoms are: a rapid rise of temperature, which is later intermittent, rigors, sweating, and all the signs of acute fever.

Septic fever Fever due to presence of pathogenic organisms or their products in blood, producing shaking chills with abrupt rise in temperature and seating.

Septoplasty Plastic surgery on nasal septum for deviated nasal septum.

Septostomy Surgical formation of an opening in septum.

Septulet Seven children in one pregnancy.

Septum A division or partition.

Atrial septum, atrioventricular septum Along with ventricular septum, the partitions dividing the various cavities of the heart.

Nasal septum The structure made of bone and cartilage which separates the nasal cavities.

Ventricular septum (See Atrial septum above).

Sequela A morbid condition occurring after a disease and resulting from it.

Sequestration Formation of sequestrum.

Sequestration pulmonary A nonfunctioning area of the lung receiving blood from systemic circulation.

Sequestrum A piece of dead bone. Inflammation in bone leads to thrombosis of blood vessels, resulting in necrosis of the affected part, which separates from the living structure.

Serine An amino acid found in urine of healthy humans.

Serious incident Abbreviated SI. SIs include acts or omissions in care that result in unexpected or avoidable death, unexpected or avoidable injury resulting in serious harm-including those where the injury required treatment to prevent death or serious harm, abuse, never events, incidents that prevent (or threaten to prevent) an organization's ability to continue to deliver an acceptable quality of health care services and incidents that cause widespread public concern resulting in loss of confidence in health care services.

Seroconversion Appearance of antibodies to an infecting agent or vaccine.

S

Serodiagnosis Diagnosis from tests involving patient's serum.

Seroepidemiology Epidemiological study of a disease by investigating for presence of diagnostic characteristic in the serum.

Serological Relating to serum.

Serological tests Those that are dependent on the formation of antibodies in the blood as a response to specific organisms or proteins.

Serology The scientific study of serum.

Serosa A serous membrane. It consists of two layers: the visceral, in close contact with the organ, and the parietal, lining the cavity.

Serosanguinous Discharge containing serum and blood.

Serositis Inflammation of serous membrane.

Serotherapy Treatment of disease by antibodies thereby conferring passive immunity.

Serotonin An amine present in blood platelets, the intestine and the central nervous system, which acts as a vasoconstrictor. It is derived from the amino acid tryptophan and is inactivated by monoamine oxidase.

Serotype A classification of microorganisms based on antigenic structure of cell.

Serous Related to serum.

Serous cavity Cavity lined by serous membrane like pleural, pericardial and peritoneal cavities.

Serous effusion An effusion of serous exudate.

Serpiginous Creeper like course.

Serpin Serine-protease inhibitor involved in coagulation, complement activation, fibrinolysis, etc. They include alfa2, antitrypsin, alfa 3, antiplasmin, PAI-I, CI inhibitor, etc.

Serrate Tooth like, notched.

Serratia Gram-negative facultative anaerobic entero bacteria producing white, pink or red pigment; cause nosocomial bacteremia, endocarditis and pneumonia in immune compromised.

Sertoli's cells Supporting cells in the seminiferous tubules that nourish the spermatids.

Sertraline Antipsychotic agent.

Serum The clear, fluid residue of blood, from which the corpuscles and fibrin have been removed.

Serum hepatitis Jaundice caused by hepatitis B virus, usually after a blood transfusion or an inoculation with contaminated material.

Serum sickness An allergic reaction usually 8–10 days after a serum injection. It may manifest by an irritating urticaria, pyrexia and painful joints. It readily responds to adrenaline and antihistaminic drugs *(See Anaphylaxis)*.

Sesamoid bone A bone of developing under a cartilage, e.g., patella.

Severe acute respiratory syndrome Abbreviated SARS. A serious acute respiratory illness caused by the SARS coronavirus known as SARS Co-V. The WHO monitors countries throughout the world for outbreaks; there have been none since 2004. Infected persons develop high fever (>38°C) and cough and/or dyspnea followed by rapidly progressive respiratory compromise. Infected persons may also experience chills, muscle aches, headache and loss of appetite. The SARS virus is highly contagious and is predominantly transmitted by droplets or by direct and indirect contact. Shedding of the virus in feces and urine also occurs. Mortality rates vary depending on age and underlying medical conditions. Treatment is symptomatic and intensive respiratory support including mechanical ventilation maybe required.

Sewer gas Methane and hydrogen sulphide produced in sewage, maybe used as fuel.

Sex 1. Either of the two divisions of organisms described respectively as male and female. 2. To discover the sex of an organism.

Sex chromosome A chromosome that determines sex. Women have two X chromosomes and men have one X chromosome and one Y chromosome.

Sex hormone A steroid hormone produced by the ovaries or the testes and controlling sexual development.

Sex limited Pertaining to a characteristic found in only one sex.

Sex linked Pertaining to a characteristic that is transmitted by genes that are located on the sex chromosomes, e.g., hemophilia.

Sexism A belief in the intrinsic superiority of one sex over the other often accompanied by prejudice, stereotyping and discrimination on the basis of sex.

Sextuplet Six children in one pregnancy.

Sexual Pertaining to sex.

Sexual development The biological and psychosocial changes that lead to sexual maturity.

Sexual deviation Aberrant sexual activity: expression of the sexual instinct in practices which are socially prohibited or unacceptable, or biologically undesirable.

Sexual intercourse Coitus.

Sexual dysfunction Sexual dissatisfaction due to defective arousal, orgasm, pain or penetration.

Sexual reflex Erection and ejaculation from sexual stimulation (whether direct or indirect) irrespective one is asleep or awake.

Sexuality 1. The characteristic quality of the male and female reproductive elements. 2. The constitution of an individual in relation to sexual attitudes and behavior.

Sexually transmitted infection Abbreviated STI. An infection transmitted either by means of sexual intercourse between heterosexual or homosexual individuals, or by intimate contact with the genitals, mouth and rectum. STIs include syphilis, gonorrhea, human immunodeficiency virus (HIV) infection, acquired immunodeficiency syndrome (AIDS), chlamydial infection, genital herpes, nonspecific urethritis, trichomoniasis, genital lice, scabies, genital warts, hepatitis B infection and yaws. 'Sexually transmitted infection' is now the preferred term for what was formerly known as sexually transmitted disease (STD).

Sezary cells An atypical mononuclear cell containing mucopolysaccharide filled cytoplasmic vacuoles.

Sezary syndrome Exfoliative skin disease characterized by infiltration of skin by sezary cells; a variant of mycosis fungoides.

SGA Small for gestational age.

SGOT Serum Glutamic-Oxaloacetic Transaminase, an enzyme excreted by damaged heart muscle. A raised serum level occurs in myocardial infarction.

SGPT Serum Glutamic-Pyruvic Transaminase, an enzyme excreted by the parenchymal cells of the liver. There is a raised blood level in infectious hepatitis.

Shakes Shivering or tremulousness.

Shaken baby syndrome The presence of unexplained fractures in the long bones, together with evidence of a subdural hematoma (bleeding under the membrane surrounding the brain) in a baby. These injuries, a result of child abuse, are caused by the violent shaking of the baby which produces a whiplash effect and a rotational movement of the head resulting in vomiting, convulsions, irritability, coma and death.

Shared care In obstetrics, a term used to describe antenatal care carried

S

out by an obstetrician and a general practitioner. The latter usually carries out the care from the time of the booking until sometime in the third trimester.

Shaking palsy Parkinson's disease.

Shaman A traditional healer who while in a trance, uses spirits to cure diseases.

Shagreen patch Thick granular grayish green skin of tuberous sclerosis.

Shear A force applied parallel to the planes of an object but opposite in direction to existing force.

Shearing force A strain produced by pressure in the structure of a substance so that each layer slides over the next. In the body, this may occur when any part is on a gradient; the deeper tissues slide towards the lower gradient and the skin remains with the supporting contact, e.g., sheets on a bed or on a chair. In the presence of moisture, this friction is exacerbated and the deeper tissues become ischemic. *(See Pressure Ulcer).*

Sheath 1. An enveloping tubular structure or part. 2. A condom, worn on the erect penis during sexual intercourse to trap seminal fluid, preventing the transmission of human immunodeficiency virus (HIV) and other viruses and also reducing the risk of pregnancy.

Shedding Casting off surface layer of epidermis.

Sheehan's syndrome Hypopituitarism secondary to pituitary infarction following postpartum hemorrhage and shock.

Sheep cell agglutination test (SCAT) A test for rheumatoid factor when sheep erythrocytes sensitized with rabbit anti-sheep RBC immunoglobulin are agglutinated by patient's serum containing rheumatoid factor.

Sheet Linen.

Draw sheet Folded linen placed under a patient which can be withdrawn without lifting the patient.

Shiatsu A form of manipulation in which the practitioner uses the thumbs, fingers and palms of the hands, knees, forearms, elbows and feet to apply pressure to the client's body in order to promote and maintain health.

Shield A protective device.

Shigella A genus of Gram-negative rod-like bacteria. Some species cause bacillary dysentery. *Shigella flexneri* and *Shigella shigae* are common in Asia, *Shigella dysenteriae* in the USA and *Shigellasonnei* in Western Europe.

Shigellosis Disease produced by *Shigella*.

Shin The bony front of the leg below the knee. The tibia.

Shingles Herpes zoster.

Shirodkar's suture *Shirodkar, Indian obstetrician.* A "purse-string" suture that is placed round an incompetent cervix during pregnancy to prevent abortion. It is removed at the 38th week.

Shiver Involuntary muscle contraction during cold, fear or at onset of some fevers.

Shock A condition produced by severe illness or trauma in which there is a sudden fall in blood pressure. This leads to lack of oxygen in the tissues and greater permeability of the capillary walls, so increasing the degree of shock by greater loss of fluid. The patient has a cold, moist skin, a feeble pulse and a low blood pressure, and is distressed, thirsty and restless.

Allergic or anaphylactic shock Shock produced by the injection of a protein to which the patient is sensitive.

Cardiogenic shock Shock as a result of an acute heart condition such as myocardial infarction.

Endotoxic shock Shock from endotoxins of Gram-negative bacteria.

Hypovolaemic shock Shock resulting from a reduction in the volume of blood in the circulation after hemorrhage or severe burns.

Neurogenic shock Shock due to nervous or emotional factors.

Shell shock A psychoneurotic condition caused by the stresses of warfare.

Spinal shock Acute flaccid paralysis with loss of all sensations and reflexes following complete transaction of spinal cord.

Shohl's solution Solution of citric acid and sodium citrate used for acidosis.

Short bowel syndrome Poor absorption of nutrients following resection of sizeable length of small intestine.

Short-sightedness Myopia

Shot A subcutaneous injection.

Shoulder The junction of the clavicle and the scapula where the arm joins the body.

Show The blood-stained discharge that occurs at the onset of labor.

Sharpnell's membrane The triangular portion of tympanic membrane lying above the malleolar fold. *SYN* – pars flaccid.

Shred Thin strand of mucus.

Shrink To reduce in size.

Shudder Convulsive tremor from fear, aversion.

Shunt A diversion, particularly of blood, due to a congenital defect, disease or surgery.

Shy drager syndrome Chronic orthostatic hypotension due to primary autonomic failure.

Sialism Excessive salivary secretion.

Sialoadenitis Inflammation of salivary gland.

Sialogogue An agent that promotes salivary secretion.

Sialography Radiographic examination of the salivary ducts after the introduction of a radiopaque contrast medium.

Sialolith A salivary calculus.

Sialoporia Deficient secretion of saliva.

Siamese twins (Named after Chang and Eng joined Chinese twins born in Siam), congenitally joined twins.

Sib A blood relative, brother or sister.

Sibilant Hissing or whistling sound.

Sibilismus A hissing sound.

Sibling One of a family of children having the same parents. Applied in psychology to one of two or more children of the same parent or substitute parent figure.

Sibling rivalry Jealousy, compounded of love and hate of one child for its sibling.

Sibutramine Antiobesity agent.

Siccus Dry.

Sick Not well, ill.

Sickle cell Crescent shaped RBC.

Sickle-cell anemia An inherited blood disease *(See Anemia)*.

Sickle-cell disease (SCD) A group of inherited red blood cell disorders. People with SCD have abnormal hemoglobin, in the red blood cells. SCD is particularly common in people with an African or Caribbean family background. *(See also Anemia)*.

Sickle cell crisis Capillary plugging by sickle cells causing joint pain, abdominal pain, renal pain, etc. due to infarction.

Sickling Tendency of RBC to assume sickle shape.

Sickness illness Sickness motion. Nausea and vomiting experienced during motion by road, air or water.

Morning sickness Nausea and vomiting of early pregnancy.

Mountain sickness Nausea, anorexia, insomnia and dyspnea of high altitude due to oxygen lack.

Sleeping sickness 1. Trypanosomiasis involving CNS (Chaga's disease), transmitted by tsetse. 2. Encephalitis lethargic.

S

Serum sickness Joint pain, fever, lymphadenopathy following injection of serum.

Sick-sinus syndrome SA node dysfunction manifesting as excessive bradycardia, brief period of sinus arrest or tachybrady syndrome.

Side effect Undesirable effects of a drug.

Sidenafyl A phosphodiesterage inhibitor used in impotency (Viagra).

Sideroblast Ferritin containing normoblast in bone marrow that constitute 20–90% of bone marrow normoblasts. The ferritin gives Prussian blue reaction indicating presence of ionized iron.

Siderocyte RBC containing iron in any form other than hemoglobin.

Siderophile A cell having affinity for iron.

Siderosis 1. Chronic inflammation of the lung due to inhalation of particles of iron. 2. Excess iron in the blood. 3. The deposit of iron in the tissues.

Siderosome A reticulocyte with iron-containing granules.

SIDS Sudden infant death syndrome.

Sieve A mesh with uniform sized pores.

Sigh A deep inspiration followed by a slow but loud expiration.

Sight Vision.

Sigmoid Shaped like the Greek letter sigma, *Sigmoid colon* or *flexure* Part of the colon in the left iliac fossa just above the rectum.

Sigmoid proctectomy Artificial communication of sigmoid flexure with colon.

Sigmoidoscope An instrument by which the interior of the rectum and sigmoid colon can be seen.

Sigmoidoscopy Examination of recto sigmoid by sigmoidoscope.

Sigmoidostomy Artificial creation of communication between two segments of colon.

Sign 1. Any objective evidence of disease or dysfunction. 2. An observable physical phenomenon so frequently associated with a given condition as to be considered indicative of its presence.

Sign language Hand and body language used by totally deaf people to communicate with others.

Vital signs The signs of life, namely pulse, respiration and temperature.

Significant other A person designated by the patient as the person who should be consulted in the event of an emergency or to contact when making arrangements for discharge.

Siliastic Silicone material which are usually inert and hence compatible with body and used in reconstructive surgery.

Silent Mute.

Sildenafil A phosphodiesterage 5 inhibitor, vasodilator used for impotency and pulmonary hypertension.

Silent angina Angina pectoris without subjective symptoms like precordial pain.

Silent period Period in a tendon reflex immediately following muscle contraction when another neural impulse entering the reflex center cannot excite efferent motor neurone.

Silica Silicon dioxide.

Silicate A salt of silicic acid.

Silicon A nonmetallic element constituting 25% of earth's crust.

Silicone A group of polymeric organic compounds used in adhesives, lubricants and prosthesis.

Silicosis Fibrosis of the lung due to the inhalation of silica dust particles. It occurs in miners, stone masons and quarry workers.

Silo-filler's disease Hypersensitive pneumonitis in workers working in silos caused by nitric acid and nitrogen dioxide that are produced by fermenting organic matter.

Silver White malleable metal used for a stringent and antiseptic effect.

Silver amalgam Alloy of silver with tin or copper used as a dental restorative material.

Silver halide The coating on radiographic films which when exposed to radiant energy forms the image.

Silver sulfadiazine Used for topical application on burn.

Silver-fork deformity Malunited Colles fracture resembling back of the fork.

Silver nitrate A germicide and local astringent used for throat cauterization; causes grayish discoloration of mucous membranes.

Silvester's method A method of artificial respiration where patient lies on back with arms raised to the sides of head, then brought down and pressed against the chest.

Silymarin Hepatoprotective agent.

Simethicone Dimethylpolysiloxanes, an antifoaming agent used to treat intestinal gas.

Simian crease A single transverse crease on palm as in monkeys. Its presence may signify Down's syndrome, Rubella syndrome, Turner's syndrome or Klinefelter's syndrome.

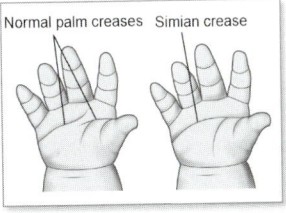

Normal palm creases   Simian crease

Simian Crease

Similimum A therapeutic concept in homeopathy where a medicine produces symptoms similar to that of the disease for which it is prescribed.

Simmond's disease Hypopituitarism due to pituitary atrophy.

Sims' position *JM Sims, American gynecologist, 1813–1883.* A semiprone position *(See Position)*.

Simulation Imitation, pretention.

Simulator Any device that creates a situation similar to one that might be encountered, a technique useful in teaching in flying practice, engine testing.

Simulium A genus of insects that includes black flies, *Simulium damnosum*, serves as intermediate host of *Onchocerca volvulus.*

Simvastin Lipid lowering agent.

Sinciput Front and upper part of head.

Sinemet Combination of levodopa and carbidopa.

Singer's node A swelling between arytenoid cartilages in singers.

Singultus Hiccups.

Sinister Evil, wickedness; in anatomy present on left side of body.

Sinistrous Awkward, clumsy, unskilled, opposite to dexterous.

Sinoatrial Situated between the sinus venosus and the atrium of the heart.

Sinoatrial node The pacemaker of the heart *(See Node)*.

Sinogram X-ray of sinus after radioopaque dye injection.

Sinuous Winding, wavy, tortuous.

Sinus 1. A cavity in a bone. 2. A venous channel, especially within the cranium. 3. An unhealed passage leading from an abscess or internal lesion to the surface.

Air sinus A cavity in a bone containing air.

Cavernous sinus A venous sinus of the dura mater which lies along the body of the sphenoid bone.

Coronary sinus The vein that returns the blood from the heart muscle into the right atrium.

Ethmoidal sinus Air spaces in the ethmoid bone.

Frontal sinus Air spaces in the frontal bone.

S

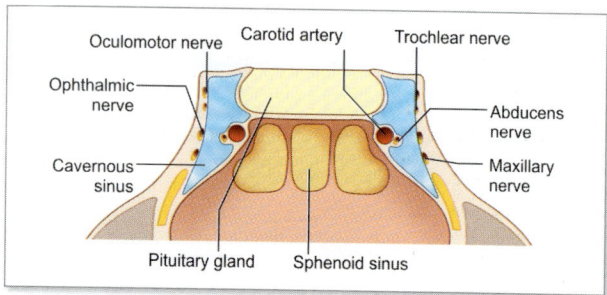

Oculomotor nerve
Carotid artery
Trochlear nerve
Ophthalmic nerve
Abducens nerve
Cavernous sinus
Maxillary nerve
Pituitary gland
Sphenoid sinus

Cavernous Sinus

Sinus arrhythmia (See Arrhythmia).

Sinus thrombosis Clotting of blood in a cranial venous channel. In the lateral sinus it is a complication of mastoiditis.

Sphenoidal sinus Air spaces in the sphenoid bone.

Sinusitis Inflammation of the lining of a sinus, especially applied to the bony cavities of the face.

Sinusoid A large blood channel with reticuloendothelial lining found in liver, spleen, adrenal and bone marrow.

Sinus rhythm The normal cardiac rhythm originating from SA node.

Siphon A tube bent at an angle with two unequal parts for transferring liquids from one container to another.

Sipple syndrome Multiple endocrine neoplasia type III.

Sirolimus Immunosuppressant.

Sitagliptin Antidiabetic.

Site Position or location.

Sitophobia Abnormal psychic aversion for particular food.

Sitosternols A mixture of saturated sterols that increase fecal elimination of cholesterol and therefore used as lipid-lowering agent.

Sitting height In anthropometry a vertical height taken from the table on which patient is sitting to the vertex.

Situational crisis In psychiatry any brief transient period of psychological stress.

Situs A position.

Inversus situs An anomaly where visceral positions are reversed.

Sitzbath Emersion of patient's buttocks and perineal region in hot water.

Six sigma Set of tools and techniques for improvement of processes.

Sixth cranial nerve Abducens nerve that supplies the external rectus.

Sjogren's syndrome A combination of rheumatoid arthritis with xerostomia, kerato conjunctivitis sicca and parotid enlargement.

Sjogren-Larsson syndrome Mental retardation, ichthyosis, spastic diplegia, inherited as an autosomal recessive trait.

Skatole A nitrogenous decomposed product of protein formed from tryptophan with bad odor.

Skeletal muscle A muscle attached to bone and involved in body movements.

Skeletal survey X-ray of entire skeleton to detect any metastasis or disease.

Skeletal traction Traction applied directly to bone through inserted pins and needles.

Skeleton The bony framework of the body, supporting and protecting the organs and soft tissues.

S

Skene's glands Paraurethral glands opening to the floor of terminal urethra. Constantly involved in gonococccal infection.

Skew Asymmetrical, to slant.

Skew deviation A condition where one eyeball is deviated upward and outward, the other being inward and downward.

Skewed distribution In statistics, the degree to which the distribution is asymmetric around the mean. The normal distribution is symmetric, thus having zero skewness.

Skill mix The ratio of staff employed in an area of health care activity, whether qualified, trained or untrained, representing the availability of skills possessed by these staff.

Skin The outer protective covering of the body. It consists of an outer layer, the epidermis or cuticle, and an inner layer, the dermis or corium, which is known as "true skin".

Skin grafting Transplantation of pieces of healthy skin to an area where loss of surface tissue has occurred.

Skin patch A drug impregnated adhesive patch which is applied to the skin. The drug is slowly absorbed, allowing its level in the blood to be maintained over a given period of time.

Skin test Application of a substance to the skin, or intradermal injection of a substance, to permit observation of the body's reaction to it.

Skin clip An alternative to sutures to close the skin wound.

Skin fold thickness Measuring thickness of subcutaneous fat over triceps, in upper abdomen and in subscapular region to assess the nutritional status.

Skull The bony framework of the head, consisting of the cranium and facial bones.

Slapped cheek syndrome Also known as fifth disease. A viral infection most commonly seen in children resulting in a bright red rash on the cheeks. It will usually clear up in 1-3 weeks.

Sleep A period of rest for the body and mind, during which volition and consciousness are in partial or complete abeyance and the bodily functions partially suspended. It occurs in a 24-hour biological rhythm. Sleep occurs in cycles which have two distinct phases. Each phase lasts approximately 60–90 minutes: orthodox or nonrapid eye movement sleep (NREM), and paradoxical or rapid eye movement sleep (REM). Sleeping requirements vary, with each individual averaging between 4 and 10 hours in a 24-hour period. The purpose of sleep is unknown but sleep deprivation is harmful.

Sleep paralysis Transient paralysis with spontaneous recovery occurring while falling asleep or on awakening.

Sleep spindle In electroencephalography, the bursts of about 14 per second waves occurring during sleep.

Sleeping sickness Trypanosomiasis. A tropical fever occurring in parts of Africa, caused by a protozoal parasite *(Trypanosoma)* which is conveyed by the tsetse fly.

Slide A piece of glass on which specimens are examined under microscope.

Sliding hernia A variety of indirect irreducible inguinal hernia in which a section of viscus forms one wall of the sac.

Slim disease A term primarily used in Africa and other tropical countries for a progressive wasting disease associated with human immunodeficiency virus infection resulting in a loss of 10% or more of the baseline body weight. *(See Aids and Human Immunodeficiency Virus).*

Sling A bandage usually slung from neck to support the arm.

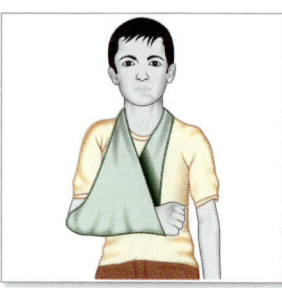

Sling

Slipped disk (slipt) A prolapsed intervertebral disk which causes pressure on the spinal nerves. It maybe very painful.

Slipped epiphysis Displacement of upper femoral epiphysis, common in children.

Slit A narrow opening.

Slit lamp A special light source so arranged with a microscope that examination of the interior of the eye can be carried out at the level of each layer.

Slough Dead tissue caused by injury or inflammation. It separates from the healthy tissue and is ultimately washed away by exuded serum, leaving a granulating surface.

Slow reacting substance of anaphylaxis A chemical substance (leukotriene) produced by mast cell degranulation in allergic conditions. It causes smooth muscle contraction, e.g., bronchospasm.

Slow virus infection Virus infection manifesting after long latency period, e.g., kuru.

Slow Taking a long time before acting or showing signs of activity.

   S.-acting drugs Those that are absorbed in the small intestine and have a sustained release over a period of time. Many of these drugs are now incorporated into skin patches.

S. viruses Those infective agents that produce infection after a latent period in the body, which may last weeks to months. *(See Prion).*

Sludge Any solid, semisolid or liquid waste arising from municipal, commercial or industrial waste water treatment, gall-bladder sludge.

Slurry A thin watery mixture.

Small for gestational age Abbreviated SGA. Term for a baby who is smaller or lighter in weight than expected for its gestational age. There is some variance in definition, from inclusion of babies below the 10th percentile to only those below the 5th percentile.

Smallpox Variola. Eradicated from the world in 1980. Smallpox vaccination is no longer required for travelers to any part of the world.

Smear A specimen for microscopic examination that has been prepared by spreading a thin film of the material across a glass slide.

Smegma The secretion of sebaceous-glands of the clitoris and prepuce.

Smell One of the five senses. Air-borne particles are deposited and dissolved in the mucous membrane lining the nose, stimulating the endings of the olfactory nerve. The nose is able to distinguish a wide range of odors.

Smellies forceps Obstetric forceps for delivery of after coming head in breech presentation.

Smellies scissors Special scissors with external cutting edges for fetal craniotomy.

Smelling salt A preparation containing ammonium carbonate and stronger ammonia water scented with aromatic substances.

Smelter's chills Zinc poisoning.

Smith–Lemli–Opitz syndrome Small stature, mental retardation, cryptorchidism, and failure to thrive.

Smith-Hodge pessary A retroversion pessary.

S

Smith fracture Fracture of lower end of radius with forward displacement of lower segment.

Smith-Petersen nail *MN Smith-Petersen, American surgeon, 1886–1953.* A metal nail used to fix the fragments of bone in intracapsular fracture of the head of the femur.

Smog Dense fog combined with smoke.

Smokeless tobacco Tobacco used for chewing or as snuff. They irritate oral mucosa and increase the risk of oral cancer.

Smoking The act of drawing into the mouth and puffing out the smoke of tobacco contained in a cigarette, cigar or pipe. A close relationship between smoking and lung cancer, heart disease and bronchitis and emphysema has definitely been established. Smoking is also harmful in pregnancy because the inhaled carbon monoxide reduces oxygen transportation in the body and the nicotine causes vasoconstriction of the arterioles. The result is a diminished supply of food and oxygen to the fetus, leading to fetal growth retardation.

Snake A limbless reptile; a serpent. The bites of many snakes are poisonous to humans.
  Snake venom antitoxin Antivenin. A serum made from animals, usually horses, which have been immunized against the venom of a specific type of snake.

Snap A sharp cracking sound.
  Snap opening A high pitched sound heard during opening of diseased valves, e.g., mitral stenosis.

Snapping jaw An audible and palpable snap on closing and opening of mouth due to displaced meniscus of temperomandibular joint.

Snapping knee An audible snapping sound on sudden extension of knee caused by slipping of biceps femoris tendon or displaced menisci.

Snare An instrument with a wire loop to remove polyps, tonsils and small growths with a pedicle.

Sneeze A sudden spasmodic expiration through nose.

Snellen's test letters *H Snellen, Dutch ophthalmologist, 1834–1908.* Square-shaped letters on a chart, used for sight testing.

Snore The noise produced while breathing through mouth during sleep.

Snout reflex A variant of sucking reflex in which sharp tapping of mid upper lip results in exaggerated contraction of the lips, positive in infants and in diffuse brain disease.

Snuff Powdered form of tobacco inhaled through nose.

Snuff box anatomical Triangular area at the base of thumb. Tenderness in this area indicates scaphoid fracture.

Snow Frozen water vapor.
  Carbon dioxide snow Solid CO_2 which is used as a refrigerant; "dry ice".
  Snow blindness Photophobia due to the glare of snow.

Snuffles A chronic discharge from the nose, occurring in children, as a result of infection of the nasal mucous membrane.

Soap A salt of one or more higher fatty acids with an alkali or metal. Soluble soaps are detergents and are prepared from alkali metals sodium and potassium.
  Soap liniment A solution of soap and camphor in alcohol and water. Used as a stimulant and rubefacient.

Social In health care, the prefix 'social' denotes a role, function or description to do with society, its peoples and its organization.
  S. anxiety disorder Fear of social situations.

S

Snellen's Test Letters

S. class A category arising from the division of society into economic or occupational groupings. The most widely used grouping of social class or occupational scale in the UK was the Registrar General's Classification designed originally for use in the 1911 Census but extensively modified for use in later censuses. Occupations are now coded to be comparable with the International Standard Classification of Occupations.

S. drift The movement of people from one social class to another usually as a result of socioeconomic circumstance or as a result of morbid processes. Sometimes referred to as social mobility.

S. exclusion People from groups, which for a variety of reasons are not able to participate in community and mainstream activities, e.g., refugees and homeless people.

S. norms Socially accepted patterns of behavior within a community or population.

S. worker A professional qualified in the treatment of individual and social problems of patients and their families. *(See also Medical (Social Worker))*

Socialization The process by which society integrates the individual, and the individual learns to behave in socially acceptable ways.

Sociology The scientific study of the development of human social relationships and organization, i.e., interpersonal and intergroup behavior as distinct from the behavior of an individual.

Sociopath A person with an antisocial personality; a psychopath.

Socket A hollow in a joint or bone.

Alveolar socket The bony space occupied by tooth and periodontal ligament.

Soda Salts of sodium.

Baking soda Sodium bicarbonate.

Caustic soda Sodium hydroxide.

Lime soda Mixture of calcium hydroxide and sodium hydroxide used to absorb carbon dioxide.

Soda ash Commercial sodium carbonate.

Soda water A solution of carbon dioxide under pressure.

Sodium Symbol Na. A metallic alkaline element widely distributed in nature, and forming an important constituent of animal tissue.

Sodium aminosalicylate An antituberculous drug used in conjunction with streptomycin and isoniazid.

Sodium bicarbonate An antacid widely used to treat digestive disorders, especially flatulence. Repeated use can cause alkalosis.

Sodium chloride Common salt. Its presence in the diet is necessary to health.

Sodium citrate Compound used to prevent clotting of blood during blood transfusions.

Sodium cromoglycate A drug used as an inhalant in the treatment of asthma.

Sodium fluoride A salt used in the fluoridation of water and also in toothpastes to prevent the formation of caries.

Sodium hydroxide Caustic soda. A powerful corrosive drug used to destroy warts. It can cause severe chemical burns.

Sodium hypochlorite A compound with germicidal properties used in solution to disinfect utensils, and diluted as a topical antibacterial agent.

Sodium phosphate A purgative.

Sodium salicylate An antipyretic drug used in the treatment of rheumatic fever.

Sodium sulphate A purgative; also used in 25% solution as a wound dressing.

Sodium valproate A drug used in the treatment of epilepsy.

Soft palate The posterior portion of roof of mouth.

Soft sore Venereal ulcer caused by Ducrey's bacillus.

Soft tissue mobilization *(See Massage)*.

Software Computer data and programs containing instructions that detail how to use a specific computer facility.

Solar keratoses Rough patches of skin caused by damage from repeated exposure to the sun.

Solar plexus Celiac plexus. A network of sympathetic nerve ganglia in the abdomen; the nerve supply to abdominal organs, below the diaphragm.

Soleus The flat broad muscle at back of calf of leg.

Solitary Single or lonely.

Solubility Capable of being dissolved.

Solute The substance that is dissolved in a solution.

Solution A liquid in which one or more substances have been dissolved.

Solution aqueous Solution containing water as the solvent.

S

Buffer solution Solution of weak acid and its salt solvent for maintaining constant pH.

Hypertonic solution Solution with greater osmotic pressure than that of body fluids.

Hypotonic solution Solution with osmotic pressure less than that of body fluids.

Isotonic solution Solution with similar osmotic pressure as that of body fluids.

Ringer's solution Solution containing chlorides of sodium, calcium and potassium.

Solvent A liquid that dissolves or has power to dissolve.

Solvent abuse (See Abuse).

Soma 1. The body as distinct from the mind. 2. The body tissue as distinct from the germ cells.

Somatesthesia The consciousness of the body.

Somatic 1. Relating to the body as opposed to the mind. 2. Relating to the body wall as distinct from the viscera.

Somatization Expression of emotional conflicts as bodily ailment.

Somatoform disorders A group of disorders in which there are symptoms of a disease but no objective evidence to explain the symptoms.

Somatomedin Insulin like growth factors derived from liver (Somatomedin C and A) that stimulate growth under influence of growth hormone.

Somatostatin A hypothalamic hormone that inhibits release of somatotropin, insulin and gastrin.

Somatotropin Growth hormone.

Somite Paired masses of mesoderm arranged segmentally alongside neural tube of the embryo.

Somnambulism Walking and carrying out other complex activities during a state of sleep.

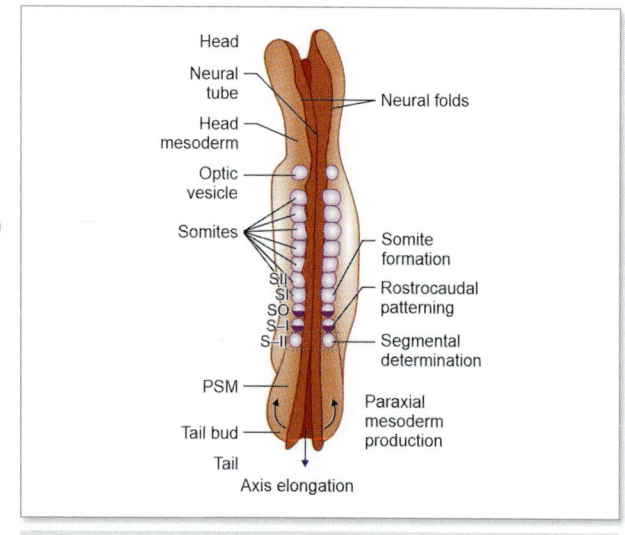

Head
Neural tube
Head mesoderm
Optic vesicle
Somites
Neural folds
Somite formation
Rostrocaudal patterning
Segmental determination
S+IV
S+III
SO
S+I
S+II
PSM
Tail bud
Tail
Paraxial mesoderm production
Axis elongation

Somite

Somniferous Promoting sleep.

Somniloquism Talking during sleep.

Somnolence Sleepiness.

Somogyi effect *M Somogyi, American biochemist, 1883–1971.* A rebound phenomenon occurring in diabetes mellitus; overtreatment with insulin induces hypoglycemia, resulting in rebound hyperglycemia and ketosis.

Sonne dysentery *CO Sonne, Danish bacteriologist, 1882–1948.* Bacillary dysentery which is common in the UK. The symptoms are diarrhea, vomiting and abdominal pain. The causative agent is *Shigella sonnei.*

Sonogram Ultrasonography record.

Sonography *(See Ultrasonography).*

Sonolucent Condition of not reflecting the ultrasound wave back to the source.

Sonorous rale Low pitched rale caused by mucous secretion in bronchus.

Soporific A drug producing sleep, narcotic.

Sorbitol A sweetening agent which is converted into sugar in the body although it is slowly absorbed from the intestine. It is used in some diabetic foods and in intravenous feeding.

Sordes Brown crusts which form on the teeth and lips of unconscious patients, or those suffering from acute or prolonged fevers.

Sore A general term for any ulcer or open skin lesion.

Cold sore Herpes simplex.

Hard sore A syphilitic chancre.

Pressure sore A sore caused by pressure from the bed (decubitus ulcer) or a splint.

Soft sore A chancroid ulcer.

Sore throat Inflammation of the larynx or pharynx, including tonsillitis.

Sotalol Beta-adrenergic blocking agent used as antihypertensive agent, anti-arrhythmic too.

Souffle A blowing sound heard on auscultation.

Uterine souffle A sound due to the blood passing through the uterine arteries of the mother, particularly over the placental site. It is synchronous with the maternal pulse.

Sound An instrument shaped like a probe for exploring cavities, detecting the presence of foreign bodies or dilating a stricture.

Souque's phenomenon A phenomenon seen in incomplete hemiplegia, consisting of involuntary extension and separation of the fingers when the arm is raised.

Southey's tube Fine caliber tubes used to drain fluid from the subcutaneous tissue in the condition of edema or anasarca.

Soybean A legume that contains high-quality protein and litter starch. *S. milk* Historically used as a milk substitute for babies who could not tolerate constituents of breast or cow's milk. Other substitutes are now available and used instead

Space dead In respiratory physiology, the area from nose to bronchioles which do not take part in exchange of oxygen and carbon dioxide.

Space medicine Branch of medicine dealing with pathological and physiological problems encountered by humans in the space.

Spam Unsolicited advertising or 'junk' mail sent to an individual address via e-mail.

Spansule Trade name for a delayed release form of capsule.

Sparfloxacin Quinolone, used for enteric fever.

Spargosis 1. Swelling of skin as in elephantiasis. 2. Distention of lactating breast with milk.

Spasm A sudden involuntary muscle contraction.

Carpopedal spasm Spasm of the hands and feet. A sign of tetany.

Clonic spasm Alternate muscle rigidity and relaxation.

Habit spasm A tic.

Nicttitating spasm Spasmodic twitching of the eyelid.

Tetanic spasm Violent muscle spasms, including opisthotonos.

Tonic spasm A sustained muscle rigidity.

Spasmophilia A tendency towards spasm and convulsion as in rickets.

Spastic 1. Caused by spasm; convulsive. 2. One affected by spasticity; often applied to persons suffering from congenital paralysis due to some cerebral lesion or impairment.

Spastic colon Irritable bowel syndrome.

Spastic paralysis Paralysis associated with lesions of the upper motor neuron, as in cerebral vascular accidents, and characterized by increased muscle tone and rigidity.

Spasticity Marked rigidity of muscles.

Spatial Pertaining to space.

Spatula 1. A flexible, blunt blade used for spreading ointment. 2. A rigid blade-shaped instrument for depressing the tongue in throat examination, etc.

SPC Statistical process control.

Special health authorities Provide services on behalf of the National Health Service in England. They operate nationally rather than serve a specific geographical area. They are independent but can be subjected to ministerial direction. Examples include the NHS Litigation Authority and NHS Blood and Transplant Authority (NHS BT).

Special needs A term generally used to describe the educational or learning needs of a child or adult with a learning disability. The expression may also be used in a wider context to describe the special educational needs of any child, e.g., one who is musically gifted.

Specific 1. Relating to a species. 2. A remedy that has a distinct curative influence on a particular disease, e.g., quinine in malaria. 3. Related to a unit mass of a substance.

Specific gravity The density of fluid compared with that of an equal volume of water.

Specimen A sample or part taken to show the nature of the whole, e.g., for chemical testing or microscopic survey.

Spectacles A frame containing lenses worn in front of the eyes to correct errors of vision or to protect from glare.

Spectinomycin Injectable antibiotic used for gonorrhea.

Spectrometer An instrument for measuring the strength and wavelengths of visible or invisible electromagnetic radiations.

Spectrophotometry Estimation of depth of color by using spectrophotometer.

Spectroscope An instrument used for analyzing the spectra of light and other radiations.

Spectrum The series of components or images obtained when a beam of electromagnetic wave is dispersed and the constituent waves are arranged according to their frequencies or wavelengths.

Specular reflection Reflecting as from a surface. A term used in ultrasound to describe an interface which gives a strong reflection or echo, e.g., the fetal skull or bony prominence

Invisible spectrum Spectral portion below the red (infrared) or above violet (ultraviolet) which is invisible to the eyes lying below 3900 a AU units and above 7700 AU units.

Visible spectrum Colors from red to violet with wavelengths of 3900–7700 AU.

Speculum Instrument for examination of canals, e.g., ear speculum, vaginal speculum.

S

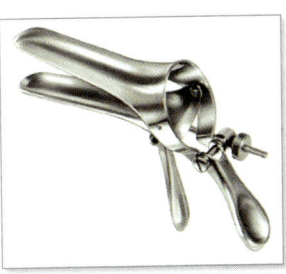

Speculum

Speech The act of communicating through sounds by means of a linguistic code.

Clipped speech Speech in which the words are cut short.

Deaf speech The characteristic utterance of people with severe hearing loss.

Explosive speech Loud, sudden utterances; a sign of mental disorder.

Incoherent speech Disconnected utterances made when the sequence of thought is disturbed, as in delirium.

Esophageal speech Speech produced after laryngectomy by swallowing air and using it to vibrate within the esophagus against the closed cricopharyngeal sphincter.

Scanning speech Speech in which the syllables are inappropriately separated from each other and are evenly stressed. Characteristic of cerebellar damage.

Speech therapist A professional trained to identify, assess and rehabilitate persons with speech or language disorders and feeding difficulties.

Staccato speech Speech in which each syllable is separately pronounced. Characteristic of multiple sclerosis.

Sperm 1. A spermatozoon. 2. The semen.

Sperm count A method of determining the concentration of spermatozoa in a semen sample.

Sperm donation The act of giving seminal fluid provided by donors for the fertilization of women whose partners are sterile.

Spermatic vein The vein draining the testis. The left vein drains into left renal vein while the right vein empties into inferior vena cava.

Spermatid A precursor cell of spermatozoon derived from secondary spermatocyte.

Spermatin A mucilaginous substance present in semen.

Spermatocele A cystic swelling in the epididymis, containing semen.

Spermatocyte The cell arising from spermatogonium that forms the spermatids.

Spermatogenesis The process of formation of mature spermatozoa, i.e., spearmatogonium –primary spermatocyte – secondary spermatocyte spermatid motile functional spermatozoa.

Spermatorrhea Involuntary loss of semen without orgasm.

Spermatozoon A mature male germ cell consisting of a flat-shaped head, a short middle part and a long tail. There are 300–500 billion sperms in a normal ejaculate.

Spermaturia Semen passed with urine.

Spermicide Any agent that will destroy spermatozoa.

Sphenoid Wedge-shaped.

Sphenoid bone The central part of the base of the skull.

Sphenoiditis Inflammation of sphenoidal sinus cells.

Sphenoid spine Downward projection from the posterior extremity of greater wing of sphenoid, giving attachment to sphenomandibular ligament.

Sphenosis Condition in which fetus becomes wedged in the pelvis.

Sphere Globe-like structure.

S

Spherocyte Erythrocyte assuming globular shape.

Spherocytosis The presence of erythrocytes in the blood that are more nearly spherical than biconcave. Characteristic of a choluric jaundice. It may also be hereditary.

Spherule A very small sphere; the structure present in tissues infected with *Coccidiodesimitis*, each spherule containing hundreds of endospores.

Sphincter A ring-shaped muscle, contraction of which closes a natural orifice.

Sphincterectomy 1. The excision of a sphincter. 2. In ophthalmology, an operation to free the sphincter of the iris when it has become attached to the back of the cornea.

Sphingolipid Lipid containing sphingosine bases.

Sphingolipidosis Hereditary disease with defective metabolism of sphingolipids. Included in this group are Tay-Sach's disease, Fabry's disease, Kufs' disease, Krabbe's disease and Niemann-Pick disease.

Sphingomyelins Phosphorus containing sphingolipids principally found in nervous tissue. They are derived from choline phosphate and a ceramide.

Sphygmo Pulse.

Sphygmograph Instrument for recording shape and force of pulse wave.

Sphygmomanometer An instrument for measuring the arterial blood pressure.

Spica A bandage applied to a joint in a series of "figures of eight".

Spicule Small, needle shaped.

Spider black widow Black female spider with four pairs of legs and poison fangs. Its bite causes excruciating abdominal pain and ascending motor palsy.

Spider finger Abnormally long phalanges of hand.

Spider nevus Branched capillary growth in the skin resembling a spider as in cirrhosis of liver.

Spigelian line The line in abdomen, that marks lateral border of rectus.

Spigot A small peg or bung to close the opening of a tube.

Spike Overflow.

Spillway The contour of teeth allowing food to escape from the cusps during mastication.

Spina Spine; a slender, thorn-like projection that occurs on many bones.

Spina bifida A congenital defect of nonunion of one or more vertebral arches, allowing protrusion of the meninges and possibly their contents *(See Meningocele and Meningomyelocele)*.

Spinal Relating to the spine.

Spinal anesthesia (See Anesthesia).

Spinal canal The hollow in the spine formed by the neural arches of the vertebrae. It contains the spinal cord, meninges and cerebrospinal fluid.

Spinal caries Disease of the vertebrae, usually tuberculous *(See Pott's disease)*.

Spinal column The backbone; the vertebral column.

Spinal cord (See Cord).

Spinal curvature Abnormal curving of the spine. If associated with caries, it is known as Pott's disease *(See Kyphosis, Lordosis and Scoliosis)*.

Spinal fluid Cerebrospinal fluid lying in the central canal and around the spinal cord within the subarachnoid space.

Spinal jacket A support for the spine, made of plaster of Paris or other material, used to give rest after injury to or operation on the spine.

Spinal nerves The 31 pairs of nerves which leave the spinal cord at regular intervals throughout its length. They pass out in pairs, one on either side between each of the vertebrae, and are distributed to the periphery.

Spinal puncture Lumbar or cisternal puncture.

Spinal shock Complete arcflexic flaccid palsy following complete transaction of spinal cord.

Spinal stenosis Narrowing of spinal canal due to trauma or degeneration of vertebral column.

Spindle A fusiform shaped body.

Spine 1. The backbone or vertebral column, consisting of 33 vertebrae, separated by fibrocartilaginous disks, and enclosing the spinal cord. 2. A sharp process of bone.

Spinhaler A nebulizing device which delivers a preset dose of the contained drug.

Spinnbarkeit [Ger.] A thread of mucus secreted by the cervix uteri. Used to determine ovulation as this usually coincides with the time at which the mucus can be drawn out on a glass slide to its maximum length.

Spiral Cooling around a center like the thread of screw.

Spiramycin Antibiotic used in toxoplasmosis, respiratory infections.

Spirillium minus A flagellated aerobic bacteria in blood of rats causing rat bite fever.

Spirochaete One of a group of microorganisms in the form of a spiral, some of which are found in impure fresh or salt water. The group includes the species *Treponema, Borrelia* and *Leptospira*

Spirogram A record made by a spirograph depicting respiratory movements.

Spirograph An instrument for registering respiratory movements.

Spirometer An instrument for measuring the air capacity of the lungs.

Spironolactone A diuretic drug used when there is excess secretion of aldosterone. It promotes the excretion of sodium and water but the retention of potassium.

Spissated Thickened.

Split To expectorate.

Spitz-Holter valve *Spitz, American engineer, JW Holter, American engineer.* A device used in the treatment of hydrocephalus to drain the cerebrospinal fluid from the ventricles into the superior venacava or the right atrium.

Splanchnic Pertaining to the viscera.

Splanchnic nerves Sympathetic nerves to the viscera.

Spleen A large, vascular, gland-like but ductless organ, colored reddish purple and situated in the left hypochondrium under the border of the stomach. It manufactures lymphocytes and breaks down red blood corpuscles.

Splenectomy Excision of the spleen.

Splenic flexure Junction of transverse colon with descending colon.

Splenitis Inflammation of the spleen, acute or chronic, hypertrophic or suppurative.

Splenium of corpus callosum The thickened posterior end of corpus callosum.

Splenius A flat muscle in upper back on either side.

Splenomegaly Enlargement of the spleen.

Splenoportogram Radiographic picture of spleen and portal vein after injection of radiopaque material into spleen.

Splenorenal Relating to the spleen and the kidney.

Splenorenal anastomosis An operation carried out to treat portal hypertension. The spleen is excised and the splenic vein is inserted into the renal vein.

Splenorenal shunt Anastomosis of splenic vein to renal vein as in portal hypertension.

Splenorrhagia Bleeding from ruptured spleen.

Splenorrhaphy Suturing of any splenic wound.

S

Splint An appliance used to support or immobilize a part while healing takes place or to correct or prevent deformity.

Thomas splint A long wire splint with a proximal ring that fits into upper thigh, used for fracture femur.

Splinter hemorrhage Small linear bleeding under the nail as in subacute bacterial endocarditis.

Splinting Fixation of injured part with a splint.

Split Division or fissure.

Split tongue Bifid tongue.

SPO$_2$ Saturation of arterial blood with oxygen.

Spondylos Vertebra.

Spondylitis Inflammation of the vertebrae.

Ankylosing spondylitis A rheumatic disease, chiefly of young males, in which there is abnormal ossification with pain and rigidity of the intervertebral, hip and sacroiliac joints.

Spondylolisthesis A sliding forward or displacement of one vertebra over another, usually the fifth lumbar over the sacrum, causing symptoms such as low back pain, as a result of pressure on the nerve roots.

Spondylosis Ankylosis of the vertebral joints, usually caused by a degenerative disease of the intervertebral disks, such as osteoarthritis.

Spondylotherapy Spinal manipulation in treatment of disease.

Sponge An absorbent pad made up of cotton and gauze to absorb fluids and blood, used in wound dressing.

Gelatin sponge Spongy substance of gelatin used to stop internal bleeding.

Spongiform Having appearance or quality of a sponge.

Spongioblast The precursor cell of astrocytes and ependymal cells that develop from neural tube.

Spongioblastoma A rapidly growing brain tumor that is highly malignant. A glioma.

Spontaneous Occurring without apparent cause. Applied to certain types of fracture and to recovery from a disease without any specific treatment.

Spontaneous fracture Fracture of an osteoporotic bone.

Spoon nail Concave nail in iron deficiency anemia.

Sporadic Pertaining to isolated cases of a disease that occurs in various and scattered places (compare Endemic and Epidemic).

Spore 1. A reproductive stage of some of the lowest forms of vegetable life, e.g., molds. 2. A protective state which some bacteria are able to assume in adverse conditions, such as lack of moisture, food or heat. In this form the organism can remain alive, but inert, for years.

Sporocyst A reproductive cell containing spores.

Sporogony Reproduction by development of spores.

Sporothrix A genus of fungi.

Sporotrichosis A chronic granulomatous fungal infection involving skin and lymph nodes with abscess formation, nodularity and ulceration.

Sporozoa A subdivision of protozoa that includes plasmodia, toxoplasma and is ospora.

Sporozoite Infective form of malarial parasite injected by mosquito bite.

Sports medicine Application of medical knowledge for treatment and prevention of sports injuries and improvement of training methods.

Sporulation Production of spores.

Spot A small area distinguishable from surrounding area.

Blind spot The optic disk containing opaque optic nerve fibers.

Cherry-red spot Red spot in retina in Tay-Sach's disease.

Koplik spot Bluish white spots on oral mucous membrane before appearance of rash of measles.

S

Mongolian spot Blue or mulberry colored spots in sacral region present at birth that disappear later.

Spotted fever A febrile disease characterized by a skin eruption, such as Rocky Mountain spotted fever, and other infections due to tick-borne rickettsiae.

Spotting Appearance of blood tinged discharge from vagina in between periods or at onset of labor.

Sprain Wrenching of a joint, producing laceration of the capsule or stretching of the ligaments, with consequent swelling, which is due to effusion of fluid into the affected part.

Sprain fracture Separation of a tendon or ligament from its bony insertion site taking along with it a piece of bone.

Spray A jet of fine medicated vapor.

Spreadsheet A computer program that aligns data in tables, rows and columns.

Spring ligament Calcaneoscaphoid ligament in the sole of foot.

Sprue A disease of malabsorption in the intestine, which maybe tropical or nontropical in form. There is steatorrhea, diarrhea, glossitis and anemia.

Spur A sharp bony outgrowth.

Calcaneal spur An exostosis from calcaneous.

Spurious False, adulterated.

Spurling's maneuver Manuever used to assess the nerve root pain by putting axial load on head with neck extension and lateral rotation toward each shoulder.

Sputum Material expelled from the air passages through the mouth. It consists chiefly of mucus and saliva; in diseased conditions of the air passages it maybe purulent, blood stained and frothy and may contain many bacteria. It must always be regarded as highly infectious.

Rusty sputum That in which altered blood permeates the mucus. Characteristic of acute lobar pneumonia.

Numular sputum Round coir shaped flat forms of sputum sinking in water as seen in bronchiectasis.

Squalene An unsaturated carbohydrate present in vegetable oils, precursor of cholesterol.

Squamous Scaly.

Squamous bone The thin part of the temporal bone which articulates with the parietal and frontal bones.

Squamous cell carcinoma A malignancy of the squamous cells of the bronchus.

Squamous epithelium Epithelium composed of flat and scale-like cells.

Square knot Double knot in which ends and standing parts are together and parallel to each other.

Squatting Sitting on one's haunches and heels.

Squint *(See Strabismus)*.

Staccato speech Jerky pronunciation with separation of each syllable and word by pauses.

Stachyose A nonabsorbable carbohydrate present in beans; hence causing flatulence.

Staging 1. The determination of distinct phases or periods in the course of a disease. 2. The classification of neoplasms according to the extent of the tumor.

TNM staging Staging of tumors according to three basic components: primary tumor (T), regional nodes (N) and metastasis (M). Subscripts are used to denote size and degree of involvement; for example, 0 indicates undetectable, and 1, 2, 3 and 4 a progressive increase in size or involvement.

Stain A dye used to color objects for microscopic examination

Acid-fast stain Staining for mycobacteria which retain carbolfuschin even when washed with acid-alcohol.

Dental stain Staining of enamel or denture due to tea, coffee or tobacco or inhalation of metals like copper (green) manganese (black), iron (brown).

Stalk An elongated structure that attaches or supports an organ.

Infundibular stalk Stalk connecting diencephalon with pituitary.

Stamina Strength, endurance.

Stammering Stuttering; a speech disorder in which the utterance is broken by hesitation and repetition or prolongation of words and syllables.

Standard deviation A measure of the dispersion of a random variable: the square root of the average squared deviation from the mean. For data that have a normal distribution, about 68% of the data points fall within one standard deviation from the mean and about 95% fall within two standard deviations.

Standard error A measure of variability; the difference between means of two samples.

Standard precautions The current model of best practice in infection control, a synthesis of Universal Precautions and Body Substance Isolation (published 1999). Standard precautions are designed to reduce the risk of transmission of blood-borne and other pathogens in hospital, from both recognized and unrecognized sources of infection, and apply to all patients at all the time. Their implementation requires that nurses and other health care professionals take appropriate measures, e.g., wear gloves, to avoid contact with (a) Blood; (b) All body fluids, secretions and excretions except sweat, regardless of whether or not they contain visible blood; (c) Nonintact skin; (4) Mucous membranes. Standard precautions are used in association with new concepts of transmission-based precautions *(See also Infection control and Appendices)*.

Standards Statements of the levels of service of care related to specific topics which staff agree to provide. Often accompanied by a description of the structure (staff, equipment, etc.) and process needed to attain specified observable outcomes.

Standards of care A measure by which a professional's conduct is compared, comprises a list of those acts that a prudent professional practitioner would have carried out (or not performed) in similar circumstances within health care.

Standstill Cessation of activity.

Stannous fluoride A fluoride compound in toothpaste that prevents dental caries.

Stanolone Anabolic steroid.

Stanozolol Anabolic steroid, used for muscle building.

Stapedectomy Removal of the stapes and insertion of a vein graft or other device to reestablish conduction of sound waves in otosclerosis.

Stapediolysis An operation in which the foot piece of the stapes is mobilized to aid conduction in deafness from otosclerosis.

Stapedius A small muscle in the middle ear attached to stapes.

Stapes The stirrup-shaped bone of the middle ear.

Staphyle Uvula, the fleshy mass hanging from soft palate.

Staphylococcus A genus of Gram-positive nonmobile bacteria which, under the microscope, appear grouped together in small masses like bunches of grapes. They are normally present on the skin and mucous membranes. *Staphylococus pyogenes (or Staphylococcus aureus)* is a common cause of boils, carbuncle and abscesses.

Staphyloderma Cutaneous infection with staphylococci.

Staphyloma A protrusion of the cornea or the sclerotic coat of the eyeball as the result of inflammation or a wound.

Staphylopharyngeus Muscle of soft palate whose contraction narrows the fauces and occludes the nasopharynx.

Staphylotoxin Toxins produced by staphylococci, e.g., the enterotoxin, hemotoxin, dermonecrotic toxin, etc.

Staple food Any principal food item of a community supplying more than 25% of calorie and eaten regularly.

Stapling Fastening of incised wounds by metal staples.

Starch A plant polysaccharide of high molecular weight which on absorption is reduced to simple sugars to provide energy. Starch is converted to sugar when some fruits ripen while peas and corn change sugar into starch as their seeds develop.

Stare Fixed gaze at any object.

Starling's law Starling law of heart depicts that the force of contraction of heart muscle is directly related to length of muscle fiber at beginning of contraction.

Startle reflex *(See Moro Reflex).*

Starvation Food deprivation.

Stasis The stagnation or stoppage of flow of a fluid.

Intestinal stasis Sluggish movement of feces through the bowel, owing to partial obstruction or to impairment of the action of the intestinal muscles.

Venous stasis Congestion of blood in the veins.

State A condition.

Statementing The provision by a local authority of a statement following formal assessment of the special educational needs of a child with mental or physical stream school with extra help, or a special school.

Static electricity Electricity produced by friction.

Stationary Fixed.

Statistical process control Abbreviated SPC. The use of statistical concepts which place the emphasis on the continuous monitoring of a process rather than the reliance on a single outcome as the sole measure for quality assurance in the delivery of a service.

Statistical significance In research, a conclusion that the results achieved have little probability of occurring by chance alone. If the result is statistically significant, e.g., below 1 in 20 or the 0. 05 level, then something other than chance produced the result.

Statistics 1. Numerical facts pertaining to a particular subject or body of objects. 2. The science dealing with the collection, tabulation and analysis of numerical facts.

Statoconia Minute beats of calcium adhering to the hair cells of macule and utricle responsible for maintenance of posture. *SYN* – statolith.

Stature Height of body in standing position.

Status Condition.

Status asthmaticus A severe and prolonged attack of asthma.

Status epilepticus A condition in which there is rapid succession of epileptic fits.

Status lymphaticus A condition in which all lymphatic tissues are hypertrophied, especially the thymus gland.

Statutory bodies Those bodies which have the statutory control of the practice of nurses, midwives and health visitors. E.g., Indian Nursing Council.

STD Sexually Transmitted Disease.

Steapsin The fat-splitting enzyme (lipase) of the pancreatic juice.

Stearate Salt of stearic acid.

Stearic acid A fatty acid mainly found in animal fats.

Stearin Ester of stearic acid and glycerine.

Steatoma 1. A sebaceous cyst. 2. Alipoma; a fatty tumor.

Steatorrhea The presence of an excess of fat in the stools owing to malabsorption of fat by the intestines.

Stein-Leventhal syndrome *IF Stein, American gynecologist, 1887–1976; ML Leventhal, American gynecologist, 1901–1971.* Condition affecting females in which obesity, hirsutism and sterility are associated with polycystic ovaries and menstrual irregularities.

Steinmann's extension *F Steinmann, Swiss surgeon, 1872–1932.* Traction applied to a limb by applying weight to a pin placed through the bone at right angles to the direction of pull of the traction force.

Steinmann pin A fine metal rod, passed through a bone, by which extension is applied to overcome muscle contraction in certain fracture *(See Kirschner wire).*

Stellate Star-shaped.

Stellate fracture A radiating fracture of the patella.

Stellate ganglion The inferior cervical ganglion. A star-shaped collection of nerve cells at the base of the neck.

Stellwag's sign Widening of palpebral fissure with infrequent blinking, a feature of Grave's disease.

Stem Stalk like structure.

Stem cell The cell which is initial precursor of specific differentiated red blood cells.

Stem cell transplant Replacement of damaged blood cells caused by conditions such as leukemia and lymphoma. An allogeneic transplant involves transplanting cells from a healthy compatible donor. An autologous stem cell transplant involves taking and later replacing cells from the host after any damaged or diseased cells have been removed.

Stenosis Abnormal narrowing or contraction of a channel or opening.

Aortic stenosis Narrowing of the opening of the aortic valve due to scar tissue formation as the result of inflammation.

Mitral stenosis Narrowing of the orifice of the mitral valve, usually following rheumatic fever.

Pulmonary stenosis A congenital narrowing of the opening from the right ventricle of the heart into the pulmonary artery.

Pyloric stenosis Narrowing of the pyloric orifice of the stomach due to scar tissue, new growth or congenital hypertrophy.

Stensen's duct *H Stensen, Danish physician, 1638–1686.* The duct of the parotid gland, opening into the mouth opposite the second upper molar.

Stent A device or splint of rubber, stainless steel or plastic mesh or a coil of wire placed inside a canal, duct or artery to keep the passage way open.

Stercobilin A brown-orange pigment derived from bile and present in feces.

Sterocolith A fecal concretion.

Stercus Feces.

Stereognosis The ability to visualize the shape of an object by touch alone.

Stereoisomerism Compounds having same number of atoms but in differing arrangement, e.g., dextrose and levulose.

Stereophotography Photography that gives depth, i.e., three-dimensional picture.

Stereoscope Instrument that gives three dimensional view of objects seen by combining images of two pictures.

Stereotaxis A method of precisely locating areas of brain concerned with a particular function by moving a probe or electrode along coordinates for measured distances from certain external landmarks.

S

Stereotype An oversimplified generalization about a group or class of people, which is often then applied to an individual. May form a basis for discrimination and prejudice.

Stereotypy Repetitive actions carried out or maintained for long periods in a monotonous fashion.

Sterets A proprietary brand of swabs impregnated with 70% isopropyl alcohol. These swabs are rubbed onto a skin site before an injection.

Steri-strips A proprietary brand of skin closure strips which are placed across a wound with a space between the edges to allow for drainage. A final strip is placed on either side parallel to the wound.

Sterile 1. Aseptic; free from microorganisms.
2. Barren; incapable of producing young.

Sterility 1. The state of being free from microorganisms.
2. The inability of a woman to become pregnant, or of a man to produce potent spermatozoa.

Sterilization 1. Rendering dressings, instruments. etc. aseptic by destroying or removing all microbial life.
2. Rendering incapable of reproduction by any means.

Sterilizer An apparatus in which object scan be sterilized *(See Autoclave)*.

Sternal puncture Removal of bone marrow for examination by pressing wide bore needle into sternum.

Sternoclavicular Relating to sternum and clavicle.

Sternocleidomastoid Muscle arising from sternum and clavicle, attached to the mastoid, helps in rotation of the head.

Sternohyoid Muscle attached to medial end of clavicle and sternum and the hyoid bone.

Sternotomy The operation in which the sternum is cut through to enable the heart to be reached.

Sternum The breast bone; the flat narrow bone in the center of the anterior wall of the thorax.

Steroid One of a group of hormones chemically related to cholesterol. They include estrogen and androgen, progesterone and the corticosteroids. They maybe naturally occurring or maybe synthesized.

Steroidogenesis Production of steroid hormones.

Sterol One of a group of steroid alcohols which includes cholesterol and ergosterol.

Stertorous Snore-like; applied to a snoring sound produced in breathing during sleep or in coma.

Stertorous respiration Respiration characterized by a heavy snoring or gasping sound.

Stethoscope The instrument used for listening to internal body sounds, especially from the heart and lung. It consists of a hollow tube, one end of which is placed over the part to be examined and the other at the ear of the examiner.

Stevens-Johnson syndrome *AM Stevens, American pediatrician, 1884–1945; FC Johnson, American pediatrician. 1894–1934.* A severe form of erythema multiforme in which the lesions may involve the oral and anogenital mucosa, eyes and viscera, associated with such constitutional symptoms as malaise, headache, fever, arthralgia and conjunctivitis.

STI Sexually Transmitted Infection.

Stibium Antimony.

Stibophen Trivalent antimony compound used in treatment of schistosomiasis.

Stiff-man syndrome A disease of unknown etiology manifesting with muscle stiffness that limits voluntary movements.

S

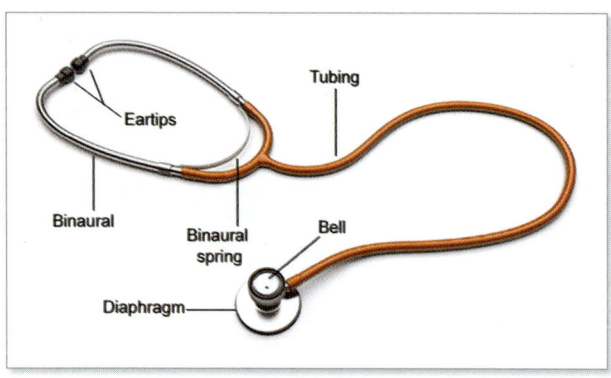

Stethoscope

Stigma 1. A small spot or mark on the skin. 2. Any mark characteristic of a condition or defect, or of a disease. It refers to visible signs rather than symptoms.

Stilboestrol A synthetic estrogen preparation used in the treatment of cancer of the prostate and less commonly for postmenopausal breast cancer.

Stillbirth A baby which has issued forth from its mother after the 24th week of pregnancy and has not, at any time after being completely expelled from its mother, breathed or shown any sign of life.

Stillbirth certificate A certificate issued to the parents by a registered medical practitioner who was present at the birth or examined the body.

Still's disease *Sir GP Still, British pediatrician, 1868–1941.* A form of rheumatoid arthritis in children, sometimes associated with enlargement of the lymph glands.

Stimulant An agent that causes increased energy or functional activity of any organ.

Stimulus Pl. Stimuli (L.). Any agent, act or influence that produces functional or trophic reaction in a receptor or an irritable tissue.

Conditioned stimulus A neutral object or event that is psychologically related to a naturally stimulating object or event and which causes a conditioned response *(See also Conditioning)*.

Discriminative stimulus A stimulus, associated with reinforcement, which exerts control over a particular form of behavior; the subject discriminates between closely related stimuli and responds positively only in the presence of that stimulus.

Eliciting stimulus Any stimulus, conditioned or unconditioned, that elicits a response.

Structured stimulus A well organized and unambiguous stimulus, the perception of which is influenced to a greater extent by the characteristics of the stimulus by those of the perceiver.

Threshold stimulus A stimulus that is just strong enough to elicit a response.

Unconditioned stimulus Any stimulus that is capable of eliciting an unconditioned response *(See also Conditioning)*.

Unstructured stimulus An unclear or ambiguous stimulus, the perception of which is influenced to a greater extent by the characteristics of the perceiver than by those of the stimulus.

Sting Punctured wound made by an insect.

S-T interval Time between completion of QRS complex and beginning of T-wave and represents the initial slow phase of ventricular repolarization.

Stippling Spotted appearance.

Stitch 1. A popular term used to describe a sudden sharp pain usually due to spasm of the diaphragm. 2. A suture.

Stitch abscess Pus from a formation where a stitch has been inserted.

Stockinet Tubular woven elastic material to place uniform pressure around a body part.

Stock The original individual or tribe from which others have descended.

Stoke A unit of viscosity.

Stokes-Adams syndrome *Sir W Stokes, Irish surgeon, 1804–1878; R Adams, Irish physician, 1791–1875.* Attacks of syncope or fainting due to cerebral anemia in some cases of complete heart block. The heart stops temporarily but breathing continues. The syndrome is treated by using an artificial pacemaker.

Stokes' law Paralysis of muscle lying adjacent to inflamed serous or mucous membrane.

Stoma 1. A mouth or mouth-like opening. 2. An artificial opening in the skin surface leading into one of the tubes forming the alimentary canal *(See Colostomy and Ileostomy).*

Stomach The dilated portion of the alimentary canal between the esophagus and the duodenum, just below the diaphragm.

Bilocular or hourglass stomach One divided into two parts by a constriction.

Stomach pH electrode Apparatus used to measure gastric contents in situ.

Stomach pump A pump that removes the contents of the stomach by suction.

Stomach tube A flexible tube used for washing out the stomach or for the administration of liquid food.

Stomachic Medicine that stimulates actions of stomach.

Stomatitis Inflammation of the mouth, either simple or with ulceration, caused by a vitamin deficiency or by a bacterial or fungal infection.

Angular stomatitis Cracking at the corners of the mouth, usually due to riboflavin deficiency.

Aphthous stomatitis That characterized by small, white, painful ulcers on the mucous membrane.

Ulcerative stomatitis Painful shallow ulcers on the tongue, cheeks and lips. A severe type that may produce serious constitutional effects.

Stone A calculus.

Stool A motion discharge from the bowels.

STP Sustainable transformation partnerships. Partnerships between local authorities and all local health providers aimed at improving health and social care in England by ensuring there are inclusive plans to meet the needs of the local population and that there is optimum efficiency across health systems

Fatty stool That which contains undigested fat.

Hunger stool Stool passed by underfed infants: frequent, small and green.

Rice water stool The water stool, containing small white flakes, seen in cholera.

Tarry tool A black tarry stool due to the presence of blood from a peptic ulcer.

S

Strabismus Squint; heterotropia. A deviation of the eye from its normal direction. It is called convergent when the eye turns in toward the nose, and divergent when it turns outward.

Concomitant strabismus A squint in which the angle of deviation stays constant.

Strabometer Instrument for measuring degree of strabismus.

Strabotomy The division of ocular muscles in the treatment of strabismus.

Strachan syndrome Neuropathy and orogenital lesions in avitaminosis.

Strain 1. Overuse or stretching of a part, e.g., a muscle or tendon. 2. A group of microorganisms within a species. 3. To pass a liquid through a filter.

Strait A narrow passage.

Strangle To choke or suffocate.

Strangury Painful and interrupted urination.

Strangulated Compressed or constricted so that the circulation of the blood is arrested.

Strangulated hernia (See Hernia).

Strangulation 1. Choking caused by compression of the air passages. 2. Arrested circulation to a part, which will result in gangrene.

Strangury A painful, frequent desire to micturate, but in which only a few drops of urine are passed with difficulty.

Strap A band to hold parts together.

Stratified Arranged in layers.

Stratified tissue A covering tissue in which the cells are arranged in layers. The germinating cells are the lowest, and as surface cells are shed there is continual replacement.

Stratum A layer applied to structures such as the skin and mucous membranes.

Stratum corneum The outer, horny layer of the epidermis.

Strawberry tongue Red papillated tongue.

Streak A line or stripe.

Streptobacillus Bacilli found in chains.

Streptococcus A genus of Gram-positive spherical bacteria occurring in chains or pairs. Divided into various groups. The first group includes the beta hemolytic human and animal pathogens; the second and third include alpha-hemolytic parasitic forms occurring as normal flora in the body; and the fourth is made up of saprophytic forms.

Streptococcus mutans Implicated in dental caries.

Streptococcus pneumoniae Pneumococcus, the most common cause of lobar pneumonia; also causes serious forms of meningitis, septicemia, empyema and peritonitis.

Streptococcus pyogenes Betahemolytic, toxigenic, pyogenic streptococci causing septic sore throat, scarlet fever, rheumatic fever, puerperal fever and acute glomerulonephritis.

Streptodornase Enzyme secreted by hemolytic streptococci which along with streptokinase is used for enzymatic debridement of infected tissue.

Streptokinase An enzyme derived from a streptococcal culture and used to liquefy clotted blood and pus.

Streptolysin Hemolysin (O and S) produced by *Streptococcus pyogenes.*

Streptomyces A genus of soil bacteria from which a large number of antibiotics are derived.

Streptomycin An antibiotic drug derived from *Streptomyces griseus;* used particularly in the treatment of tuberculosis, when treatment is combined with other drugs to reduce drug resistance.

Stress Any factor, mental or physical, the pressure of which can adversely affect the functioning of the body.

Stress disorders Those resulting from an individual's inability to withstand stress.

Stress fracture Hairline fracture often only visible 3–4 weeks after undue muscle stress as in runners.

Stress incontinence Incontinence, usually of urine, when the intraabdominal pressure is raised, such as in coughing, sneezing or laughing.

Stress test Method of evaluating cardiovascular fitness by exercise on treadmill or bicycle ergometer or after drugs (dipyridamole, dobutamine).

Stress ulcer Peptic ulcer caused by excessive stress as in burn, head trauma.

Stretch To lengthen.

Stretcher A litter or carriage for patients.

Stretch receptor Proprioceptors in muscle or tendon that are stimulated by stretch or pull.

Stretch reflex Contraction of a muscle as a result of pull exerted on its tendon.

Stria Pl. striae. A line or stripe.

Striae gravidarum The lines that appear on the abdomen of pregnant women. They are red in first pregnancy, but white subsequently, and are due to stretching and rupture of the elastic fibers.

Striatal epilepsy A form of epilepsy characterized by tonic seizure of arm and leg due to disease of corpus striatum.

Striated Striped.

Striated muscle Voluntary muscle *(See Muscle).*

Striatum The caudate and lentiform nuclei of brain taken together.

Stricture A narrowing or local contraction of a canal. It maybe caused by muscle spasm, new growth, or scar tissue formation after inflammation.

Stridor A harsh, vibrating, shrill sound, produced during respiration when there is partial obstruction of the larynx or trachea.

Strionigral Tract arising from put a men and caudate nucleus and ending in substantia nigra.

Stroboscope A device by which moving object may appear to be at rest; a rapid motion may appear to be slowed.

Stroke A popular term to describe the sudden onset of symptoms, especially those of cerebral origin affecting movement, sensation, speech and vision. There maybe paralysis and loss of sensation down one side of the body or one side of the face.

Apoplectic stroke Cerebral hemorrhage.

Heat stroke A hyperpyrexia accompanied by cerebral symptoms. It may occur in someone newly arrived in a very hot climate.

Stroke volume Amount of blood ejected from ventricle during systole.

Stroma The connective tissue forming the ground substance, framework or matrix of an organ, as opposed to the functioning part or parenchyma.

Stromatosis Presence of mesenchyma like tissue throughout the endometrium of uterus.

Strongyloides A genus of nematode worms, one of which,

Strongyloides stercoralis, is common in tropical countries and causes diarrhea and intestinal ulcers.

Strontium Symbol Sr. A metallic element. Isotopes of strontium are used in bone scanning to detect abnormalities.

Strontium-90 A radioactive isotope used in radiotherapy in the treatment of skin and eye malignancies.

Struma Enlarged thyroid gland.

Struma ovarii Form of ovarian teratoma composed of thyroid follicles filled with colloid.

Strumpell's sign Dorsiflexion of foot when thigh is flexed on abdomen.

Struvite Crystals of magnesium ammonium phosphate.

Strychnine A highly poisonous alkaloid made from the seeds of *Strychnosnux vomica.* Formerly used in small amounts in "tonics".

Stryker frame An apparatus specially designed for care of patients with injuries of the spinal cord or paralysis. It is constructed of pipe and canvas and is designed so that one nurse can turn the patient without difficulty.

Stupe Counter irritant for topical use.

Stupor A state of semi unconsciousness, occurring in the course of many varieties of mental illness, in which the patient does not move or speak, and makes no response to stimuli.

Sturge-Weber syndrome *WA Sturge, British physician, 1850–1919; Sir RD Weber; British physician, 1824–1918.* A congenital abnormality in which there is a port wine stain on the face with an angioma of the meninges on the same side. Common symptoms are epilepsy, hemiplegia and associated learning difficulties.

Stuttering *(See Stammering).*

Stye *(See Hordeolum).*

Stylet A wire or rod for keeping clear the lumen of catheters, cannulae and hollow needles.

Styloglossus Muscle connecting tongue and styloid process that helps to retract and raise the tongue.

Styloid Like a pen.

    Styloid process A long pointed spine, particularly one projecting from the temporal bone. Also processes on the ulna and radius.

Stylopharyngeus Muscle that elevates and opens up the pharynx.

Stylus A probe or slender wire for stiffening or clearing a canal or catheter.

Styptic An astringent which, applied locally, arrests hemorrhage, e.g., alum and tannic acid.

Sub Under, beneath, less in quantity.

Subacute Moderately acute. Applied to a disease that progresses moderately rapidly, but does not become acute.

Subacute myelo-optic neuropathy Neurological disease characterized by sensory motor disturbances, impaired vision, abdominal pain and ataxia occurring as a toxicity of chinoquinol (iodochlorhydroxyquin).

Subacute sclerosing panencephalitis A cerebral degenerative disease with decreasing mental function, and myoclonic jerks and rigidity. Probably related to chronic measle virus infection of CNS.

Subarachnoid Below the arachnoid.

    Subarachnoid hemorrhage Bleeding into the subarachnoid space (the area between the arachnoid membrane and pia mater surround the brain).

    Subarachnoid space Between the arachnoid and pia mater of the brain and spinal cord, and containing cerebrospinal fluid.

Subclavian Beneath the clavicle.

    Subclavian artery The main vessel of supply to the neck and arms.

    Subclavian steal syndrome Shunting of blood away from cerebral circulation via vertebral artery to subclavian when subclavian is occluded at is origin. Exercise of involved arm then produces dizziness due to cerebral anoxia.

    Subclavian triangle Triangle shaped part of neck formed by clavicle and the omohyoid and sternomastoid muscles.

Subclavius A tiny muscle from first rib to under surface of clavicle.

Subclinical Without clinical manifestations; said of the early stages or a very mild form of a disease.

Subconscious 1. Not conscious yet able to be recalled to consciousness. 2. In psychoanalysis, the part of the mind that retains memories which cannot without much effort be recalled to mind.

S

Subcutaneous Beneath the skin.
Subcutaneous injection One given hypodermically.
Subdural Below the dura mater.
Subdural hematoma A blood clot between the arachnoid and dura mater. It maybe acute or arise slowly from a minor injury.
Subdural space Space between dura and arachnoid.
Suberosis Hypersensitive pneumonitis in workers exposed to cork.
Subfamily In taxonomy between family and a tribe.
Subinvolution Incomplete or delayed return of the uterus to its pregravid size during the puerperium, usually as the result of retained products of conception and infection.
Subjective Related to the individual.
Subjective symptoms Those of which the patient is aware by sensory stimulation, but which cannot easily be seen by other *(See also Objective)*.
Sublimate A substance obtained by sublimation.
Sublimation 1. The vaporization of a solid and its condensation into a solid deposit. 2. In psychoanalysis, a redirecting of energy at an unconscious level. The transference into socially acceptable channels of tendencies that cannot be expressed. An important aspect of maturity.
Subliminal Below the threshold of perception.
Sublingual Beneath the tongue.
Sublingual glands Two small salivary glands in the floor of the mouth.
Subluxation Partial dislocation of ajoint.
Submaxillary Beneath the lower jaw.
Submaxillary glands Two salivary glands situated under the lower jaw.
Submerge To dip in water.
Submucous Beneath mucous membrane.
Submucous resection An operation to correct a deflected nasal septum.

Subnormal Below normal.
Subphrenic Beneath the diaphragm.
Subphrenic abscess One that develops below the diaphragm, usually after peritonitis or from postoperative infection.
Subscription That part of prescription containing directions for compounding ingredients.
Subsidence Gradual disappearance of symptoms of disease.
Subsistence Minimum or barely needed essentials for life.
Substance P A 11 amino acid peptide acting as neurotransmitter in pain fiber system.
Substitution The act of putting one thing in place of another. In psychology, this maybe the nurse or foster mother in the place of the child's own mother. In psychotherapy, the nurse or therapist maybe substituted for someone in the patient's background.
Subthalamic nucleus An elliptical mass of gray matter lying in ventral thalamus above the cerebral peduncle and rostral to substantia nigra.
Subtle Very fine or delicate; causing injury without attracting attention.
Substrate A substance on which an enzyme acts.
Subtraction A method of removing overlying shadows in radiography.
Succedaneum Something which can be used as a substitute.
Succenturiate Acting as a substitute.
Succinyl choline A neuromuscular blocking agent used as muscle relaxant during anesthesia.
Succus A juice.
Succus entericus A digestive fluid secreted by intestinal glands.
Succus gastricus Gastric juice.
Succussion A method of determining when free fluid is present in a cavity in the body. A sound of splashing is heard when the patient moves or is deliberately moved.
Suck To draw fluid into mouth.

Suckle Breastfeed.

Sucralfate Drug used in peptic ulcer.

Sucrase Enzyme present in intestinal juice which splits cane sugar into glucose and fructose.

Sucrose A disaccharide obtained from cane or beet sugar.

Suction 1. The process of sucking. 2. The removal of gas or fluid from a cavity or other container by means of reduced pressure.

Post-tussive suction A sucking noise heard in the lungs just after a cough.

Sudamen A small white vesicle formed in the sweat glands after prolonged sweating.

Sudan Biological stain for fat.

Sudanophilic Staining easily with sudan stain.

Sudeck's atrophy Acute atrophy of bone at the site of injury.

Sudden infant death syndrome Abbreviated SIDS. The sudden and unexpected death of an apparently healthy infant, typically occurring between the ages of 3 weeks and 5 months, and not explained by careful postmortem studies. Called crib or cot death because the infant often is found dead in the cot. The prone position, tobacco smoke and over heating have been found to increase the risk of cot death, so these should be avoided.

Sudor Sweat; perspiration.

Sudorific Diaphoretic; an agent causing sweating. Suffocation asphyxiation; a cessation of breathing caused by occlusion of the air passages, leading to unconsciousness and ultimately to death.

Sufentanil An opioid analgesic.

Suffocation Feeling choked.

Suffusion A process of diffusion or over spreading, as in flushing of the skin; blushing.

Sugar A group of sweet carbohydrates classified chemically as monosaccharides or disaccharides. The following are included: *beet sugar* obtained from sugar beet; *cane sugar* obtained from sugarcane; *fructose* fruit sugar; *grape sugar* dextrose, *glucose; milk sugar* lactose.

Muscle sugar Inclination to act on suggestions of others.

Suggestibility Inclination to act on suggestions of others.

Suggestion A tool of psychotherapy in which an idea is presented to and accepted by a patient.

Posthypnotic suggestion One implanted in a patient under hypnosis, which lasts after return to a normal condition.

Suicide The intentional taking of one's own life. Legally, a death suspected of being due to violence that is self inflicted is not termed a suicide unless the victim leaves positive evidence of the intention to commit suicide, or the method of death is such that a verdict of suicide is inevitable. Some religious faiths consider it to be a sin and may refuse a consecrated burial.

Suit An outer garment.

Sulbactam Beta lactamase inhibitor.

Sulbatiamine Rejuvenating agent.

Sulcus A furrow or fissure; applied especially to those of the brain.

Sulfacetamide An antibacterial sulphonamide used as eye drops to treat corneal and conjunctival infections.

Sulfadiazine A slow-acting sulphonamide drug which is relatively nontoxic. Used in the treatment of meningococcal meningitis.

Sulfadimidine A sulphonamide of which a high blood level can be obtained with reduced incidence of side effects. Used in the treatment of urinary tract infections.

Sulfadoxine Sulfa used in malaria.

Sulfamerazine A derivative of sulfadiazine.

Sulfamethizole A sulphonamide used in urinary infection as it is rapidly excreted in an active form.

Sulfamethoxazole Sulfa usually combined with trimethoprim for broad spectrum action and complimentary bactericidal effect.

Sulfanilamide A formerly used coaltar product for infections.

Sulfapyridine Sulfonamide used in the treatment of dermatitis herpetiformis.

Sulfasalazine A sulphonamide used in the treatment of ulcerative colitis.

Sulphatase An enzyme that hydrolyzes sulfuric acid esters.

Sulfathiazole A rapidly absorbable sulfa.

Sulfatide Any cerebroside with a sulfate radical esterified to galactose.

Sulfemoglobin A form of greenish hemoglobin formed by action of hydrogen sulfide on blood, causes cyanosis if in excess.

Sulfinpyrazone Antigout agent.

Sulfisoxazole Sulfa used in urinary tract infection.

Sulfonamide The generic term for all aminobenzene sulphonamide preparations, including the bactericidal sulpha drugs.

Sulfone One of a group of drugs which with prolonged use have been successful in treating leprosy. Dapsone is the most widely used.

Sulfonyl urea One of a group of oral hypoglycemic agents used in the treatment of diabetes mellitus.

Sulfoxone sodium A drug for treatment of leprosy and dermatitis herpetiformis.

Sulfur Yellow inflammable element.

Sulfur dioxide A bactericide and disinfectant.

Sulfur precipitated A keratolytic agent.

Sulfur sublimed A scabicide and keratolytic agent.

Sulfuric acid 10% solution used as an astringent and for gastric hypoacidity.

Sulindac Norsteroidal anti-inflammatory drug.

Sulpiride Agent used in peptic ulcer.

Sulthiame An anticonvulsant drug used in the treatment of epilepsy.

Summary care record *(See SCR)*

Summation Cumulative action or stimuli.

Sunburn A dermatitis due to exposure to the sun's rays, causing burning and redness.

Sunscreen Agents like PABA used for protection against solar dermatitis.

Sunscreen protective factor index The ratio of the amount of exposure needed to produce minimal erythema response with the sunscreen in place divided by amount of exposure required to produce the same reaction without the sunscreen.

Sunstroke A profound disturbance of the body's heat regulating mechanism caused by prolonged exposure to excessive heat from the sun. Persons over 40 and those in poor health are most susceptible to it.

Superego Part of the personality that is concerned with moral standards and ideals that are derived unconsciously from parents, teachers and environment, and influence the person's whole mental make-up, acting as a control on impulses of the ego.

Superfecundation The fertilization of two or more ova, produced during the same menstrual cycle, by spermatozoa from separate coital acts.

Superfetation The fertilization of a second ovum when pregnancy has already started, producing two fetuses of different maturity.

Superinfection A new infection caused by a different organism from that which caused initial infection.

Superior Above; the upper of two parts.

Supernatant The clear liquid remaining at top as the heavy particles settle down below.

Supernumerary In excess of regular number, e.g., supernumerary teeth and supernumerary breast.

Superoxide A highly reactive form of oxygen (oxygen with single electron) produced during phagocytosis and bacterial digestion by neutrophils, lipid metabolism.

Superoxide dismutage Enzyme that destroys superoxide, being tried in myocardial infarction.

Superscription The beginning of prescription marked by letter Rx meaning "you take."

Superstructure Any visible part external to the main structure.

Supination Turning the palm or foot upward, lying on the back.

Supinator Muscle causing supination of forearm.

Supine 1. Lying on the back, with the face upward. 2. With the palm of the hand upward *(See Prone)*.

Support In the health care setting, the assistance and aid that is provided to patients and their families. This support maybe physical, e.g., in assisting a patient to walk, or psychological, as when listening to the concerns of relatives.

S. worker Fulfilling a supporting role such as a health care assistant, physiotherapy assistant or foot care assistant. In clinical areas, the support workers work under the supervision of a registered practitioner who is responsible for the support worker's practice and activities.

Suppository A medicated solid substance, prepared for insertion into the rectum or vagina, which will dissolve at body temperature.

Suppression 1. Complete cessation of a secretion. 2. In psychology, conscious inhibition as distinct from repression, which is unconscious.

Suppression of urine No secretion of urine by the kidneys.

Suppurate To form or generate pus.

Suppuration The formation of pus.

Supra Meaning above, beyond.

Supraclavicular fossa Depression on either side of neck above the clavicle.

Supracondylar Above the condyles.

Supracondylar fracture One above the lower end of the humerus or femur.

Suprahyoid muscles The digastric, geniohyoid, myohyoid and stylohyoid mucles.

Supraorbital Above the orbit of the eye.

Suprapubic Above the pubic bones.

Suprapubic cystotomy Surgical incision of the urinary bladder just above the pubic bones.

Suprarenal Above the kidney.

Suprarenal gland Adrenal gland. One of a pair of triangular endocrine glands situated on the upper surface of the kidneys *(See Adrenal)*.

Supraventricular tachycardia (SVT) Abnormally fast heartbeat of over 100 beats per minute not connected with exercise

Sura Calf or calf muscles.

Suramin A urea derivative used in treatment of trypanosomiasis.

Sure start Children's center, which gives help and advice on child and family health, parenting, money, training and employment. *(See Children's Caters)*.

Surfactant A surface-active agent. A mixture of phospholipids that is secreted into the pulmonary alveoli and reduces the surface tension of pulmonary fluids, thus contributing to the elastic properties of pulmonary tissue. Surfactant can be instilled via a tracheal catheter as treatment for respiratory distress syndrome *(See also Respiratory (Distress syndrome of newborn))*.

Surgeon A medical practitioner who specializes in surgery.

S

Surgery The branch of medicine that treats disease by operative measures.

Surgical dressing Sterile gauze or other materials for wound dressing.

Surgical neck Constricted part of shaft of humerus below the tuberosities, the common site for fracture.

Surrogate A real or imaginary substitute for a person or object in someone's life.

Surrogate mother A woman who carries a child for another (the commissioning parent) with the intention that the child be handed over after birth.

Survey The systematic collection of information, not forming part of a scientific epidemiological study.

Surveillance The monitoring of some program.

Susceptibility Lack of resistance to infection. The opposite to immunity.

Suscitate To stimulate or reactivate.

Suspensory Supporting a part.

Suspensory bandage One applied to support a part of the body, particularly the scrotum or the lower jaw.

Suspensory ligament A ligament that supports or suspends an organ, e.g., that of the lens of the eye.

Suture 1. A stitch or series of stitches used to close a wound. 2. The jagged line of junction of the bones of the cranium.

Atraumatic suture A suture fused to the needle to obtain a single thickness through each puncture of the needle.

Continuous suture A form of oversewing with one length of suture.

Coronal suture The junction between the frontal and parietal bones.

Everting suture A type of mattress stitch that turns the edges outwards to give a closer approximation.

Fascial suture A strip of fascia taken from the patient and used to form a suture.

Interrupted suture A series of separate sutures.

Lambdoid suture The junction between the parietal and occipital bones.

Mattress suture One in which each suture is taken twice through the wound, giving a loop one side and a knot on the other.

Purse-string suture A circular continuous suture round a small wound or appendix stump.

Sagittal suture The junction between the two occipital bones.

Subcuticular suture A continuous suture placed just below the skin.

Tension suture or *relaxation suture* One taking a large bite and relieving the tension on the true stitch line.

Suxamethonium A short-acting muscle relaxant drug primarily used in intubation of a patient.

Swab 1. A small piece of cotton wool or gauze. 2. In pathology, a dressed sterile stick used in taking bacteriological specimens.

Swallowing The taking in of a substance through the mouth and pharynx and into the esophagus. It is a combination of a voluntary act and a series of reflex actions. Once begun, the process operates automatically. Also called deglutition.

Swan-Ganz catheter A soft flexible catheter with a balloon at its tip. The balloon helps to guide the catheter into pulmonary artery. The balloon is inflated in distal pulmonary artery and the pressure is recorded which is pulmonary wedge pressure equivalent to left atrial pressure.

Swan-neck deformity Deformity of hand in rheumatoid arthritis with hyperextension of proximal interphalangeal joints due to tight interossei. Swan-neck deformity in renal tubules is a feature of adult Fanconi syndrome.

S

Sweat Perspiration; a clear watery fluid secreted by the sweat glands.

Sweat glands Coiled tubular glands situated in the dermis with long ducts to the skin surface.

Sweet's syndrome Painful skin plaques due to neutrophilic infiltration.

Swelling Enlargement mostly localized.

Swimmer's itch Itchy eruptions on skin due to swim in water containing cercariae of schistosomes.

Swine influenza A highly contagious respiratory disease of pigs caused by infection with the swine fever influenza viruses, A (H1N1) pdm09 virus (shortened to H1N1). Infected swine can infect and cause symptomatic disease in humans, with fever of sudden onset, cough or shortness of breath associated with headache, tiredness, aching muscles, sneezing and runny nose. The virus was first identified in 2009. The regular flu vaccine protects against H1N1. *(See Influenza, Avian Influenza and Orthomyxovirus).*

Sycophant Flatterer, praiser of persons in command of wealth or influence.

Sycosis A pustular inflammation of the hair follicles, usually of the beard and moustache.

Sydenham's chorea T Sydenham, British physician, 1624–1689. A disorder of the central nervous system closely linked with rheumatic fever; called also Saint Vitus' dance. The condition, usually self-limited, is characterized by purposeless, irregular movements of the voluntary muscles that cannot be controlled by the patient.

Sylvian fissure The fissure separating temporal lobe from frontal and parietal lobes.

Symbiosis In parasitology, an intimate association between two different organisms for the mutual benefit of both.

Symblepharon Adhesion of an eyelid to the eyeball.

Symbolism In psychology, an abnormal mental condition in which events or objects are interpreted as symbols of the patient's own thoughts. In psychiatry, the re-entry into consciousness of repressed material in an acceptable form.

Syme's amputation Amputation just above ankle joint with removal of malleoli.

Sympathectomy Division of autonomic nerve fibers which control specific involuntary muscles. An operation performed for many conditions, among them Raynaud's disease.

Sympathetic 1. Exhibiting sympathy. 2. Relating to the autonomic nervous system.

Sympathetic nervous system One of the two divisions of the autonomic nervous system. It supplies involuntary muscle and glands; it stimulates the ductless glands and the circulatory and respiratory systems, but inhibits the digestive system.

Sympathetic ophthalmia Inflammation leading to loss of sight in the opposite eye after a perforating injury in the ciliary region.

Sympathomimetic Pertaining to drugs that produce effects similar to those caused by a stimulation of the sympathetic nervous system.

Symphsis A cartilaginous joint along the line of union of two bones.

S. pubis The cartilaginous junction of the two pubic bones.

Symphysiotomy Section of symphysis pubis to increase capacity of contracted pelvis to facilitate childbirth.

Symptom Any indication of disease perceived by the patient.

Cardinal Symptoms 1. Symptoms of greatest significance to the doctor, establishing the identity of the illness. 2. The symptoms shown in the temperature, pulse and respiration.

Dissociation symptom Anesthesia to pain and to heat and cold, without impairment of tactile sensibility.

Objective symptom One perceptible to others than the patient, such as pallor, rapid pulse or respiration, restlessness, etc.

Presenting symptom The symptom or group of symptoms about which the patient complains or from which relief is sought.

Signal symptom A sensation, aura or other subjective experience indicative of an impending epileptic or other seizure.

Subjective symptom One perceptible only to the patient, as pain, pruritus, vertigo, etc.

Withdrawal symptoms Symptoms that follow sudden abstinence from a drug on which a person is dependent.

Symptomatology 1. The study of the symptoms of a disease. 2. The symptoms of a particular disease, taken together.

Synalgia Pain felt in one part of the body but caused by inflammation of or injury to another part. Referred pain.

Synapse The junction between the termination of an axon and the dendrites of another nerve cell. Chemical transmitters pass the impulse across the space.

Synarthrosis A type of joint where skeletal elements are joined by a continuous intervening cartilage, fibrous tissue or bone. Hence movement is limited or absent and joint cavity is lacking, e.g., chondrosis, suture joints.

Synchondrosis A joint in which the surfaces are connected by plate of cartilage.

Synchysis Degenerative condition of vitreous.

Syncope A simple faint or temporary loss of consciousness due to cerebral ischemia, often caused by dilatation of the peripheral blood vessels and a sudden fall in blood pressure.

Syncytiotrophoblast Outer layer of chorionic villi.

Syncytium A mass of cytoplasm with numerous nuclei but no division into separate cells.

Syndactylism Possessing webbed fingers or toes. A condition in which two or more fingers or toes are joined together.

Syndactyly Persistence of web between fingers/toes, an autosomal dominant trait.

Syndesmology Study of ligaments, joints, their movements and disorders.

Syndesmosis A form of articulation where bones are united by cartilages.

Syndrome A group of signs or symptoms typical of a distinctive disease, which frequently occur together and form a distinctive clinical picture.

Synechia Adhesion of iris to lens and cornea.

Synergist 1. A muscle that works in conjunction with another muscle. 2. A drug that works in combination with another drug, the two drugs having a greater effect when taken together than when taken separately.

Synergism Harmonious action of two agents to produce an effect greater than that produced by either agents singly.

Synergist A muscle acting in cooperation with another.

Synergy Coordinated action of two or more agents.

Syngamy Union of gametes in fertilization.

Syngeneic Individual or cells without tissue incompatibility.

Synkaryon A nucleus resulting from fusion of two pronuclei.

Synkinesis An involuntary movement of one part occurring simultaneously with reflex or voluntary movement of another part.

Synonym Having the same or similar meaning.

Synopsis A summary; general review.

Synorchidism Partial or complete fusion of two testicles within scrotum or abdomen.

Synovectomy Excision of a diseased synovial membrane to restore joint movement.

Synovia A colorless viscid lubricating fluid in the joint cavity, bursae and tendon sheaths.

Synovial cyst Accumulation of synovial in a bursa.

Synovial fluid The fluid that surrounds a joint and is secreted by the synovial membrane. It is a thick, colorless, lubricating substance.

Synovial membrane A serous membrane lining the articular capsule of a movable joint and terminating at the edge of the articular cartilage.

Synovioma A tumor of synovial membrane.

Synovitis Inflammation of a synovial membrane, usually with an effusion of fluid within the joint.

Synthesis The building up of a more complex structure from simple components. This may apply to drugs or to plant or animal tissues.

Synthetase An enzyme that acts as a catalyst to unite two molecules.

Syphilis An infectious venereal disease leading to many structural and cutaneous lesions; called also lues. Syphilis is caused by a spiral shaped bacterium (spirochaete), *Treponema pallidum*. It is a sexually transmitted infection, with the exception of congenital syphilis acquired by an infant from the mother in utero. There is an early infectious stage, followed by a latent period of many years before the noninfectious late stage, when serious disorders of the nervous and vascular systems arise.

Congenital syphilis That transmitted by the mother to the fetus; it is preventable if the mother receives a full course of penicillin during her pregnancy.

Nonveneral syphilis A chronic treponemal infection mainly seen in children, occurring in many areas of the world; it is caused by an organism in distinguishable from *Treponema pallidum* and transmitted by direct nonsexual contact. Lesions are usually oral mucous patches; subsequent lesions occur in the axillae, inguinal region and rectum. Then, after a latent period, destructive lesions of the skin and bones develop.

Syphilitic macules Small red non-itchy eruptions all over the body in secondary syphilis.

Syringe An instrument for injecting fluids or for aspirating or irrigating body cavities. It consists of a hollow tube with a tight-fitting piston. A hollow needle or a thin tube can befitted to the end.

Syringomyelia The formation of cavities filled with fluid inside the spinal cord. Impairment of muscle function and sensation result at the level of and below the lesion. Painless injury maybe the first symptom. It is a progressive disease.

Syringomyelitis Inflammation of the spinal cord, as the result of which cavities are formed in it.

Syringomyelocele A type of spina bifida in which the protruded sac of fluid communicates with the central canal of the spinal cord.

Syrinx Eustachian tube; pathological cavity within spinal cord, a fistula.

Syrup Concentrated sugar in water.

System A group of cells/organs that perform a particular function.

Systematic Describing a process that is carried out according to a method or a system.

S. review A methodical approach to literature reviews that reduces random error and bias. This requires a review of clinical literature in a particular field that has set explicit tests for whether research is valuable enough to be included in an overview of the area. This is often combined with a statistical meta-analysis of clinical trial results.

S. sampling A type of sampling in which a convenient number is chosen, e.g., every tenth or fourth member of the population is selected into the sample.

S. lupus erythematosus (See Lupus).

Systeme international d'Unites SI units. The international system for measurement in science, industry and general use. It was agreed in 1960, and it is now illegal in the UK to prescribe or dispense drugs in any other units.

Systemic Pertaining to or affecting the body as a whole.

Systemic circulation Circulation of the blood throughout the body, other than the pulmonary circulation *(See Sclerosis).*

Systole The period of contraction of the heart *(See Diastole).*

Atrial systole The contraction of the heart by which the blood is pumped from the atria into the ventricles.

Extra systole A premature contraction of the atrium or ventricle, without alteration of the fundamental rhythm of the pacemaker.

Ventricular systole The contraction of the heart by which the blood is pumped into the aorta and pulmonary artery.

Systolic Relating to a systole.

Systolic murmur An abnormal sound produced during systole in heart infections.

Systolic pressure The highest pressure of the blood reached during systole.

⊙⊙⊙

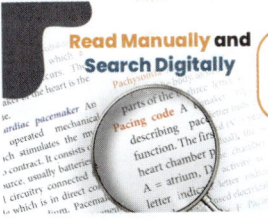
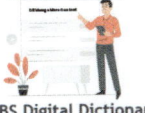

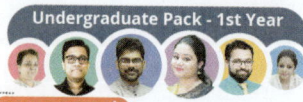
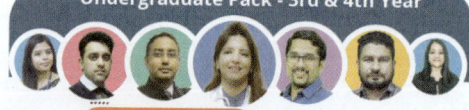
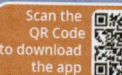

T Symbol for thymine.

T cell A lymphocyte which is derived from the thymus and is responsible for cell-mediated immunity.

TAB Typhoid-paratyphoid A and B vaccine; paratyphoid C may now be included. A sterile suspension of the killed salmonellae causing these diseases. Used as a preventative, it provides an active immunity.

Tabes A wasting away.

Tabes dorsalis Locomotor ataxia. A slowly progressive disease of the nervous system affecting the posterior nerve roots and spinal cord. It is a late manifestation of syphilis.

Tabetic crises Paroxysms of pain occurring during course of tabes dorsalis.

Tablespoon A rough measure equivalent to 15 mL.

Taboo Any ritual prohibition of certain activities, e.g., incest in many societies, or the open discussion of death and dying.

Taboparesis The presence of the symptoms of both tabes dorsalis and general paralysis of the insane in a patient suffering from late syphilis.

Tabular bone A flat bone composed of an outer and an inner table of compact bone with cancellous or diploe between them.

Tachogram A graphic tracing of rate of blood flow.

Tachyarrhythmia Abnormally rapid heart rate with or without irregularity.

Tachycardia Abnormally rapid action of the heart and consequent increase in pulse rate *(See Bradycardia).*
Paroxysmal tachycardia Spasmodic increase in cardiac contractions of sudden onset lasting a variable time, from a few seconds to hours.

Tachyphasia, tachyphrasia Extreme volubility of speech. It may be a sign of mental disorder.

Tachyphrenia Hyperactivity of the mental processes.

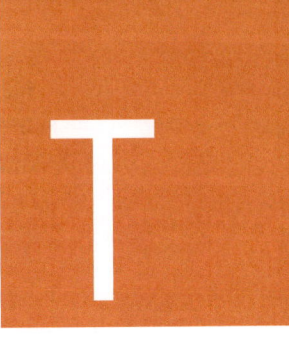

Tachypnea Rapid, shallow respirations; a reflex response to stimulation of the vagus nerve endings in the pulmonary vessels.

Tachypnea Rapid, shallow respirations; a reflex response to stimulation of the vagus nerve endings in the pulmonary vessels.

Tachysterol One of the isomers of ergosterol.

Tacrine Parasympathomimetic agent for Alzheimer's disease.

Tacrolimus Immunosuppressant.

Tactile Relating to the sense of touch.
Tactile discrimination The ability to localize two points of touch on skin surface as two discrete sensations.
Tactile localization Ability to accurately identify the site of tactile stimulation (touch, pain or pressure).

Tactometer Instrument for determining acuity of tactile sensitiveness.

Tadalafil Anti-impotency agent.

Taenia A genus of tapeworms.
T. saginata The beef tapeworm. The common type of tapeworm found in the human intestine.
T. solium The pork tapeworm. Can also be parasitic in humans, causing cysticercosis. *(See Tapeworm).*

Taenia coli Three bands in large intestine into which muscular fibers are collected.

Taeniasis An infestation with tapeworms.

Taenia

TAF Toxoid-antitoxin floccules. A vaccine used for diphtheria immunization (See Toxoid).

Tag A small polyp or growth; a label.

Tag skin Small outgrowth of skin.

Tagging Incorporating radioactive isotope into chemical compounds to trace the metabolism.

T'ai chi A system of movement. Chinese in origin, promoting general health and well-being.

Takayasu arteritis Aortic branch occlusion of unknown origin, often involving ophthalmic artery.

Takotsubo cardiomyopathy Also known as acute stress cardiomyopathy. Temporary and reversible symptoms of chest pain and breathlessness after significant emotional or physical stress.

Talc Hydrous magnesium silicate, used as dusting powder.

Talipes Club foot. A deformity caused by a congenital or acquired contraction of the muscles or tendons of the foot.
Talipes calcaneus The heel alone touches the ground on standing.
Talipes equinus The toes touch the ground but not the heel.
Talipes valgus The inner edge of the foot only is in contact with the ground.
Talipes varus The person walks on the outer edge of the foot.

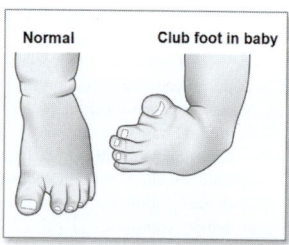

Talipes

Talus The astragalus or ankle bone.

Tamm-Horsfall mucoprotein A mucoprotein secreted from renal tubules.

Tamoxifen Antiestrogen drug used in adjuvant therapy of breast cancer.

Tampon A plug of absorbent material inserted in the vagina, the nose or other orifice to restrain hemorrhage or absorb secretion.

Tamponade The surgical use of tampons.
Cardiac tamponade Impairment of heart action by hemorrhage or effusion into the pericardium; may be due to a stab wound or follow surgery.
Temponade balloon Used to arrest variceal bleed.

Tamsulosin Alfa blocker for prostatic hypertrophy.

Tangier disease A syndrome of HDL deficiency first discovered in Tangier island. Symptoms and signs include polyneuropathy, lymphadenopathy, orange tonsils, hepatosplenomegaly.

Tannin An acid substance found in tea and an astringent, topical hemostatic and antidote for various poisons.

Tantalum Symbol Ta. A metallic element used for prostheses and wire sutures.

Tantrum An outburst of ill temper.

Temper tantrum A behavior disorder of childhood. A display of bad temper in which the child perform sun controlled actions in a state of emotional stress.

Tapeworm Any of a group of cestode flat worms, including the *Taenia* genus, which are parasitic in the intestines of humans and many animals. The adult consists of around head with suckers or hooklets for attachment (scolex). From this, numerous segments (proglottids) arise, each of which produces ova capable of independent existence for a considerable length of time. Treatment is by anthelmintic drugs.

Tapia syndrome Paralysis of pharynx, larynx and atrophy of tongue due to paralysis of tenth and twelfth cranial nerves.

Tapotement [Fr.] A tapping movement used in massage.

Tapping *(See Paracentesis).*

Tar Thick brown to black liquid obtained from distillation of carbonaceous matter.

Tardieu's spot Subpleural spots of ecchymosis following death by strangulation.

Tardive Tending to be late.

Target cell An abnormal erythrocyte which when stained shows a central and peripheral rim of hemoglobin with intermediate unstained area resembling a target.

Target cells Abnormal flat red blood cells seen in liver and spleen disease and in the hemoglobinopathies.

The hemoglobin is distributed as a small inner mass with a pale outer ring.

Tarnier's sign A sign of impending abortion; the disappearance of angle between upper and lower uterine segments of uterus.

Tarnish Discoloration.

Tarsal Relating to a tarsus.

Tarsal bones The seven small bones of the ankle and in step.

Tarsal cyst Meibomian cyst; chalazion.

Tarsal glands Meibomian glands of the eyelids.

Tarsal plates Small cartilages in the upper and lower eyelids.

Tarsal tunnel syndrome Weakness of plantar flexion of toes and numbness of sole of foot due to compression of tibial nerve in the tarsal tunnel.

Tarsalgia Pain in the foot, usually associated with flattening of the arch.

Tarsectomy Excision of one or more bones tarsus.

Tarsitis Inflammation of margin of eyelid; inflammation of tarsal bones (the seven bones of ankle).

Tarsorrhaphy Stitching of the eyelids together to protect the cornea or to allow healing of an abrasion.

Tarsus The ankle with its seven constituent bones, i.e., talus, calcaneus, cuboid, navicular and the three cuneiform bones.

Tartar A hard incrustation deposited on the teeth and on dentures.

Tartar emetic Antimony potassium tartrate. A salt used in the treatment of schistosomiasis and leishmaniasis.

Tartrazin A pyrazole aniline dye used to color foods, cloth and drugs.

Task allocation A method of organizing care whereby each specific type of care is carried out by a separate nominated nurse, e.g., for the same patient one nurse will record the blood pressure and another nurse will give the prescribed medications.

T

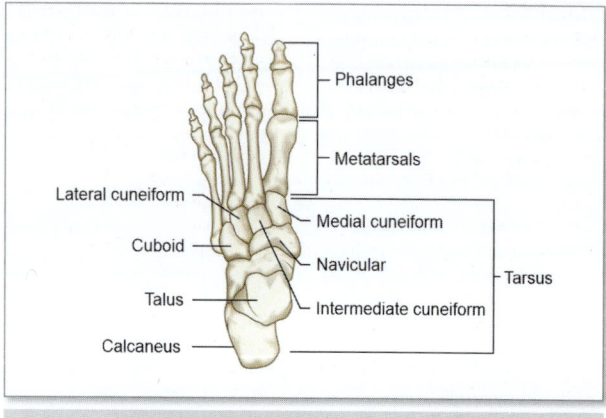

Tarsal

Taste The sense by which it is possible to identify what is eaten and drunk. Taste receptors (buds) lie on the tongue and give the sensations of sweet, sour, salt and bitter.

Tattoo A permanent discoloration of the skin due to a foreign pigment.

Tattooing The deliberate (usually for decorative purposes) or accidental insertion of colored material into the deeper layers of the skin, perhaps as a result of an explosion.

Taurocholic acid Bile acid that yields taurine and cholic acid on hydrolysis.

Taxis Manipulation by hand to restore any part to its normal position. It can be used to reduce a hernia or a dislocation.

Taxonomy The theory and practice of the classification of animals and plants.

Tay-Sachs disease *W Tay, British physician, 1843–1927; B Sachs, American neurologist, 1858–1944.* Autosomal recessive form of gliosidosis (lipid storage disease) manifesting with mental retardation, blindness, cherry-red spot in macula, etc. due to deficiency of hexosamini-

dase. Leading to accumulation of sphingolipid in CNS.

TB Tuberculosis.

T cells Thymus derived lymphocytes consisting of helper inducer cells (T4), killer T-cells and suppressor T-cells.

Tea black Tea made from the leaves that have been fermented before they are dried.

Tea green Tea made by heating the leaves in open trays.

Teaism Chronic poisoning from excessive intake of tea.

Team nursing A method of organizing care based on the allocation of each nurse to a team that cares for a group of patients, usually for a number of shifts.

Tears The watery, slightly alkaline and saline secretion of the lacrimal glands that moistens the conjunctiva.

Teaspoon Measure equivalent to 5 mL.

Teat 1. A nipple of the breast. 2. A manufactured nipple used on infants' feeding bottles.

Technetium Symbol Tc. A metallic element. Radioactive t. An isotope (99 m Tc) used in a number of diagnostic tests. As it has a short half-life (6 hours), a high dose may be given for scanning organs, but the patient receives only a low radiation dose.

Technology The scientific knowledge and its practical application.

Tectocephaly Boat-shaped head.

Tectospinal tract A descending tract from tectum of midbrain to spinal cord.

Tectum Structure resembling a roof; dorsal midbrain consisting of superior and inferior colliculi.

Teenage Age bracket of 13–19 years.

Teeth (*See Dentition*).

Tegaserol Serotonin agonist for irritable bowel syndrome (IBS).

Tegmen A structure that covers a part.

Tegmentum The dorsal portion of midbrain containing red nucleus and oculomotor nuclei.

Tegument The skin.

Teichopsia Zigzag lines bounding a luminous object in visual field as in migraine.

Teicoplanin Higher antibiotic.

Tela Any web-like structure.

Telangiectasis A group of dilated capillary blood vessels web-like or radiating in form.

Telangioma A tumor of the blood capillaries.

Telbivudine Anti-HIV drug.

Telecare Personal alarms that can be used for someone's help in the event of falls, unusual movement or hypothermia, which can allow people to live independently at home by enabling someone else to remotely monitor their safety.

Telediagnosis Diagnosis based on data transmitted electronically to the doctor.

Telemedicine Exchange of medical information from one site to another through the use of telecommunication and information technologies.

Telemetry Transmission of data to a distant place by electronic means.

Telencephalon The embryonic forebrain that develops into olfactory lobes, cerebral cortex and corpora striata.

Teleology The belief that everything in nature is directed towards some final purpose.

Teleopsia A visual perceptive disorder where objects appear to have excess depth or close objects appear to be away.

Telepaque Iopanaoic acid.

Telepathy The transmission of thought without any normal means of communication between two persons.

Teleradiography Radiography with radiation source at about 2 meters away from body.

Telereceptor A sensory nerve ending which can respond to distant stimuli. Those of the eyes, ears and nose are examples. Teleceptor.

Teletherapy Treatment of cancer in which source of radiation is placed at some distance from body.

Telmisartan ACE receptor antagonist for hypertension.

Telogen Resting stage of hair growth.

Telophase The last stage in the division of cells when the chromosomes have been reconstituted in the nuclei at either end of the cell and the cell cytoplasm divides to form two new cells.

Temper State of one's mood, disposition and mind.

Temperament The combination of intellectual, emotional and physical characteristic of an individual.

Temperate Moderate.

Temperature The degree of heat of a substance or body as measured by a thermometer.

Normal temperature (oral) The normal temperature of the human body is 37°C (98.6°F), with a slight decrease in the early morning and a slight increase at night. It indicates the balance between heat production and heat loss.

T

630

Rectal temperature More accurate than oral or axillary temperature. It is about 1°F higher than oral temperature, whereas axillary temperature is 1°F lower than oral temperature.

Template A mold or pattern. In radiotherapy, a map of the area of the patient requiring treatment and of those areas to be protected from radiation.

Temple The region on either side of the head above the zygomatic arch.

Temporal Pertaining to the side of the head.

Temporal arteritis Giant cell arteritis. A chronic inflammatory condition of the carotid arterial system, occurring usually in elderly people. There is persistent headache and partial or total blindness may result.

Temporal bone One of a pair of bones on either side of the skull containing the organ of hearing.

Temporal lobe The part of the cerebrum below the lateral sulcus.

Temporalis The muscle in tempora' fossa inserted into coronoid process of mandible, a muscle of mastication.

Temporomandibular Relating to the temporal bone and the mandible.

T. Joint The hinge of the lower jaw.

T. Joint syndrome Painful dysfunction of the temporomandibular joint, marked by a clicking or grinding sensation in the joint; commonly caused by malocclusion of the teeth. Also known as temporomandibular disorder.

Temporoparietal Relating to temporal and parietal bones.

Tenacious Thick and viscid, as applied to sputum or other body fluids.

Tenacity Condition of being tough, stubborn.

Tenaculum Sharp hook like instrument.

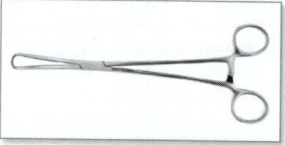

Tenaculum

Tendinitis Inflammation of a tendon and its attachments.

Tendinous synovitis Inflammation of tendon's synovial sheath.

Tendon A band of fibrous tissue forming the termination of a muscle and attaching it to a bone.

Achilles tendon That inserted into the calcaneum.

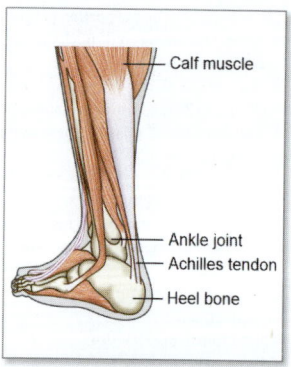

Achilles Tendon

Tendon grafting An operation which repairs a defect in one tendon by a graft from another.

Tendon insertion The point of attachment of a muscle to a bone which it moves.

Tendon reflex The muscular contraction produced on percussing a tendon.

Tendovaginitis Inflammation of tendon and its sheath.

Tenesmus A painful, ineffectual straining to empty the bowel or bladder.

Teniposide Antineoplastic agents of podophylotoxin group.

Tennis elbow A painful disorder which affects the extensor muscles of the forearm at their attachment to the external epicondyle.

Tenon's capsule *JR Tenon, French surgeon, 1724–1816.* The fibrous tissue in which the eyeball is situated.

Tenon's space Space between the posterior surface of eyeball and Tenon's capsule.

Tenonitis Inflammation of Tenon's capsule. Proptosis of the eyeball occurs, often accompanied by pain and pyrexia.

Tenorrhaphy The suturing together of the ends of a divided tendon.

Tenosynovectomy Excision of tendon sheath.

Tenosynovitis Inflammation of tendon sheath.

Tenotome Instrument for cutting tendon.

Tenotomy Surgical section of a tendon.

Tenosynovitis Inflammation of a tendon sheath.

Tenoxicam Analgesic anti-inflammatory.

TENS Abbreviation for Transcutaneous Electrical Nerve Stimulation. A method of treating persistent pain by passing small electrical currents into the spinal cord or sensory nerves by means of electrodes applied to the skin. TENS is noninvasive and nonaddictive, with no known side effects.

Tension The act of stretching or the state of being stretched.

Arterial tension The pressure of blood on the vessel wall during cardiac contraction.

Intraocular tension The pressure of the contents of the eye on its walls, measured by a tonometer.

Intravenous tension The pressure of blood within the veins.

Premenstrual tension Symptoms of abdominal distension, headache, emotional liability and depression, occurring a few days before the onset of menstruation *(See Premenstrual).*

Surface tension Tension or resistance which acts to preserve the integrity of a surface, particularly the surface of a liquid.

Tension headache Headache caused by sustained contraction of muscles of head and neck.

Tension suture Suture used to reduce pull of the edges of wound.

Tensor Any muscle that makes a part tense.

Tensor valipalatini A muscle of soft palate arising from cartilaginous medial end of auditory tube and inserted into palatal aponeurosis.

Tentacle A slender projection of invertebrates used for tactile purposes or feeding.

Tentative Provisional.

Tenth cranial nerve Vagus nerve supplying heart, lungs, abdominal viscera, esophagus, etc.

Tentorial notch An arched cavity formed by anterior and inner border of tentorium cerebella.

Tendorial pressure cone The herniation of uncus of temporal lobe and midbrain through tentorial notch due to raised intracranial pressure.

Tentorium cerebella The process of dura mater between cerebrum and cerebellum supporting the occipital lobes.

Tepid Lukewarm.

Teratoblastoma A tumor containing embryonic tissue.

Teratocarcinoma Carcinoma developing from epithelial element of a teratoma.

Teratogen An agent or influence that causes physical defects in the developing embryo.

T

Teratogenesis The development of abnormal structures in an embryo.

Teratology Scientific study of teratogens and their mode of action.

Teratoma A solid tumor containing tissues similar to those of a dermoid cyst. Found most often in the ovaries and testes, many of these tumors are malignant.

Teratosis Deformed fetus.

Terazosin Alfa-blocker, used in hypertension and benign prostate hypertrophy (BPH).

Terbinaline Antifungal agent.

Terbutaline Synthetic sympathomimetic amine used as bronchodilator.

Terconazole A ketoconazole derivative, antifungal agent.

Teres Round and smooth.

Terfenadine H$_1$ receptor blocker, antiallergic agent.

Terlipressin Synthetic antidiuretic hormone.

Term The end of pregnancy, normally calculated as 280 days or 40 weeks from the date of the last normal menstrual period but considered to be any time after the 37th week of pregnancy.

Terminal Pertains to end or placed at the end.

Terminal arteriole Arteriole without any branches which ends in capillaries.

Terminal cancer An advanced stage of cancer from which patient cannot recover.

Terminal illness Illness from which recovery is impossible, hence death is imminent.

Terminal infection An acute infection that appears at late stage of another disease and often prove fatal.

Termination of pregnancy (TOP) Abortion that is induced, legally or illegally.

Terminology Nomenclature, a system of technical terms used in arts, science and trade.

Terpene A hydrocarbon used as an expectorant.

Terracing Suturing in several rows through thick tissues in wound closure.

Terramycin Oxytetracycline, synthesized by *Streptomyces rimosus*, effective against bacteria, rickettsia and Chlamydia.

Terror Great fear.

Tertian Recurring every 48 hours *(See Malaria).*

Tertiary Third.

Tertiary prevention Prevention of ill health, mitigating the effects of illness and disease that have already occurred.

Tertiary syphilis The noninfectious stage of neurosyphilis.

Testis The male reproductive gland located in scrotum about 4 cm long 2 cm wide.

Test meal A meal of definite quality and quantity given for analysis of stomach function.

Test 1. An examination or trial. 2. Analysis of the composition of a substance by the use of chemicalreagents.

Agglutination test One whose results depend on agglutination of bacteria or other cells. Used in diagnosing certain infectious disease and rheumatoid arthritis, the cross-matching of blood and in pregnancy tests; in the latter no agglutination indicates a positive pregnancy test, whereas when agglutination occurs the result is negative.

Complement-fixation tests Tests that utilize antigen-antibody reaction, and result in hemolysis, to determine the presence of various organisms in the blood.

Concentration test A test of renal function based on the patient's ability to concentrate urine.

Creatinine clearance test A test for renal function based on the rate at which ingested creatinine is filtered through the renal glomeruli.

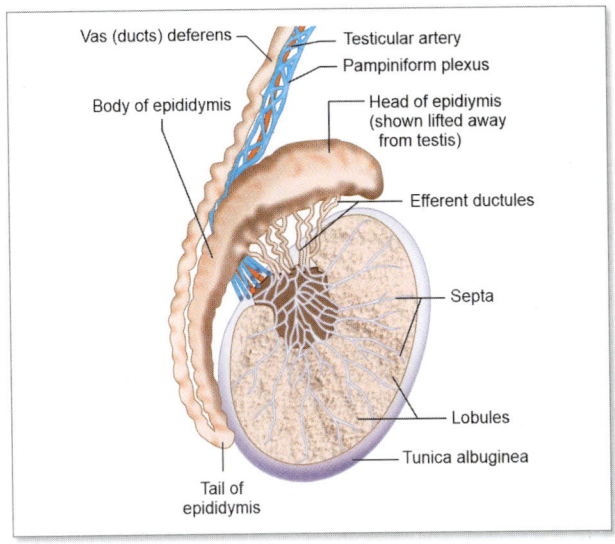

Vas (ducts) deferens — Testicular artery
— Pampiniform plexus
Body of epididymis — Head of epidiymis
(shown lifted away
from testis)
— Efferent ductules
— Septa
— Lobules
— Tunica albuginea
Tail of
epididymis

Testis

Early pregnancy test A do-it-your-self immunological test for pregnancy, performed as early as 9 days after menstruation was expected.

Glucose tolerance test A metabolic test of carbohydrate tolerance used to diagnose diabetes mellitus.

Glycosylated hemoglobin test Measurement of the percentage of hemoglobin A1 (HbA1) molecules, which helps to assess diabetic control. HbA1 is a type of adult hemoglobin where one part of the beta chain has been combined with glucose. It increases in diabetes, especially when the blood glucose control is poor.

Histamine test After a rapid intravenous injection of histamine phosphate, the blood pressure normally falls, but in patients with pheochromocytoma, after fall, there is a marked rise in blood pressure.

Pregnancy tests Laboratory procedures for early determination of pregnancy.

Sickling test A method to demonstrate hemoglobin S and the sickling phenomenon in erythrocytes, performed by reducing the oxygen concentration to which the red cells are exposed.

Test weighing A method of determining the amount of breast milk taken by weighing the baby before and after the feed without changing any of its clothes, so that the difference equals the feed. Sometimes called test feeding. With successful demand feeding there should be no need for this scheme.

Treponema pallidum hemagglutination (TPHA) test, Treponemapallidum immobilization (TPI) test Serological tests related directly to the causative organism, used in the diagnosis of syphilis.

T

VDRL test A slide flocculation test for syphilis designed by the Venereal Disease Research Laboratory, USA.

Test meal A meal of definite quality and quantity given for analysis of stomach function.

Testicle A testis; one of the two glands in the scrotum which produce spermatozoa.

Undescended testicle A condition in which the organ remains in the pelvis or inguinal canal.

Testicular self-examination Should be performed regularly once a month for the detection of early tumors of the testis, which are highly curable if detected at an early stage. Self-examination should take place after a warm bath or shower, which relaxes the scrotal skin. It is performed as follows; (a) Standing in front of a mirror, look for any swelling. One testicle may appear larger than the other or hang lower; this is usually perfectly normal, (b) Examine each testicle with both hands and gently roll each testicle between the fingers and thumb. A small lump is felt for and, if found, almost always occurs in only one testis and is usually painless, (c) A cord-like structure found on the top and back of each testicle should be found and examined for any swelling.

Testis A testicle.

Testosterone The hormone produced by the testes which stimulates the development of sex characteristics. It can now be made synthetically, and is used medicinally in cases of failure of sex function and as a palliative treatment in some cases of advanced metastatic breast cancer in females.

Test tube baby A baby born to a mother whose ovum was removed, fertilized outside her body and implanted in her uterus.

Tetanolysin A hemolytic component of the toxin produced by *Glostridium tetani.*

Tetanospasmin The toxin of *Clostridium tetani* responsible for spasm.

Tetanus An acute disease of the nervous system caused by the contamination of wounds by the spores of a soil bacterium,

Clostridium tetani. Muscle stiffness around the site of the wound occurs, followed by rigidity of face and neck muscles; hence "lockjaw". All muscles are then affected and opisthotonos may occur.

Tetanus antitoxin A serum that gives a short-term passive immunity and may be used with penicillin for immediate treatment of a case of tetanus.

Tetanus vaccine (or toxoid) Will give an active immunity.

Tetany An increased excitability of the nerves due to a lack of available calcium, accompanied by painful muscle spasm of the hands and feet (carpopedal spasm). The cause may be hypoparathyroidism or alkalosis owing to excessive vomiting or hyperventilation.

Tetracaine Local anesthetic used topically.

Tetrachlorethylene A clear colorless bitter liquid used as anthelmintic, potentially hepatotoxic.

Tetracycline An antibiotic drug belonging to the group known as the tetracyclines which are effective against many different microorganisms, including rickettsiae. Gram-negative and Gram-positive organisms and certain viruses.

Tetrad A group of four things.

Tetradactyly Having four digits on a hand or foot.

Tetrahydrocanabinol Principal active component of *Canabis indica.*

Tetrahydrozoline A vasoconstrictor used in ophthalmic and nasal drops.

Tetraiodothyronine One of the principal hormones secreted by thyroid. *SYN* –thyroxine (T_4).

Tetralogy A series of four.

Tetralogy of Fallot (See Fallot's tetralogy).

Tetramisole Anthelmintic.

Tetraparesis Paresis of all four limbs.

Tetraplegia Quadriplegia. Paralysis of all four limbs.

Thalamic nuclei The anterior, lateral, medial and posterior thalamic nuclei.

Thalamic syndrome Severe sharp boring and burning pain caused by vascular lesions of thalamus.

Thalamotomy Destruction of thalamus by several means to treat psychosis or intractable pain.

Thalamus A mass of nerve cells at the base of the cerebrum. Most sensory impulses from the body pass to this area and are transmitted to the cortex.

Thalassemia A group of hemolytic anemias mostly found in the Mediterranean region and the far East, caused by the inheritance of abnormal hemoglobin.

Thalassemia major Cooley's anemia; the severest form of thalassemia with death usually occurring before adolescence.

Thalassemia minor A mild form of the disease with few symptoms. Those suffering from it can pass the disease on to their children.

Thalassemia A group of inherited hemolytic anemias where there is interference with the synthesis of hemoglobin resulting in anemia. Several types are recognized, according to the symptoms. Thalassemia is prevalent in the Mediterranean, Middle East and Southeast Asian regions. The only possible cure is a stem cell or bone marrow transplant but this carries significant risks so is not often performed. Genetic counselling is advised for the parents or other close relatives of a child with thalassemia and also for any person with thalassemia trait.

Thalassotherapy Treatment involving sea bathing or a sea voyage.

Thalidomide Alfa glutarimide previously used as sedative but now only used in lepra reaction; causes severe birth defects if given to pregnant mothers.

Thallium A metallic element used as rodenticide.

Thanatology 1. The study of death and dying. 2. The forensic study of the causes of death.

Thanatophobia Morbid fear of death.

Thebaine An alkaloid present in opium.

Thebesian valve An endocardial fold at entrance of coronary sinus into right atrium.

Thebesian vein Small veins draining blood from myocardium directly into heart chambers.

Theca A sheath, such as the covering of a tendon.

Theca folliculi The covering of a Graafian follicle.

Theca vertebralis The membranes enclosing the spinal cord; the dura mater.

Thecoma A benign tumor of ovary.

Thecomatosis Increased connective tissue in the ovary.

Thelalgia Pain in the nipples of breast.

Thelarche The beginning of breast development during puberty.

Thelothism Nipple erection by contraction of its smooth muscles.

Thenar 1. The palm of the hand. 2. The fleshy part at the base of the thumb.

Thenar muscles Abductor and flexor muscles of thumb.

Theobromine A smooth muscle dilator, used as a mild stimulant and diuretic.

Theomania Religious insanity.

Theophylline An alkaloid derived from tea leaves, which increases the heart rate and the excretion of urine, thus reducing edema. Used mainly in the treatment of bronchospasm and asthma.

Theophylline ethylenediamine Aminophylline.

Theorem A proposition proved by logic or argument.

Theory An assumption based on certain evidence or certain observations but lacking scientific proof.

Therapeutic Pertaining to therapeutics or treatment of disease; curative.

Therapeutic abortion (See Abortion).

Therapeutic community Any treatment setting (usually psychiatric) which provides a living learning situation through group processes emphasizing social, environmental and personal interactions and which encourages the individual to learn socially from these processes.

Therapeutic index The ratio of toxic dose of a substance to its therapeutic dose; an index of safety of the drug.

Therapeutic use of self The ability of the psychiatric nurse to use therapy and experimental knowledge along with self-awareness and the ability to explore and use one's personal impact on others.

Therapeutics The science and art of healing and the treatment of disease.

Therapist Practitioner of some kind of therapy.

Therapy The treatment of disease.

Collapse therapy Production of pneumothorax to affect pulmonary collapse as a method of treatment of nonhealing cavitary pulmonary tuberculosis.

Electroconvulsive therapy Passing of electric current in the convulsive dose to treat psychosis or suicidal depression.

Photodynamic therapy Method of treating cancer by using light absorbing chemicals that are selectively retained by malignant cells.

Physical therapy Use of physical agents such as massage, heat, hydration, electricity, exercise in the treatment of disease.

Replacement therapy Therapeutic use of medicine as substitute for natural body substances, e.g., thyroid hormone, insulin.

Thermal Relating to heat.

Thermalgesia Pain caused by exposure to heat.

Thermesthesia Capability to perceive heat and cold.

Thermic Pertains to heat.

Thermistor An apparatus for determining small changes in temperature.

Thermoanesthesia Insensitivity to heat.

Thermocautery The deliberate destruction of tissue by means of heat *(See Cautery).*

Thermocoagulation Coagulation or destruction of tissue by passage of high frequency current.

Thermocouple Device for measuring slight temperature changes.

Thermodilution A technique for determination of cardiac output from injection of cold saline into bloodstream and measuring the temperature change downstream.

Thermogenesis Production of body heat.

Thermography A method of measuring the amount of heat produced by different areas of the body, using infrared photography. Used as a diagnostic aid in the detection of breast tumors and the assessment of rheumatic joints, also used in the study of pain.

Thermoluminescent dosimeter A monitoring device that stores energy of ionizing radiation. When heated it emits light proportional to the amount of radiation to which it has been exposed, used by radiographers and those working near radiation source.

Thermolysis The loss of body heat by radiation, by excretion and by the evaporation of sweat.

Thermometer An instrument for measuring temperature.

Clinical thermometer One used to measure the body temperature.

Electronic thermometer A clinical thermometer which works electrically. It contains electronic devices whose characteristics change with temperature. The reading is recorded within seconds and displayed visually.

Thermometry Measurement of temperature.

Thermophilic Thriving best in environment of raised temperature.

Thermoreceptor A nerve ending that responds to heat and cold.

Thermoregulation The normal regulation of body temperature by the maintenance of the balance between heat production and heat loss.

Thermoregulatory center Hypothalamic center that regulates heat production and heat loss.

Thermostasis Maintenance of body temperature.

Thermostat An apparatus which automatically regulates the temperature and maintains it at a specified level.

Thermotaxis The normal regulation of body temperature by the maintenance of the balance between heat production and heat loss.

Thermotherapy The treatment of disease by application of heat.

Thiabendazole Anthelmintic used for strongyloidiasis and cutaneous larva migrans.

Thiazolidinediones A group of antidiabetic agents.

Thiamine Vitamin B_1. An essential vitamin involved in carbohydrate metabolism. A deficiency causes beriberi. The source is liver and unrefined cereals, wheat germ and rice water.

Thiazides Any of a group of diuretics that act by inhibiting the reabsorption of sodium by the proximal renal tubule and stimulating chloride excretion, with resultant increase in excretion of water.

Thiersch skin graft *K Thiersch, German surgeon, 1822–1895.* The transplantation of areas of partial thickness skin *(See Graft).*

Thio Prefix meaning sulfur.

Thioguanine An antimetabolite used in the treatment of acute leukemia.

Thiopental sodium An ultra short acting barbiturate used for inducing surgical anesthesia.

Thiopentone A basal narcotic of the barbiturate group given intravenously as a short-acting anesthetic and in preoperative preparation.

Thioridazine Antipsychotic agent.

Thiotepa An alkylating agent, antineoplastic drug.

Thiothixene An antipsychotic drug.

Thiouracil A drug used in the treatment of thyrotoxicosis. A derivative, propylthiouracil, which is more active and less toxic, is now more often used.

Thiourea Antithyroid drug.

Third degree burn Burn involving entire thickness of skin and deeper structures.

Third heart sound Heart sound occurring at the end of rapid ventricular filling.

Thirst An uncomfortable sensation of dryness of the mouth and throat with a desire for oral fluids.

Abnormal thirst Polydipsia.

Thomas splint *HO Thomas, British orthopedic surgeon, 1834–1891.* A splint consisting of an oval iron ring that fits over the lower limb. Attached to the ring are two round iron rods which are bent into a W shape at the lower end. It is used to support the limb and move the weight from the knee joint to the pelvis.

Thoracectomy A process of making incision on chest wall and resecting a portion of rib.

Thoracentesis Puncture of chest wall to drain out pleural fluids.

Thoracic Relating to the thorax.

Thoracic cage The bony structure surrounding the chest.

Thoracic duct The large lymphatic vessel situated in the thorax along the spine. It opens into the left subclavian vein.

Thoracic outlet syndrome Compression of the neurovascular structures at the superior thoracic outlet located just above the first rib and behind the clavicle leading to various symptoms like pain in the neck and shoulder, numbness and tingling of the fingers and a weak grip.

Thoracocentesis Puncture of the wall of the thorax to allow aspiration of pleural fluid.

Thoracolumbar Relating to the thoracic and lumbar parts of the spinal cord.

Thoracoplasty Partial resection of ribs to induce collapse of underlying lung as in lung abscess, or empyema.

Thoracoscopy Examination of the pleural cavity by means of an endoscopic instrument.

Thoracostomy Surgical resection of chest wall for drainage.

Thoracostomy tube A tube inserted into the chest wall to drain air or fluid from pleural space.

Thoracotomy A surgical incision into the thorax.

Thorax The chest; a cavity containing the heart, lungs, bronchi and esophagus. It is bounded by the diaphragm, the sternum, the thoracic vertebrae and the ribs.

Barrel shaped thorax A development in emphysema, when the chest is malformed like a barrel.

Thorium Radioactive metallic substance.

Thoron A radioactive isotope of radon.

Threadworm A species of roundworm. *Enterobius vermicularis,* parasitic in the large intestine, particularly of children.

Threonine One of the essential amino acids.

Threshold 1. Point at which physiological response is produced. 2. A measure of sensitivity of an organ or function.

Threshold dose Minimum dose that will be effective.

Thrill A tremor discerned by palpation.

Thrix Hair.

Throat 1. The anterior surface of the neck. 2. The pharynx.

Clergyman's sore throat Laryngitis.

Sore throat Pharyngitis.

Throbbing Pulsatile.

Thrombasthenia A platelet disorder with prolonged bleeding time, and abnormal clot retraction.

Thrombectomy Excision of a thrombus.

Thrombin An enzyme that converts fibrinogen to fibrin during the later stages of blood clotting.

Thromboangiitis Inflammation of blood vessels with clot formation.

Thromboangiitis obliterans Inflammation of the arteries, usually of the legs of young males, causing intermittent claudication and gangrene. Buerger's disease.

Thrombocythemia Absolute increase in platelet count.

Thrombocyte A disk-shaped bloodplatelet; essential for the clotting of shed blood.

Thrombocytopenia A reduction in the number of platelets in the blood; bleeding may occur. Destruction of platelets can be caused by infections, certain drugs, transfusion related purpuras, idiopathic thrombocytopenic purpura and disseminated intravascular coagulation.

Thrombocytosis An increase in the number of platelets in the blood.

Thromboembolism A detached thrombus causing occlusion of a vessel.

Thrombogenesis The process of formation of blood clot.

Thrombokinase Thromboplastin. A lipid containing protein, activated by blood platelets and injured tissues, which is capable of activating prothrombin to form thrombin, which, combined with fibrinogen, forms a clot.

Thrombolysis The disintegration or dissolving of a clot by the infusion of an enzyme such as streptokinase into the blood.

Thrombophlebitis The formation of a clot, associated with inflammation of the lining of a vein.

Thromboplastin *(See Thrombokinase).*

Thrombosis The formation of a thrombus.

Cavernous sinus thrombosis Thrombosis of the cavernous sinus, usually the result of infection of the face, when the veins in the sinus are affected via ophthalmic vessels.

Cerebral thrombosis The occlusion of a cerebral artery, the most common cause of cerebral infarction (a 'stroke').

Coronary thrombosis The occlusion of a coronary vessel, by which the heart muscle is deprived of blood, causing myocardial ischemia and often leading to myocardial infarction (a 'heart attack').

Lateral sinus thrombosis A complication of mastoiditis when infection of the lateral sinus of the dura mater occurs and there is clot formation.

Thrombus A stationary blood clot caused by coagulation of the blood in the heart or in an artery or a vein.

Thrush An infection of the mucous membranes, most commonly of the mouth and vagina, by a fungus.
Candida albicans (See Candidiasis).

Thrust The sudden move forward.

Thumb The short thick first finger on radial side of hand having two phalanges in place of 3.

Thumb sucking Habit of sucking thumb.

Thymectomy Surgical removal of thymus.

Thymine Symbol T. One of the pyrimidine bases found in DNA.

Thymocyte A lymphocyte that migrates from bone marrow to thymus where it matures and is released in blood as T-lymphocyte.

Thymol An aromatic antiseptic used in solution as a mouth wash.

Thymoma A tumor that originates in thymus tissue.

Thymopoietin A substance produced by thymus gland that helps in differentiation of thymacytes.

Thymus A gland-like structure situated in the upper thorax and neck. Present in early life, it reaches its maximum development during puberty and continues to play an immunological role throughout life, even though its function declines with age.

Thyroepiglottic muscle Muscle arising from inner surface of thyroid cartilage and inserted into epiglottis. Acts to depress the epiglottis.

Thyroglobulin Iodine-containing protein secreted by thyroid gland and stored within the colloid.

Thyroglossal Relating to the thyroid and the tongue.
Thyroglossal cyst (See Cyst).

Thyroid 1. Shaped like a shield. 2. Pertaining to the thyroid gland.
Intrathoracic or *retrosternal thyroid* Position of neck and wholly or in part behind the sternum.

Thyroid cartilage The largest cartilage of the larynx. It forms the "Adam's apple" in the front of the throat.

Thyroid gland A ductless gland, consisting of two lobes, situated in front and on either side of the trachea. It secretes the hormones thyroxine and triiodothyronine which are concerned in regulating the metabolic rate.

Thyroid-stimulating hormone Abbreviated TSH. Thyrotrophin; a hormone, produced by the anterior pituitary gland, which controls the activity of the thyroid gland.

Thyroidectomy Partial or complete removal of the thyroid gland.

Thyroiditis Inflammation of the thyroid. Acute thyroiditis, usually due to a virus infection, is characterized by sore throat, fever and painful enlargement of the gland.

Hashimoto's thyroiditis A progressive autoimmune disease of the thyroid gland with degeneration of its epithelial elements and replacement by lymphoid and fibrous tissue.

Thyorid storm A complication of thyrotoxicosis precipitated by infection, surgery; manifests with high fever, restlessness and congestive failure.

Thyromegaly Enlarged thyroid gland.

Thyroparathyroidectomy Surgical removal of the thyroid and parathyroid glands.

Thyroptosis Downward displacement of thyroid.

Thyrotoxic Pertains to hyperactivity of thyroid gland.

Thyrotoxicosis Hyperthyroidism. The symptoms arise when there is over activity of the thyroid gland. The metabolism is speeded up and there is enlargement of the gland and exophthalmos.

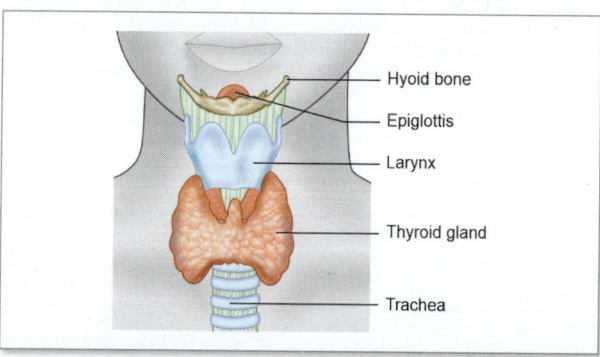

Hyoid bone

Epiglottis

Larynx

Thyroid gland

Trachea

Thyroid

Thyrotropic Agent that stimulates thyroid gland.

Thyrotropin *(See Thyroid Stimulating hormone).*

Thyroxine One of the two hormones secreted by the thyroid gland. It is used in the treatment of hypothyroidism.

TIA Transient Ischemic Attack.

Tianeptine Antidepressant agent.

Tibia The shin bone; the larger of the two bones of the leg, extending from knee to ankle.

Tic A spasmodic twitching of certain muscles, usually of the face, neck or shoulder.

Douloureux paroxysmaltic Trigeminal neuralgia.

Ticarcillin A semisynthetic penicillin effective agent pseudomonas.

Tick A blood-sucking parasite which may transmit the organisms of disease.

Tickling Gentle stimulation of sensitive surface and the reflex theory.

Ticlopidine Antiplatelet agent.

Tidal volume The amount of gas passing into and out of the lungs in each respiratory cycle.

Tietze syndrome Sternal costochondritis of unknown etiology, often requiring injection procaine and steroids locally.

Timolol Beta-blocker.

Tincture An alcoholic extraction of animal or vegetable substance.

Tincture of iodine A skin disinfectant containing a mixture of sodium iodide in an alcohol water solution. This term is not used nowadays.

Tine test A tuberculin skin test employing a multiple puncture, disposable device. It is especially useful in mass screening of children, but is less accurate than the Mantoux test.

Tinea A group of skin infections caused by a variety of fungi and named after the area of the body affected, thus: *Tinea barbae,* the beard; *Tinea capitis,* the head; *Tinea circinata* or *Tinea corporis,* the body; *Tinea cruris,* the groin; and *Tinea pedis,* the feet *(See Ringworm).*

Tinel's sign Tingling sensation on pressing or tapping a damaged or degenerating nerve.

Tingle Pricking or stinging sensation.

Tinidazole An imidazole used in amebiasis.

Tinnitus A ringing, buzzing or roaring sound in the ears.

Tinocordin Immunostimulant.

Tiotropium Antiasthmatic inhaler.

Tissue A group or layer of similarly specialized cells that together perform certain special functions.

Macrophage tissue A large wandering branched cell with single nucleus capable of ingesting particulate matter.

Plasminogen activator tissue (TPA) A thrombolytic agent that is clot specific, acting on plasminogen causing breakdown of fibrin.

Tittanium dioxide Used in solutions for protection against sunburn.

Titillation Sensation produced by tickling.

Titration Determination of a given component in solution by addition of a liquid reagent of known strength until a given endpoint, e.g., change in color, is reached, indicating that the component has been consumed by reaction with the reagent.

Titubation Unsteadiness of posture, swaying of trunk and head while sitting, staggering gait.

Tizanidine Muscle relaxant.

TNAI Trained Nurses Association of India.

TNM classification Method of classifying malignant tumors based on local characteristics of the tumor, involvement of lymph nodes and distant metastasis.

Toad skin Excessive dryness, wrinkling and scaling of skin as in vitamin A deficiency (phrynoderma).

Tobacco The dried leaves of the plant *Nicotiana tabacum,* containing the drug nicotine, which may be smoked, chewed or inhaled. All these activities are potentially dangerous to health. Cigarette smoking in particular is responsible for an increase in cancer of the lungs and mouth and bronchitis. Smoking increases the likelihood of emphysema and coronary artery disease. It is also harmful during pregnancy, leading to smaller and less healthy babies.

Tobacco withdrawal syndrome A change in mood or behavior associated with the stopping of or reduction in cigarette smoking.

642

Tobramycin An antibiotic drug used chiefly in the treatment of *Pseudomona* infection.

Tocainide A lidocaine analog, antiarrhythmic drug.

Tocodynamometer Device for estimating force of uterine contraction. *SYN* – tocometer.

Tocography The measurement of alterations in the intrauterine pressure during labor.

Tocology Science of parturition.

Tocolysis Suppression of uterine contraction.

Tocopherol Vitamin E, present in wheat germ, green leaves and milk.

Tocophobia A fear of child birth or pregnancy.

Todd's paralysis Focal weakness in a part of the body after a seizure.

Toe Any of the five digits of foot.

Clawtoe dorsal subluxation of toes 2–5 in rheumatoid arthritis.

Hammertoe proximal phalanx is extended and 2nd and 3rd are flexed.

Toilet Wound cleaning.

Toilet training Teachings for a child to achieve control over urination and defecation.

Token economy programme A behavioral approach to modifying troublesome behaviors and restoring lost self-help behaviors by the systematic rewarding of desired behavior by giving tokens which may be exchanged for goods or privileges.

Tolazamide An oral hypoglycemic drug used in the treatment of diabetes mellitus.

Tolazoline A vasodilator drug of the peripheral blood vessels, used in the treatment of peripheral vascular disease.

Tolbutamide An oral drug that stimulates the release of insulin from the pancreas. Used in the treatment of diabetes mellitus.

Tolerance The ability to endure without effect or injury.

Drug tolerance Decrease of susceptibility to the effects of a drug due to its continued administration.

Immunological tolerance Specific nonreactivity of lymphoid tissues to a particular antigen capable, under other conditions, of inducing immunity.

Tolfenamic acid A fenamate anti-inflammatory drug.

Tolnaftate Synthetic antifungal agent used topically.

Tolterodine Antimuscarinic agent.

Tomography Body section radiography in which X-rays or ultrasound waves are used to produce an image of a layer of tissue at any depth.

Tone 1. The normal degree of tension, e.g., in a muscle. 2. A particular quality of sound.

Tongue A muscular organ attached to the floor of the mouth and concerned in taste, mastication, swallowing and speech. It is covered by a mucous membrane from which project numerous papillae.

Tongue tie Congenital shortness of frenulum linguae with poor protrusion, difficulty in articulation and sucking.

Tonic 1. A term popularly applied to any drug supposed to brace or tone up the body or any particular part or organ. 2. Possessing tone in a state of contraction, e.g., muscles.

Tonic spasm A prolonged contraction of one or several muscles, as seen in epilepsy, for example *(See Clonic).*

Tonicity Property of possessing tone.

Tonography The measurement made by an electric tonometer recording the intraocular pressure and so, indirectly, the drainage of aqueous humor from the eye.

Tonometer Instrument for measuring intraocular pressure.

Tonometry Measurement of intraocular tension.

Tonsil A mass of lymphoid tissue, particularly one of two small, almond shaped bodies, situated one on each side between the pillars of the fauces. It is covered by mucous membrane, and its surface is pitted with follicles.

Pharyngeal tonsil The lymphadenoid tissue of the pharynx between the pharyngo-tympanic tubes. Adenoids.

Tonsil test A small sample of tonsil obtained in suspected cases of Creutzfeldt-Jakob disease (CID) for the identification of the prion found in new variant CJD, a spongiform encephalopathy.

Tonsillar sinus Space between the plica triangular is and anterior surface of tonsils.

Tonsillectomy Excision of one or both tonsils.

Tonsillitis Inflammation of tonsils.

Tonsillitis follicular Tonsillitis principally affecting the crypts.

Tonus The normal state of partial contraction of the muscles.

Tooth A structure in the mouth designed for the mastication of food. Each is composed of a crown, neck and root with one or more fangs. The main bulk is of dentine enclosing a central pulp; the crown is covered with a hard white substance called enamel *(See Dentition).*

Tooth brushing The act of using a soft brush for cleaning the teeth and gums.

Topagnosis Loss of ability to localize site of tactile sensation.

Tophaceous Related to tophus.

Topiramate Anticonvulsant.

Tophus A small, hard, chalky deposit of sodium urate in the skin and cartilage, occurring in gout and sometimes appearing on the auricle of the ear.

Topical Relating to a particular spot; local.

Topical lotion One for local or external application.

Topotecan Anti-cancer agent.

Topography The study of the surface of the body in relation to the underlying structures.

TORCH Acronym for toxoplasmosis, other, rubella, cytomegalo virus and herpes simplex infections.

Torpent Medicine that modifies irritation.

Torpidity Sluggishness, inactivity.

Torpor A sluggish condition in which response to stimuli is absent or very slow.

Torque A force producing rotary motion.

Torr The pressure of 1/760 of standard atmosphere pressure or simply 1 mm Hg.

Torsade de pointes Polymorphic rapid ventricular tachycardia with changing QRS configuration.

Torsemide Diuretic

Torsion Twisting: (a) Of an artery to arrest hemorrhage; (b) Of the pedicle of a cyst, which produces venous congestion in the cyst and consequent gangrene (a possible complication of ovarian cyst).

Torso The body, excluding the head and the limbs; the trunk.

Torticollis Wryneck, a contracted state of the cervical muscles, producing torsion of the neck. The deformity may be congenital or secondary to pressure on the accessory nerve, to inflammation of glands in the neck, or to muscle spasm.

Tourtuous Having many bends or twists and turns.

Torture Infliction of mental or physical pain.

Torula Yeast like organism, now called *Cryptococcus.*

Total hip replacement Replacement of acetabulum and head of femur by metallic or silicone prosthesis in the treatment of advanced disabling hip disease.

Total parenteral nutrition (TPN) Provision of total electrolyte, protein, calorie, vitamin and mineral need via intravenous route.

Total Complete, the whole number or amount.

T. body irradiation Abbreviated TBI. The complete exposure of the patient's body to radiotherapy, used in the treatment of some cancers and prior to stem cell or bone marrow transplantation.

T. burn surface area Abbreviated TBSA. A formula for predicting outcomes after a burn injury: (age + TBSA) = percentage chance of surviving. *(See Lund and Browder Chart)*.

T. lung capacity Abbreviated TLC. The volume of air held in the lungs following deep inspiration.

T. parenteral nutrition abbreviated TPN. The supplying of all essential nutrients to a patient via the intravenous route. *(See Annexure 1)*.

T. quality management (TQM) A largely superseded approach to management based upon the idea that quality of service depends upon the active involvement of all members of staff in achieving and maintaining high standards of care throughout an organization. TQM had great popularity in the 1980s and 1990s but has been replaced by LEAN and SIX SIGMA.

Totipotent A cell capable of dividing into a large variety of cells.

Touch Tactile sense or perceive from palpation.

Tourette's syndrome A neurological disorder that starts in childhood. Characterized by repetitive grimaces and tics; involuntary barks, grunts, shouting and other noises may appear as the disease progresses. Some sufferers may also use obscene language (coprolalia). Also known as Gilles de la Tourette's syndrome. Causes are unknown although there may be a genetic cause in some cases.

Tourniquet A constrictive band applied to a limb to arrest arterial hemorrhage. No longer used in first aid because its use may cause permanent damage to muscles or nerve supply.

Touton cells Giant multinucleated cells found in lesions of xanthomatosis.

Toxaemia Poisoning of the blood by the absorption of bacterial toxins.

Toxaemia of pregnancy A condition affecting pregnant women and characterized by albuminuria, hypertension and edema, with the possibility of pre-eclampsia and eclampsia developing.

Toxic 1. Poisonous, relating to a poison 2. Caused by a toxin

Toxic allergic syndrome A disease caused by ingestion of adulterated rapeseed oil with aniline producing respiratory distress, eosinophilia, hepatosplenomegaly, etc.

Toxic shock syndrome A severe illness characterized by high fever of sudden onset, vomiting, diarrhea and in severe cases, death. A sunburn—like rash with peeling of the skin occurs.

Toxicity The degree of virulence of a poison.

Toxicology The science dealing with poisons.

Toxicosis A diseased condition resulting from poisoning.

Toxiferous Containing a poison.

Toxigenic Producing toxins or poisons.

Toxigenicity The virulence of a toxin producing pathogenic organism.

Toxin Any poisonous compound, usually referring to that produced by bacteria.

Toxocara A genus of nematode worms, parasitic in the intestines of dogs and cats, which may also infest humans, especially children. The spleen, liver and lungs are most often affected but the parasite may also infest the retina, causing inflammation and granulation.

Toxoid A toxin which has been deprived of some of its harmful properties but is still capable of producing immunity and may be used in a vaccine.

Toxolysin Substance capable of destroying toxin.

Toxoplasma A genus of protozoa which infests birds and animals and maybe transmitted from them to humans.

Toxoplasmosis A disease due to *Toxoplasma gondii*. The congenital form causes system lesions, brain defects and death. The acquired infection is often asymptomatic but may result in pneumonia, skin rashes and nephritis.

TPA Total Parenteral Alimentation

TPA Total Parenteral Nutrition.

Trabecula A dividing band or septum, extending from the capsule of an organ into its interior and holding the functioning cells in position.

Trabeculectomy An operation to lower the intraocular pressure in glaucoma that cannot be controlled by medication.

Trace 1. Very small quantity. 2. A visible mark or sign.

Trace elements Organic elements normally present in minute quantity but very essential for plant or animal life.

Tracer A means by which something may be followed, as (a) A mechanical device by which the outline or movements of an object can be graphically recorded or (b) A material by which the progress of a compound through the body may be observed, e.g., a radioactive isotope tracer.

Trachea The windpipe; a cartilaginous tube lined with ciliated mucous membrane, extending from the lower part of the larynx to the commencement of the bronchi.

Trachealis Smooth muscle fibers extending between the ends of tracheal rings whose contraction narrows the lumen.

Tracheal ring C-shaped fibrous rings of trachea.

Tracheal tug The downward tugging movement of larynx in thoracic aortic aneurysm.

Tracheitis Inflammation of the trachea causing pain in the chest, with coughing.

Trachelectomy Amputation of uterine cervix.

Trachelitis Inflammation of cervix.

Trachelology Scientific study of neck, its diseases and injuries.

Tracheobronchitis Acute infection of the trachea and bronchi due to viruses or bacteria.

Tracheobronchomegaly Congenital enlargement of trachea and bronchi.

Tracheocele Protrusion of tracheal mucous membrane through its wall.

Tracheomalacia Softening of cartilaginous framework of trachea.

Tracheostomy A surgical opening into the third and fourth cartilage rings of the trachea.

Tracheostomy tubes Those used to maintain an airway after tracheotomy, either permanently or until the normal use of the air passages is regained.

Tracheotomy Surgical incision of the trachea.

High tracheotomy Superior tracheotomy.

Inferior or *low tracheotomy* That in which the opening is made below the thyroid isthmus.

Superior tracheotomy High tracheotomy. That in which the opening is made above the thyroid isthmus.

Trachitis Inflammation of trachea.

Trachoma A chronic infectious disease of the conjunctiva and cornea, producing photophobia, pain and lacrimation, caused by an organism once thought to be a virus but now classified as a strain of the bacterium *Chlamydia trachomatis.* Trachoma is more prevalent in Africa and Asia than in other parts of the world.

Tracing A graphic record of some events like respiration, electrical activity of heart and brain.

Tract 1. A pathway. 2. Bundle of nerve fibers within spinal cord or brain acting as an anatomical and functional unit.

Traction 1. The exertion of a pulling force, such as that applied to a fractured bone or dislocated joint or to relieve muscle spasm, to maintain proper position and facilitate healing. 2. In obstetrics, that along the axis of the pelvis to assist in delivery of a fetal part, or the placenta and membranes.

Hamilton-Russell traction A form of traction of the leg.

Head traction Traction exerted on the head in the treatment of cervical injury.

Skeletal traction A method of keeping the fractured ends of bone in position by traction on the bone. A metal pin or wire is passed through the distal fragment or adjacent bone to overcome muscle contraction.

Tract of Schuz Periventricular tract.

Tractotomy Surgical section of a tract in CNS, e.g., for pain relief.

Tragus Cartilaginous projection in front of external auditory meatus.

Training 1. An organized system of instruction. 2. Systematic exercise for physical development or some specialized aim.

Trait An inherited or developed physical or mental characteristic.

Tramadol Anti-inflammatory pain killer.

Trance A condition of semiconsciousness of hysterical, cataleptic or hypnotic origin. It is not due to organic disease.

Trandolapril ACE inhibitor.

Tranquilizer A drug which allays anxiety, relieves tension and has a calming effect on the patient.

Transabdominal Across the abdominal wall or through the abdominal cavity.

Transactional analysis A theory of personality structure and a psycho therapeutic method. The human personality is viewed as consisting of three ego states: the parent, the adult and the child. The aim is to allow the adult ego to take control over the child and parent egos.

Transaminase One of a group of enzymes which catalyse the transfer of an amine group from one amino acid into another. Transaminases include glutamioxalacetic transaminase (GOT) and glutamic pyruvic transaminase (GPT).

Transamination Resuscitation by mouth to mouth respiration.

Transatrial Procedure done through or across the atrium.

Transcendental meditation A technique for attaining a state of physical relaxation and psychological calm by the regular practice of relaxation procedure which entails the repetition of a mantra. Has been successfully used by some patients to reduce hypertension.

Transcortin A corticosteroid binding globulin.

Transcriptase A polymerase that transcripts by converting a DNA base sequence into its complementary RNA base sequence.

Transcription The DNA directed synthesis of messenger RNA.

Transcultural nursing Being aware of the patient's cultural health beliefs and values and incorporating these into the agreed care plan with the patient.

Transcutaneous blood gas monitors The application to a baby's skin of a probe which is heated to a temperature of 44°C and enables measurements of PO_2 and PCO_2 to be made. Accuracy depends on the quality of peripheral circulation, thus trans cutaneous blood gas monitoring is usually used in conjunction with intermittent arterial sampling.

Transcutaneous electrical nerve stimulation *(See TENS).*

Transdermal Through the skin.

T. Patch A medicated adhesive patch that is placed onto the skin to deliver a specific dose of medication through the skin and into the bloodstream. The main advantage of the transdermal patch is that it provides a controlled release of the medication into the patient. The main disadvantage is that only drugs whose molecules are small enough to penetrate the skin can be delivered by this method.

Transducer Device that converts one form of energy into another, e.g., ultrasonic transducers that convert sound energy to electrical energy.

Transection Cutting across the long axis.

Transexamic acid A factor present in antigen sensitized lymphocytes.

Transferrin Iron transporting globulin in plasma.

Transference In psychiatry, the unconscious transfer by the patient on to the psychiatrist of feelings that are appropriate to other people significant to the patient.

Transfixion The act of piercing through and through.

Transfixion sutures A method of closing a wound by the use of suture which is placed through both wound edges in a figure-of- eight fashion.

Transformation Change of shape or form, in oncology the change of one tissue into another; a type of mutation occurring in bacteria.

Transfusion The introduction of whole blood or a blood component into a vein, performed in cases of severe loss of blood, shock, septicemia, etc. It is used to supply actual volume of blood, or to introduce constituents, such as clotting factors or antibodies, that are deficient in the patient.

Direct transfusion The transfer of blood directly from a donor to a recipient.

Exchange transfusion Replacement transfusion. The removal of most or all of the recipient's blood and its replacement with fresh blood. Used with infants suffering from erythroblastosis *(See Rhesus factor).*

Intra-arterial transfusion The passing of blood into an artery under positive pressure in cases where large quantities are required rapidly, as in cardiovascular surgery.

Replacement transfusion Exchange transfusion.

Transfusion reaction A variety of reactions including fever, chill, hemolysis, jaundice, shock and anaphylaxis occurring during transfusion.

Transgrow A special medium for culture of *N Gonorrhea.*

Transient ischaemic attack Abbreviated TIA. A sudden episode of temporary or passing symptoms, caused by diminished blood flow through the carotid or vertebrobasilar blood vessels.

Transillumination The illumination of a translucent body structure by a strong light as an aid to diagnosis, particularly of tumors of the retina and of abnormalities in the ethmoidal and frontal sinuses.

Transition Passing from one state or position to another.

Translation Protein synthesis under direction of RNA.

Translocation In morphology, the transfer of a segment of a chromosome to a different site on the same chromosome or to a different chromosome. It can be a cause of congenital abnormality.

Translucent Allowing light rays to pass through indistinctly.

Transmethylation Transfer of a methyl group from a donor to a receptor compound. Methionine and choline serve as donors of methyl group.

Transmigration Movement from one place to another, as in the passage of blood cells through the walls of the capillaries. Diapedesis.

External transmigration The passage of an ovum from its ovary to the uterine tube on the opposite side.

Internal transmigration The movement of an ovum from one uterine tube to the other through the uterus.

Transmissible Capable of being transmitted from one person to another; communicable, infectious.

Transmission-based precautions Precautions, designed to be applied to patients known or suspected to be infected with pathogens that are highly transmissible or epidemiologically important, and for which additional measures beyond standard precautions are needed to interrupt transmission in hospital. There are three types of transmission-based precaution: airborne, droplet and contact precautions. They may be combined for diseases that have multiple routes of transmission. When employed either singly or in combination, they are used in addition to 'standard precautions'.

Transmural Across a wall, e.g., myocardial infarction involving full thickness of wall in a given area.

Transparent Permitting passage of light rays without obstruction.

Transpeptidase An enzyme that catalyzes the transfer of a peptide from one compound to another.

Transplacental Across the placenta. Movement may be from mother to fetus or vice versa.

Transplacental infection May affect the unborn child.

Transplant 1. An organ or tissue taken from the body and grafted in to another area of the same individual or another individual. 2. To transfer tissue from one part to another or from one individual to another.

Transplantation The transfer of living organs from one part of the body to another (autotransplant) or from one individual to another (allograft). Transplantation is often called grafting, though the latter is more commonly used to refer to the transfer of skin.

Heteroplastic transplantation Transplantation of a part from one individual to another of the same or closely related species.

Heterotopic transplantation Transplantation in which transplant is placed in a different location in host than it had in donor.

Transport Movement or transfer of substances in biological system; transport may be active, passive or carrier mediated.

Transposition 1. Displacement of any of the viscera to the opposite side of the body. 2. The operation which partially removes a piece of tissue from one part of the body to another, complete severance being delayed until it has become established in its new position.

Transposition of the great vessels A congenital abnormality of the heart in which the positions of the pulmonary artery and aorta are reversed.

Transsexualism A disturbance of gender identity; there is a persistent conviction that the person's true gender is opposite to the actual anatomical sex.

Transudate Any fluid that passes through a membrane.

Transudation Oozing of fluid through the membrane.

Transurethral An operation performed through urethra, e.g., transurethral prostatectomy.

Transverse Cross-wise.

Transverse presentation Position of the fetus whereby it lies across the pelvis; this position must be corrected before normal birth can take place.

Transverse mesocolon The transverse portion of mesentery connecting transverse colon with posterior abdominal wall.

Transverse myelitis Inflammation of spinal cord involving entire cord substance at a particular level, usually of unknown etiology.

Transverse sinus A sinus of dura mater running from internal occipital protuberance along attached margin of tentorium cerebella to reach jugular foramen.

Transvestite A person who experiences a habitual and strongly persistent desire to dress as a member of the opposite sex ('cross-dressing'), often for reasons of sexual gratification. The majority are male and have no desire to physically change sex (by surgery).

Transvestism Dressing or masquerading in the clothing of opposite sex to be accepted as a member of opposite sex.

Tranylcypromine A monoamine oxidase inhibitor used in psychiatry for the treatment of depression.

Trapezium The first bone of the second row of carpal bones.

Trapezius The muscle arising from occipital bone, nuchal ligament and the spines of thoracic vertebra and inserted into clavicle, acromion and spine of scapula.

Trauma Injury.

Birth trauma An injury to the infant sustained during the process of being born. In some psychiatric theories, the psychological shock produced in an infant by the experience of being born.

Psychological trauma An emotional shock that makes a lasting impression.

Trauma score A numerical grading system that assesses neurological and cardiopulmonary functions to assess severity of trauma and prediction of survival.

Traumatology The branch of surgery dealing with wounds and their care.

Tray A flat surface with raised edges.

Tray impression In dentistry U shaped receptacle to carry impression material and support it in contact with teeth.

Trazodone Antidepressant.

Treacher Collins syndrome Mandibulofacial dysostosis.

Treatment The mode of dealing with a patient or disease.

Active treatment That in which specific medical or surgical treatment is undertaken.

Conservative treatment That which aims at preserving and restoring injured parts by natural means, e.g., rest, fluid replacement, etc. as opposed to radical or surgical methods.

Empirical treatment Treatment based on observation of symptoms and not on science.

Palliative treatment That which relieves distressing symptoms but does not cure the disease.

Prophylactic treatment That which aims at the prevention of disease.

Trematoda A class of fluke worms, some of which are parasitic in humans. Many of them have fresh waters nails as secondary hosts.

Tremble Involuntary shaking or quivering.

Tremor An involuntary, muscular quivering which mayst be due to fatigue, emotion or disease. Tremor, first of one hand, and later affecting the other limbs, is the first symptom of Parkinsonism.

Intention tremor One that occurs on attempting a movement, as in disseminated sclerosis.

Tremulous Trembling or shaking.

Trench fever The disease caused by *Rickettsia quintana*, transmitted by body louse.

Trench foot A condition akin to frost bite due to keeping of feet in wet socks and shoes for prolonged period.

Trench mouth Painful pseudomembranous ulceration of mucous membrane of mouth.

Trend The tendency to proceed in a certain direction.

Trendelenburg's position F Trendelenburg, German surgeon, 1844–1924 (See Position).

Trendelenburg's sign A test of the stability of the hip. The patient stands on the affected leg and flexes the other knee and hip. If there is dislocation the pelvis is lower on the side of the flexed leg, which is the reverse of normal.

Trephination The process of cutting a piece of bone from skull by a trephine.

Trephine An instrument for cutting out a circular piece of bone, usually from the skull.

Corneal trephine One used to cut out a piece of cornea in keratoplasty.

Transpidation Fear, anxiety, trembling motion.

Treponema A genus of spirochaetes. Anaerobic bacteria, they are motile, spiral and parasitic in humans and animals.

Treponema carateum The causative agent of pinta.

Treponema pallidum The causative agent of syphilis.

Treponema immobilization test A serological test for syphilis.

Treponemapertenue The causative agent of yaws (framboesia).

Tretinoin Transretinoic acid used topically for acne.

Triacetin Antifungal agent used topically.

Triad Any three things having or denoting something in common.

Tri-iodothyronine A hormone produced by the thyroid gland together with thyroxine.

Triage [Fr.] 1. Choosing, classifying or sorting. 2. A process by which a patient is assessed upon arrival to determine the urgency of the problem, and to designate appropriate health care resources to care for the identified problem.

Triage nurse A registered nurse with specialists skills and knowledge who carries out the assessment and classification of casualties according to the type and severity of their injuries in order to assign them for treatment in the accident and emergency department.

Triamcinolone A glucocorticoid steroid which does not cause salt and water retention; used to treat inflammatory disorders.

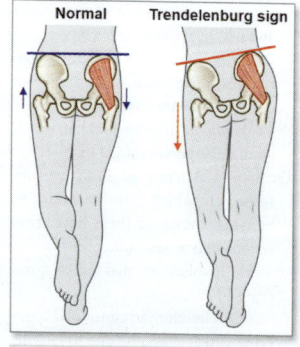

Trendelenburg's Sign

Triamterene A diuretic that acts by antagonizing aldosterone and does not cause potassium loss. Used in the treatment of edema.

Triangle An area formed by three angles and three sides.

Triangular ligament The ligaments left and right connecting right and left lobes of liver with corresponding portions of diaphragm.

Triatoma A genus of blood sucking bugs, one variety of it transmits *Trypanosoma cruzi*, causative agent of Chaga's disease.

Triazolam Benzodiazepine anxiolytic.

Tribadism A condition where women attempt to imitate heterosexual intercourse with each other.

Tribasic Composed of three replaceable hydrogen atoms.

Tribe A taxonomic division between genus and family.

Tribromoethanol An anesthetic agent.

Tricarboxylic acid cycle The metabolic cycle of pyruvic acid breakdown for production of energy; the terminal pathway where by fats, carbohydrates and proteins are utilized.

Triceps Having three heads.

    Triceps muscle That situated on the back of the upper arm, which extends the forearm.

Trichiasis 1. A condition of ingrowing hair about an orifice, or ingrowing eyelashes. 2. The appearance of hair-like filaments in the urine.

Trichinella A genus of nematode.

    Trichinella spiralis of this genus causes trichinois from ingestion of undercooked pork containing the cyst.

Trichinellosis Disease caused by *Trichinella spiralis SYN* – trichinosis. Symptoms are swelling of face, firm, tender swollen muscles, fever and eosinophilia.

Trichinosis A disease caused by eating underdone pork containing a parasite.

    Trichinella spiralis. This becomes deposited in muscle and causes stiffness and painful swelling. There may also be nausea, diarrhea and fever. Trichiniasis.

Trichlor acetic acid The caustic agent used for cauterization of warts, condylomata and hyperplastic tissue.

Trichloroethylene A weak inhalation anesthetic. Used in midwifery and for painful dressings and also in general anesthesia in combination with other anesthetics.

Trichobezoar A hair ball in the stomach.

Trichogen An agent stimulating hair growth.

Trichology The study of hair.

Tricholine Hepatic stimulant.

Trichomatosis Entangled matted hair due to fungal disease.

Trichomonas A genus of flagellate protozoa that are parasitic to humans.

    Trichomonas hominis Infests the bowel and may cause dysentery.

    Trichomonas tenax Infests the mouth and may be present in cases of pyorrhea.

    Trichomonas vaginalis Is commonly present in the vagina and may cause leucorrhea and vaginitis.

Trichomoniasis Infestation with a parasite of the genus *Trichomonas.*

Trichomycosis Any fungal disease of hair.

Trichophytobezoar A hair ball found in the stomach along with vegetable fiber and other debris.

Trichophyton A genus of fungi that affect the skin, nails and hair.

Trichophytosis Infection of the skin, nails or hair with one of the genus *Trichophyton (See Tinea).*

Trichorrhexis Splitting of hair.

Trichosis Any abnormal growth of hair.

Trichosporon A genus of fungi growing on hair.

Trichotilomania Unnatural impulse to pull out one's own hair.

Trichromatic Able to differentiate three primary colors, which means normal color vision.

Trichuriasis Infestation by the whip worm.

Trichuris A genus of nematode worms which may infest the colon and cause diarrhea. A whipworm.

Tricitratesoral solution Solution of sodium citrate, potassium citrate and citric acid.

Triclophos sodium A sedative hypnotic preparation.

Triclosan Gum antiseptic.

Tricuspid Having three flaps or cusps.

Tricuspid atresia Congenital atresia of tricuspid valve with cyanosis and clubbing.

Tricuspid valve That at the opening between the right atrium and the right ventricle of the heart.

Trident Having three prongs.

Tridihexethyl chloride An anticholingergic agent.

Triethylenemelamine One member of nitrogen mustard group of antineoplastic agent.

Triethylenethiophosphoramide An alkylating agent used in cancer chemotherapy. *SYN* – thiotepa.

Trifluoperazine A potent tranquilizing drug that is used in the treatment of schizophrenia and of psychoneuroses.

Trifluperidol Antipsychotic.

Triflupromazine Antipsychotic agent used mainly for nausea and vomiting (Siquil).

Trifocal Pertaining to a spectacle lens that has three foci, one for distant, one for intermediate and one for near vision.

Trifurcation Division into three branches.

Trigeminal Divided into three.

Trigeminal nerves The fifth pair of cranial nerves, each of which is divided into three main branches and supplies one side of the face.

Trigeminal neuralgia Pain in the face which is confined to branches of the trigeminal nerve. Tic douloureux.

Trigger To initiate with suddenness. An event or impulse that initiates other events or actions.

Trigger finger A stenosing of the tendon sheath at the metacarpophalangeal joint, allowing flexion of the finger but not extension without assistance, when it "clicks" into position.

Trigger zone Any area of hyperexcitability in the body which when stimulated precipitates a specific response, e.g., epileptic fit or an attack of neuralgia.

Triglyceride "Human fat", an ester of glycerol and three fatty acids.

Trigone A triangular area.

Trigone of the bladder The triangular space on the floor of the bladder, between the ureteric openings and the urethral orifice.

Trigonitis Inflammation of mucous membrane of the trigone of bladder.

Trihexyphenidyl hydrochloride An anticholinergic drug used in parkinsonism.

Tri-iodothyronine T_3, the active form of thyroid hormone.

Trikates A mixture of potassium acetate, potassium bicarbonate and potassium citrate.

Trilabe A three pronged forceps for removing foreign body from bladder.

Trilaminar Three layered.

Trilobate Having three lobes.

Trilocular Having three compartments.

Trilogy A series of three events.

Trimeprazine A sedative drug used for preoperative medication, in the treatment of pruritus and to sedate children.

Trimester A period of 3 months.

First trimester of pregnancy The first 3 months during which rapid development is taking place.

Trimetazidine Antianginal coronary vasodilator.

Trimethadione An anticonvulsant.

Trimethaphan Ganglion blocking agent used for treatment of hypertension.

Trimethobenzamide An anti-emetic drug.

Trimethoprim Anti-bacterial agent used for urinary tract infection; when combined with sulfamethoxazole causes sequential block in enzyme synthesis within a wide range of bacteria.

Trimethylaminuria A rare genetic disorder that causes a strong body odor due to the inability to process trimethylamine. Also known as fish odor syndrome.

Trimethylene Cyclopropane, the general anesthetic agent.

Trimipramine An antidepressant drug used particularly when anxiety and insomnia accompany depression.

Trimmer Instrument used to cut and shape things like gingival, dental plaster.

Trimorphous Having three different forms like larva, pupa and adults as in insects.

Trinitroglycerol Nitroglycerin, the vasodilator.

Trinitrophenol *SYN* – Picric acid, reagent.

Trinitrotoluene *SYN* – TNT, an explosive.

Triose A monosaccharide with 3 carbon atoms.

Trioxsalen Agent that induces repigmentation, hence used in vitiligo.

Trip Hallucinatory experience produced by various drugs.

Tripelenaminecitrate An antihistaminic agent.

Tripier's amputation Amputation of toot with part of calcaneous.

Triple response The three basic response of skin to injury like redness, flare and wheal.

Triplet Three children in one pregnancy.

Triplets Three children carried in the uterus at once and born at one labor.

Triploidy Having three supports or legs.

Triplopia A condition in which three images of an object are seen at the same time.

Tripod Having three sets of chromosomes.

Tripolidine hydrochloride An antihistaminic drug.

Tripotassium dicitratobismuthate Bismuth compound used in peptic ulcer.

Triptorelin GnRH analog.

Triradiate Radiating in three directions.

Trismus Lockjaw; a tonic spasm of the muscles of the jaw.

Trisomy The presence of an extra chromosome in each cell in addition to the normal paired set of 46. The cause of several chromosome disorders including Down's syndrome and Klinefelter's syndrome.

T13 Trisomy of chromosome 13 manifest with hypertelorism, low set ears, mental retardation and death during infancy.

T21 Down's syndrome with simian crease, sloping forehead, epicanthic folds, Brush field's spots, flat nose and mental retardation.

Trisulfapyrimidines A combination of sulfamerazine, sulfamethazine and sulfadiazine.

Tritanopia Blue blindness.

Tritium Heavier form of hydrogen.

Trituration The act of making a substance into powdered form.

Trivalent Combining with or replacing three hydrogen atoms.

Trocar A pointed instrument used with a cannula for performing paracentesis.

Trochanter Either of two bony prominences below the neck of the femur.

Greater trochanter That on the outer side forming the bony prominence of the hip.

Lesser trochanter That on the inner side at the neck of the femur.

Troche Solid cylindrical form containing medicine. SYN – Lozenge.

Trochlea Any pulley-shaped structure, but particularly the fibro cartilage near the inner angular process of the frontal bone through which passes the tendon of the superior oblique muscle of the eye.

Trochlear Relating to nutrition.

Trochlear nerves Those that control the nutrition of a part.

Trochlear ulcer One arising from a failure in the nutrition of apart.

Trombicula A genus of mite that may serve as vectors for various diseases.

Tromethamine *SYN* – THAM. A systemic alkalizer used in lactic acidosis.

Trophic Relating to nutrition of a part particularly when denervated.

Trophoblast The layer of cells surrounding the blastocyst at the time of and responsible for implantation.

Trophocyte The supporting cells of Sertoli which nourish the developing spermatozoa.

Trophology The science of nutrition.

Trophozoite The active mobile feeding state of protozoa.

Tropia A manifest squint, one that is present when both eyes are open.

Tropicamide An anticholinergic drug used for producing mydriasis as 2% lotion.

Tropical Relating to the areas north and south of the equator, termed the tropics.

Tropical medicine That concerned with diseases that are more prevalent in hot climates.

Tropin When suffixed indicates stimulating effect especially of a hormone on target tissue.

Tropism Involuntary response of an organism like turning towards or away from a stimulus.

Tropomyosin A muscle protein involved in the formation of cross bridges during muscle contraction.

Troponin A muscle protein that attaches to actin and myosin. It binds to calcium and inhibits actin-myosin cross bridge formation. Elevated troponin T/I occurs in myocardinal infarction.

Trousseau's sign *A Trousseau, French physician, 1801–1867.* 1. Spontaneous peripheral venous thrombosis. 2. A sign for tetany in which carpal spasm can be elicited by compressing the upper arm and causing ischemia to the nerves distally.

True conjugate (diameter of pelvic inlet) The distance from posterior surface of symphysis pubis to sacral promontory (11 cm).

Truancy Absence of a child from school without leave. A disorder of conduct which may result from emotional insecurity or a feeling of unfairness.

Truncus A trunk; the main part of the body, or a part of it, from which other parts spring.

Truncus arteriosus The arterial trunk connected to the fetal heart which develops into the aortic and pulmonary arteries.

Trunk The main stem of lymphatic, nerve or blood vessel.

Truss An apparatus in the form of a belt with a pressure pad for retaining a hernia in place after reduction.

Trypanosoma A genus of protozoan parasites, which pass some of their life cycle in the blood of vertebrates, including humans.

T. gambiense and *T. rhodesiense* are transmitted by the bite of the tsetse fly, and are the causes of sleeping sickness.

Trypanosomiasis A disease caused by infestation with *Trypanosoma.* Sleeping sickness.

Tryparsamide An arsenic compound used in sleeping sickness.

Trypsin A digestive enzyme that converts protein into amino acids.

Trypsinogen The precursor of trypsin. It is secreted in the pancreatic juice and activated by the enterokinase of the intestinal juices into trypsin.

Tryptophan One of the essential amino acids.

Tsetse fly A fly of the genus *Glossina* which transmits the parasite *Trypanosoma* to humans, causing trypanosomiasis.

TSH Thyroid-stimulating hormone.

Tsutsugamushi disease Scrub typhus, which occurs in Japan and is transmitted by the bite of a mite.

Tubal Relating to a tube.

Tubal ligation Tying of the fallopian tubes as a method of female sterilization.

Tubal pregnancy Extrauterine pregnancy where the embryo develops in the uterine tube. Ectopic pregnancy.

Tube feeding Administration of liquid and semisolid foods through a nasogastric, gastrostomy or enterostomy tube. Tube feeds are administered to patients who are unable to take foods by mouth.

Tubectomy Surgical removal of a part or whole of fallopian tube.

Tubegauz A proprietary brand of woven circular bandage applied with a special applicator.

Tuber A swelling or enlargement.

Tuber cinereum A part of base of hypothalamus connected to posterior lobe of pituitary by an infundibulum.

Tubercle 1. A small nodule or a rounded prominence on a bone. 2. The specific lesion (a small nodule) produced by the tubercle bacillus.

Tubercular Pertaining to tubercles.

Tuberculin The filtrate from a fluid medium in which *Mycobacterium tuberculosis* has been grown and which contains its toxins.

Old tuberculin Prepared from the human bacillus and used in skin tests in diagnosing tuberculosis *(See Mantoux test and Heaf test).*

Tuberculin test A test to know if a patient has been exposed to tubercle bacilli in the past. 5 or 10 TU is injected intradermally and induration is measured after 72 hours. When induration exceeds 10 × 10 mm the test is termed positive.

Tuberculoma A tuberculous abscess.

Tuberculum A small eminence.

Tuberculum adductor A projection from medial condyle of femur to which abductor magnus is attached.

Tuberculum dental Elevation on crown of a tooth due to excess enamel formation.

Tuberculosis An infectious, inflammatory, notifiable disease, produced by the tubercle bacillus

Mycobacterium tuberculosis, that is chronic in nature.

Bovine tuberculosis A form found in cattle and spread by infected milk.

Miliary tuberculosis A severe form with small tuberculous lesions spread throughout the body and severe toxemia.

Open tuberculosis Any type of tuberculosis in which the organisms are being excreted from the body.

Pulmonary tuberculosis That affecting the lungs; also termed phthisis.

Tuberculosis of the spine Pott's disease.

T

Tuberosity An elevation or protuberance on a bone to which tendons are attached.

Tuberous Covered with tubers.

Tuberous sclerosis A familial disease with tumors on the surfaces of the lateral ventricles of the brain and sclerotic patches on its surface; marked by mental deterioration and epileptic attacks.

Tubocurarine A preparation of curare used to secure skeletal muscle relaxation.

Tubo-ovarian Relates to fallopian tube and the ovary.

Tuboplasty Plastic surgery or repair of fallopian tubes in order to restore fertility.

Tubule A small tube.

Renal or *uriniferous tubule* The essential secreting tube of the kidney.

Tubulin A protein present in the microtubules of cell.

Tubulodermoid A dermoid tumor in the persistent remnant tubular structure.

Tuft A small coiled mass or cluster.

Tugging Drag or pull e.g., tracheal tug, the sign of aortic aneurysm.

Tularemia A plague-like disease of rodents, caused by *Francisella (Pasteurella) tularensis*, which is transmissible to humans. The illness can be contracted by handling diseased animals or their hides, eating infected wild game or being bitten by insects that have fed on infected animals. It causes fever and headache; the lymph glands enlarge and may suppurate.

Tumefaction A swelling or the process of becoming swollen. Tumescence.

Tumescence 1. A swelling or enlarging of a part. 2. A swollen condition. 3. A penile erection.

Tumor An abnormal swelling. The term is usually applied to a morbid growth of tissue which may be benign or malignant. A neoplasm.

Benign or innocent tumor One that does not infiltrate or cause metastases, and is unlikely to recur if removed.

Malignant tumor One that invades and destroys tissue, and can spread to neighboring tissues, and to more distant sites via the blood and the lymphatic systems.

Tumor angiogenesis factor A protein factor present in all cancerous tissue which stimulates capillary growth.

Tumoricidal Having killing effect on tumor cells.

Tumor markers Certain substances present in blood that indicate possible presence of malignancy, e.g., carcinoembryonic antigen in tumors of colon, lungs and breast; alfa-fetoprotein in hepatoma, acid phosphatase in prostatic malignancy.

Tumor necrosis factor A lymphokine produced by macrophages.

Tumor viruses Viruses causing malignant neoplasms, e.g., EB virus linked to Burkitt's lymphoma; HSV_2 in cancer cervix, AIDS virus in Kaposi sarcoma.

Tunga A genus of fleas.

Tungsten A metallic element used in X-ray tube.

Tunica A coat, a covering, or the lining of a vessel.

Tunica adventitia, Tunica media, Tunica intima The outer, middle and inner coats of an artery, respectively.

Tunica vaginalis The membrane covering the front and sides of the testis.

Tuning fork A metal instrument used for testing hearing by means of the sounds produced by its vibration.

Tunnel In anatomy, a canal through a structure.

Carpal tunnel The osteofibrous channel in the wrist between the carpal bones and tissue covering the flexor tendons.

Carpal tunnel syndrome Pain and tingling in the hand and fingers caused by compression of the median nerve in the carpal tunnel.

Tunnel vision Vision that is restricted to the central field. Occurs in chronic glaucoma and in retinitis pigmentosa.

Tuohy needle A needle used for inserting epidural catheters. It is slightly curved at the end.

Turbid Cloudy.

Turbidity The quality of not having transparency of liquid due to contamination of suspended particles.

Turbinate Scroll-shaped.

Turbinate bone One of the three long thin plates that form the walls of the nasal cavity.

Turgid Swollen or distended.

Turner syndrome *H.H. Turner, American physician, 1892-1970.* A chromosomal defect in females, causing short stature. Classically, an absence of one X chromosome and affects 1 in 2000 live female births. The majority have streak ovaries (a form of ovarian dysgenesis) leading to an absence of puberty and infertility. Other features may include webbing of the neck, cubitus valgus, nail abnormalities and coarctation of the aorta. Intelligence is usually normal.

Turpentine A pine plant derivative containing mixture of terpenes and other hydrocarbon used in liniments and counter irritants.

Tutamen Tissue with protective action, e.g., tutamen oculi, i.e., eyebrows, eyelashes, etc.

Tutamen wave The positive or negative wave representing repolarization of heart muscle in electrocardiogram.

Twig A final branch of a nerve or vessel.

Twilight sleep A state of partial anesthesia where perception of pain is greatly reduced.

Twilight state Partial disturbance of consciousness, a state that may follow an epileptic fit and may be associated with alcoholism and some confusional states. The person can still carry out some routine activities but has no awareness or memory of doing so.

Twin One of a pair of individuals who have developed in the uterus together.

Binovular (dizygotic) twin Each twin has developed from a separate ovum; fraternal twins.

Uniovular (monozygotic) twin Both twins have developed from the same cell; identical twins.

Twitch Sudden spasmodic muscle contraction.

Tyloxapol A detergent used to reduce viscosity of bronchopulmonary secretions.

Tympanic membrane Membrane at the junction middle ear and external ear.

Tympanectomy Excision of the tympanic membrane.

Tympanites Distension of the abdomen by accumulation of gas in the intestine or the peritoneal cavity.

Tympanitis Inflammation of the middle ear; otitis media.

Tympanography Radiographic examination of Eustachian tubes and middle ear after introducing contrast material.

Tympanometry Procedure for objective evaluation of mobility of tympanic membrane and diagnosis of middle ear diseases.

Tympanoplasty An operation to reconstruct the eardrum and restore conductivity to the middle ear. Myringoplasty.

Tympanosclerosis Fibrosis and the formation of calcified deposits in the middle ear, which lead to deafness.

Tympano sclerosis Fibrosis and the formation of calcified deposits in the middle ear which lead to deafness.

T

Tympanum 1. The middle ear. 2. The eardrum or tympanic membrane.

Tympany 1. Abdominal distension with gas. 2. Tympanic resonance on percussion.

Type The general or prevailing character of any particular case of disease, person/substance, etc.

Asthenic type A type of physical constitution, with long limbs, small trunk, flat chest and weak muscles.

Athletic type A type of physical constitution with broad shoulders, deep chest, flat abdomen, thick neck and good muscular development. *Blood type Blood* group.

Phage type A subgroup of a bacterial species susceptible to a particular bacteriophage and demonstrated by phage typing *(See Phage)*. Also called lysotype and phagotype.

Pyknic type A type of physical constitution marked by rounded body, large chest, thick shoulders, broad head and short neck.

Type A behavior A behavior pattern associated with the development of coronary heart disease, characterized by excessive competitiveness and aggression and a fast-paced lifestyle. Research has shown that this type of behavior is associated with coronary artery disease and myocardial infarction. The opposite type of behavior, exhibited by individuals who are relaxed, unhurried and less aggressive, is called type B and is associated with a lower risk of heart disease.

Typhlectomy Excision of cecum.

Typhlitis Inflammation of cecum.

Typhlology Study of blindness and its causes.

Typhlopexy Suturing of movable cecum to anterior abdominal wall.

Typhloureterostomy Implantation of ureters into cecum.

Typhoid fever Enteric fever. A notifiable infectious disease caused by *Salmonella typhi,* which is transmitted by water, milk or other foods, especially shellfish, that have been contaminated. There is high fever, a red rash, delirium and sometimes intestinal hemorrhage. Recovery usually begins during the fourth week of the disease. A person who has had typhoid fever gains immunity from it but may become a carrier. Although perfectly well, the person harbours the bacteria and passes them out in the feces. The typhoid bacillus often lodges in the gallbladder of carriers.

Typhoid vaccine Vaccine containing killed *Salmonella typhi.*

Typhus An acute, notifiable, infectious disease caused by species of the parasitic microorganism *Rickettsia.* There is high fever, a widespread red rash and severe headache. Typhus is likely to occur where there is overcrowding, lack of personal cleanliness and bad hygienic conditions, because the infection is spread by bites of infected lice or by rat fleas.

Scrub typhus A form spread by mites and widespread in the Far East. Tsutsugamushi disease.

Typing Identification of types, e.g., 1. Bacteriophage typing, i.e., determination of bacterial species by bacteriophages. 2. Tissue typing, i.e., testing for histocompatibility of tissues to be used in transplant or graft.

Tyramine An enzyme present in cheese, broad-bean pods, yeast extracts, wine and strong beer, which has a similar effect in the body to that of adrenaline. Foodstuffs containing tyramine should be avoided by patients taking monoamine oxidase inhibitors.

Tyrosine An essential amino acid which is the product of phenylalanine metabolism. In some diseases, especially of the liver, it is present as a deposit in the urine. It is a precursor of catecholamines, melanin and thyroid hormones.

Tyrosinemia Increased tyrosine concentration in blood due to deficiency of enzyme tyrosine aminotransferase manifested with mental retardation, keratitis, dermatitis, etc.

Tyrosinosis A congenital condition in which there is an error of metabolism and phenylalanine cannot be reduced to tyrosine. Hepatic failure may occur.

Tyrothricin Antibacterial agent.

Tysons' glands Modified sebaceous glands in prepuce secreting smegma.

Tzanck test Examination of tissue from base of an intact bulla to demonstrate degenerative changes as in pemphigus.

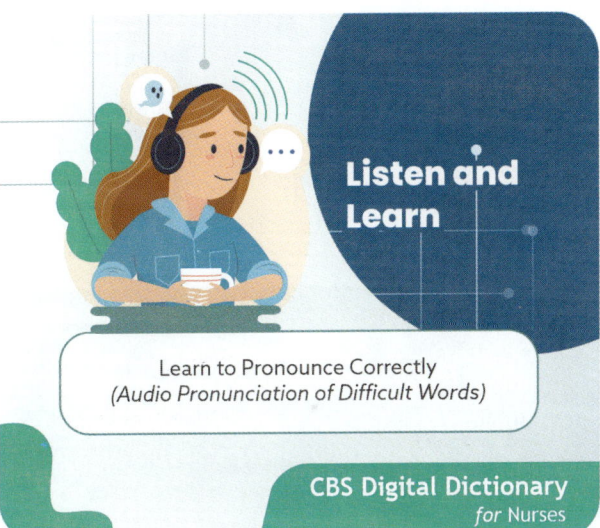

Listen and Learn

Learn to Pronounce Correctly
(Audio Pronunciation of Difficult Words)

CBS Digital Dictionary
for Nurses

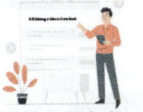

Dil Mange
More Content

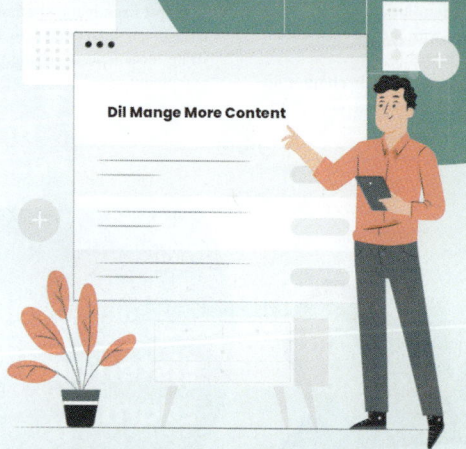

Dil Mange More Content

- Get additional explanations of Important Terminologies
- Word Quiz on Day-To-Day Basis on Scientific and General Terminology (One New Word Every Day with example)
- **50+** Animated & Interactive Videos on various important Topics and Concepts on nursing students' day-to-day interactions/daily needs.
- 4 Hybrid Updates (Every Quarter) covering New Words, Recent Topics & Interactive Videos

CBS Digital Dictionary
for Nurses

UGC University Grants Commission

UIP Universal Immunization Programme

UKCC United Kingdom Central Council for Nursing, Midwifery and Health Visiting.

Ubiquinone Coenzyme Q, important for intracellular respiration.

Ulcer An erosion or loss of continuity of the skin or of a mucous membrane, often accompanied by suppuration.

Decubitus ulcer A pressure sore caused by lying immobile for long periods of time.

Duodenal ulcer A peptic ulcer in the duodenum.

Gastric ulcer One in the lining of the stomach.

Gravitational ulcer A varicose ulcer of the leg which heals with difficulty because of its dependent position and the poor venous return.

Gummatous ulcer One arising in late noninfective syphilis; it is slow to heal.

Indolent ulcer One that is painless and heals slowly.

Peptic ulcer One that occurs on the mucous membrane of either the stomach or duodenum.

Perforating ulcer One that erodes through the thickness of the wall of an organ.

Rodent ulcer A slow-growing epithelioma of the face which may cause much local destruction and ulceration, but does not give rise to metastases. Basal cell carcinoma.

Trophic ulcer One due to a failure of nutrition of a part.

Varicose ulcer Gravitational ulcer.

Ulceration Formation of ulcer on surface such as skin, cornea or mucous membrane.

Ulcerative Characterized by ulceration (the formation of ulcers).

Ulcerative colitis Inflammation and ulceration of the colon and rectum of unknown cause.

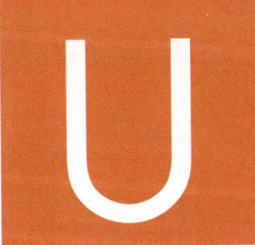

Ulna The inner and larger bone of forearm.

Ultra vires A change made beyond powers. An NHS organization must behave reasonably and in accordance with its powers. If an organization acts beyond its powers (ultra vires), it lays itself open to judicial review.

Ultrafiltration A filtration process that separates colloidal particles from the suspending liquid.

Ultrasonic Relating to sound waves having a frequency range beyond the upper limit perceived by the human ear. These waves are widely used instead of X-rays, particularly in the examination of structures not opaque to X-rays.

Ultrasonogram An echo picture obtained from using ultrasound.

Ultrasonography Radiological technique in which deep structures of the body are visualized by recording the reflections (echoes) of ultrasonic waves directed into the tissues.

Ultrasound Ultrasonic waves used to examine the interior organs of the body. These waves can also be used in the treatment of soft-tissue pain, and to break up renal calculi or the crystalline lens when cataract is present.

Ultrasound screening A method of body imaging based on the reflectivity of sound. Ultrasound scanning is noninvasive and is widely used in obstetrics to detect the site of the placenta, the presence of fetal abnormalities and the sex of the fetus; it will reveal a multiple

pregnancy at an early stage. Also used by other medical disciplines.

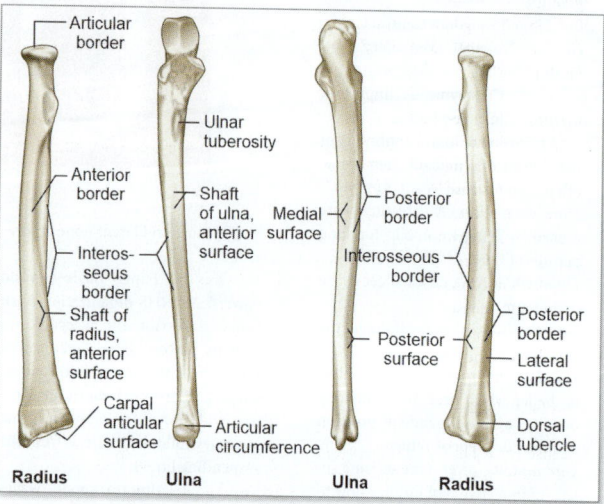

Radius	**Ulna**	**Ulna**	**Radius**

Labels: Articular border, Anterior border, Interosseous border, Shaft of radius, anterior surface, Carpal articular surface, Ulnar tuberosity, Shaft of ulna, anterior surface, Articular circumference, Medial surface, Posterior border, Interosseous border, Posterior surface, Posterior border, Lateral surface, Dorsal tubercle

Ulna

Ultrastructure Structure of tissue as visible only under electron microscope but not to normal eye.

Ultraviolet light Used to promote vitamin D formation and for treatment of certain skin conditions.

Ultraviolet rays Short wavelength electromagnetic rays. They are present in sunlight and cause tanning and sunburn.

Ultraviolet therapy Treatment with ultraviolet radiation.

Umbilical cord Arises from the placenta and enters the fetus at the site of the future navel, providing the nutritional, hormonal and immunological link between mother and fetus during pregnancy.

Umbilication Formation at the apex of a vesicle or pustule a depression (e.g., in small pox), any depression resembling the navel.

Umbilicus The navel; the circular depressed scar in the center of the abdomen where the umbilical cord of the fetus was attached.

Umbo Projecting center of a round surface.

Umbrella filter A filter placed in a vein to prevent passage of emboli as in prevention of pulmonary infarction in deep vein thrombosis.

Uncal herniation Transtentorial herniation of uncus.

Unciform Shaped like a hook.

Unciform fasciculus The bundle of fibers connecting frontal lobes with temporal lobes (uncinate fasiculus).

Unciform process Anterior end of hippocampal gyrus.

Uncinate Hook shaped

Uncinate bundle of Russel Fibers from cerebellum passing into vestibular nuclei via superor cerebellar peduncle.

U

Uncinate fits Periodic episodes of olfactory and gustatory hallucinations usually disagreeable or loss of taste and smell.

Uncinate gyrus Rostral portion of hippocampal gyrus.

Unconditioned response An unlearned response, i.e., one that occurs naturally.

Unconscious 1. Insensible; incapable of responding to sensory stimuli and of having subjective experiences. 2. Part of mental activity which includes primitive or repressed wishes, concealed from consciousness by the psychological censor.
Collective unconscious In Jungian psychology, the portion of the unconscious which is theoretically common to human beings.

Unconsciousness The state of being unconscious. This may vary in depth from deep unconsciousness, when no response can be obtained, through to lesser degrees of unconsciousness when the patient can be roused by painful stimuli, to a level when the patient can be roused by speech or non-painful stimuli. Deep prolonged unconsciousness is known as coma.

Uncus Hooked anterior end of hippocampal gyrus.

Undecylenic acid An antifungal agent used in the treatment of such infections as athlete's foot. May be used in powder, ointment, lotion or spray form.

Undernutrition Malnutrition occurring either due to inadequate food intake or body's inability to utilize the nutrients.

Underweight Weight more than 1-0% less than the ideal weight for height and age.

Undine A glass flask with a spout used for irrigation of the eye.

Undine curse Sleep apnea.

Undulant Rising and falling like a wave.
Uudulant fever (See Brucellosis).

Undulation Continuous wave like motion or pulsation.

Ungual Resembling nails.

Unguentum An ointment.

Unicorn Having a single horn or cornu as in uterus.

Unicuspid Having a single cusp, e.g., tooth or valve.

Uniform resource locator Abbreviated URL. Commonly informally referred to as a web address used in the location of a specific website.

Unilateral On one side only.

Uninucleated Having a single nucleus.

Uniocular Pertains to one eye.

Union 1. A joining together. 2. The repair of tissue after separation by incision or fracture *(See Callus and Healing).*

Uniovular From one ovum.
Uniovular twins Identical twins, developed from one ovum.

Unipara A woman who has had only one child.

Unipolar Having a single process, e.g., unipolar neurone.

Unit 1. A single thing. 2. A standard of measurement.
Intensive care unit A hospital department reserved for those with severe medical or surgical disorders.
International insulin unit A measurement of the pure crystalline insulin arrived at by biological assay.
SI unit One of the various units of measurement making up the système International d' Unités *(International System of Units).*

Univalent Capable of combining with or replacing one atom of hydrogen.

Universal antidote Two parts of activated charcoal, one part magnesium oxide and one part tannic acid used in poisoning by unknown agents by oral route.

U

Universal cuff An adaptive device fitted on the palm to hold items such as utensils when normal grasp is not present.

Universal donor A person of blood group 'O' Rh-ve

Universal precautions Abbreviated UP. A concept developed by nurse during the mid-1980s (largely as a response to human immunodeficiency virus, or HIV, epidemics) that assumes all patients are potentially infected with blood-borne viruses; consequently, universal blood and body fluid infection control precautions are used for all patients, all the time. This concept has been further developed and is known as standard precautions.

Universal recipient A person of blood group AB, Rh positive.

Unmedullated A nerve without myelin sheath. SYN-unmyelinated.

Unna's paste 15% Zinc oxide in glycogelatin base.

Unsaturated Not combined to the full extent or capable of dissolving or absorbing more.

Upper motor neuron lesion Damage to corticospinal or pyramidal tracts in the brain or spinal cord causing paraplegia, hemiplegia or quadriplegia upon location of lesion.

Upper respiratory infection Infection involving nasopharyngeal tissues and bronchi.

Uptake Absorption of nutrient or radioactive material.

Urachal Referring to the urachus.

Urachal cyst A congenital abnormality in which a small cyst persists along the course of the urachus.

Urachal fistula One that forms when the urachus fails to close. Urine may leak from the umbilicus.

Urachus A tubular canal existing in the fetus, connecting the bladder with the umbilicus. In the adult it persists in the form of a solid fibrous cord.

Uracil A pyrimidine base of ribonucleic acids.

Uraemia 1. An excess in the blood of urea, creatinine and other nitrogenous End products of protein and amino acid metabolism; sometimes referred to as azotaemia. 2. In current usage, the entire complex of signs and symptoms of chronic renal failure. Depending upon the cause it may or may not be reversible. Uremia leads to vomiting and nausea, headache, weakness, metabolic disturbances, convulsions and coma *(See Renal (Failure))*.

Uranium A radioactive element.

Urate A salt of uric acid.

Sodium urate A compound generally found in concentration around joints in cases of gout.

Urea Carbamide. A white crystalline substance which is an end-product of protein metabolism and the chief nitrogenous constituent of urine. It is a diuretic. The normal daily output is about 33 g.

Urea cycle The metabolic process of urea formation from metabolism of nitrogen containg foods.

Urea frost Deposits of urea particle on skin in patients of advanced uremia.

Urea plasma A microorganism is sexually transmitted and causes urogenital infection in both partners.

Blood urine That which is present in the blood. Normal value is 20–40 mg/100 mL.

Urease An enzyme that breaks down urea into ammonia and carbondioxide.

Uremia A complex biochemical abnormality in kidney failure, characterized by azotemia, acidosis, anemia and many systemic symptoms.

Uremia prerenal Uremia occurring not primarily due to kidney disease but due to fluid loss.

Ureter One of the two long narrow tubes that convey the urine from the kidney to the bladder.

Ureterectomy The surgical removal of a ureter.

Ureteric Relating to the ureter. *Ureteric catheter (See Catheter).*

Ureteric transplantation An operation in which the ureters are divided from the bladder and implanted in the colon or loop of ileum. Congenital defects or malignant growth may make this necessary.

Ureterocele A cystic enlargement of the wall of the ureter at its entry into the bladder.

Ureteroileostomy Anastomosis of ureter into a segment of small intestine.

Ureterolithiasis Formation of stone in ureter.

Ureterovesicostomy Re-implantation of ureters in bladder.

Ureterolith A calculus in a ureter.

Ureterolithotomy Removal of a calculus from the ureter.

Ureteronephrectomy Surgical removal of a kidney and its ureter.

Ureterostomy The surgical creation of a permanent opening through which the ureter discharges urine.

Ureterovaginal Relating to the ureter and vagina.

Ureterovaginal fistula An opening into the ureter by which urine escapes via the vagina.

Urethane Compound with diuretic, hypnotic and cytostatic properties, often used in leukemia.

Urethra The canal through which the urine is discharged from the bladder. The male urethra is about 18 cm long and the female about 3.5 cm.

Urethritis Inflammation of the urethra. The condition is frequently a symptom of gonorrhea but may be caused by other infectious organisms.

Nonspecific urethritis Abbreviated NSU. A sexually transmitted inflammation of the urethra caused by a variety of organisms other than gonococci *(See Non-specific (Urethritis)).*

Urethrocele A prolapse of the female urethral wall which may result from damage to the pelvic floor during childbirth.

Urethrography Radiographic examination of the urethra. A radiopaque contrast medium is inserted by catheter.

Urethroscope An instrument for examining the interior of the urethra.

Urgency A sudden, irresistible need to urinate.

Uric acid Lithic acid, the end-product of nucleic acid metabolism, a normal constituent of urine. Its accumulation in the blood produces uric acidemia. Renal calculi are frequently formed of it.

Uricase An enzyme present in most mammals excluding man that breaks uric acid into allantoin and carbon dioxide.

Uricemia Excess uric acid in blood.

Uricosuria Excessive excretion of uric acid in urine.

Uricosuric Any drug that promotes the excretion of uric acid in the urine.

Uridine A nucleoside of ribonucleic acids, consisting of uracil and D ribose.

Urinalysis The bacteriological or chemical examination of the urine.

Urinary Relating to urine.

Urinary calculus Concretions formed in urinary passage of calcium carbonate/phosphate/oxalate, uric acid and cystine.

Urinary incontinence Inability to control urination.

Urinary pigments Urochrome, urosilin, uroerythrin and hematoporphyrin.

Urinary retention Inability to empty the bladder of urine.

Urinary sediment Deposits in urine like bacteria, phosphates, uric acid, calcium oxalate/phosphate/carbonate, etc.

Urinary tract The system that conducts urine from the kidneys to the exterior, including the ureters, the bladder and the urethra.

Urinary tract infection Infection involving urethra, bladder, ureter and renal pelvis.

Urination Micturition. The act of passing urine.

Urine The clear fluid of a varying straw colour secreted by the kidneys and excreted through the bladder and urethra. It is composed of 96% water and 4% solid constituents, the most important being urea and uric acid. Specific gravity = 1.003-1.0035; slightly acidic. *Residual u.* that remains in the bladder after micturition. *U. retention* The inability to urinate voluntarily or to empty a full bladder.

Urinoma A cyst containing urine.

Urinometer An instrument used for measuring the specific gravity of urine.

URL Uniform resource locator.

Urobilin The main pigment of urine, derived from urobilinogen.

Urobilinogen A pigment derived from bilirubin which, on oxidation, forms Urobilin.

Urobilinuria Excess of urobilin in the urine.

Urocele Swelling of scrotum with urine.

Urochesia Act of passing urine from the anus.

Urochrome The yellow pigment which colors urine.

Urocyanin A blue pigment in urine in certain diseases like scarlet fever.

Urodynamics The dynamics of the propulsion and flow of urine in the urinary tract.

Urodynia Pain while passing urine.

Uroerythrin A red pigment found in urine.

Uroflavin A fluorescent compound present in persons taking riboflavin.

Urofuscin A red-brown pigment in urine of patients of porphyria.

Urogastrone A polypeptide present in urine that inhibits gastric acid secretion.

Urogenital Relating to the urinary and genital organs. Urinogenital.

Urogenital diaphragm The sheet of tissue stretching across the pubic arch, formed by deep transverse perineal and sphincter urethrae muscles. *SYN* – triangular ligament.

Urogram A radiographic image obtained by urography.

Urography Radiographic examination of the urinary tract after the injection of a radiopaque, water-soluble, iodine containing medium.

Urokinase An enzyme in urine which is secreted by the kidneys and causes fibrinolysis. In certain diseases it may cause bleeding from the kidneys.

Urolith A calculus in the urinary tract.

Urolithiasis Formation of calculi in urinary tract and the associated symptoms thereof.

Urology The study of diseases of the urinary tract.

Uroporphyrin A red pigment present in urine and feces in porphyria.

Urostomy An artificial urinary conduit for deflecting urine from the ureters to the abdominal wall.

Urticaria Nettle-rash or hives. An acute or chronic skin condition characterized by the recurrent appearance of eruption of weals, causing great irritation. The cause may be certain foods, infection, drugs or emotional stress. *(See Allergy)*.

Usher's syndrome Congenital deafness and retinitis pigmentosa progressing to complete blindess.

Uta Infection with *Leishmania brazilliensis* causing nasopharyngeal and mucocutaneous lesions.

Uterine Relating to the uterus.

Uterine soufflé The sound of blood flow in uterine vessels in gravid uterus.

Uterine subinvolution Failure of uterus to return to its normal size after childbirth.

Uterosalpingography Radiographic examination of the uterus and the uterine tubes.

Uterovesical Referring to the uterus and bladder.

Uterivesucal pouch The fold of peritoneum between the two organs.

Uterus The womb; a triangular, hollow, muscle organ situated in the pelvic cavity between the bladder and the rectum. Its function is the nourishment and protection of the fetus during pregnancy and its expulsion at term.

Bicornuate uterus One having two horns. A congenital fallopian tube malformation *(See Bicornuate).*

Gravid uterus The pregnant uterus.

Uterus didelphys A double uterus caused by the failure of union of the two Müllerian ducts from which it is formed.

Utilitarianism A philosophical or ethical view, which holds that utility entails the greatest happiness of the greatest number of people and therefore that an action should always produce more benefits than harm.

Utricle The delicate membranous sac in the bony vestibule of the ear.

Uvea Uveal tract. The pigmented layer of the eye, consisting of the iris, ciliary body and choroid.

Uveitis Inflammation of the uveal tract.

Uveoparotitis Inflammation of uvea and parotid glands as in sarcoidosis.

Uviometer An instrument for measuring the intensity of ultraviolet light.

Uvula The small fleshy appendage which is the free edge of the soft palate, hanging from the roof of the mouth.

Uvulotome Instrument for performing uvulotomy.

U wave A low-amplitude positive wave that follows T-wave in ECG. U-wave inversion indicates coronary artery disease.

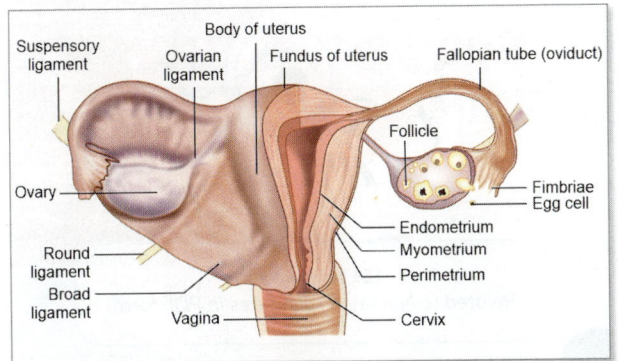

Uterus

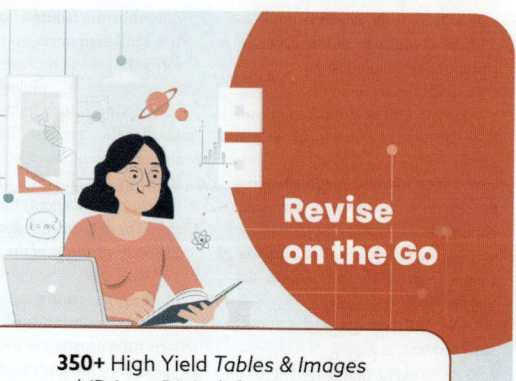

Revise on the Go

350+ High Yield *Tables & Images covered (Print + Digital) for Quick Reference*

CBS Digital Dictionary
for Nurses

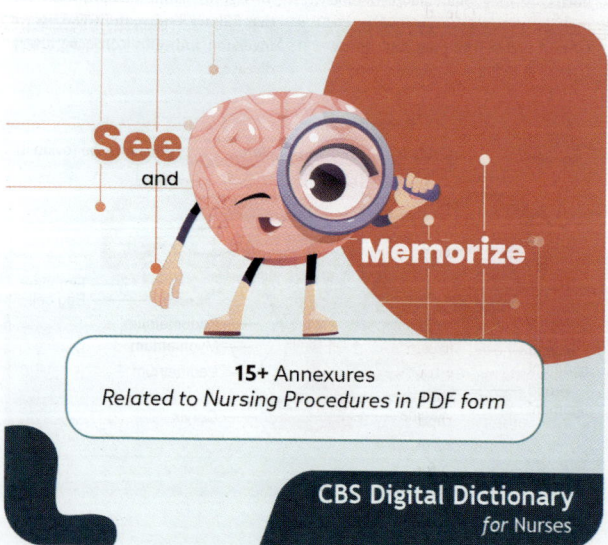

See and Memorize

15+ Annexures
Related to Nursing Procedures in PDF form

CBS Digital Dictionary
for Nurses

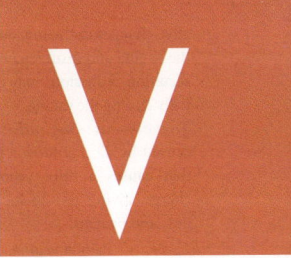

Vaccination The introduction of vaccine into the body to produce immunity to a specific disease.

Vaccine A suspension of killed or attenuated organisms (viruses, bacteria and rickettsiae), administered for prevention, amelioration or treatment of infectious diseases.

Attenuated vaccine One prepared from living organisms which, through long cultivation, have lost their virulence.

Bacille Calmette Guerin vaccine An attenuated bovine bacillus vaccine giving immunity from tuberculosis.

Sabin vaccine An attenuated poliovirus vaccine that can be administered by mouth, in a syrup or on sugar.

Salk vaccine One prepared from an inactivated strain of poliomyelitis virus.

TAB vaccine A sterile solution of the organisms that cause typhoid and paratyphoid A and B. Paratyphoid C may now be included.

Triple vaccine One that protects against diphtheria, tetanus and whooping cough.

Pentavalent vaccine Is a conjugate vaccine that protects against five major infections in one shot: Diphtheria, pertusis, tetanus, hepatitis B and haemophilus influenza type b (Hib). Route of administration - intramuscular

Vaccine therapy A therapy in which infectious organisms, particles, or antigens are injected in body to develop immunity against a disease.

Vaccinia Cowpox; a virus infection of cows, which may be transmitted to humans by contact with the lesions. A local pustular eruption is produced. Also known as cowpox.

Vacuole A clear space in the cell protoplasm.

Vacuum A space from which air or gas has been extracted.

Vacuum extractor An instrument known as a ventouse is used to assist delivery of the fetus. A suction cup is attached to the head and a vacuum created slowly. Gentle traction is applied, which is synchronized with the uterine contractions.

Vacuum aspiration A method of termination of pregnancy by applying suction to a catheter placed in uterine cavity.

Vagabond's disease Body louse infection causing itching and skin discoloration.

Vagal Relating to the vagus nerve.

Vagal tone Cardiac inhibitory effect by vagus.

Vagina The canal, lined with mucous membrane, that leads from the cervix of the uterus to the vulva.

Vaginal bulb Small erectile tissue on each side of vestibule.

Vaginal hysterectomy Surgical removal of uterus through vagina.

Vaginal lubricant An ointment or cream which is used for reduction of dryness in vagina.

Vaginal vibrator A vibrator placed in vagina for erotic stimulation.

Vaginismus A painful spasm of the muscles of the vagina, occurring usually when the vulva or vagina is touched, resulting in painful sexual intercourse or dyspareunia.

Vaginitis Inflammation of the vagina.

Atrophic or *postmenopausal vaginitis.* Inflammation caused by degenerative changes in the mucous lining of the vagina and insufficient oestrogen secretion. Adhesions may occur, partially closing the vagina.

Trichomonas vaginitis Infection caused by *T. vaginalis*, a protozoon that causes a thin, yellowish discharge, giving rise to local tenderness and pruritis.

Vaginodynia Pain in vagina.

Vaginoplasty Plastic surgery of the vagina.

Vagitus First cry of newborn child.

Vagotomy Surgical incision of the vagus nerve or any of its branches. A treatment for gastric or duodenal ulcer.

Highly selective vagotomy Division of only those vagal fibers supplying the acid-secreting glands of the stomach.

Medical vagotomy Interruption of impulses carried by the vagus nerve by administration of suitable drugs.

Vagus The tenth cranial nerve, arising in the medulla and providing the parasympathetic nerve supply to the organs in the thorax and abdomen.

Vagus resection Vagotomy.

Valacyclovir L-valyl ester of acyclovir, antiviral for herpes.

Valdecoxib Anti-inflammatory, analgesic.

Valenthamate Uterine relaxant.

Valgus A displacement outwards, particularly of the feet *(See Genu, Hallux, Talipes).*

Validity The extent to which a measure, indicator or method of data collection possesses the quality of being sound or true, as far as can be judged.

Valine An essential amino acid formed by the digestion of dietary protein.

Valium Trade name for the preparation of diazepam, an anxiolytic and skeletal muscle relaxant.

Valproic acid Anticonvulsant.

Valsalva's manoeuvre *AM Valsalva, Italian anatomist, 1666–1723.* Technique for increasing the intrathoracic pressure by closing the mouth and nostrils and blowing out the cheeks, thereby forcing air back into the nasopharynx. When the breath is released, the intrathoracic pressure drops and the blood is quickly propelled through the heart, producing an increase in the heart rate (tachycardia) and the blood pressure. Immediately after this event a reflex bradycardia ensues. Valsalva's manoeuvre occurs when a person strains to defecate or urinate, uses the arm and upper trunk muscles to move up in bed, or strains during coughing, gagging or vomiting. The increased pressure, immediate tachycardia and reflex bradycardia can bring about cardiac arrest in vulnerable heart patients.

Valsalva sinuses The dilatations in the root of aorta behind the semilunar cusps where the coronary arteries originate.

Valsartan ACE receptor inhibitor.

Valve 1. A means of regulating the flow of liquid or gas through a pipe. 2. A fold of membrane in a passage or tube, so placed as to permit passage of fluid in one direction only. Valves are important structures in the heart, in veins and in lymph vessels.

Semilunar valve Either of two valves at the junction of the pulmonary artery and aorta, respectively, with the heart.

Valves of Houston Mucosal folds of recturm.

Valve ileocecal Valve between ileum and large intestine (cecum) composed of two membranous folds.

Valvethebesian Valves at the entrance of coronary sinus into right atrium.

Valvoplasty Dilatation of valve.

Valvotomy Valvulotomy. A surgical operation to open up a fibrosed valve, e.g., mitral valvotomy to relieve mitral stenosis.

Valvulae conniventes Circular membranous folds in the lumen of small intestine that retard the passage of food thereby promoting absorption of nutrients. *SYN*–plica circularis.

Valvulitis Inflammation of a valve, particularly of the heart.

Vancomycin An antibiotic highly effective against Gram-positive bacteria, especially staphylococci. The toxic effects are quite severe and may include damage to the eighth cranial (vestibulocochlear) nerve, and renal disorders.

Vancomycin hydrochloride Antibiotic, 1-2 g daily, specific for resistant staphylococcal infection.

Vanguard Sites across England where new models of care are tested.

Van den Bergh's test Blood test for detection of bilirubin.

Vanilla Obtained from tropical orchid, an aromatic substance used for flavoring.

Vanilylmandelic acid (VMA) Metabolite of epinephrine and norepinephrine in urine, amount increased in pheochromocytoma.

Vapor Gaseous state of a substance.

Vaporizer An apparatus for producing a very fine spray of a liquid.

Variable In social research, a characteristic which can be measured and which may vary along a continuum (e.g., recording of foot size in a population being studied), be more discrete (e.g., in family size) or be bipolar (e.g., sex).

Variance Used in statistics. The distribution range of a set of results around a mean. *(See Standard Deviation).*

Variant Having some different characteristic from the original.

Varicella Chicken pox. An infectious disease of childhood with an incubation period of 12–20 days. There is slight fever and an eruption of transparent vesicles in the chest, on the first day of disease; these appear in successive crops all over the body. The vesicles soon dry up, sometimes leaving shallow pits in the skin. The disease is usually mild, but may be severe in neonates, adults and those who are immune-compromised. Chicken pox is a notifiable disease.

Varicella zoster virus Abbreviated VZV. A human herpes virus that causes chickenpox during childhood and may reactivate later in life to cause shingles.

Varicella-zoster immune globulin An immunoglobulin isolated from human volunteers with high antibody titer against varicella-zoster virus.

Varices Alternative name for enlarged.

Varicocele Dilated pampiniform plexus in the spermatic cord, commonly on left side, feeling like a bag of worms.

Varicose Swollen or dilated.

Varicose ulcer Gravitational ulcer *(See Ulcer)*

Varicose veins A dilated and twisted condition of the veins (usually those of the leg) caused by structural changes in the walls or valves of the vessels.

Varicosity The condition of varicose.

Varicotomy Excision of varicose vein.

Variola Small pox.

Varix An enlarged or varicose vein.

Varus A displacement inwards *(See Genu, Hallux, Talipes).*

Vas Pl. vasa. A vessel or duct.

Vas deferens One of a pair of excretory ducts conveying the semen from the epididymis to the urethra.

Vas efferens One of the many small tubes that convey semen from the testis to the epididymis.

Vasa vasorum The minute nutrient vessels that supply the walls of the arteries and veins.

Vascular Relating to, or consisting largely of, blood vessels.

Vascular system The cardiovascular system.

Vascularization The development of new blood vessels within a tissue.

Vascular ring A form of congenital anomaly where an arterial ring surrounds trachea and esophagus often causing compression.

Vasculature The arrangement and interrelationship of blood vessels.

Vasculitis Angiitis; inflammation of a blood vessel.

Allergic vasculitis A severe allergic response to drugs or to cold. Arising in small arteries or veins, with fibrosis and thrombi formation.

Vasculopathy Any disease of blood vessels.

Vasectomy Excision of a part of the vas deferens. If performed bilaterally, sterility results. Employed as a method of contraception.

Vasoactive Causing either constriction or dilation of blood vessels.

Vasoactive intestinal polypeptide A peptide of GI tract that inhibits gastric acid secretion but promotes intestinal secretion, excess secretion causing diarrhea.

Vasoconstrictor Any agent that causes contraction of a blood vessel and therefore a decrease in the blood flow and a rise in the blood pressure.

Vasodepressor An agent that depresses circulation, i.e., lowers blood pressure by dilating blood vessels.

Vasodilator Any agent that causes an increase in the lumen of blood vessels and therefore an increase in the blood flow and a fall in the blood pressure.

Vasointestinal polypeptide A gut hormone increasing gut motility and secretion.

Vasomotor Controlling the muscles of blood vessels, both dilator and constrictor.

Vasomotor center Nerve cells in the medulla oblongata controlling the vasomotor nerves.

Vasomotor nerves Sympathetic nerves regulating the tension of the blood vessels.

Vasomotor system Part of the nervous system which controls the constriction or dilation of blood vessels.

Vasopressin Antidiuretic hormone (ADH). A hormone from the posterior lobe of the pituitary gland which causes constriction of plain muscle fibers and reabsorption of water in the renal tubules. Used in the treatment of diabetes insipidus and bleeding from esophageal varices.

Vasopressor Agent bringing about contraction of blood vessels.

Vasovagal Vascular and vagal.

Vasovagal attack Fainting or syncope, often evoked by emotional stress associated with tear and pain. There is postural hypotension.

Vasovagal syncope Sudden fainting due to hypotension caused by emotional stress, pain or trauma.

Vasovasostomy Rejoining of torn vas deferens of testis.

Vastus Large or great; one of the three muscles of the thigh.

VDU Visual display unit.

Vector 1. An animal that carries organisms or parasites from one host to another, either to a member of the same species or to one of another species. 2. A quantity with magnitude and direction.

Electrocardiographic vector The area of the heart that is monitored during electrocardiographic investigation.

Vecturonium A muscle relaxant used in general anesthesia.

Vegan A vegetarian who excludes all animal protein from the diet.

Vegetarian A person who eats only food of vegetable origin.

Vegetarian diet One in which no meat is eaten. A lactovegetarian diet prohibits the intake of meat, poultry, fish and eggs. An ovo-lactovegetarian diet allows any foods from plants plus eggs, milk and other dairy products. An ovovegetarian diet allows eggs and foods of plant origin, but prohibits all animal and dairy products.

Vegetation In pathology, a plant-like outgrowth.

Adenoid vegetation Overgrowth of lymphoid tissue in the nasopharynx.

Vegetative Quiscent, passive.

Vehicle In pharmacy, a substance or medium in which a drug is administered.

Vein A vessel carrying blood from the capillaries back to the heart. It has thin walls and a lining endothelium from which the venous valves are formed.

Velamentous Expanding like a veil or sheet.

Velamentum Membranous covering.

Vellus The fine hair left on the body after the lanugo hair disappear in the newborn.

Velpeau's bandage A special form of roller bandage incorporating shoulder, arm and forearm.

Vemer A thin plate of bone forming the posterior septum of the nose.

Veneer In dentistry, materials like acrylic resin which is bonded to surface of tooth.

Venepuncture The insertion of a needle into a vein for the introduction of a drug or fluid or for the withdrawal of blood.

Venereal Pertaining to or caused by sexual intercourse.

Venereal disease A disease transmitted by sexual intercourse or other genital contact. The term venereal disease (VD) is being replaced by the term Sexually Transmitted Infection (STI).

Venereal wart Moist reddish elevations on genitals and anus.

Venereologist A specialist of study of the causes and treatments of sexually transmitted diseases.

Venereology The study and treatment of venereal diseases.

Venesection Phlebotomy. Surgical blood-letting by opening a vein or introducing a wide-bore needle. Performed on blood donors and occasionally to relieve venous congestion.

Venipuncture Puncture of a vein for drawing out blood or introducing any substance.

Venlafaxine Antidepressant.

Venogram 1. A graphic recording of the pulse in a vein. 2. A radiograph taken during venography.

Venography Radiographic examination of a vein after the instillation of a contrast medium to trace its pathway.

Venom A poison secreted by an insect, snake or other animal. *Russell's viper venom* The venom of the Russell viper *(Vipera ruselli)* which acts in vitro as an intrinsic thromboplastin and is useful in defining deficiencies of clotting factor X.

Venemous Poisonous.

Venoocclusive Pertains to obstruction of veins, e.g., veno-occulsive disease of liver.

Venotomy Act of making incision in vein.

Venous Pertaining to the similar to veins. *Venous sinus* One of 14 channels, similar to veins, by which blood leaves the cerebral circulation. *Venous hum* A continuous murmur heard on veins of neck.

Vent An opening in any cavity.

Ventilation 1. The process or act of supplying a house or room continuously with fresh air. 2. In respiratory physiology, the process of exchange of air between the lungs and the ambient air.

Pulmonary ventilation (Usually measured in litres per minute) refers to the total exchange, whereas *alveolar ventilation* Refers to the effective ventilation of the alveoli, where gas exchange with the blood takes place. 3. In psychiatry, the free discussion of one's problems or grievances.

Ventilation coefficient the amount of air that must be respired for each liter of oxygen to be absorbed.

Ventilator An apparatus designed to qualify the air that is breathed through it either intermittently or continuously. Ventilators provide an intermittent flow of air and/or oxygen under pressure and are connected to the patient by a tube inserted through the mouth, the nose or an opening in the trachea.

Ventimask An oxygen mask that provides oxygen enrichment of the inspired air while eliminating the need to re-breathe the expired carbon dioxide.

Ventolin Trade name for a salbutamol metered-dose inhaler; a bronchodilator.

Ventouse *(See Vacuum extractor).*

Ventral Anterior or front side or lower or underneath.

Hernia Hernia through anterior abdominal wall.

Ventricle A small pouch or cavity; applied especially to the lower chambers of the heart and to the four cavities of the brain.

Ventricular Pertaining to a ventricle. *Ventricular folds* The outer folds of mucous membrane forming the false vocal cords.

Ventricular septal defect Abbreviated VSD. Congenital abnormality in which there is communication between the two ventricles of the heart as a result of maldevelopment of the intraventricular septum.

Ventriculitis Inflammation of ependymal lining of cerebral ventricles.

Ventriculoatriostomy Establishment of communication between cerebral ventricle and right atrium by placement of a shunt to treat hydrocephalus.

Ventriculocisternostomy Establishing communication between cerebral ventricle and cistern magna.

Ventriculography 1. Radiographic examination of the ventricles of the heart using a radiopaque contrast medium. 2. Radiographic examination of the ventricles of the brain after the injection of air or a contrast medium through a burr hole.

Ventriculostomy Establishing communication between third ventricle and cistern interpeduncularis to treat hydrocephalus.

Ventrolateral Both ventral and lateral.

Ventromedial Both ventral and medial.

Ventrosuspension Fixation of displaced uterus to anterior abdominal wall.

Venturi mask GB. Venturi, Italian physicist, 1746-1822. A type of disposable mask used to deliver a controlled oxygen concentration to a patient. The flow of 100% oxygen through the mask draws in a controlled amount of room air (21% oxygen). Commonly available masks deliver 24%, 28%, 35%, 40% or 60% oxygen. At concentrations above 24%, humidification may be required.

Venturi nebulizer A type of nebulizer used in aerosol therapy. The pressure drop of gas flowing through the nebulizer draws liquid from a capillary tube. As the liquid enters the gas stream, it breaks up into a spray of small droplets.

Venule A minute vein which collects blood from the capillaries.

Verapamil A coronary dilator used in the treatment of tachycardia and of supraventricular angina pectoris.

Verbigeration The monotonous repetition of phrases or meaningless words.

Verge An edge or margin, e.g., anal verge, i.e., the transitional area between smooth perianal area and the hairy skin.

Verility Sexual potency in male; state of possessing masculine qualities.

Vermicide An agent that destroys intestinal worms; an anthelmintic.

Vermicular Resembling a worm, e.g., vermicular movement.

Vermiform Worm-shaped.

Vermiform appendix The worm-shaped structure attached to the cecum.

Vermifuge An agent that expels intestinal worms; an anthelmintic.

Vermilion border The junction between the skin and oral mucous membrane at the lips.

Vermin Small insects and animals.

Verminous Infested with worms or other animal parasites, such as lice.

Vermination Infestation with worms.

Vermis A worm, median lobe of cerebellum between the lateral lobes.

Vernet's syndrome Paralysis of 9th, 10th and 11th cranial nerves due to injury to jugular foramen.

Vernix [L.] Varnish.

Ver nix caseosa The fatty covering on the skin of the fetus during the last months of pregnancy. It consists of cells and sebaceous material.

Verruca A wart. Hypertrophy of the prickle cell layer of the epidermis and thickening of the horny layer. A virus is the causative organism.

Verruca acuminata A venereal wart that appears on the external genitalia.

Verruca plana A small, smooth, usually skin colored or light-brown, slightly raised wart, sometimes occurring in great numbers; seen most often in children.

Verruca plantaris A viral epidermal tumor on the sole of the foot.

Versicolor Having many colors or change in colors.

Version The turning of a part; applied particularly to the turning of a fetus inorder to facilitate delivery.

External version Manipulation of the uterus through the abdominal wall in order to change the position of the fetus.

Internal version Rotation of the fetus by means of manipulation with one hand in the vagina.

Podalic version Turning of the fetus so that the head is uppermost and the feet presenting.

Spontaneous version One that occurs naturally without the application of force.

Vertebra One of the 33 irregular bones forming the spinal column: 7 cervical, 12 thoracic, 5 lumbar, 5 sacral (sacrum) and 4 coccygeal (coccyx) vertebrae.

Vertebral Pertaining to a vertebra. *Vertebral canal* The cavity within spinal column containing the spinal cord.

Vertebral column The spine or backbone.

Vertebral pedicle The portion of bone projecting backward from each side of body of vertebra and connecting the lamaina with body.

Vertebrobasilar Pertaining to the vertebral and the basilar arteries.

Vertebrobasilar disease A condition affecting the flow of blood through the vertebral and basilar arteries which may cause recurrent attacks of blindness, diplopia, vertigo, dysarthria and hemiparesis.

Vertebrate Those having a vertebral column.

Vertex The crown of the head.

Vertex presentation Position of the fetus such that the crown of the head appears in the vagina first.

Vertical Perpendicular to the horizontal plane, upright.

Side view   Back view

C1
C2
C3
C4
C5
C6
C7 — 7 Cervical vertebrae
T1
T2
T3
T4
T5
T6
T7
T8 — 12 Thoracic vertebrae
T9
T10
T11
T12
L1
L2
L3 — 5 Lumbar vertebrae
L4
L5
Sacrum 5 fused vertebrae
Coccyx (3 fused vertebrae)

Vertebral Column

Vertical transmission Transmission of an infection from an infected mother to her newborn child during pregnancy, delivery or in the postpartum period through breast milk. Also called perinatal or mother-to-child transmission.

Vertiginous Afflicted with vertigo.

Vertigo A feeling of rotation or of going round, in either oneself or one's surroundings, particularly associated with disease of the cerebellum and the vestibular nerve of the ear. It may occur in diplopia or Meniere's syndrome.

Verumontanum An elevation on the floor or the prostatic urethra where seminal ducts open.

Very Low-density lipoprotein (VLDL) The least dense plasma lipid.

Vesica A bladder.

Vesical Shaped like a bladder.

Vesical reflux Desire to urinate once bladder is distended.

Vesicant Agent that produces blisters.

Vesicle 1. In anatomy, a small bladder, usually containing fluid. 2. A very small blister, usually containing serum.

Seminal vesicle One of a pair of sacs which arise from the vas deferens near the bladder and contain semen.

Vesicoureteric Relating to the urinary bladder and the ureters.

Vesicle reflux The passing of urine backwards up the ureter during micturition. A cause of pyelonephritis in children.

Vesicopustule A vesicle in which pus has formed.

Vesicostomy Surgical opening into bladder.

Vesicouterine pouch Extension of peritoneal cavity downwards between bladder and uterus.

Vesicovaginal Relating to the bladder and vagina *(See Fistula)*.

Vesicular Relating to or containing vesicles.

Vesicular breathing The soft murmur of normal respiration, as heard on auscultation.

Vesicular mole Hydatidiform mole.

Vesiculectomy Partial or complete excision of seminal vesicle.

Vesiculitis Inflammation of a vesicle, particularly the seminal vesicles.

Vesiculogram X-ray of seminal vesicles.

Vessel A tube, duct or canal for conveying fluid, usually blood or lymph.

Vestibular Relating to a vestibule.

Vestibular apparatus The anatomical parts including saccule, utricle, semicircular canals, vestibular nerve and nuclei, concerned with body equilibrium.

Vestibular area A triangular area lateral to sulcus limitans, beneath which lie the terminal nuclei of vestibular nerve.

Vestibular bulbs Two saculated collection of veins lying on either side of vagina homologous to make corpus spongiosum.

Vestibular glands Those in the vestibule of the vagina, including Bartholin's glands.

Vestibular nerve A branch of the auditory nerve supplying the semicircular canals and concerned with balance and equilibrium.

Vestibule A space or cavity at the entrance to another structure.

Vestibule of the ear The cavity at the entrance to the cochlea.

Vestibule of the vagina The space between the labia minora at the entrance to the vagina.

Vestibulocochlear Pertaining to the vestibule of the ear and the cochlea.

Vestibulocochlear nerve The eighth cranial nerve. Also known as the auditory nerve.

Vestigial Rudimentary. Referring to the remains of an anatomical structure which, being of no further use, has atrophied.

Vestige A small incompletely developed structure.

Veterinary Pertains to animal diseases and their treatment.

Viable Capable of independent life.

Viagra A trade name for the oral drug sildenafil citrate, used for the treatment of erectile dysfunction. Viagra increases the man's ability to achieve and maintain a penile erection during sexual stimulation. It is given by mouth and is only available on medical prescription after appropriate assessment.

Vial A small glass bottle for medicines and chemicals.

Vibrator Device that produces vibration and chemicals.

Vibratory sense The ability to perceive vibrations or that transmitted through skin and bone from a vibrating tuning fork.

Vibrio A genus of Gram-negative bacteria, curved and motile by means of flagellae.

Vibrio cholerae That which causes cholera.

Vibrometer 1. A device that produces rapid vibrations of tympanic membrane, a form of massage to treat deafness. 2. Device used to measure vibratory sensation threshold, useful in judging clinical status of peripheral neuropathy.

Vicarious 1. Obtained or undergone at second hand through sympathetic participation in another's experiences. 2. Substituted for another; used when one organ functions instead of another.

Vicarious menstruation Blood loss during menstruation at sites other than vagina like nose, breast.

Vidarabine Antiviral agent effective against herpes simplex and zoster.

Vidian artery Artery passing through pterygoid canal.

Vidian canal A canal in the medial pterygoid plate of sphenoid bone for passage of vidian vessels and nerve.

Vidian nerve A branch from sphenopalatine ganglion.

Vigil Wakefulness.

Vigilant Being attentive, watchful and alert.

Vigor Force or strength of body and mind.

Villiferous Having villi or tuft of hair.

Villus A small finger-like process projecting from a surface. *Chorionic villus (See Chorionic).*

Intestinal villi Those of the mucous membrane of the small intestine, each of which contains a blood capillary and a lacteal.

Vinblastine A vinca alkaloid used as an antineoplastic in the treatment of Hodgkin's disease and testicular germinal cell cancer, usually in combination with other antineoplastic agents.

Vincent's angina *JH Vincent, French physician, 1862–1950 (See Angina).*

Vincristine A vinca alkaloid used as an antineoplastic in the treatment of acute leukaemias, Hodgkin's disease, non-Hodgkin's lymphomas and some solid tumors, usually in combination with other antineoplastic agents.

Vincristine sulfate A cytotoxic agent extracted from plant vinca rosea.

Vindesine Vinca alkaloid, antineoplastic agent.

Vinegar A weak solution of acetic acid.

Vinorelbine Anticancer agent.

Vinyl A plastic material now used extensively for medical equipment.

Vinyl chloride A chemical often causing lung malignancy.

Vinyl ether A short-acting inhalation anesthetic drug used mainly for inducing anesthesia and for minor surgery.

Violaceous Violet, said of a discoloration of skin.

Violent Great force, fierceness.

Viomycin Antibiotic produced by *Streptomyces griseus,* used in tuberculosis.

Vipoma A rare tumor of pancreas secreting vasoactive polypeptide causing diarrhea, achlorhydria.

Virchow cell Lepra cell.

Virchow's node Supraclavicular lymphnode.

Virchow-Robin space Perivascular spaces.

Virchow's angle The angle formed by joining the nasofrontal suture and the most prominent point on superior alveolar process with the line joining the same point and superior border of external auditory meatus.

Viraemia The presence of viruses in the blood.

Virgin Woman who has had no sexual intercourse; uncontaminated, fresh.

Virginity The state of being virgin.

Viricide Destructive to viruses.

Virile reflex Contraction of bulbocavernosus muscle on percussing dorsum of penis or compressing the glans penis.

Virilism Masculine traits exhibited by a female owing to the production of excessive amounts of androgenic hormone either in the adrenal cortex or from an ovarian tumor. *(See Arrhenoblastoma).*

Virilization Masculine changes in female like appearance of moustache and beard, atrophy of breast, enlarged clitoris, male voice and male type baldness.

Virion A fully developed complete infectious viral particle consisting of its nucleic acid and a surrounding coat of protein (capsid); the extracellular (cell-free) form of a virus.

V

Viroids Small naked virus genome without a dormant phase.

Virology The scientific study of viruses, their growth and the diseases caused by them.

Virtual ward Operates like a hospital ward but the patient stays at home and is cared for by a team based in the community.

Virulence The power of a microorganism to produce toxins or poisons. This depends on (a) the number and power of the invading organisms, and (b) the power of the microorganism to overcome host resistance.

Virulent Dangerously poisonous.

Virus Any member of a unique class of infectious agents, which were originally distinguished by their smallness and their inability to replicate outside a living host cell; because these properties are shared by certain other microorganisms (rickettsiae, chlamydiae), viruses are now characterized by their simple organization and their unique mode of replication. A virus consists of genetic material, which may be either DNA or RNA, and is surrounded by a protein coat and, in some viruses, by a membranous envelope. They cause many diseases, including chicken pox (varicella), herpes zoster (shingles), herpes infections, measles (rubeola), German measles (rubella), mumps, infectious mononucleosis, hepatitis A and B, yellow fever, the common cold, acquired immune deficiency syndrome (AIDS), influenza, certain types of pneumonia and croup and other respiratory infections, poliomyelitis, and several types of encephalitis. There is evidence that certain viruses may be capable of causing cancer.

Viscera Pl. of viscus.

Visceral Relating to viscera.

Visceroptosis Downward displacement of a viscus.

Viscid Sticky and glutinous.

Viscosity Resistance to flowing. A sticky and glutinous quality.

Viscus Any of the organs contained in the body cavities, especially in the abdomen.

Vision The faculty of seeing. Sight.

Visual Relating to sight.

Visual acuity Sharpness of vision. It is assessed by reading test types.

Visual cells The rods and cones of the retina.

Visual display unit Abbreviated VDU. The monitor screen attached to a computer.

Visual field The area within which objects can be seen when looking straight ahead.

Visual purple The pigment in the outerlayers of the retina. Rhodopsin.

Visualization The technique of using the imagination and relaxation to create any desired changes in an individual's life.

Vital Relating to life.

Vital capacity The amount of air that can be expelled from the lungs after a full inspiration.

Vital signs The signs of life, namely pulse, respiration and temperature.

Vital statistics The records kept of births and deaths among the population, including the causes of death, and the factors that seem to influence their rise and fall.

Vitality The state of being alive, vigor.

Vitallium A metal alloy used in dentistry and for prostheses in bone surgery.

Vitamin Any of a group of accessory food factors which are contained in foodstuffs and are essential to life, growth and reproduction.

Vitamin A Fat soluble vitamin derived from carotenes (alpha, beta and gamma) in food, responsible for growth, development and integrity of epithelial tissues, and functioning of Rhods, the visual sensory cells that contain visual purple for dim vision.

Vitamin B$_1$ Thiamine, an essential coenzyme for decarboxylation of pyruvate to acetyl coenzyme.

Vitamin B$_2$ Riboflavin; constituent of flavoproteins responsible for tissue oxidation.

Vitamin B$_6$ Pyridoxine, a coenzyme for over 60 different enzyme systems, required for heme synthesis and neuro excitability.

Vitamin B$_{12}$ Cyanocobalamin, essential for cytoplasmic maturation of red cells and intactness of neurons.

Vitamin C Ascorbic acid, a factor essential for integrity of intercellular cement in many tissues, especially capillaries.

Vitamin D One of several vitamins (D$_2$, D$_3$, D$_4$, D$_5$) that have antirachitic property. Vitamin D$_2$ (Calciferol) D$_3$ (irradiated 7 dehydrocholesterol), D$_4$ irradiated 22 dihydro ergosterol, D$_5$ (irradiated dehydrositosterol), all are essential for calcium and phosphorus metabolism.

Vitamin E Tachysterol (alpha tocopherol), which prevents oxidation of polyunsaturated fatty acids in cell membranes.

Vitamin K Naphthoquinone derivative that helps in synthesis of prothrombin in liver.

Vitamin supplement A tablet or capsule comprising of one or several vitamins.

Vitellin An egg yolk protein containing lecithin.

Vitelline duct The duct connecting yolk sac with the embryonic gut.

Vitelline veins Two veins carrying blood from yolk sac.

Vitellus The yolk of an ovum.

Vitiligo A skin disease marked by an absence of pigment, producing white patches on the face and body. Leukoderma.

Vitrectomy Surgical extraction of the vitreous humour and its replacement by a physiological solution in the treatment of vitreous hemorrhage in diabetic retinopathy.

Vitreous Glassy.

Vitreous humour The transparent jelly-like substance filling the posterior of the eye, from lens to retina.

Viviparous Giving birth to young alive offspring rather than larvae or embryo.

Vocal Pertaining to the voice, or the organs that produce the voice.

Vocal apparatus Parts of human body that produce speech. These include the lips, tongue, teeth, hard and soft palates, uvula, larynx and pharynx.

Vocal cords The two folds of tissue in the larynx, formed of fibrous tissue covered with squamous epithelium.

Vocal resonance The normal sounds of speech heard through the chest wall by means of a stethoscope.

Vocal fold The thin edges of vocal cords.

Vocal fremitus Palpable vibration on chest wall while patient speaks.

Vocal muscle The inner portion of thyroarytenoid muscle which lies in contact with vocal ligament.

Vocal process The part of arytenoids cartilage to which are attached the vocal cords.

Voice Sound produced in human beings by vibration of vocal cords.

Void To evacuate bladder and bowel.

Volar Relates to palm of hand and sole of foot.

Volatile Having a tendency to evaporate readily.

Volition The conscious adoption by the individual of a line of action.

Volkmann's canals Vascular channels in compact bone, not surrounded by concentric lamellae as are haversian canals.

Volkmann's ischemic contracture R. Von Volkmann, German surgeon, 1830-1889, Contraction of the fingers and sometimes of the wrist or

V

of analogous parts of the foot, with loss of power, after severe injury or improper usage of a tourniquet or cast

Volley The discharge of a number of nerve stimuli in quick succession.

Volsella Forceps with one or more hooks at the end of each blade.

Volt The unit of electromotive force which when applied to a conductor with resistance of one ohm produces a current of one ampere.

Voltage Difference in potential expressed in Volts.

Volume The space occupied by a substance.

Minute volume The total volume of air breathed in or out in 1 min.

Packed cell volume That occupied by the blood cells after centrifuging (about 45% of the blood sample).

Residual volume The amount of air left in the lungs after breathing out fully.

Voluntary Under the control of the will *(See Involuntary)*.

Voluntary muscle Any muscle whose contraction and relaxation is controlled by will. SYN –Stripped, Skeletal muscles.

Voluptuous Pleasures of senses.

Volvulus Twisting of a loop of bowel causing obstruction. Most common in the sigmoid colon.

Vomer A thin plate of bone forming the posterior septum of the nose.

Vomit 1. Matter ejected from the stomach through the mouth (vomitus). 2. To eject material in this way.

Bilious vomit Vomit mixed with bile. The vomit is stained yellow or green.

Coffee ground vomit Ejected matter that contains small quantities of altered blood, which has the appearance of coffee grounds.

Faecal or *stercoraceous vomit* Vomit mixed with faeces. Occurs in intestinal obstruction when the contents of the upper intestine regurgitate back into the stomach. It is dark brown with an unpleasant odor.

Vomiting A reflex act of expulsion of the stomach contents via the esophagus and mouth. It may be preceded by nausea and excess salivation if the cause is local irritation in the stomach.

Cyclical vomiting Recurrent attacks of vomiting often occurring in children and associated with acidosis.

Projectile vomiting The forcible ejection of the gastric contents, usually without warning. Present in hypertrophic pyloric stenosis and in cerebral diseases.

Vomiting of pregnancy Vomiting occurring in the months of pregnancy. Morning sickness.

Vomitus Material ejected by vomiting.

Van Gierke's disease Glycogen storage disease due to absence of glucose-6-phosphate resulting in hypoglycermia and acidosis.

Von Graefe's sign Failure of lid to roll downward on looking down as in thyrotoxicosis.

Von Recklinghausen's disease 1. Neurofibromatosis. 2. Hemochromatosis. 3. Generalized osteitis fibrosa cystica.

Von Willebrand's disease *E.A. von Willebrand, Finnish physician, 1870-1949.* A bleeding disorder inherited as an autosomal dominant trait (rarely recessive), characterized by a deficiency of a blood protein called von Willebrand factor (VWF). VWF binds factor VIII, which is involved in the clotting process. Symptoms include epistaxis and increased bleeding after trauma or surgery, menorrhagia and postpartum bleeding.

VSD Ventricular Septal Defect.

Voracious Having insatiable appetite.

Voriconazole Antifungal.

Vorinostat Antilymphoma drug.

Vortex A structure having whorled or spiral appearance.

Vorticose veins Four veins receiving all blood from choroid and emptying into posterior cilliary and superior ophthalmic veins.

Voyeurism Satisfaction obtained from observing nude persons or sexual activity of others.

Vuerometer Apparatus for measuring interpupillary distance.

Vulgaris Common or ordinary.

Vulnerable Susceptible to injury of any kind.

Vulnerability Weakness. Susceptibility to injury or infection.

Vulnerate To wound.

Vulsellum A forcep with hook on each blade.

Vulva The external female genital organs.

Vulvectomy Excision of the vulva.

Vulvitis Inflammation of the vulva.

Vulvodynia Non-specific pain around vulva with itching and difficult intercourse.

Vulvovaginitis Inflammation of the vulva and vagina.

VZ Varicella zoster virus.

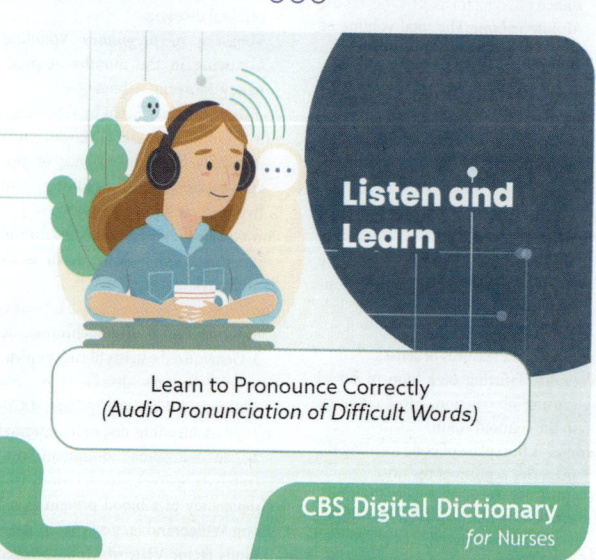
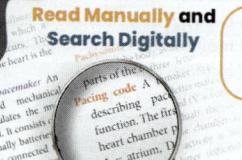

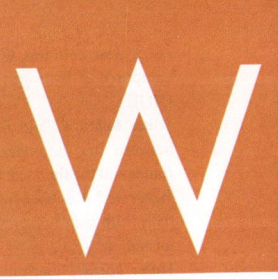

Waardenburg syndrome A congenital pigmentary disorder with vitiligo, heterochromic irides, and often congenital deafness.

Wafer A flat vaginal pessary.

Waist The part of human body between trunk and hips.

Wakefulness Sleeplessness.

Wald cycle Metabolic cycle of breakdown and synthesis of rhodopsin.

Waldenstrom's disease Osteochondritis deformans juvenilis.

Waldeyer's ring *HWG van Waldeyer-Hartz, German anatomist, 1836–1921.* The circle of lymphoid tissue in the pharynx formed by the lingual, faucial and pharyngeal tonsils.

Walk Locomotion of upright posture.

Walk-in centers Establishments that deliver accessible health care services on a drop-in basis. They offer NHS consultations and provide treatment for minor injuries and illnesses, general health information, self-treatment advice, information about out-of-hours general practitioner/ dental services and local pharmacy services, and are situated in major towns and cities. They generally operate during the day and at weekends, in times and places that people find convenient and are usually nurse-led, though a number of other health professionals and social care staff may be involved. Centers are managed by an NHS body or general practitioner federation and funded by the local health commissioners.

Wall The limiting material/substance of a cell, artery, vein, bladder.

Wallenberg's syndrome Occulsion of posterior inferior cerebellar artery syndrome manifest with dysphagia, cerebellar dysfunction, sensory-motor disturbances.

Wallerrian degeneration Degeneration of nerve fiber along with myelin sheath. The neurillema does not degenerate but forms a tube to guide growth of severed axons.

Wandering Not fixed, moving about.

Wangensteen tube *OH Wangensteen, American surgeon, 1898–1981.* A gastrointestinal aspiration tube with a tip that is opaque to X-rays.

Warburg apparatus A capillary manometer employed for O_2 consumption and CO_2 production studies.

Ward A large hospital room accommodating more than 4 patients.

Warfarin An oral anticoagulant drug that depresses the prothrombin level. Used mainly in the treatment of coronary and venous thrombosis.

Wart An elevation of the skin often of a brownish color, caused by hypertrophy of papillae in the dermis due to a virus infection *(See Verruca and Condyloma)*.

Wash Hypertrophied epidermis due to papilloma virus infection.

Wasp A form of insects.

Wasp sting Injection of wasp venom into skin.

Wasserman test *AP von Wassermann, German bacteriologist, 1866-1925.* A complement fixation test, rarely used today that enables the diagnosis of syphilis.

Waste Loss of strength; refuse no longer useful to the body; waste product.

Wasting A process of loss of weight and decreased physical vigor, appetite and mental activity.

Water A clear, colorless, tasteless liquid composed of hydrogen and oxygen (HO).

Water balance Fluid balance. That between the fluid taken in by all routes and the fluid lost by all routes.

Water bed A rubber bed filled partially with water to prevent bedsore formation.

Water borne Descriptive of certain diseases that are spread by contaminated water.

Water brash The eructation of dilute acid from the stomach to the pharynx, giving a burning sensation. Pyrosis. Heartburn.

Water hammer pulse Pulse marked by a forceful beat but sudden collapse.

Water seal drainage A closed method of drainage from the pleural space allowing the escape of fluid and air but preventing air entering because the drainage tube discharges under water.

Waterhouse - Friderichsen syndrome *R Waterhouse, British physician, 1873–1958; C Friderichsen, Danish physician, b. 1886.* A rare disorder. Meningococcal meningitis, which is marked by sudden onset and short course fever, coma, cyanosis, hemorrhages from the skin and mucous membranes, and hemorrhage into the adrenal glands.

Waterlow scale *(See Pressure Ulcer Assessment Scales).*

Watson-Crick helix *JD Watson, American geneticist, b. 1928; F Crick, British biochemist, b. 1916.* Double helix; a representation of the structure of deoxyribonucleic acid (DNA), consisting of two coiled chains, each of which contains information completely specifying the other chain.

Watson-Schwartz test A test used to acute porphyria to differentiate porphobilinogen from urobilinogen.

Watt Unit of electrical power, i.e., power produced by one ampere of current flowing with electromotive force of one volt.

Wave An undulating or vibrating motion; an oscillation seen in ECG, EEG or other graphic recordings.;

Wave 'a' A wave in jugular venous pulse produced by atrial conctraction and absent in atrial fibrillation.

Wave 'c' A wave in jugular venous pulse that reflects closure of tricuspid valve.

Wave excitation The excitatory impulse originating from SA node of heart and spreading to ventricles via A-V node.

Wave pulse The ejection of blood into root of aorta that causes the impact to be transmitted along the arterial wall.

Wavelength The distance of a single wave cycle measured from top of one wave to top of next wave.

Wax Any substance of animal, plant or mineral origin consisting a mixture of high molecular weight fatty acids, high molecular weight monohydric alcohols, esters of fatty acids and alcohols and solid hydrocarbons. Waxes are usually hard, brittle solid that become pliable on warming and melt on further heating.

Waxy cast Dense highly refractile urinary cast composed of amyloid material as in chronic renal disease.

Waxy degeneration 1. Amyloid degeneration. 2. Zenker's degeneration.

Waxy flexibility A cataleptic state in which a patient's limbs are held indefinitely in any position in which they have been placed *(See Catatonia).*

Weal A raised stripe on the skin, as is caused by the lash of a whip. Typical of urticaria.

Wean 1. To discontinue breast or bottle feeding and substitute other feeding habits, e.g., solid foods. This should be effected gradually from 6th month. 2. In respiratory therapy, to gradually decrease dependence on assisted ventilation until the patient is able to breathe spontaneously.

Wear and tear theory The concept of aging that equates the human body with a machine, and that as body parts and organs wear out physiological functions deteriorate affecting the quality of life.

Web A membrane extending across a space, e.g., esophageal web causing dysphagia.

Webbing The state of being connected by a membrane or a fold of skin.
Webbing of the hands (or feet) Congenital abnormality in which the digits are not separated from each other. Syndactyly.
Webbing of the neck Folds of skin in the neck, giving it a webbed appearance. Occurs in certain congenital conditions, e.g., Turner's syndrome.

Weber's test A tuning fork test for unilateral deafness. A vibrating tuning fork is placed on middle of forehead. In conductive deafness the diseased ear perceives the vibrations better.

Wegener's syndrome Glomerulitis, vasculitis, granulomatous lesions of respiratory tract which respond to corticosteroids and cyclophosphamide.

Weil's disease *A Weil German physician, 1848–1916.* Spirochaetal jaundice. The organism, *Leptospira-icterohaemorrhagiae*, is harboured and excreted by rats and enters through a bite or skin abrasion, or infected food or water.

Weil-Felix reaction *E Weil, Austrian physician, 1880–1922: A Felix, Czech bacteriologist, 1887–1956.* An agglutination test of blood serum used in the diagnosis of typhus.

Well-baby clinic Mothers are encouraged to bring their infants to these clinics for assessment and monitoring of the child's health. Immunization is available and there are opportunities for 'family' health promotion.

Well-man clinic A health promotion clinic available for men to screen for health problems and to promote health, e.g., self-examination of the testicles *(See Testicular selfexamination)*.

Well-woman clinic A health promotion clinic available to screen women for breast and cervical cancer, anaemia, diabetes and hypertension and to promote health, e.g., self-examination of the breasts *(See Breast)*.

Wellness The development of a personal lifestyle that promotes feelings of well-being, achieves the highest level of health within one's capability, and minimizes chances of becoming ill. It is guided by a developing sense of self-awareness and self-responsibility encompassing emotional, mental physical, social, spiritual and environmental health.

Wen A small sebaceous cyst; a steatoma.

Wenckebach's phenomenon A form of incomplete heart block where there is progressive lengthening of P-R interval ending in a dropped test.

Werdnig-Hoffmann disease *G Werdnig, Austrian neurologist, 1844–1919; J E Hoffmann, German neurologist, 1857–1919.* Disease characterized by progressive spinal muscular atrophy affecting the shoulder, neck, pelvis and eventually the respiratory muscles of infants.

Werner's syndrome *CWO Werner German physician, 1879–1936.* A hereditary condition characterized by cataracts, osteoporosis, stunted growth and premature graying of the hair.

Wernicke's encephalopathy Encephalopathy with memory deficit, ocular palsy, delirium associated with thiamine deficiency of chronic alcoholism.

Wernicke-Korsakoff syndrome *K Wernicke, German neurologist, 1848–1905; SS Korsakoff, Russian neurologist, 1854–1900.* A disorder of the central nervous system, usually associated with chronic alcoholism, nutritional deficiency, and severe deficiency of vitamin B1. It is characterized by a combination of motor and sensory disturbances and disordered memory function. One form is Wernicke's encephalo-pathy, a neurological condition due to vitamin B1 deficiency. Untreated, it progresses from mental confusion and double vision to lethargy and coma.

Wertheim's operation *E Wertheim, Austrian gynecologist, 1864–1920 (See Hysterectomy).*

West Nile virus A virus spread by mosquitoes occurring across the world. In around 1 in 100 it can be serious with encephalitis developing that can be fatal

Western blotting A technique for analyzing protein antigens and detecting small amount of antibodies as in test of AIDS.

Westphal-Edinger nucleus A parasympathetic nucleus rostral to motor nucleus of third nerve in midbrain whose efferent fibers innervate the ciliary muscles of eye.

Wet dream Nocturnal emission of semen.

Wet nurse A lactating woman who breast-feeds another woman's child.

Wharton's duct Duct of submandibular salivary gland opening by side of frenum linguae.

Wharton's jelly *T Wharton, British physician, 1614–1673.* The connective tissue of the umbilical cord.

Wheal An elevation of skin with white center and pale red periphery accompanied by itching as seen in urticaria, anaphylaxis, insect bite.

Wheelchair A chair with four wheels – two small and two big for mobility of partially paralyzed patient or transporting sick.

Wheezing Breathing with a rasp or whistling sound. It results from constriction or obstruction of the throat, pharynx, trachea or bronchi.

Whiplash injury Injury to the spinal cord, nerve roots ligaments or vertebrae in the cervical region due to a sudden jerking back of the head and neck. Common in road traffic accidents where there is sudden acceleration or deceleration of the vehicle.

Whiplash shake syndrome A constellation of injuries to the brain and eye that may occur when a young child is shaken vigorously with the head unsupported. This causes stretching and tearing of the cerebral vessels and brain substance commonly leading to subdural haematomas and retinal hemorrhages. It may result in paralysis, blindness and other visual disturbances, convulsions and death *(See Shaken baby syndrome).*

Whipple's operation *AO Whipple, American surgeon, 1881–1963.* Radical pancreato-duodenectomy performed for carcinoma of the head of the pancreas.

Whipworm *(See Trichuris).*

Whirl To feel giddy, to revolve rapidly.

Whisky An alcoholic drink with ethyl alcohol content of 45–50%.

Whisper To speak in a low, soft voice.

Whitfield ointment Benzoic acid + salicylic acid, keratolytic, antifungal.

White cell A white blood cell.

White leg Milk leg *(See Phlegmasia).*

White line The midline (linea alba) of abdomen representing the white tendinous attachments of external oblique and transverses muscles.

White matter Part of central nervous system composed of myelinated nerve fibers.

White softening Softening of any tissue in which affected area becomes white and anemic.

Whitlow A felon; a suppurating inflammation of a finger near the nail.

Melanotic whitlow A malignant tumor of the nail bed characterized by formation of melanotic tissue.

Subperiosteal whitlow One in which the infection involves the bone covering.

Superficial whitlow A pustule between the true skin and cuticle *(See Paronychia).*

WHO World Health Organization.

Whole bowel irrigation Flushing large volumes of fluid through the gastrointestinal tract; done for treatment of poisoning.

Whole system planning Strategic planning and commissioning across a range of service and organizational boundaries. Deals with the impact that changes one part of the system whether health and social care or housing, and are likely to have impact on other parts.

Whole systems approach The consideration of the interrelatedness of various elements, which come together for a common purpose and continually have impact upon one another. The comprehension of complex systems, e.g., health care and social care, requires understanding of a diverse range of perspectives, and an appreciation that change will often be required across a number of areas to meet needs.

Whole time equivalent Total weekly contracted hours of full-and part-time staff expressed as a multiple of the standard working week.

Whoop The inspiratory crowing sound following the cough paroxysm in whooping cough.

Whooping cough A notifiable infectious disease characterized by catarrh of the respiratory tract and paroxysms of coughing: ending in a prolonged whooping respiration; called also pertusis. The causative organism is *Bordetella pertussis.* Whooping cough is a serious disease; most cases occur in children. All babies should be immunized against whooping cough unless there is a sound medical objection.

Whorl 1. A type of fingerprint. 2. Spiral arrangement.

Widal reaction *GFL Widal, French physician, 1862–1929.* A blood agglutination test for typhoid fever.

Will The mental faculty for control of one's actions, emotions, thoughts and deciding the actions.

Willi's circle An arterial arrangement at base of brain encircling the optic chiasma and hypophysis formed by internal carotids, anterior cerebrals, posterior cerebrals and basilar arteries.

Willis-Ekbom syndrome Also known as restless leg syndrome, results in an uncontrollable urge to move the legs, possibly associated with dopamine. In some people, it is temporary and in others permanent and debilitating. The temporary form is very common in pregnancy.

Wilm's tumor *M. Wilms, German surgeon, 1867-1918.* A highly malignant tumor of the kidney occurring in young children. A nephroblastoma.

Wilson's disease *SAK Wilson, British neurologist, 1878–1937.* Hepatolenticular degeneration. A congenital abnormality in the metabolism of copper leading to neurological degeneration.

Window An aperture for admission of light and air.

Window oval The fenestra vestibule.

Window round The fenestra cochlea.

Windpipe *(See trachea).*

Wine Fermented juice of any fruit with alcohol content of 1-5%.

W

Wing Any structure resembling wings of bird, e.g., greater and lesser wings of sphenoid.

Winking jaw Involuntary simultaneous closure of the eyelids as the jaw is moved.

Wintergreen oil Methyl salicylate used as counter irritant.

Wire Kirschner Steel wire placed through long bone for traction.

Wiring The fixing together of a broken or split bone by the use of a wire. Commonly used for the jaw, the patella and the sternum.

Wisdom teeth The back moral teeth, the eruption of which is often delayed until maturity.

Wish fulfillment A desire, not always acknowledged consciously by the person, which is fulfilled through dreams or by day-dreaming.

Wiskott-Aldrich syndrome Sex linked recessive disorder of immune function with impaired T and B-cell activity, thrombocytopenia, eczema and propensity to infection.

Witch's milk Milk secreted from breast of newborn infant from stimulation by maternal LH.

Withdrawal 1. A pathological retreat from reality. 2. Abstention from drugs to which one is habituated or addicted; also denoting the symptoms occasioned by such withdrawal. *Withdrawal symptoms* Symptoms brought about by abrupt withdrawal of a narcotic or other drug to which a person has become addicted; called also abstinence syndrome. The usual reactions to withdrawal may include anxiety, weakness, gastrointestinal symptoms, nausea and vomiting, tremor, fever, rapid heartbeat, convulsions and delirium.

Wolffian body An embryonic organ on each side of vertebral column, the mesonephros.

Wolffian cyst A cyst present in the broad ligament.

Wolffian duct Duct from mesonephros to cloaca in fetus.

Wolff-Parkinson-White syndrome *L Wolff, American cardiologist, 1898– 1972; Sir J Parkinson, British physician, 1885–1976; P D White, American cardiologist, 1886–1973.* Abnormal heart rhythm caused by an accessory bundle between the atria and ventricles. A congenital disorder.

Wolman's disease An inherited metabolic disease in infants with hepatosplenomegaly, adrenal calcification and foam cells in bone marrow.

Womb The uterus.

Wood alcohol Methyl alcohol distilled from wood is highly poisonous causing blindness.

Wood's light *RW Wood, American physicist, 1868–1953.* Ultraviolet light transmitted through a glass filter containing nickel oxide. It produces fluorescence of infected hairs when placed over a scalp affected with ringworm.

Wool fat Anhydrous lanolin obtained from sheep wool, used as base for ointment.

Woolsorter's disease Pulmonary anthrax.

Word blindness *(See Dyslexia).*

Word salad Rapid speech in which the words are strung together without meaning.

World Health Organization Abbreviated WHO. The specialized agency of the United Nations that is concerned with health at an international level. WHO organizes health campaigns against infectious diseases and sponsors research in medical laboratories. It also provides expert advice on all matters directly or indirectly concerned with physical or mental health to all member states.

World wide web Abbreviated WWW. An information space where documents and other resources are stored

W

and interlinked and accessed via the internet.

Worm Any one of a number of groups of long soft-bodied invertebrates, some of which are parasitic to humans.

Wormian bone Small irregular bones along cranial sutures.

Wound A cut or break in continuity of any tissue, caused by injury or operation. It is classified according to its nature.

Abrased wound The skin is scraped off, but there is no deeper injury.

Contused wound With bruising of the surrounding tissue.

Incised wound Usually the result of operation, and produced by a knife or similar instrument. The edges of the wound can remain in apposition and it should heal by first intention.

Lacerated wound One with torn edges and tissues, usually the result of accident or injury. It is often septic and heals by second intention.

Open wound A gaping wound on the body surface.

Penetrating wound Often made by gunshot, shrapnel, etc. There may be an inlet and outlet hole and vital organs are often penetrated by the missile.

Punctured wound Made by a pointed or spiked instrument.

Septic wound Any type into which infection has been introduced, causing suppurative inflammation. It heals by second intention.

Wound healing The restoration of integrity to injured tissues by replacement of dead tissue with viable tissue. The process starts immediately after an injury and may continue for months or years *(See Healing)*.

Wright's stain Combination of eosin and methylene blue to stain blood slides.

Wright's syndrome A neuromuscular syndrome caused by prolonged hyper- abduction of arm leading to occlusion of subclavian artery and stretching of trunks of brachial plexus.

Wrinkles A furrow or ridge of skin.

Wrist The point of the carpus and bones of the forearm.

Wrist drop Loss of power in the muscles of the hand. It may be due to nerve or tendon injury, but can result from lack of sufficient support by splint or sling.

Writer's cramp A colloquial term for painful spasm of the hand and forearm, caused by excessive writing and poor posture.

Wryneck *(See torticollis)*

Wuchereria A genus of nematode-worms which are the principle vectors of filariasis.

Wuchereria bancrofti The most common species in tropical and subtropical areas.

Wylie's operation Shortening of round ligament of uterus for retroflexion in combating prolapsed uterus.

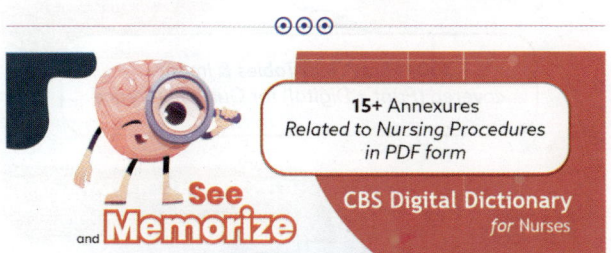

Dil Mange More Content

- Get additional explanations of Important Terminologies
- Word Quiz on Day-To-Day Basis on Scientific and General Terminology (One New Word Every Day with example)
- **50+** Animated & Interactive Videos on various important Topics and Concepts on nursing students' day-to-day interactions/daily needs.
- 4 Hybrid Updates (Every Quarter) covering New Words, Recent Topics & Interactive Videos

CBS Digital Dictionary
for Nurses

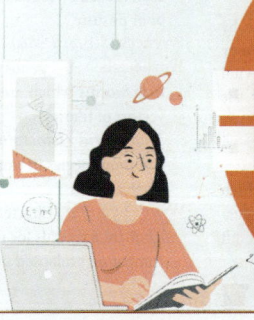

Revise on the Go

350+ High Yield *Tables & Images* covered (Print + Digital) for Quick Reference

CBS Digital Dictionary
for Nurses

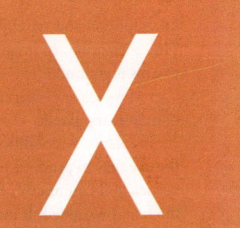

Xanthelasma A disease marked by the formation of flat or slightly raised yellow cholesterol deposits on the eyelids.

Xanthine A compound found in plant and animal tissues; the forerunner of uric acid in nucleoprotein metabolism.

Xanthine calculi Brown to red, hard and laminated calculi in urinary tract.

Xanthine oxidase A flavor-protein enzyme catalyzing oxidation of certain purines.

Xanthochromia 1. The presence of yellow patches on the skin. 2. The yellow coloring of cerebrospinal fluid seen in patients who have had a subarachnoid hemorrhage.

Xanthoderma Yellow coloration of skin.

Xanthodont Yellowness of teeth.

Xanthogranuloma A tumor having characteristics of both xanthoma and granuloma

Xanthoma The presence in the skin of flat areas of yellowish pigmentation due to deposits of lipids. There are several varieties.

Xanthoma palpebrarum Xanthelasma.

Xanthomatosis Appearance of multiple xanthomas in skin due to cholesterol deposit within histiocytes and reticuloendothelial cells.

Xanthophyll The yellow pigment of egg yolk.

Xanthopsia A disturbance of vision in which all objects appear yellow.

Xanthosis A yellow skin pigmentation, seen in some cases of diabetes and poliomyelitis.

Xanthuria Excretion of excess of xanthine in urine.

X-chromosome The female sex chromosome, being present in all female gametes and only half the male gametes. When union takes place two X chromosomes result in female child

(XX) but one of each results in a male child (XY) *(See Y chromosome)*.

X-disease Poisoning caused by ingestion of nuts contaminated with aspergillus aflatoxin.

Xenobiotic An antibiotic not produced by body, i.e., foreign antibiotic.

Xenograft Graft from one species to another *SYN* – heterograft.

Xenology Study of parasites, their relationship to each other.

Xenomenia Menstruation from a part other than vagina.

Xenon An inert gas whose radio isotope Xe^{133} is used to image the heart, lungs and brain.

Xenophobia Abnormal fear for strangers.

Xenophthalmia Inflammation of the eye due to presence of foreign body.

Xephoiditis Inflammation of the xiphoid process.

Xenopsylla A genus of fleas, some of which are vectors of plague.

Xenopsylla cheopis The rat flea, which transmits bubonic plague.

Xerasia A condition of abnormal dryness and brittleness of hair resulting in hair loss.

Xerocheilia Dryness of lips.

Xeroderma A hereditary condition in which there is excessive dryness of the skin. A mild form of ichthyosis.

Xeroderma pigmentosum A rare hereditary and often fatal disease in which there is extreme sensitivity of the skin and eyes to light. It begins in childhood and rapidly progresses. The formation of malignant neoplasms is common.

Xeromammography Xeroradiography of mammary glands.

Xerophthalmia A condition in which the eye fails to produce tears and the cornea and conjunctiva become dry, thick and wrinkled. It maybe caused by deficiency of vitamin A. Also known as xeroma.

Xeroradiography An X-ray technique involving dry process where selenium covered plates are altered by the X-ray producing the image.

Xerosis A condition of dryness, especially of the eyes, mouth, vagina or skin.

Xerostomia Dryness of mouth due to poor salivary secretion.

Xerotocia Dry labor caused due to diminished amount of amniotic fluid.

Xiphisternum The pointed lower end of sternum.

Xiphoid Sword shaped.

Xiphoid process The lowest portion of sternum with a sword shaped cartilaginous process supported by bone.

X-linked Pertaining to the genes, or the effect of these genes, situated on the X chromosome. X-linked disorders are those caused by the genes on the X chromosome.

X-rays Electromagnetic waves of short length which are capable of penetrating many substances and of producing chemical changes and reactions in living matter. They are used both to aid diagnosis and to treat disease. Also called Roentgen rays.

XXY A syndrome where boys are born with an additional X chromosome. *(See Klinefelter syndrome).*

Xylene Di-methyl benzene, used as a solvent and cleansing agent in microscopy.

Xylenol Di-methyl phenol, used in preparation of coaltar disinfectants.

Xylitol An alcohol with chemical properties similar to sucrose.

Xerostomia Dryness of the mouth due to a failure of salivary gland secretion.

Xylocaine A proprietary preparation of lignocaine used for local anesthesia.

Xylometazoline A vasoconstrictor used in nasal decongestant drops.

Xylose A pentose sugar, found in connective tissue and sometimes in urine, which is not metabolized in the body.

Xylulose A pentose sugar occurring in nature.

Xyrospasm Spasm of wrist and forearm muscles in professionals like barbers.

Xysma The flocculent pseudomembrane seen in diarrheal stool.

XYY syndrome An extremely rare condition in males in which there is an extra Y chromosome, making a total of 47 chromosomes in each body cell *(See Klinefelter's syndrome).*

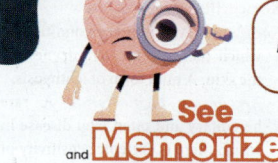

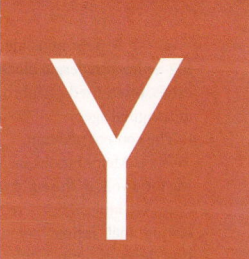

Y chromosome The male sex chromosome, being present in half the male gametes and none of the female. It carries few major genes *(See X chromosome)*.

Yawning An involuntary act in which the mouth is opened wide and air is drawn in and exhaled. It may accompany tiredness or boredom.

Yaws Framboesia. A skin infection common in tropical countries. Caused by *Treponema pertenue,* it is common among people, especially children, who live under primitive conditions in equatorial Africa, South America, and the East and West Indies.

Yeast Any of the fungi of the genus *Saccharomyces.* They produce fermentation in malt and in sweetened fruit juices, resulting in the formation of alcoholic solutions such as beer and wines.

Yellow body Corpus luteum.

Yellow card scheme A system of reporting side effects from taking or using any prescription medicine, herbal remedy, an over the counter (OTC) medicine or medical device; to report a defective or counterfeit medicine; or to report safety concerns about e-cigarettes. A patient, parent, carer or health care professional can report a suspected side effect by telephone or email. This reporting scheme is available in the UK and is monitored and managed by the Medicines and Healthcare products Regulatory Agency (MHRA).

Yellow fever An acute, notifiable, infectious disease of the tropics caused by a virus and transmitted by a mosquito *(Aedes aegypti).* The virus attacks the liver and kidneys and the symptoms include rigor, headache, pain in the back and limbs, high fever and black vomit. Hemorrhage from the intestinal mucous membrane may occur. There is a high mortality rate.

Yellow spot 1. Anterior end of vocal cord. 2. Central point of retina, the sight of the clearest vision.

Yersinia A genus of Gram-negative bacteria.

Yersinia enterocolitica Producing mesenteric lymphadenitis and dysentery.

Yersinia pestis Causative agent of plague.

Yersinia pseudotuberculosis Produces pseudotuberculosis.

Yersinia ligament The y-shaped ligament on anterior capsule of hip joint.

Yersiniosis Infection caused due to Yersinia organisms.

Yin and yang The two complementary principles of Chinese philosophy incorporated into traditional Chinese medicine. Yin is feminine, dark and negative; Yang is masculine, bright and positive. Together, the Yin-Yang interaction and balance is believed to maintain the harmony of the body and, in a healthy person, maintain a state of dynamic balance.

Yoga One of the six systems of Indian philosophy which emphasizes personal physical preparation using isometric exercises, relaxation, breathing techniques and the attainment of defined body positions to achieve relaxation, with physical and emotional harmony and wellbeing.

Yogurt A form of curdled milk by lactobacilli, useful in patients with lactase deficiency.

Yohimbine A poisonous alkaloid having alpha-adrenergic blocking properties, often used as aphrodisiac and antianginal agent.

Yolk The content of ovum.

Yolk sac Membranous sac surrounding food yolk in the embryo.

Young Helmoholtz theory Theory stating that retinal colour perception depends upon 3 different sets of fibers responsible for red, green and violet.

Young's rule The formula for calculating dose of a medicine for child from known adult dose, i.e., Child's dose = (Age of child/(Age of child + 12)) × Average adult dose.

Yttrium Symbol Y. A rare chemical element, which in its radioactive form is sometimes used in cancer therapy and the treatment of severe arthritis.

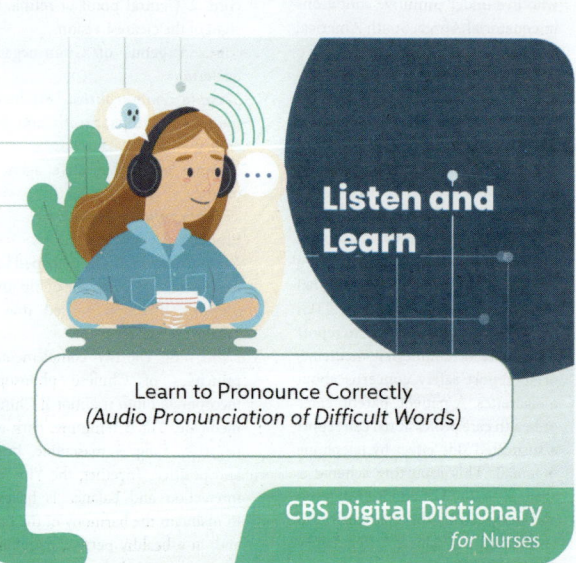

Listen and Learn

Learn to Pronounce Correctly
(Audio Pronunciation of Difficult Words)

CBS Digital Dictionary
for Nurses

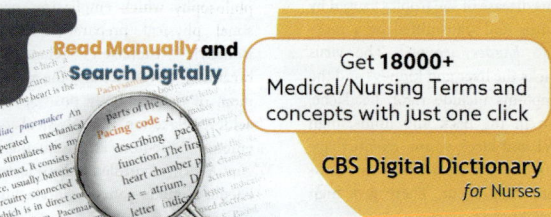

Read Manually and Search Digitally

Get **18000+** Medical/Nursing Terms and concepts with just one click

CBS Digital Dictionary
for Nurses

Y

Z-plasty A plastic operation for removing and repairing deformity resulting from a contraction scar.

Z-track injection An intramuscular injection technique, which allows a medication, e.g., an iron preparation, to be given but which prevents the leakage and the staining of tissues surrounding the site. See injection.

Zafirlukast Leukotriene antagonist for asthma.

Zaleplon Benzodiazepine antianxiety agent.

Z disk In striated muscle the dark band that bisects I bands. Actin filament is attached to Z disk and area between two Z disks in the sarocomere.

Zein A maize protein deficient in tryptophan and lysine.

Zeis' gland Sebaceous glands on eyelid margin.

Zen Zen Buddhism is the teaching that a form of medication consisting of the contemplation of one's essential nature to the exclusion of everything else is the way to true enlightenment.

Zenith The highest point. The opposite is NADIR.

Zero Nought; symbol 0. In the Celsius thermometer, 0°C is the melting point of ice; in the Fahrenheit thermometer, 0°F is 32° below the melting point of ice. *(See Celsius and Fahrenheit)*.

Z line A thin dark line that transversely bisects the clear zone of a muscle fiber; the distance between two z lines constitutes a sarcomere.

Zenker degeneration A waxy hyaline degeneration of skeletal muscles in acute infectious diseases like typhoid fever.

Zenker's diverticula Herniation of mucous membrane of esophagus through a defect in its wall often swelling with food to cause esophageal obstruction.

Zidovudine An antiviral drug used to retard the progress of AIDS. Also known as azidothymidine or AZT.

Ziehl-Neelsen method F Ziehl, German bacteriologist, 1857–1926; FKA Neelsen, German pathologist, 1854–1894. A method of staining tubercle bacilli for microscopic study.

Zieve's syndrome Transient hyperlipidemia, hemolytic anemia and jaundice following consumption of large amounts of alcohol.

Zika virus (also known as Zika fever) A viral disease mainly spread by mosquitoes, serious for pregnant women as it is thought to cause birth defects, particularly microcephaly (small head). There is currently no vaccine.

Zimmer The trade name of a metal, light-weight walking aid, commonly applied to other products of similar design and weight. Predominantly, used by the elderly to assist in rehabilitation.

Zinc Symbol Zn. A trace element which is essential in the body for cell growth and multiplication. The recommended daily intake of zinc is 15 mg for an adult. A severe deficiency of zinc can retard growth in children, cause a low sperm count in adult males, and retard wound healing.

Zinc-eugenol cement Used in dentistry for impression material, cavity liner, temporary restoration.

Zinc ointment 20% zinc oxide ointment for external application.

Zinn's ligament Connective tissue in eye to which recti are attached.

Ziprosidone Anticonvulsant.

Z

Zirconium A metallic element used as a white pigment in dental porcelain.

Zn Symbol of zinc.

Zollinger-Ellison syndrome *RM Zollinger, American physician. b. 1903; EH Ellison. American physician, 1918–1970.* A rare condition in which a pancreatic tumor causes excessive outpouring of gastric juice. Peptic ulcers may occur.

Zona A zone.

   Zona facialis Herpes of the face.

   Zona glomerulosa The outer layer of adrenal cortex.

   Zona pellucida The membrane surrounding the ovum.

   Zona reticularis The innermost layer of adrenal cortex.

Zonary placenta Placenta arranged like a broad ring around the chorion.

Zonula A zonule. In anatomy, a small, usually circular, area.

   Ciliary zonula The area surrounded by the suspensory ligaments of the eye.

Zonesthesia Constricting cord like sensation.

Zonule A small zone.

Zonules of zinn Suspensory ligament of the lens.

Zonulysin A proteolytic enzyme that maybe used in eye surgery to dissolve the suspensory ligament.

Zoogeny The development and evolution of animals.

Zoogony Animal breeding.

Zoology The science dealing with animal life.

Zoonosis A disease of animals that is transmissible to humans, e.g., anthrax, cat scratch fever, etc.

Zoonotic Concering zoonoses.

Zoophilia Sexual gratification by intercourse with animals.

Zoophobia Abnormal fear for animals.

Zoster *(See Herpes).*

Zuclopenthixol Antipsychotic agent.

Zygoma The arch formed by the union of the temporal bone with the malar bone in front of the ear.

Zygote A single fertilized cell formed from the union of a male and a female gamete.

Zygomaticoauricularis Muscle that draws pinna of ear forwards.

Zygomatic process 1. A thin projection from temporal bone at its squamous portion, articulating with zygomatic bone. 2. A strong prominent lateral projection from the supraorbital margin of the frontal bone articulating with maxillary process of zygomatic bone.

   Zygomatic reflex When zygoma is percussed the lower jaw moves towards percussed side.

Zygomycosis A form of mycoses that predominanty affects the face, the lungs and paranasal sinuses with thrombosis of blood vessels and infarction, common to diabetics, SYN-mucormycosis.

Zygospore The spore resulting from union of two similar gametes, as in certain algae and fungi.

Zymase An enzyme found in yeast, bacteria and plants that can convert carbohydrate into H_2O and CO_2 aerobically or ferment it to alcohol anaerobically.

Zyme An enzyme or ferment.

Zymogen The inactive precursor of an enzyme.

Zymologist The person who specializes in the study of enzymes.

Zymology The science of fermentation.

Zymosis Fermentation.

Zymosterol A sterol from yeast.

Z

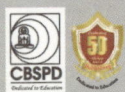

CBS NURSING DRUG GUIDE 2024–2025

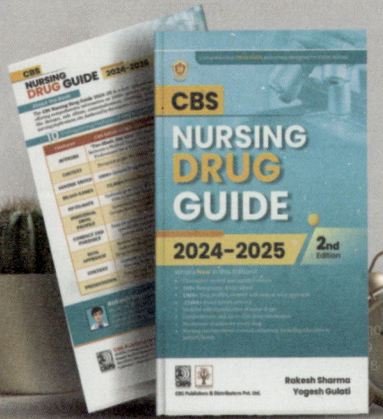

2nd Edition

Rakesh Sharma, Yogesh Gulati

ISBN	Pages	MRP
9789390619511	**1724**	**₹1295**/-

CBS **Dictionary** for Nurses

English English Hindi

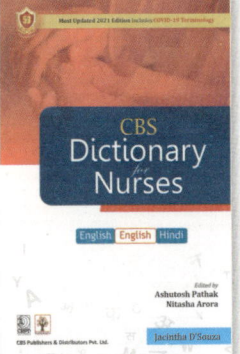

Jacintha D'Souza

ISBN	Pages	MRP
9789390619061	**952**	**₹595**/-